Library of
Davidson College

Library of
Davidson College

LAW AND PSYCHIATRY

Law and Psychiatry
RETHINKING THE RELATIONSHIP

MICHAEL S. MOORE
University of Southern California Law Center

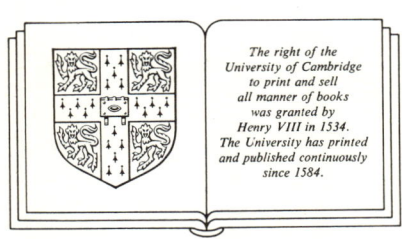

CAMBRIDGE UNIVERSITY PRESS
Cambridge
London   New York   New Rochelle   Melbourne   Sydney

Published by the Press Syndicate of the University of Cambridge
The Pitt Building, Trumpington Street, Cambridge CB2 1RP
32 East 57 Street, New York, NY 10022, USA
296 Beaconsfield Parade, Middle Park, Melbourne 3206, Australia

© Cambridge University Press 1984

First published 1984

Printed in the United States of America

Library of Congress Cataloging in Publication Data
Moore, Michael, 1943–
Law and psychiatry.
Bibliography: p.
Includes index.
1. Forensic psychiatry. 2. Insanity—Jurisprudence.
I. Title. [DNLM: 1. Forensic psychiatry. W 740
M823L]
K487.P75M66 1984 614'.1 83-7264
ISBN 0 521 25598 8 hard covers
ISBN 0 521 31978 1 paperback

FOR DOROTHY AND FOR LYNN

Contents

Preface	*page* xi
Acknowledgments	xiii
Introduction	1

Part I *Law and psychiatry: competing views of persons?*
1. The idea of practical reason and explanation in the social sciences 9
   Reason-giving explanations and practical reasoning 9
   Contrasting mentalistic explanations and interpretations 14
   Functional attributions 26
   Mechanistic explanations 32
2. The legal view of persons 44
   Persons in law, morals, and metaphysics 44
   Persons as the subjects of legal and moral responsibility 49
   Persons as the holders of legal and moral rights 90
   The legal view of persons 100
3. The challenge of psychiatry 113
   The human being as the universally sick animal 114
   The omnipresent unconscious 126
   The corporate self 142

Part II *Rationality and madness*
4. Does madness exist? 155
   The mythology of radical psychiatry 156
   Conclusion 180
5. Psychiatry and the concept of mental illness 182
   The ordinary meaning of mental illness 182

Contents

	The purposes behind psychiatric redefinition of mental illness	198
	The expansive psychiatric definitions of mental illness	204
	A more moderate psychiatric definition of mental illness	210
6.	The legal concept of insanity	217
	The insanity tests and their underlying moral bases	218
	Two experiments in merging legal and psychiatric definitions of mental illness	224
	The purposes behind a legal definition of mental illness	232
	Defining mental illness so as to give just deserts	243

Part III *Practical reason and the unconscious*

7.	Does the unconscious exist?	249
	The senses of unconscious revisited	249
	The existence of unconsciousness as a property	250
	The existence of the unconscious as an entity	267
8.	The nature of psychoanalytic explanation in terms of the unconscious	281
	A sketch of the psychoanalytic theory of dreams	282
	Motives for dreaming	285
	Conclusion	308
9.	The unconscious as the source of an increased responsibility	310
	Are accidents explained by unconscious mental states really actions?	311
	Are accidental actions explained by unconscious mental states really intentional?	322
	Are intentional actions explained by unconscious mental states really attempts at unconscious aims?	331
	Is one responsible for unconsciously acting intentionally or for acting with certain unconscious reasons?	337
	Persons, the unconscious, and the body	348
10.	The unconscious as the source of a decreased responsibility	350
	Do unconscious mental states diminish responsibility simply because they are causes of behavior?	351

Contents

Can unconscious mental states show an apparently intentional action to be unintentional?	365
The unconscious and rationality	372
Unconscious mental states as compulsions	374
Conclusion	381

Part IV *Legal persons and psychiatric subagents*

11. The unity of the self	387
The psychoanalytic challenge to the unity of the self	387
The psychoanalytic challenge to the unity of the self reconsidered	398
The disunities of self and psychoanalytic structuralism	410
Conclusion: Toward a philosophical rethinking of law and psychiatry	416
The methodological thesis: the need for philosophy in law and psychiatry	416
The substantive thesis: the shared view of persons in law and psychiatry	423
Notes	426
References	495
Index	514

Preface

THIS BOOK GREW out of a series of articles I have written over the last thirteen years. They were not originally produced with the intent of joining them as a book with a single theme. In revising them, I faced the task of looking at the articles "from the outside" and asking myself what in general I had been about all these years. Work on the book consequently involved the development of something like a theory of my own past thinking.

The theme that became clear to me as important to all of the essays, and important to me personally, was a view of what persons are like: a view that we are responsible for who we are and what we do because we have the capacities rationally to will our fate in this world. Such a view entails ultimate metaphysical faith in our reason and its power to control our actions. The unity of the previous essays was that each dealt, in one way or another, with an apparent challenge by psychiatry to this conception of what we are like. I thus came to write the book in its present form as an explicit defense of this view of persons. I developed Chapters 2 and 3 especially to lay out this theme and to link the other essays together by virtue of it. The remaining chapters are by and large derived from earlier articles, although each has been adapted extensively.

The book appears at a time when the relationship between law and psychiatry is being publicly reexamined. This ferment is in large part due (as it has often been throughout English and American history) to an unpopular insanity acquittal, that of John Hinckley, Jr., for his attempted assassination of President Reagan in 1981. One of my wishes for the book is that it may help to shape the present debate about psychiatry's role in the law away from the political rhetoric of those wanting to be "tough on crime" and toward a more reflective reconsideration of the relationship between psychiatry and our legal institutions. In any case, however matters stand when the public furor inevitably dies down, the most general concern of the book should remain of interest to each of us: how we do and should think of ourselves. Law and psychiatry each have many things to

Preface

say on this topic that will always be worth listening to, as, I hope, will a book that asks whether, on this topic, they are saying the same thing.

Michael S. Moore

Berkeley, California

Acknowledgments

CHAPTER 8, and portions of Chapters 1 and 7, are derived from a paper I gave in 1978 as part of the Eighteenth Annual Lecture Series in the Philosophy and History of Science at the University of Pittsburgh. This appeared as The Nature of Psychoanalytic Explanation, initially published in *Psychoanalysis and Contemporary Thought,* vol. 3(1980), pp. 459–543 (copyright 1980, Michael S. Moore) and reprinted in revised form in Larry Laudan (ed.), *Mind and Medicine: Problems of Explanation and Evaluation in Psychiatry and the Biomedical Sciences* (Berkeley: University of California Press, 1983). Chapter 4 stems from a paper I presented in 1975 to colloquia of the philosophy departments of the University of Kansas and the University of Nebraska and to a meeting of the Fellows in Law and the Humanities of Harvard University. It appeared in article form as Some Myths About "Mental Illness," in *Inquiry,* vol. 18(1975), pp. 233–65, and in the *Archives of General Psychiatry,* vol. 32(1975), pp. 1483–97 (copyright 1975, American Medical Association). Portions of Chapter 5 are based on a commentary I gave at the 1977 annual meeting of the American Psychopathological Association in New York City. This commentary (which concerns several proposed definitions of mental illness) appeared in R. Spitzer and D. Klein (eds.), *Critical Issues in Psychiatric Diagnosis* (New York: Raven Press, 1978). Other portions of Chapter 5, and the bulk of Chapter 6, are derived from a paper I delivered in 1976 to the Institute of Medical Humanities of the University of Texas Medical School and to the Department of Philosophy at Rice University. This appeared as an article, Legal Conceptions of Mental Illness, in B. Brody and T. Engelhardt (eds.), *Mental Illness: Law and Public Policy* (Dordrecht: Reidel, 1980) (copyright 1980, Reidel, Dordrecht, the Netherlands). The remainder of Chapter 6 appeared as an article in *Cites,* entitled Closet Retributivism (spring-summer, 1982), pp. 5–15.

Chapters 9 and 10 are derived from a paper I presented to the Third Annual Congress on Law and Psychiatry held in British Columbia in 1979, to a faculty workshop at the University of Southern California Law

Acknowledgments

Center, and to a seminar for law teachers sponsored in 1979 by the National Endowment for the Humanities at the University of California at Los Angeles. The preliminary version of the paper appeared as Responsibility for Unconsciously Motivated Action, *International Journal for Law and Psychiatry*, vol. 2(1979), pp. 323–47; the much longer version appeared as Responsibility and the Unconscious, *Southern California Law Review*, vol. 53(1980), pp. 1563–1675 (copyright 1980, Michael S. Moore).

Chapter 11 originated as a paper given initially at the Third Annual Conference of the International Union for the History and the Philosophy of Science, held in Montréal in 1980. In revised form the paper was later delivered to the Department of Philosophy at Stanford University, and it was published under the title, The Unity of the Self, in M. Ruse (ed.), *Nature Animated* (Dordrecht: Reidel, 1982) (copyright 1982, Michael S. Moore). The conclusion was given by me to a colloquium of the faculty of the School of Law (Boalt Hall), University of California, Berkeley, and to the Ninth International Congress on Law and Psychiatry at Santa Margherita, Italy, in 1983. It will appear as part of an article, Philosophical Perspectives on Law and Psychiatry, in a forthcoming issue of the *International Journal of Law and Psychiatry*.

Grateful acknowledgment is made to the editor of the *Archives of General Psychiatry*, the American Medical Association, and the D. Reidel Publishing Company for permission to reprint the material from two of the aforementioned articles.

I also wish to thank the participants at the preceding conferences for their many helpful comments. In particular, Robert Audi, Alan Garfinkel, Michael Green, Adolf Grunbaum, Herbert Morris, and Stephen Morse gave my earlier papers the careful criticism that has made them better than they otherwise would have been. Special thanks also go to Christopher Boorse, Susan Levy, Herbert Morris, and Stephen Morse, who read and commented on all or part of the manuscript.

The research assistants who helped to make manageable the otherwise unmanageable number of references in both the earlier papers and in the present volume were Liza Atkins, Amy Forbes, Lisa McCabe, Carol Tsuchida, David Vieweg, and Jan Zager. The index was prepared by Carol Voeller.

Last, special thanks go to Jan Rugolo and Esther Robertson for their typing of the original papers and of the manuscript itself. Their extraordinary dedication to the task has been an act of friendship.

Introduction

THIS BOOK IS about the relationship between two disciplines, law and psychiatry. It seeks to defend two overall theses, one methodological and the other substantive. The overall methodological thesis is that neither lawyers nor psychiatrists have been philosophical enough and that the relationship between the disciplines needs to be rethought in light of some greater philosophical understanding. As things now stand, lawyers and psychiatrists often talk past each other because neither discipline appreciates the degree to which they share common philosophical presuppositions. A prominent example is provided by the century-old debate between psychiatrists and lawyers about determinism and responsibility. Psychiatry is often painted (by both lawyers and psychiatrists) as a scientific, deterministic world view that leaves no room for free will and responsibility, whereas law is often painted (again, by both groups) as a system of thought that takes free will as its unquestionable first postulate.[1] Given these supposedly contradictory starting points the disciplines are often thought to be incommensurable.

The overall methodological thesis stems from the perception that debates between lawyers and psychiatrists are as fruitless as they are because both sides fail to perceive accurately the true presuppositions of each discipline. These presuppositions may be called "philosophical," because they have to do with issues traditionally the subject matter of philosophy. In the example given earlier, such presuppositions have to do with the meaning of free will, the relation of determinism to excuses in both law and morals, and the extent to which any theory of the mind and persons (psychiatry included) must be committed to an idea of personal freedom. More philosophical attention to these particular presuppositions need not leave one viewing law and psychiatry as incommensurable systems of thought, because it may turn out (as I believe it does) that psychiatry presupposes free will no less than does the law, and the law presupposes causation of behavior no less than does psychiatry. One can see this, however, only by working through the philosophy.

Introduction

Most of these philosophical presuppositions of both law and psychiatry have to do with the mind and mental states. Because a theory of the mind is the most essential ingredient in any theory of the person,[2] such presuppositions also have to do with the idea of a person. Both law and psychiatry should be viewed as systems of thought that possess theories about minds and persons. Psychiatry (at least when it leaves purely taxonomic concerns) rather explicitly contains a theory of mind and persons. The legal theory of mind is more implicit, to be found in legal doctrines and principles that make extensive use of concepts such as voluntariness, intention, desire, and motivation. Implicit though it is, the law too has a theory of mind and persons that is revealed by its systematic use of such mental concepts.

The overall substantive thesis of the book is that the legal and psychiatric views of minds and persons do not contradict one another. Such theories are not the same in all respects, but they do not differ in those respects most relevant to the issues that have traditionally divided lawyers and psychiatrists. The thesis is that if lawyers and psychiatrists would but look (in a philosophical way), they would see that nothing in the psychiatric view of persons contradicts the law's presupposition that a person is an autonomous and a rational agent.

I will proceed to develop these two theses as follows. In Part I I discuss the view of mind implicit in the law and seek to pinpoint where psychiatry seems to differ most dramatically from the legal view of minds and persons. This discussion proceeds in three chapters. In Chapter 1 I discuss the basic scheme of explanation of the actions of persons in ordinary thought and the social sciences. This scheme of explanation is in terms of reasons for action, which itself involves the idea of an agent using "practical reason," in the classical phrase. This form of explanation is contrasted with other kinds of explanations in the social sciences with which it is often confused, namely, functional accounts, mental cause accounts, and hermeneutic interpretations. This form of explanation is also contrasted with explanations of behavior that at least purport to make no use of mental or personal concepts, explanations such as those offered by behaviorism or physiological psychology.

Chapter 2 seeks to delineate the legal theory of persons as one in which practical reason is central. This theory is approached in three steps. The first is to begin with two quite broad legal contexts in which the concept of a person appears: Legal persons are the appropriate agents both to be assigned various kinds of legal *responsibility* and to be the holders of various types of legal *rights*. The second step is to note that agents can be legal persons in either of these contexts only if they are moral agents. Legal liability is seen to depend on moral responsibility, and legal rights are seen to depend on moral rights. The third step is to see that beings are moral

Introduction

agents only if they are "practical reasoners," that is, they act for reasons. Considerable attention is directed throughout the chapter to showing that the legal and moral concepts in terms of which rights and responsibilities are assigned—concepts such as action, intention, rationality, and justification or excuse—presuppose the concept of persons as practical reasoners.

Chapter 3 outlines the challenge that psychiatry appears to present to this legal theory of persons. That challenge is seen to come principally from three aspects of psychiatric theory: (1) the hypothesis that we are all somewhat crazy and thus sick rather than bad; (2) the hypothesis that none of us is free from the "grip" of our unconscious; and (3) the hypothesis that none of us is a truly unified agent in the way the law supposes, but that each of us is better conceptualized as consisting of a community of subagents, each with its own concerns and intentions. Such apparent psychiatric views seem to conflict with the presuppositions necessary in law to view persons as the holders of rights and responsibilities.

Each of these three seeming differences between the legal and the psychiatric theories of minds and persons forms the subject matter of the succeeding parts of the book. In Part II I explore the relationship between the law's presupposition of a person as a rational agent, and modern psychiatry's extended view of madness that "all of us are a little bit crazy." In the first chapter of Part II, Chapter 4, I explore and then reject the easy response to modern psychiatry's extended view of mental illness. This is the response of Thomas Szasz and his lawyerly following that there is no problem here because there is no such thing as mental illness. Beginning afresh, Chapter 5 attempts to articulate the popular view of mental illness enshrined in our ordinary usage of terms such as "madness," "crazy," or "mentally ill." Reasons are then explored why psychiatrists in the twentieth century have sought to give definitions of mental illness that are much broader than this popular notion. The chapter closes with a critical examination of the broader definitions psychiatrists have offered us, concluding that even for psychiatric purposes these definitions are too broad.

Chapter 6 analyzes the legal concept of insanity. The chapter proceeds, first, by showing that essential to any viable concept of legal insanity is some concept of mental illness; second, that lawyers cannot simply adopt psychiatric definitions of mental illness in light of the probable different purposes the concept serves in the two disciplines; and third, that the purpose for which the criminal law defines mental illness is the retributive one of giving just deserts. The chapter closes by attempting to work out a more restrictive, legal view of mental illness that does not allow the collapse of all bad behavior into sick behavior. This more restrictive legal conceptualization of mental illness is presented as being a return to the popular notion of mental illness as madness, a concept shared by both law and psychiatry in the early nineteenth century.

Introduction

In Part II I seek to defuse the potentially disruptive consequences of enriching the legal view of mind with the second challenging idea from psychiatry, namely the idea of the unconscious. The first chapter of this part, Chapter 7, explores and then rejects an easy response to the challenge to the legal view of mind presented by the unconscious. This is the response that denies sense to the idea that there could be such a thing as an unconscious. Although this response is popular with lawyers (good empiricists all), it has been more forcefully articulated by two generations of philosophers, and the chapter proceeds by considering and rejecting their arguments. Beginning afresh, Chapter 8 seeks to explicate the kinds of explanations psychiatry is capable of delivering in terms of unconscious mental states. The chapter focuses on the psychoanalytic theory of dreams as its example. The essential thesis of the chapter is that although each of the various levels of explanation in the psychoanalytic theory of dreams is cast in terms of unconscious reasons for action, there is almost no case in which psychoanalysts can make out that form of explanation. Rather, each of these levels of explanation is shown to be better conceptualized in terms of causes, functions, or nonexplanatory interpretations.

Chapter 9 applies the insights of Chapter 8 to the assessment of moral and legal responsibility. If the form of explanation psychoanalysts proferred were in terms of unconscious reasons for action, then what we take to be accidents should really be seen as intentional actions for which we are responsible. Given the pervasiveness of the unconscious, the extension of responsibility in such a case would be dramatic. However, by having reconceived the kind of explanation psychoanalysis has in fact provided, such extension of responsibility can be seen to be unwarranted, which is the overall thesis of Chapter 9.

Chapter 10 begins with a common assertion among psychiatrists in general, and psychoanalysts in particular, that the unconscious, far from extending responsibility, contracts it to the vanishing point. We are never responsible, in this view, because our conscious will is in the grip of the unconscious. Chapter 10 separates four strands of this argument, and shows how the correct conception of the unconscious supports none of these strands. That we are responsible for our consciously intentional actions, despite our possession of an unconscious, is the general thesis of this chapter.

In Part IV I examine the last of the three challenging ideas of psychiatry, namely, the fragmentation of the self threatened by any partitioning scheme such as Freud's that would urge that "we" are best conceived as communities of subagents rather than as unified persons. Chapter 11, the only chapter in this part, proceeds in two steps. I first organize the insights about human behavior that might tempt one to subdivide a person into multiple selves. Very generally, these insights are three: Persons are con-

Introduction

flict-ridden creatures, they have a mind that can be given a functional organization, and they have an unconscious. The second step is to examine various senses in which one might say that we lack unity of self and to conclude that in no harmful sense can psychoanalytic theory or the data on which it is based show that most of us are not one, unified self presupposed by law and morality.

In the conclusion I shall return to the ultimate theses of the book: first, that both lawyers and psychiatrists need to know more about the philosophy of science, the philosophy of mind, and the philosophy of law if either group is to get straight the relationship between the two disciplines; and second, that a rethinking of the relationship in terms of such knowledge should show that neither the legal nor the psychiatric theory of the person departs significantly from the ancient and commonsense idea that persons are beings who are sufficiently rational, "in charge" of their actions, and unified in their purposes, that they may justly be the subjects of praise and blame, justly the holders of rights and of responsibilities.

A word of warning may be in order to the nonphilosophical readers of this book. Chapters 1 and 2 may well be slow going for those unfamiliar with the recent philosophy of action/philosophy of mind or with that part of moral philosophy dealing with the concepts in terms of which we ascribe responsibility. Such readers may find it profitable to delay reading Chapters 1 and 2 and begin with Chapter 3, which sets forth the three challenges of psychiatry described earlier. In doing this one will have to rely on one's intuitive understanding of the concepts of rationality and autonomy and their relation to the law's views about persons, but since each of us has some intuitive understanding of such concepts this may not be too serious a disadvantage. Those readers who do bypass Chapters 1 and 2 may wish to return to those chapters as they find it necessary in pursuing the topics of the later chapters. Chapter 8, for example, presupposes that the reader has ready to hand the typology of explanatory accounts developed in Chapter 1, for that typology is used in the later chapter to clarify psychoanalytic explanations. Chapters 9 and 10, as another example, similarly presuppose that the reader has rather clearly in mind the conditions under which responsibility is ascribed, the main subject of Chapter 2, for the unconscious is discussed in the later chapters as it affects those conditions.

Chapters 1 and 2 are included early in the book, despite their density, because they are logically prior to the later discussion. The reader who wishes to build the argument from the ground up will thus wish to read straight through, holding the author to make good his promise that each of the philosophical distinctions discussed in the early chapters will have its payoff in understanding the relations between law and psychiatry addressed in the later chapters.

I Law and Psychiatry: Competing Views of Persons?

1 The Idea of Practical Reason and Explanation in the Social Sciences

A CONCEPT CENTRAL to our understanding of ourselves is the idea of practical reason. Before exploring the relation between personhood and practical reason (the burden of Chapter 2), the preliminary task undertaken in this chapter is to understand the idea of practical reason itself. This I shall do in terms of a notion that runs throughout the social sciences, the idea of explaining human behavior by "reasons for action."

Reason-Giving Explanations and Practical Reasoning

One might say a host of seemingly distinct things in response to the question of why one performed a certain action. One might open a window, for example, because one is too hot, or in order to chill the wine, or because one believes that the English guests present prefer a cooler room temperature, and so on. Despite the appearances, all such explanations fit a relatively straightforward pattern of explanation that philosophers today call "reasons for action."[1] Although in ordinary speech we often cite only one of the premises (and sometimes give only an elliptical expression of this premise), a full explanation in terms of reasons for action requires two premises: the major premise, specifying the agent's desires (goals, objectives, moral beliefs, purposes, aims, wants, etc.), and the minor premise, specifying the agent's factual beliefs about the situation he is in and his ability to achieve, through some particular action, the object of his desires.

Thus, if X opens the window in order to chill the wine (alternatively, because he believes the wine is warm or because he wants to chill the wine), we will have explained his action by citing explicitly or implicitly:

1. his desire that the wine be chilled and
2. his belief that opening the window will chill the wine.

Knowing this desire and belief set of X, we can understand his action in the fundamental way in which we understand all human actions, in terms of the agent's reasons or motives for acting.

There are two quite distinct components to the understanding generated by this mode of explanation, which have given rise to much confusion in contemporary philosophy. Reasons for an action both *rationalize* the action and causally explain it.

Taking these aspects in order, a belief/desire set rationalizes an action in the sense that it portrays the action as the rational thing to do, given the agent's beliefs and desires. We understand the action in this sense because we can understand that a rational agent would so act, that had we a similar belief/desire set, we too would so act. We can see the action as a means to something the agent wants. As long as the object of the agent's desire is intelligible as something a person in our culture could conceivably want, and so long as the factual beliefs are not themselves irrational, we can empathize with the action, even if we disagree with it morally or aesthetically. We can empathize because, knowing the belief/desire set, we perceive the activity to be the rational thing for an agent with such beliefs and desires to do.

This aspect of reasons for acting, or motives, is sometimes confusingly expressed by saying that there is a *logical* connection between the sentences describing the belief/desire set and the sentence describing the action.[2] Yet without supplementation with further premises[3] there is no logical connection between sentences describing a desire and a belief of an agent, and a sentence describing the agent's action. Still, there is some connection between the *content* of the beliefs and desires and the action they explain. The content of X's belief about means (constituting the minor premise) will necessarily include the same description of the action to be explained (opening the window), as is given in the conclusion, and the content of this belief will also necessarily include the same description of the object of the desire (chilling the wine), as is given in the major premise. One may schematize this practical syllogism as follows:

1. $D(q)$
2. $B(p \supset q)$
   p

Here $D(q)$ means "X desires that the wine be chilled"; $B(p \supset q)$ means "X believes if he opens the window, then the wine will be chilled"; and p means "X opens the window."

To specify with any precision the kinds of relationships that must obtain between each of the occurrences of p, between each of the occurrences of q, and between p and q in the second premise in the foregoing schema is a matter of surprising complexity. For there are deep philosophical difficulties about the semantics of those sentence fragments describing the content of mental states such as beliefs and desires.[4] Nonetheless, for our purposes it may suffice to say, first, that p and q name the same proposition in each of their occurrences in the explanation schema; this means that the p, p and q, q relationship required for a belief/desire set to constitute a reason-giving form of explanation are those of propositional identity: $p = p$ and $q = q$. Second, it may also suffice to say that the relationship between p and q in the second premise is that of material implication, so that the action described by p is taken to be a sufficient condition for obtaining the state of affairs described by q. That all three of these relationships hold for belief/desire sets that are reasons for actions is but to say that we presuppose the rationality of the agent who will see these relationships in selecting a means to the desired end. To say there is a "logical relationship" in such patterns of explanation is really to say that an action is *rationalized* in the fashion just outlined.

The second sense in which we understand an action when we understand its reason is that we understand which of an agent's many beliefs and desires actually caused this action. When we say that X opened the window because of his beliefs and desires, the "because" is necessarily causal. For X might have had any number of belief/desire sets that would equally well rationalize his actions. He might have desired, for example, to offend his guests and believed that intentionally opening the window would accomplish that; yet even if he has such a desire, and even if he intentionally opens the window, it need not be for the latter reason at all. He may be much too polite for that. His reason may be simply as stated earlier: to chill the wine. Which reason is his reason for opening the window is a straightforwardly causal hypothesis: Whichever belief/desire set caused him to act as he did explains his action. Thus the etymology of "motive": something that moves us to action.

Often it is the case that we act for mixed motives. On the causal account of reasons for action such cases should be analyzed in the same way as are concurrent cause problems generally. Just as there are two sorts of concurrent causes in a wide variety of explanatory contexts, there are two sorts of mixed motives: (1) where each belief/desire set was sufficient (the overdetermination cases), and (2) where each set was necessary but only jointly sufficient. Irrespective of which kind of mixed motives one has when one acts, it remains true that of all the belief/desire sets the actor may have had that would rationalize his action, only those that (jointly or singly) cause it are the motives or reasons for that action.

An explanation in terms of reasons for action requires that both the rationalization and the causation features be satisfied. A belief/desire set will be a reason for action if and only if it both rationalizes and causes the action it is supposed to explain. It is perhaps clarifying to consider briefly two philosophical traditions that favor one of these functions to the exclusion of the other in their account of reason-giving explanations.

There is, first of all, a well-entrenched body of philosophical literature that has urged that reasons cannot be causes.[5] The early versions of this position have been nicely set forth and demolished in a seminal work by Donald Davidson.[6] One later version has been to urge that reasons cannot be causes because reasons serve *exclusively* a rationalizing function. As put forward by A. R. Louch, for example, reasons are seen as justifying warrants for action and thus cannot serve as causes.[7]

The problem with this view is that it reconstrues reason-giving *explanations* as if they were nonexplanatory *justifications*. In such a view it only looks as if we are giving explanations in terms of causally efficacious belief/desire sets when we give reasons for our actions; really, we are only justifying our actions by exhibiting them as necessary means to some end we and our audiences share. In short, this view would collapse explanation by reasons into what are popularly known as "rationalizations."

The term rationalization was coined by Ernest Jones,[8] Freud's biographer and one of his inner circle, to describe the citing of belief/desire sets for action when the sets cited were not reasons for acting. Belief/desire sets cited in this way are often given to justify an action, by showing it to be the rational thing to do relative to the (presumably good) end cited. Such sets do not explain an action, however, because they did not cause it. Rationalization in Jones's sense is an attempt to parade as the reasons explaining an action those belief/desire sets that would justify the action if they were the reasons for which it was performed. In other words, rationalization is justification, or an attempt at it—not explanation at all. Motives must explain as well as justify in Jones's sense of "rationalize," or else they are not the reasons for an action.

Another philosophical position would urge the opposite mistake.[9] In this view, a belief or a desire can be the reason for an action if such belief or desire—or the two together—causes the action in question. It need not be the case that the belief or the desire *rationalize* the action for such mental states to be reasons for acting. To test such a view, consider two examples of causation by desires or by beliefs without rationalization:[10]

1. His desire to beat Bobby Fisher caused his heart attack.
2. His belief that a murderer was prowling in the hall caused his heart to palpitate.

It is plain that such mental states of belief and desire do not explain their respective behaviors in the way reasons explain actions. In such cases the desire or the belief causes the event to be explained, but the belief or desire does not rationalize the event. We do not, in such examples, come to see the heart attack or palpitation as the action of a rational agent pursuing an end that is intelligible to us. The desires and beliefs accordingly do not operate in such explanations as reasons for action. For that matter, the events explained are not actions at all. The desires or beliefs simply cause these nonaction events.

To summarize the result of this discussion: A desire that some state of affairs q obtain is the reason for an intentional action p by action X if and only if:

1. X desired q; and
2. X believed that doing p would produce q; and
3. X's doing p was caused by a desire for q and the belief that doing p would produce q.

The event to be explained, the action, is both exhibited as the rational thing to do (because of its relationship to the content of the beliefs and desires in the first two criteria) and explained (because of the causal hypothesis in the third criterion).

Having outlined a relatively standard account of reasons for action, it remains to relate that account to the ideas of practical reason and practical reasoners. Reasons for acting is a form of explanation in terms of states that exist at a time in the world and that enter into causal relations with themselves and actions. Often confused with this form of *explanation* is the kind of *logic* or patterns of valid inferences that rational agents employ as or before they act.[11] Logic deals with timeless propositions (not states or events) and with the logical (not causal) relations between them. The kind of inference-drawing patterns that deal with action have, since Aristotle, been called "practical syllogisms," and the kind of reasoning one does who employs such practical syllogisms Aristotle called "practical reasoning."[12]

Practical reasoning involves the formulation of ends and the selection of means to the attainment of those ends. Practical reasoning thus takes the *content* of one's desires or moral beliefs and the *content* of one's factual beliefs to be premises in an argument. The actor worrying about chilling the wine might reason:

1. Let it be the case that the wine is chilled.
2. If I open the window, then the wine is chilled.

Therefore:

3. I open the window.

Such practical reasoning is practical in that it aims at telling us what to do. In this it is to be distinguished from what Aristotle called "theoretical reasoning," which aims at telling us what to believe. The conclusion of a practical syllogism is accordingly a directive to action, not the more typical proposition about how the world is, the conclusion of true logical syllogisms. Moreover, apart from the differing form of their conclusions, practical syllogisms do not fit any of the patterns of valid inference of standard deductive logic. The conclusion that I should open the window does not follow deductively from the two premises stated.

The relation of practical reasoning to reason-giving explanations should be relatively apparent: The premises of a valid practical argument leading to some directive to action as its conclusion are just the contents of a belief/desire set that could rationalize the action in question. In terms of the example given, the validity of a practical syllogism consists in three relations obtaining: first, that the proposition in premise 1 (the wine is chilled) is identical to the proposition contained in the consequent clause of premise 2 (the wine is chilled); second, that the proposition in the antecedent clause of premise 2 (I open the window) is identical to the proposition in the conclusion (I open the window); and third, that the state of affairs described in the antecedent clause of premise 2 (the window is opened) is a sufficient condition for the occurrence of the state of affairs described in the consequent clause of premise 2 (the wine is chilled).

The extent to which agents must actually reason through a valid practical argument before we are entitled to explain their actions as having been done for reasons is somewhat less apparent. In Chapter 7 I shall examine and reject the argument that one must *consciously* reason through such practical arguments for reason-giving explanations to be appropriate. But despite the conclusion of that discussion, it still must be the case that a belief/desire set can be the reason for which an action was done only if the actor (consciously or unconsciously) reasoned through a valid practical syllogism. Practical reasoning at some level of consciousness is a presupposition of reason-giving explanations.

What kinds of agents can be practical reasoners? I shall argue in the succeeding chapter that the preeminent practical reasoners with which we are familiar are persons. Before addressing the connection between personhood and practical reason, however, other forms of explanation require some discussion.

Contrasting Mentalistic Explanations and Interpretations

Reason-giving accounts are not the only kind of explanations social scientists give to explain human behavior. It is my purpose here to distinguish two kinds of explanations with which reasons for action are often confused. I shall call these "mental cause explanations" and "hermeneutic interpretations." The first is to cite a belief, desire, or other mental state that *causally explains* a human action but does not rationalize it; the second is to cite a belief/desire set that *rationalizes* but does not causally explain some human action. One might thus view these two forms of explanation as partial or incomplete reason-giving accounts in that they each perform only one of the defining functions of the reason-giving form of explanation.

MENTAL STATE CAUSATION

Mental cause explanations that do not amount to reasons for action were mentioned briefly before.[13] The examples given were of two kinds: where a desire alone caused an event ("His desire to beat Bobby Fisher caused his heart attack"), and where a belief alone did so ("His belief that a murderer was prowling in the hall caused his heart to palpitate"). Because it turns out to be more pertinent to the psychoanalytic explanations of behavior later examined, I shall focus on the first kind of mental cause explanation alone, that is, where desires cause events.

From the examples of such explanations that most readily come to mind, there seems to be a lack of two characteristics of a truly motivational explanation. First, the minor premise is missing entirely. Our ambitious chess player did not *believe* that having a heart attack would get him what he wanted (beating Bobby Fisher in chess). Second, the chess player did not perform an *action* in having a heart attack; it was something that happened to him, not something he did.

Lack of each of these features is sufficient to disqualify such explanations as motivational in character. With respect to the first, without the belief that action p leads to object of desire q, the desire for q will not rationalize p in any of the senses shortly to be explored. For it is the content of the belief that makes the action the rational thing to do in order to obtain the object of the desire. Without such a belief, a desire with any object may be cited as the cause of any event. A desire to be an artist may cause one to live a long time, to kill one's mother, or to cut off an ear. Without the belief, the object of the desire need have no "rationalizing" connection to the action; the desire with such an object need only be a cause of the action.

With respect to the second deficiency—the lack of an action to be explained—there is a long-noticed conceptual connection between the concept of reasons and that of an action. Indeed, in contemporary accounts of action the one often is used as a sufficient criterion for the other.[14] If an event is motivated, then that event is an action, on this account. This of course means that if some event is *not* an action, then whatever is cited to explain it *cannot* be a reason. The range of items reasons explain is limited to actions. Accordingly, to cite a desire as an explanation of a heart attack, which is not an action, cannot be a reason-giving explanation.

There is, I think, nothing wrong with this traditional analysis of the connection between the concepts of acting and of acting for reasons. Reasons are reasons *for acting*. If we acted for a reason, necessarily we acted. What is overlooked by those who use reasons as their criterion of action is the Freudian possibility: The discovery of hidden reasons ipso facto transforms the events explained by them into full-fledged human actions. If one has as one's only criterion of action that it be explicable by reasons, then there is nothing to prevent a Freudian from expanding the extension of "action" by discovering hidden motives. What one needs is some criterion of action, other than reasons, in order to make the objection here interposed—no action—a significant objection. I defer discussion of this until Chapter 2, where I attempt to draw out an account of action that is independent of the explanation-by-reasons theory of action.

Assuming we have some criterion of action independent of the appropriateness of reason-giving explanations, the earlier chess player example remains distinguishable on both grounds, no belief and no action. It turns out that the first is the more crucial of the distinctions in any event. For there are explanations of events that are admittedly actions, but that nonetheless are not motivational explanations.[15] Suppose X is a prisoner who wants very much to get out of prison. He rattles the bars of his cell "because he wants out." His rattling the cage is an action he performs, and his desires cause it; yet he does not rattle the bars in order to get out because he does not believe for an instant that he can shake loose the bars. His desire, in other words, is not his reason for acting. He must adopt his action as a means to attain the object of his desire, which he does not do because he does not have the requisite belief in the causal efficacy of his action. His action expresses his desire, if you like, but he does not act on it as a reason.

Although in the example given the distinction seems intuitive enough, the way to blur the distinction is to allow that *invalid* practical reasoning could be the reasons for which one acted.[16] If belief/desire sets the contents of which form invalid practical syllogisms could nonetheless be reasons for acting, then the distinction between reason-giving explanations and mental cause explanations would not evaporate. It would, however, become a matter of degree: At some point, one would say, the reasoning is too defective to rationalize the behavior that it causes so that the desire/belief set should be seen only as a mental cause and not as a reason.

Examples of such "imperfect practical reasoning" are more difficult to come by than it has seemed to some philosophers. Let me begin with a case of weakness of will, since weakness of will is often the kind of case thought to require the notion of invalid practical reasons.[17] Suppose that the prisoner of a moment ago wants more than anything else to escape from prison; he is in a situation such that he believes that if he shoots the guard standing between him and freedom, he will successfully escape for good. He further believes that shooting the guard is the *only* way he will escape. Nonetheless, he cannot bring himself to do it. So he ends up shooting near the guard, but not at him, knowing full well that this will not only *not* let him escape but will get him into further trouble.

What is the form of the explanation for this seemingly irrational action? If the belief/desire set already described explains the prisoner's action, it may seem to be an example of invalid practical reasoning operating as a reason for action, for the prisoner's reasoning would be:

1. Let it be the case that I escape.
2. If I shoot at the guard, then I will escape.

Therefore:

3. I will *not* shoot at the guard but only near him.

The problem for this kind of example is the doubt one should have that the cited belief/desire set explains the prisoner's action at all. For although by hypothesis the prisoner has the desire to escape and the belief about shooting the guard as the necessary means to escape, prima facie these do not cause him to shoot near the guard. Rather, a second belief/desire set seems to explain the prisoner's action: He does not want to be a murderer and believes that if he shoots the guard, he will be. This second belief/desire set adequately rationalizes his action (i.e., its contents form a valid practical syllogism); assuming that it causes him to shoot near the guard rather than at him, the second belief/desire set explains his action. And this second set is unproblematically of the reason-giving form.

In order to get the desire to escape back into the picture, suppose one shifted the question slightly. Rather than asking, Why did he shoot *near* the guard rather than at him? suppose one asked, Why did he shoot at all?[18] A truthful answer to this latter question might well be: He wanted to escape very much. Now, however, although the desire to escape explains the action, there is little temptation to regard such desires as a reason for action. The desire that explains the action operates in a purely causal way, with *no* rationalization of the action. There does not seem to be even an *invalid* practical inference by the prisoner in such a case.

So suppose that we ask a third question: Why did the prisoner shoot near the guard, rather than shooting in the air or doing something else that would equally well express his frustration? The explanation for this kind of expression of frustration might well be: He believed that by shooting *at* the guard he could have escaped, which he very much wanted to do. It was because shooting *near* the guard was much like shooting *at* the guard that it, rather than some other action, was the way in which he expressed his frustration.

To answer this third question, it is his desire to escape and his belief that shooting at the guard would allow him to escape that cause the action; yet the action done is still not rationalized by the belief/desire set because the action is not a believed means to the satisfaction of the desire. Should we classify this nonetheless as a reason-giving account? I think the answer is still no. Only if the actor has another belief—that if he shoots near the guard he is really shooting at the guard—can one make this into a reason-giving account.[19] As it stands, because the belief and desire do not rationalize the action they cause, they are not the reason for which it is done. Mental cause accounts, no matter how closely they approximate a fully rationalizing practical syllogism, remain non-reason-giving accounts. This is true even when, as in this last example, both a belief and a desire cause the act, and when the act that is caused is "very close" to an action that would be rationalized by the belief/desire set in question.

HERMENEUTIC INTERPRETATIONS

Explanations in the social sciences are often said to be different from explanations in the natural sciences because in social sciences explanations are discoveries of the *meaning* of certain behavior.[20] The first thing one wants to see here is the variety of things that can be meant by this claim *short of saying* that a social scientist uses a reason-giving form of explanation. The most natural way to order this variety is by starting with a likely consequence of an action and seeing what else has to be said before that consequence would be eligible to fully rationalize that action, in the way that reasons do.

Suppose an actor (X) strikes another (Y) and that the likely consequence of this (R) is that there will be violent retaliation. One sense in which we may say that X's action has meaning is the sense of meaning in which we might say, "This means that Y will retaliate."[21] An action has meaning in this sense only because we, the observers, perceive that R is a likely consequence of the action. There is no implication that X in any sense perceived this meaning or acted because of that perception.

This "observer meaning" can be what one discovers when one "finds the meaning" of a painting or other work of art. Often the motives with which the artist painted the painting are judged totally irrelevant to what the painting means. The (observer) meaning of the painting is what we, the observers, think to be a plausible interpretation of its elements, and our interpretive judgments are guided by what we think to be the likely impressions produced by various elements of the painting.

There is undoubtedly more to art interpretation than this, but the example, even when supplemented by a more adequate analysis, is illustrative of the basic distinction proposed: between the meaning the painting may have for us as we observe the effects its elements produce within us, and the meaning it had for the actor who produced it. Much of our finding meaning in phenomena consists only of our perceiving likely consequences of those phenomena.

If we are to move beyond the minimal sense of (observer) meaning to begin to rationalize the action, we must come to see some likely consequence as a "possible motive" for an action.[22] This involves two steps: First, we must judge that it would not be irrational for an actor in X's position to have believed that striking Y would lead to retaliation;[23] second, we must judge that it would be an intelligible thing to want, that Y retaliate.[24] If the belief is widely irrational—for example, that saying "storks" rather than "stocks" will make one a mother—then we cannot fully understand the action as that of a rational agent. Similarly, if the desire is so bizarre as to be unintelligible to us—say, a desire to keep one's elbow in the mud all afternoon for no further reason—we also cannot understand the action as that of a fully rational agent. Only if there is a set of rational beliefs promoting intelligible desires can we exhibit an action as fully rational.

It is true that any set of beliefs and desires that fits the general form, X desires q, X believes that if he does p, then q will be obtained, will exhibit action p as rational in some sense.[25] Let us say of such cases that an action is exhibited as being *minimally* rational if we can hypothesize a set of beliefs and desires the content of which exhibits the form of a valid practical syllogism, no matter how bizarre or irrational those beliefs and desires themselves may be. Let us say that an action is *fully* rational only if the beliefs are themselves rational and the desires are themselves intelligible.

Notice that to say any of these things about an action is still not to say anything about the actor. To say that an action may be seen as either minimally or fully rational is only to say that we, the observers, can hypothesize a set of beliefs and desires that, if the actor had them and acted on them, would render the action rational. Hence, to say that an action has meaning in this second sense still says nothing about the actor.

In order to transform these interpretations of the meaning of behavior into reason-giving explanations of behavior, three things are necessary. First, it must be the case that the desire we discovered is not only intelligible to us as an end on which a person might act; it must also have been a desire that the actor in question must have possessed. It must have been the actor's desire. Second, the belief we posit in interpreting the behavior must not only be a rational belief to hold; it must also have been a belief the actor actually possessed. Again *the actor's* belief. And third, for this belief and this desire to have been the reason for acting, they must have *caused* the action in question.

To say all of this is to maintain a sharp distinction between *interpreting* human action by finding its meaning and *explaining* human action by finding the reasons for which it was done. Interpretation is only the discovery that there is an intelligible end and a set of rational beliefs in light of which the action would be a rational thing to do. Such interpretive accounts do not explain actions.

This distinction will later become important to us in understanding the nature of psychoanalytic theory, because it will allow us to separate Freud's interpretive ambitions (for dreams and the like) from his explanatory ambitions. In the present context the distinction is important to us in understanding the nature of reason-giving explanations in terms of what they are *not:* They are not mere rationalizations.

Rather remarkably an entire tradition has grown up that, if it does not deny this distinction altogether, at the very least blurs it beyond recognition. This tradition has quite diverse strands. One strand I have adverted to before, consisting of that group of analytic philosophers who believed that reasons explained actions *only* by showing actions to be warranted in light of a set of ends they served.[26] Any such view makes meaning interpretation indistinguishable from reason-giving explanation. Another strand of this tradition stemmed from the philosophy of the later Wittgenstein.[27] Richard Peters,[28] the early Melden,[29] and Peter Winch,[30] among others,[31] were much impressed with Wittgenstein's discussions of games and rituals as the basis of understanding social behavior. They accordingly wished to view acting for reasons as an instance of "rule-following" behavior. In response to the crucial question of whether there was any difference between behavior that happened to be in accordance with some regularity an observer could discover, and rule-following behavior, such philosophers urged that the difference was to be found more in the observer than in the phenomena. As Peter Winch put it, "It is only in a situation in which it makes sense to suppose that *somebody else* could in principle discover the rule which I am following that I can intelligibly be said to be following a rule at all."[32] Only if it is possible for the observer to grasp what regularities the actor is following "by being brought to the pitch of himself going on in that way,"[33] can the actor be said to be following a rule.

With such a viewpoint it becomes impossible to distinguish mere interpretations by meanings from true explanations by reasons. For in such an account acting from reasons is no more than behavior in accordance with regularities about which we, the observers, are willing to take a certain point of view (namely, to interpret it as rule *following* and not merely being "rule governed").

Practical Reason and Explanation

Two other strands of this tradition are to be found in two groups of historians and philosophers of history. The first group, led by the work of Michael Oakeshott[34] and William Dray,[35] urged that history does not proceed by the discovery of general laws, as is the case in the natural sciences. Rather, history explains particular events with the aid of other particular events. Because of this, it was thought, history could not be seen as providing causal accounts of human behavior. (This would have to be true if Carl Hempel's famous analysis of causal accounts in terms of general, "covering" laws were correct.[36]) History accordingly was seen as providing noncausal interpretations—what Dray calls "rational explanations"—of human actions. Since history, like other social sciences, uses the language of reasons for action in its explanations, this group's construal of historical explanations as consisting of noncausal interpretations collapses any distinction between meaning interpretations and reason-giving explanations.

The second group in the philosophy of history tending to blur the meaning/reasons distinction is that flowing from the work of R. G. Collingwood.[37] Collingwood urged that historical explanation (in terms of the reasons of historical agents) could not be approached solely from its "external" aspect; rather, historians had to be "internal" in the sense that they needed empathetic understanding of the historical agent's reasons. Historians needed to be able to recapitulate the practical inferences of their subjects, and they could do this only if they could see as desirable the major premises of such practical reasoning. Collingwood's admirers would put this by saying that historians cannot *understand* the subject's reasons except by this act of imagination, wherein what is meant by "understand" is a special sense of the word much like the Droysen–Dilthey–Weber idea of *verstehen*.[38]

Where those sympathetic to the *verstehen* tradition in history usually end up is in collapsing reason-giving explanations into mere interpretations of the meaning of social phenomena. For "empathetic understanding" again emphasizes the *observer's* role in explaining historical events to the exclusion of the role of the historical actor's actual psychological states. One would not have to say that empathy is any more than a heuristic device to get at what were *really* the causally operative reasons of some historical agent; but admirers of Collingwood, Weber, et al. typically claim much more than this for empathy, namely, that the *truth* of an historical explanation in terms of reasons itself depends on whether this empathetic understanding is attainable. This again collapses reason-giving explanations into mere meaning interpretations.

Yet another strand contributing to the interpretive tradition is those contemporary philosophers who are much impressed with artificial intelligence and the seeming intentionality of computers. Dan Dennett, for example, treats reason-giving explanations as a matter of interpretive strategy.[39] According to Dennett, we are very pragmatic in deciding whether to explain the behavior of a person, an animal, or a computer in terms of beliefs and desires: If doing so aids us in predicting the behavior of the entity, then we should treat it as an "intentional system" that acts for reasons. There appears to be for Dennett no fact of the matter about whether the entity *really* has the beliefs and desires with which we explain its behavior. Rather, framing belief/desire sets in the form of practical syllogisms is an interpretation we place on the facts, an explanatory strategy whose only limits appear to be the pragmatist's slogan, "Do so as long as it is useful." In such a view there is little room for a distinction between explanations in terms of causally operative beliefs and desires, on the one hand, and interpretations in terms of beliefs and desires that the agent did not have, on the other.

The last of the strands supporting the interpretivist tradition comes from an offshoot of continental phenomenology, hermeneutics. Hermeneutics is the art (sometimes said to be the science) of interpretation. Although it would be difficult to characterize this burgeoning literature in a short space,[40] the aspect of hermeneutics that has captured the adherence of such analytic admirers as G. H. Von Wright[41] and Richard Rorty[42] is its holistic approach to explanations. Von Wright, for example, thinks that we attribute belief/desire sets to individuals when doing so best comports with the entire story we can tell about those individuals and the community in which they (and we) live. "Behavior gets its intentional character from being *seen* by the agent himself or by an outside observer in a wider perspective, from being *set* in a context of aims and cognitions."[43]

Because the larger story we choose to tell about human beings is that they are by and large rational (in the sense of acting on valid practical syllogisms), we interpret human behavior in terms of belief/desire sets of the required form: "We turn the validity of the practical syllogism into a standard for interpreting the situation. . . . The necessity of the practical inference schema is, one could say, a necessity conceived *ex post actu*."[44] If one attributes beliefs and desires to an individual in this way—not because he *really* had them, but rather because his having them fits one's narrative or story—then again reason-giving "explanation" is really just interpretation in terms of rationalizing reasons. To the extent which hermeneuticists make Von Wright's kinds of claims, they join him in collapsing explanation by reasons into interpretation by meanings.

All of the quite diverse strands of the tradition I have been considering have in common their denial of two points: (1) that to explain an action by reasons is to claim that the actor really possessed the belief/desire set that was his reason for acting; and (2) that to explain an action by reasons is to claim that some belief/desire set of the actor's *caused* that action. To argue against the interpretive tradition will accordingly be to argue for these two propositions, which I now propose to do.

To argue for the second of these propositions is very straightforward, so I shall address it first. The argument simply is that for any given action there will always be more than one set of beliefs and desires that could fully rationalize it. Without the requirement that a belief/desire set must *cause* the action in question, how could we prefer one set to any other as "the reasons" for which the action was done? Certainly one cannot do so simply on the basis that the belief/desire set must rationalize the action, be intelligible in our culture, make or fit a good story, and the like.

I know of no halfway respectable answer that an interpretivist has to this question. Von Wright's entire treatment of the problem, for example, is as follows:

> A problem which we have not considered here is which of alternative sets of premises should be accepted for a given conclusion. This is the problem of testing the correctness (truth) of the "material," as distinct from "formal," validity of a proposed teleological explanation. *It will not be discussed in the present work.*[45]

Without a better answer than this the interpretivist has not accounted for a fundamental feature of reason-giving explanations, namely, that motives move us to action.

Arguing for the reality of beliefs and desires requires more extended treatment. There are various reasons that might convince one that mental states such as beliefs and desires do not exist except as some kind of fictional posits in the interpretive stance of an observer. Behaviorist suspicions about the public verifiability of mental states are well known. More pertinent here is the kind of skepticism about mental states stemming from one of their long-noticed features, namely, their Intentionality. Franz Brentano made famous the notion that mental states are directed upon Intentional *objects*.[46] Although Brentano meant real objects (albeit not existing in space), modern philosophy reconstrues his insight to be about *language:* Mental states are directed toward some kind of linguistic (either sentential or propositional) object.[47] One does not just desire or believe; one desires that something be the case or believes that something is the case. "Belief" and "desire" are incomplete without some linguistic object. Moreover, what counts as one desire or belief rather than another is a matter of the linguistic objects of those desires or of those beliefs. A belief that it is raining is different from a belief that the weather forecaster is a fool, because the statements believed—"It is raining" and "The weather forecaster is a fool"—are different. Furthermore, the relation between the statement that is the object of belief or desire, and the statement expressed by the overall sentence, is a nontruth–functional relation. For example, the truth of the statement, "John believes that Mary is a hard worker," does not depend on the truth of the statement, "Mary is a hard worker." The latter statement may be true or false without affecting the truth about

John's beliefs. And finally, one can see that such "objects" are essentially linguistic in character by asking questions of reference: Who is referred to when we say, "John believes that Mary is a hard worker"? The obvious answer may seem to be that Mary, the person, is referred to, until we realize that there are other names or descriptions with which we can pick out Mary, for example, "the laziest worker in the office" (if, in fact, Mary is very lazy). If "Mary" names Mary when part of the object of John's belief, then we ought to be able to substitute another equally good name or description for Mary, thus: "John believes that the laziest worker in the the office is a hard worker." Yet this is not at all what John believes. Certain names or descriptions of Mary are what we use to individuate John's beliefs about Mary. We do not use Mary herself. It is in this way that the objects of mental states are essentially linguistic, because it is the language used (rather than the things seemingly referred to by that language) that is important in characterizing the objects of belief or of desire.[48]

Because the objects of the mental states of belief and desire are essentially linguistic, it might seem inevitable that the necessary linguistic characterization of those objects could come from nowhere else *but* the linguistic efforts of the interpreter. The only seeming alternative would be to think that the *actor* explicitly says to himself the sentence that forms the content of his beliefs and desires. Yet such silent soliloquies surely cannot be the source of such contents, because the observer often rewords the actor's own explicit formulation of his beliefs and desires into the observer's own language and his own idiom, and we think it quite legitimate that he do so. Hence, the interpretivist concludes, the *only* way such objects or contents can be formulated is by the observer's empathetic understanding, the desire to fill out a story so it makes sense, and so on.

If I am right, the basic motivation for believing that ascribing "real" beliefs or desires to an agent makes no sense lies in the difficulties one has in formulating the objects of mental states without observer interpretation.[49] That this is an insufficient motive for being an interpretivist can be seen by repairing to another essentially linguistic context, that of reported speech. Suppose an observer reports: "John said that Mary is a hard worker." Such indirect speech, which does not quote the original speaker but paraphrases what he meant, is much like the sentences that describe mental states in that both take linguistic objects. In addition, in neither context is the connection between the dependent clause and the overall sentence truth—functional. The truth of the overall sentence, "John said that Mary is a hard worker," does not depend on the truth of the enclosed sentence, "Mary is a hard worker." For John could have said it without Mary's being a hard worker, just as John could have believed that Mary is a hard worker without Mary's in fact being a hard worker. Moreover, just as before, simply because John said that Mary is a hard worker, it is not true that John said that the laziest worker in the office is a hard worker—even if "Mary" and "the laziest worker in the office" both refer to one and the same person. From these three features one may conclude that the objects of indirect speech are essentially linguistic, just as they are for beliefs, desires, and other mental states.

The truth of the overall sentence, "John said that Mary is a hard worker," is a function of two items: (1) that there was some uterance U by John, and (2) that "Mary is a hard worker" is an accurate interpretation of U. It thus is the case that there is an interpretive task bound up in verifying the truth of the sentences of indirect speech. Yet no one, I should think, would be tempted to assert that because some interpretation is required for the truth of sentences reporting indirect speech, there is no fact of the matter about what the utterance really was.[50] It is true that the observer must characterize (interpret) that utterance—itself a bit of language used by John—but surely the necessity of such interpretation is no argument at all that utterances do not exist except in the observer's "story" or "interpretive stance" or whatever. Utterances are real-world speech acts by real-world people that unproblematically exist.

An interpretivist's response to this might well be that beliefs and desires are unlike utterances in a crucial way. Although both beliefs and utterances take linguistic objects that require interpretation, with utterances there is an established text to be interpreted. For beliefs or desires, the interpretivist might ask, what is *the* authoritative formulation of their objects that can serve as the text against which all interpretations are to be judged for accuracy? One might urge that "the text" forming the objects of beliefs and desires is to be found in the actor's speech to himself about what he wants and what he believes on certain occasions. But this idea—that we have beliefs or desires only when we have engaged in some such silent soliloquy—is a very inaccurate view of mind. We unproblematically explain behavior by reasons when there is no such explicit recital by the actor of the premises of his practical reasoning.

I shall urge in Chapter 7 that the text for beliefs or desires is to be found in two sources: first, in the abilities of the actor to avow the objects of his beliefs and desires. Such abilities do not depend on any silent sayings to oneself, nor need such abilities be readily exercisable by an agent—they may be "repressed." Second, the text may be found in whatever physiological events may turn out to be "the language of thought" in the brain.[51]

Hence, although finding the text is a more complicated affair for beliefs and desires than for utterances, it is not the case that there is *no* text save that which an external observer brings with him when he seeks to explain the behavior. Because there is a text, the need for interpreting that text—the object of beliefs and desires—no more commits one to the interpretivist tradition than a similar need commits one to interpretivism about utterances. Some interpretation is involved in formulating the objects of beliefs, of desires, and of utterances; in all cases, however, there is a fact of the matter about what was *really* believed, desired, or uttered.

Functional Attributions

The word "purpose" has two distinct senses: In one sense it is a member of the family of concepts used in reason-giving explanations (motive, intention, desire, etc.); in the other it specifies the function some process, object, or action may serve. If I distribute leaflets protesting the continuation of nuclear testing, my purpose (reason) in doing so can be to end the tests. A social scientist, however, might describe my action as serving the purpose (function) of alienating local law-enforcement officials, if in fact that is what occurs as a result of my activity. The apparent discrepancy between my statement of purpose and the social scientist's is not like the disagreement an actor sometimes has with an observer as to the actor's motives. Rather, two different kinds of statement have been made. Both of them could be correct, and yet I still may not have acted from mixed motives.

Function statements share an overlapping vocabulary with reason-giving explanations. The word purpose can mean either, as the leaflet example illustrates; the phrasing "in order to" or "for the sake of" is equally appropriate with either type of statement. Both types of statements are often thought to give teleological explanations. Both concepts may share a common historical origin in primitive animism.[52] Because of these superficial grammatical similarities and historical background, it is common to find one kind of statement being confused with the other. This is particularly true of both popular and psychoanalytic talk of unconscious purposes. Because of this potential and actual confusion, a brief examination of the meaning of function statements and of the ways in which they differ from statements giving reasons will be pursued.

THE LOGIC OF FUNCTIONAL ATTRIBUTIONS

As an example of a function statement, consider the statement, "The function of the heartbeat is to circulate the blood."[53] Four elements are commonly found in the unpacking of such statements: (1) a system (S) is tacitly assumed; (2) an endstate or goal of the system (ES) is also tacitly assumed; (3) an identifiable part of the system or a process (P) occurring within the system (which is the item for which an explanation is sought) is expressly mentioned; and (4) an effect (E) of the process or part (that is also a state of the system) is expressly mentioned.

In such an explanation the information content is that the activity of the part or process P causally contributes to the occurrence of the effect E; the tacit assumptions further assert that E itself causally contributes to the attainment or to the maintenance of the system as a whole in some general end state ES. Thus, "the function of the heartbeat is to circulate the blood" presupposes the existence of a system (the human body), labels an identifiable part (the heart) or process (the heart's beating), and specifies an immediate effect of that process, namely, a state of the system in which the blood circulates. The function assigned to the heart is the effect named in the statement (the circulation of blood), and the information content is that in certain living systems with which we are familiar (namely, vertebrates), the heart's beating causes the circulation of blood. This effect (the circulation of blood) is only of interest to us because it itself in turn causally contributes to the survival of such organisms. Hence, the ultimate implication of such a functional statement will be that the beating of the heart causally contributes to the survival of the organism.

It is important to stress that it is only relative to some end state ES in system S that a function may be assigned. For if one did not have in view a certain end state of a certain system such as physical health, one would be free to designate any consequence of the heart's beating as its function. Carl Hempel's example of another effect of the heart's beating is the noise it makes in the chest cavity. Freed of the requirement that E itself causally contribute to the maintenance of some general end state ES, the one consequence of the heartbeat is as good as the other to be emphasized as *the* function of the heart.

Thus, although the statement with which we began did not expressly mention either a system or an end state, both must be tacitly assumed if anything significant is to be asserted by such statements. In fact, of course, the contexts in which such statements are made will often expressly provide definitions of S and ES.

Such function statements tell us that there is a causal connection between the part or process to which a function is attributed and the existence of the end state. In vertebrates, the heart's beating causes the blood to circulate. Thus, functional explanations involve causal laws, but "in reverse." Rather than explaining the heart's beating by reference to its causes, a function statement mentions one of its effects (the circulation of blood). The relationship of cause and effect is asserted in such statements, but we are told what has been *caused by* the part or process about which we are curious, not what *causes* it to be or to do what it does.

It has struck many people as decidedly peculiar that an effect of an event should be cited to explain it; it sounds much like the Aristotelian notion of a "final cause," where some end causally determines the events that are its means. Yet nothing of the sort need be asserted in one's use of "purpose" in the sense of function. For much of the use of function statements, such as that about heartbeats, is not explanatory of the heartbeat at all; the attribution of functions in such statements is merely a description of the heart or heartbeat that emphasizes one of its capacities. Where scientists share a common concern for a particular system and maintenance of some particular end state in the system, such attribution of functions is a useful descriptive task. Thus, in medicine one is concerned with the human body, and there is widespread agreement among doctors on the desirability of maintaining that system in the particular end state we call health. In such circumstances it is useful for medical texts to attribute functions to organs and other physical structures, or to their activities. Formulating medical information in this way serves to emphasize the causal contribution each such organ or process makes and can make to the maintenance of an end state that it is the business of doctors to preserve. It is a way of referencing a great deal of information in such a way that one knows immediately the contribution of each part of the system to some end state of that system in which one is interested.

The referencing of a good deal of causal information in this way, so as to emphasize just those features relevant to a particular undertaking, does not constitute an explanation of why, for example, a heart beats.[54] Functional statements in such situations are simply a mode of organizing information about parts of a system and their relationship to each other around a central concern. Such functional organization of the parts of a system allows us to see immediately what must be done to keep that system in some desired end state *ES*. It tells us that, if in general we are interested in maintaining system *S* in state *ES*, we must make certain process *P* occurs. If we wish to keep patients healthy, for example, we must keep their hearts beating.

It is sometimes thought that functional attributions make sense only with regard to systems that are self-regulating, that is, that tend naturally to maintain themselves in some end state or that tend naturally to engage in behavior that seeks a goal. Examples of such self-regulating systems can be human artifacts, such as thermostats for furnaces or guidance mechanisms for missiles, or they can be natural systems, such as those subsystems that maintain bodily temperature in vertebrates.

It is true that we are perhaps more comfortable in giving such self-regulating systems a functional organization, because in a sense they seem already to have one. This is because self-regulating systems already seem to define by their behavior the goal or end state around which a functional organization can be built. And insofar as scientists, such as biologists, wish to study such self-regulating systems, there is nothing illegitimate about treating as *the* goal of the system that goal or end state toward whose maintenance the system's parts in fact contribute. It is, however, important to see that functions can meaningfully be attributed within systems that are not self-regulating. One assigns functions, in such a case, not by the causal role each part plays in the system's achieving some natural goal or equilibrium; rather, one assigns functions relative to some goal or end state that one thinks desirable to achieve or maintain in such systems. A chair, for example, could be given a functional organization different from that which normally would suggest itself if one defined the goal of the chair to be other than for sitting by persons; if one referenced the contribution each part made to the ability of a chair to be used as a paperweight, for example, one would assign functions to the parts of the chair quite different from those that would be assigned to it if the chair's purpose is the more normal one.

We fail to perceive this freedom that we have to give any object alternative functional organizations because often (for self-regulating systems) the designed or naturally maintained goal for the system is just the goal we are interested in maintaining in such systems anyway. Physical medicine provides one such example. It is concerned with a well-defined system in which numerous homeostatic balances are maintained (e.g., body temperature), each of which contributes to health and survival; and the maintenance of that same state of that system (health and survival) is one about which doctors are much concerned. The latter is a sufficient basis on which doctors may attribute functions to parts and processes in the body; the former allows biologists, whose profession is not to maintain health or any other end state in human bodies, nonetheless to attribute functions in a similar way. Physical medicine is built on biology, not because doctors cannot give the body a different functional organization than do biologists, but because their own professional concerns (in maintaining just the end state that biologists study) dictate that they do not do so.

The suspicions functional explanations engender outside of medicine or biology are largely due to the fact that functions are assigned without any attention being paid to the interests that guide an intelligent selection of an end state. Rather, some effect of a social practice or habit is singled out as "the function" of the practice in question (and worse, even treated as an explanation of such practice) without any reason being given as to why we should be concerned about the particular end state of the system relative to which the function is assigned. We may be told, for example, that the function of a ceremonial rain dance among certain tribes is to reinforce group solidarity. Although the reinforcement of group solidarity may be an effect of the practice in question, so are many other things—tired feet, satisfaction at the completion of exercise, and relaxation of group anxieties. Without some stipulation of an end state about which we are most concerned to maintain in such systems (societies), or which is in fact maintained in such systems and is therefore worthy of study, there is little to be gained by selecting this one effect of the action in question over a host of others for emphasis as *the* function. It is about as useful as saying that the function of the heart is to produce sounds in the chest cavity. Functions can be assigned only relative to end states, and they are usefully assigned only when such end states are a matter of great interest to us to preserve, or are preserved irrespective of our interests in nature.

REASONS AND FUNCTIONS

The difference between functional attributions and reason-giving explanations should be relatively apparent from the foregoing exposition. Function statements do not give explanations of an event, and in any case they do not explain it in either of the two ways that reasons explain human actions: (1) Assigning a function to an event is not to render that event intelligible in the same way that a possible motive renders an action intelligible, that is, by exhibiting it as the rational thing to do; (2) nor does the function an action may serve in any way involve the mind of the actor — the actor need not believe the action will have the effect called its function, nor need the actor desire (in any sense) to bring about this effect. Each of these two fundamental distinctions is amplified in the following discussion.

Actions are rendered intelligible to us by motivational explanations because the latter presuppose a set of beliefs and desires that are intelligible in a given culture (because they are familiar to the members of that culture), and because such explanations exhibit the action in question as the rational thing to do in light of such intelligible beliefs and desires. Explaining an action by reference to some function it serves, however, is not to show the action as intelligible in this way. This is true, first, because one is not exhibiting the activities of hearts and of individuals in societies as rational when one assigns them a function. One is simply stating in rather peculiar form a causal connection between certain events and the maintenance of certain states in a larger system. Second, the effects that are labeled functions are often not the kinds of affairs people intelligibly desire, in any culture. As Richard Peters once noted, "End-states are not goals like hunting a man, marrying a girl, or becoming Prime Minister. They are more mysterious states of quiescence, satisfaction, tension-reduction, and so on."[55]

Even more fundamentally, assigning a function to an action does not entail anything about the mind of the actor. To say that the function of my distributing leaflets is to aggravate local law-enforcement officials is to assert that such alienation was in fact a consequence of my action — a causal assertion that says nothing about my state of mind (although it has some other implications for further effects on some larger system, as already discussed). For such a result to have been my reason I must have *believed* that such a causal connection existed; whether such an event *is* a consequence of my action is not only insufficient, but also irrelevant, for I could well act with such a reason on the basis of a mistaken belief about a causal connection that does not exist. It is my beliefs and not the objective facts of the matter that are relevant to reason-giving explanations, although not to functional attributions. Similarly, for police baiting to have been my reason I must also have desired that it come about. Unless we all desire all those consequences of our actions that have some conservative impact on some system, the fact that my action has a function is irrelevant to whether I desired one effect the function picks out for emphasis over all the other effects of my action. In short, functions have nothing to do with the actor's mind, and function is not a mental word at all.

To these two differences may be added the highly related point that the scope for appropriate functional attributions is considerably different from the scope of reason-giving explanations. As examined in Chapter 2, reasons explain the actions of persons. Function, however, shares no such restriction. Although functions may be assigned to human actions (usually as having some contributing role in some larger social system), they are also assigned to purely physiological processes, or the movements of parts in man-made machines, or in fact any natural, unintelligent phenomenon with an end state meeting the criteria set forth earlier.

For each of these three reasons, then, functional attributions differ markedly in character from explanations in terms of reasons. None of this is to say that in certain cases the function an action serves may not also be the actor's reason for so acting. Thus, for example, a historian writing about John Stuart Mill might assert that Mill's writing of his autobiography served the function of placing before numerous readers the story of an unusual education. By implicit reference to a system (nineteenth-century English society), and to an end state for that system (a better-educated society, itself thought of as a necessary condition for democracy to work perhaps), a significant functional attribution might be made out here. Yet even if it could, the function served by Mill's action might also turn out to be his reason for having written the book. If Mill adopted an outlook whereby he thought it desirable for society to be educated, and if he believed that publishing the tale of his own education would serve that purpose, and if in fact his beliefs and desires in this respect were the cause of his action, then the education of society was also his reason for writing his autobiography. All that is necessary for such a coincidence of function and motive is that the actor adopt the end state of the system as a personal goal. The most obvious type of motive where such overlap may be most expected is in the moral sphere, where goals may be adopted as a social duty, that is, for social (i.e., systemic) reasons. For well-socialized individuals, the functions served by their actions in society (relative to certain end states such as public order) will often be their reasons in fact for those actions. Such coincidences, of course, do not affect the differences in the two types of explanation. They do make more comprehensible the confusion between them.

Mechanistic Explanations

In both ordinary life and the social sciences we often explain human behavior in ways that prima facie have little to do with the actor's reasons for acting. One may explain X's earlier opening of the window, for example, as being due to various environmental or genetic factors that made X the person that he is, or to various goings-on within his body and brain that cause him to open the window. I propose to call such explanations "mechanistic explanations," and to contrast reason-giving explanations with them.

The distinctive feature of mechanistic explanations is not their dependence on some distinctive notion of the causal relation. It may be the case that there is "one fairly definite meaning associated with the word [cause] in many areas of science as well as in ordinary discourse," as Ernst Nagel once suggested,[56] and that this notion is distinct from the kind of causal relation that connects reasons to the action they explain. My own view is that the causal relation between belief/desire sets and actions is the same as the causal relation between physiological events and action. If so, the distinction between reason-giving explanations and mechanistic explanations is not to be sought here.

The distinctive features of mechanistic explanations are to be found in the range of events eligible to serve as causes or effects. A mechanical cause, as I shall use the phrase, is not a mental state (unless it can be shown that such mental state is identical to some physical state). Explaining that a person went through a window because a truck hit him and pushed him through it would be a mechanistic explanation; explaining that the person went through the window because he was very angry would not be a mechanistic explanation because the cause is a mental state. Events and states of a nonmental sort eligible to serve as mechanical causes are things like the possession of an extra Y chromosome, a tumor in the brain, a low level of neurotransmitters in the brain, or a high level of blood sugar in the bloodstream.

The kinds of events that can be explained by mechanistic explanations also differ somewhat from the kinds of events that can be explained by reason-giving accounts. The kinds of events that reasons can explain are actions by persons or personlike entities. The kinds of events that mechanical causes explain include not only actions by persons, but also all sorts of mental or physical events. The range of items potentially explicable by mechanistic accounts thus overlaps with reason-giving accounts, but is much larger.

A large body of not very persuasive literature in philosophy urges that the domains of events properly explainable by reasons or by mechanical causes are *exclusive* of one another.[57] Often this is put by saying that mechanically caused actions are inconceivable or a contradiction in terms, or even more simply, that actions cannot be caused. I need claim nothing this strong (nor do I believe it to be true). My second distinction between reason-giving and mechanistic explanations does not claim an "exclusive jurisdiction" for each form of explanation; only, that what mechanical causes can explain includes human actions, but much else besides.

Mechanistic explanations are thus distinguishable from reason-giving explanations on two grounds: first, by the kinds of events capable in each case of doing the explaining (the causes), and second, by the kinds of events each form of explanation is capable of explaining (the effects). Intuitively, I think we easily grasp whether a particular explanation is of one kind or the other (or neither). What I now wish to examine is whether reason-giving explanations, despite their commonsense separation from mechanistic explanations, are not in reality a subset of the latter. There are two kinds of reductionist schemes here: physicalist schemes, which would reduce reason-giving explanations to mechanistic accounts in terms of neurophysiological goings-on; and behaviorist schemes, which (when they do not seek to discredit reason-giving accounts entirely) seek to reduce them to the status of a kind of shorthand for overt behavior. In closing this chapter, I shall consider briefly each of such reductionist interpretations of practical reason.

REASONS AND NEUROPHYSIOLOGY

The question here is not whether behavior is determined ("determinism"), nor even whether behavior is determined by those kinds of causes called mechanical causes ("mechanism"). My own determinist and mechanist assumptions are that human behavior is fully determined by mechanistic kinds of happenings in the human body. Even with such strong assumptions the question remains whether reason-giving explanations can be reduced to mechanistic explanations.

As Alan Garfinkel observes in his recent work on explanations, reductionist claims about explanations are often expressed as ontological claims about what there really is. "The claim that psychology is reducible to physics or chemistry is expressed as the statement that people 'are just' physical objects. To claim that actions are reducible to primitive drives is put as the statement that human behavior 'is just' the expression of those drives."[58] With this popular idea of reduction, the question of whether reason-giving explanations could be reduced to neurophysiological explanations would devolve into the question of whether human actions were identical to bodily movements and whether beliefs and desires were identical to certain kinds of brain states.

Each of these questions of identity has spawned an enormous literature in the philosophy of action and the philosophy of mind, respectively. Even if we knew as much of the physiology of musculature as we liked, and even if we knew as much about the brain and central nervous system as we liked, it is far from clear that it would turn out that actions were "just the same as" (i.e., identical to) bodily movements or that beliefs and desires were just the same as certain brain states.

In fact, there have been numerous arguments in philosophy purporting to show that these identities are not logically possible. One popular argument of this kind depends on the differential knowledge we each have of our mental states that we do not have of our brain states. As Norman Malcolm once put it:

> We know that our daughter is afraid of the neighbor's shaggy dog, but we do not know anything about the condition of her brain. We know that our dinner companion just this moment decided to order beef instead of fish, but we know nothing, and care nothing, about what physical processes may be going on inside his skull. As youngsters we learn to use the verbs of sensation, cognition, or intention, without having any knowledge, or even any beliefs, about the inner physiology of human beings. We say that we know that our friend is crying from pain, because we saw him crack his shin on the porch step. But if we were asked whether we are sure that such-and-such a process is taking place in his brain, we should not understand the relevance of the question: it would be an irritating change of subject. Our common procedures of *verifying* that someone feels cold, sees an afterimage, heard the warning gun, suddenly recognized a face in the crowd, are not connected with investigations of inner physiology.[59]

Since we do know what we are talking about when we talk about actions for reasons and yet do not know any physiology, beliefs and desires are not (the argument is supposed to conclude) physiological states.

The problem with this argument is that it uses what we presently know as the touchstone of what there is. Suppose we did not know that water was H_2O. Malcolm's kind of argument could be constructed to show that water was not H_2O because we did not know that it was. Yet scientific discoveries about what is identical to what cannot be foreclosed in this way by our present ignorance. Beliefs and desires might *be* brain states even if we do not know it.

Philosophy is replete with much more sophisticated arguments against identifying acts with movements or beliefs and desires with brain states.

Because of the force of such arguments, many have sought some account of mind that does not commit one to some identity thesis yet allows one to hang on to one's deterministic and mechanistic assumptions about the connection of brain states and behavior. One way of doing this is to adopt a "functionalist" perspective on what mental states are.[60] In such a perspective beliefs and desires are functional states of the person. The existence of such states is *not* dependent on how (or whether) they are physically realized in a person, but rather on the role such states play in that person's intelligent functioning. The analogy is often drawn to the kinds of states posited by researchers in artificial intelligence, who care and know little about the physical structure that may realize the various functionally defined subroutines they have devised.

A functionalist view about mental states leaves the question of reduction unresolved. Functionalism justifies granting "provisional independence" to reason-giving accounts from underlying neurophysiological accounts because it makes intelligible how belief/desire states could cause behavior even if such states do not turn out to be physical states of the brain. As Alan Garfinkel puts it, functionalism makes possible "a style of explanation in which explanations of the upper-level phenomena proceed independently of any reduction. The idea is that no matter what the substratum turns out to be, we can proceed independently to construct upper-level [i.e., mentalistic] explanations."[61]

Provisional independence, however, is all such a view of mind can justify. It cannot justify the much more strident declaration of full independence claimed for reason-giving accounts by the generation of "conceptual analysts" of the 1950s and 1960s.[62] It may turn out that beliefs and desires are states of the brain, despite the difficulties of characterizing the *contents* of such states in the language of neurophysiology. No amount of "category-mistake" type arguments can deny this possibility, so that the best we can do is leave open the question of reduction and proceed nonetheless to treat reason-giving accounts as a distinct and legitimate form of explanation.

Although it is arguable from the historical record, this kind of provisional independence of reason-giving accounts was Freud's own view: "All of our provisional ideas in psychology will someday be based on an organic substructure."[63] Many contemporary psychoanalytic theorists share Freud's reductionist hopes in this regard. David Rapaport, for example, did not question that "motives, just like any other psychological processes, have a (neuro-) physiological substrate in the organism."[64] Despite such reductionist hopes, Freud was wise enough to see that his speculations about the physiological referents of mental terms were just that—speculations—and he refrained from even publishing his *Project for a Scientific Psychology*,[65] which contained them. What Freud and the Freudians have done is grant provisional independence to psychological concepts, including belief and desire, in that they have utilized such concepts as *psychological* concepts, admitting that it could not yet be shown (and indeed, it might not turn out) that they were reducible to physiological concepts.

REASONS AND BEHAVIORISM

The second sort of mechanistic scheme that seeks to reduce reason-giving accounts to mechanistic accounts is behaviorism. Behaviorism consists of an assortment of views, some of which I shall shortly distinguish. In general, however, it should be identified as the view that human behavior is best explained by environmental causes (stimuli), rather than by mentalistic or neurophysiological accounts. Behaviorist explanations are mechanistic in that the events doing the explaining are not mental states, but are natural events occurring in the history of the individual whose behavior they explain.

Not all forms of behaviorism are reductionist in character. What are called "methodological behaviorists" simply put mentalistic explanations to the side, urging that mental states are too private, internal, inferred, or in some other way unfit for a (methodologically) proper science of human behavior.[66] Likewise, B. F. Skinner, although not classifying himself as a methodological behaviorist, is most consistently construed to be nonreductionist in his treatment of mental states.[67] For Skinner, concepts such as belief or desire are to be shunned for a variety of reasons, the most important of which is that such explanations presuppose some kind of "homunculus" who resides "inside" the brain.

Although we shall have occasion to return briefly to Skinner when we look at determinism in psychiatry, for now both he and the methodological behaviorists may be put to the side. This is because, for such nonreductionist behaviorists, there is a clear distinction between reason-giving explanations and mechanistic explanations in terms of environmental causes. I shall now pursue two forms of behaviorism for which the distinction is much less clear.

The first of these is what is often called philosophical, logical, or analytical behaviorism. Philosophical behaviorism is reductionist in character, for it asserts that mental words such as belief or desire name, not behavior itself, but *dispositions* to behave in certain ways. In such an account, to say that X believes that it is raining can be reduced to statements about what X is disposed to do, for example, carry an umbrella, not take long walks, or say "it is raining." To explain an action by citing a belief or a desire, accordingly, will not be to name a set of states *causing* the action; rather, it will be to say that X was disposed to an act of that type, much in the way that to explain a lump of sugar dissolving by citing the sugar's solubility will be to say that it was disposed to do that under certain conditions.

Such a reduction is mechanistic in character because the dispositions to which mental states are reduced are themselves mere theoretical stand-ins ("behavioral constructs") for the real causes of action, environmental stimuli. It is because of our past conditioning that we are disposed, for example, to avoid painful things; so that to explain that X avoided the fire because he did not want to get burned is ultimately to say that events in his past caused him to engage in such pain-avoidance behavior.

Philosophical behaviorism has had its share of prestigious proponents. The tough-minded version of philosophical behaviorism had its origins in the logical positivist philosophy of Rudolph Carnap, who held that "all sentences of psychology describe physical occurrences, namely, the physical behavior of humans and other animals."[68] Psychologists too, influenced by the verificationist theory of meaning of logical positivism, shared this tough-minded view. Clark Hull, for example, held that the "basic elements" out of which a science of psychology was to be constructed were "colorless movements and mere receptor impulses" to which statements about purposes and reasons were to be reduced.[69] There are also many suggestions in Skinner to the effect that such reductions of reason-giving explanations to the nonpurposive language of movements and impulses are possible and desirable.[70]

A less tough-minded reductionist analysis of belief and desire is the philosophical behaviorism of Gilbert Ryle.[71] Unlike Carnap, Hull, and Skinner, Ryle did not seek to reduce talk of desires and so forth to talk of mechanical, "colorless" movements. Ryle's program was to reduce such mentalistic talk to dispositions, including prominently dispositions to behave. The difference for Ryle was that such dispositions need not themselves be further reducible to mechanistic causes in the environment.

Despite its famous proponents, philosophical behaviorism is virtually dead among philosophers, psychologists, artificial intelligence specialists, linguists, and others currently worrying about the nature of mental states such as belief and desire. This is in part due to a variety of philosophical attacks on philosophical behaviorism. These included Norman Malcolm's epistemic arguments, based on the oddness of behavioral translations of first-person psychological reports.[72] ("I am in pain" is a statement whose truth is not inferred by the actor from observing his own pain behavior.) The likes of Richard Peters and others also urged that behavioral reductions could not bridge the "logical gulf" or "categorical difference" between intelligent, rule-following, purposive action, on the one hand, and colorless movements and other "dumb" phenomena, on the other.[73] More recently, Quine and others have urged that certain logical peculiarities of mentalistic language—having to do with belief and other mental words taking *objects* or contents—preclude any kind of reduction, whether of a behavioral or a neurophysiological kind. For Quine, as for Skinner, this means one should *avoid* belief, desire, and other Intentional idioms, in formulating a truly scientific (and behaviorist) science of human behavior; one should avoid such idioms precisely because one could *not* reduce them to scientifically respectable (i.e., non-Intentional) speech.[74]

The death knell for philosophical behaviorism has not come from any of these arguments, however (some of them, indeed, are not persuasive), but from other considerations. One is the erosion of the logical positivist theory of meaning underlying philosophical behaviorism. The main temptation to seek to reduce belief or desire to behavior comes from a logical positivist view about meaning according to which all nonanalytic expressions must have currently verifiable conditions that can serve as the criteria for the correct use of those expressions. For mental terms such as belief, the only public evidence we have is the behavior of the person whose belief it is, which leads directly to the reductionist analysis of philosophical behaviorism. Few persons today would subscribe to such a logical positivist theory of meaning, for reasons which I have gone into in detail elsewhere.[75] Briefly, belief can be a meaningful term even if we have no criteria for its application. Beliefs, desires, and the like may be real physiological states of the brain, or they may be nonreducible functional states, as already discussed. This scientific question cannot be foreclosed by enshrining our present indicators of mental states in people (behavior of certain sorts) as if such indicators were analytically necessary or sufficient conditions. It is good evidence that one is in pain, for example, that one engages in pain-expressing behavior; such evidence, however, cannot be said to be an analytically necessary or sufficient *criterion* for being in pain. For an individual could learn the pain behavior, act just as if he were in pain, and yet not be in pain; alternatively he could be in pain but not engage in any behavior symptomatic of pain (e.g., he could be under the influence of curare, which paralyzes but does not eliminate the painful feelings). Only in light of our best theory of what sort of state pain is can we answer whether someone is in pain. One cannot foreclose the development of such scientific theories by positing that there are fixed connections (meaning connections) of "pain" to certain kinds of behaviors.

Aside from this erosion of the meaning-theory foundations of philosophical behaviorism, the position can be seen to be untenable simply by examining carefully attempted behaviorist reductions of mental terms such as belief. It is no accident that nowhere in *The Concept of Mind* does Ryle give more than a sketch of what a translation of mental terms into "multitrack" dispositions would look like. The kind of translations Skinner casually throws off from time to time throughout his work are not persuasive even to his admirers, who regard them as loose paraphrases but not reductions.[76] Just as logical positivism's attempted reduction of object language to phenomenal language failed in large part because no adequate translations were ever proposed, so philosophical behaviorism has foundered in large part because of the reductionists' similar failure to deliver the promised translations.

For these reasons we can put philosophical behaviorism to the side as an attempted reduction of reason-giving explanations to mechanistic ones. A second kind of reductionist behaviorism is to be found in an offshoot of the neobehaviorist theory of motivation in terms of *drives*. As used by stimulus–response reinforcement theorists, drives appear to serve two explanatory functions: First, they explain why a response occurs on a particular occasion—they "activate" or "energize" the behavior. Second, drives explain why certain responses are reinforced—because such responses produce a reduction in drive, a state the organism is postulated to seek.[77] Drives are thought to be capable of fulfilling both of these explanatory roles because they are conceptualized as a kind of psychic energy that both causes behavior and whose elimination reinforces the behavior that eliminates it. In such a theory human beings are conceptualized as kinds of energy-minimizing mechanisms.

Such drive theorists were mainly concerned with replacing reason-giving (or teleological) explanations with the mechanistic accounts in terms of stimuli, psychic energy, and drive discharge. For this reason they conceived of drives as essentially undirected toward any goals. Because such theorists would *replace* commonsense explanations in terms of reasons with explanations in terms of the discharge of undirected drive energies, rather than *reduce* such explanations to mechanistic ones, such theorists are not themselves our main concern. Of interest to us here is an offshoot of such drive theorists, namely, those who seek to link the mechanistic notions of undirected energy and drive to the more ordinary (and necessarily object-directed) ideas of desire and belief. A good example of this attempted reduction is David Rapaport's theory of motivation.[78] Rapaport is a useful example because, despite his recognition that psychoanalysis has been "written off by most psychologists as the product of Freud's 'mechanistic' bent,"[79] he nonetheless outdoes even Freud in seeking a mechanical translation of mental terms such as "motive." Rapaport does so, moreover, while explicitly taking work in philosophy and behaviorist psychology into account. This systematic treatment of motive is thus particularly worth attention.

Rapaport begins by acknowledging the behaviorist's problem of explaining purposive behavior in terms of mechanistic causes, such as undirected psychic energy: "One of the central problems of all psychology is how to resolve the paradox that as a science it is to give an explanation, in terms of causes, of behavior, which is purposive, i.e., teleological phenomenon in its very nature."[80] Rapaport's resolution of this paradox is to treat psychic energy as having direction, namely, the directions posited for it in Freud's theory of the instincts:

Freud's solution is to postulate the object as a defining characteristic. The instinctual drive energy tending towards discharge provides an explanation in terms of causes of the changes we refer to as behavior. However, unlike the direction of other (e.g., physical) causes the direction of instinctual drive discharge is not unequivocally determined, but rather is contingent on the presence of the instinctual drive object.[81] This, we are told, "is the outstanding conceptual invention in Freud's theory of the instinctual drive."[82]

This attempt to reduce motives to directed psychic energy takes place in the following steps. Rapaport's general definition is that *"motives are appetitive internal forces."*[83] By "appetitive," Rapaport has in mind four defining characteristics: peremptoriness, cyclic character, selectiveness, and displaceability.

By "peremptoriness," Rapaport first appears to mean some urgency experienced by the subject: "In contradistinction to voluntary behavior which we can 'take or leave', motivated behaviors are those which we cannot help doing. It is this mandatory character of behavior that we designate by the term 'peremptoriness.' "[84] "Cyclic character" means no more than that the "peremptoriness of motives has a cyclic rise and fall," the rise taking place before behavior is initiated leading toward some goal, the fall after the goal is attained. "Selectiveness" is introduced to bring the psychoanalytic conception of "motive" in line with the ordinary notion of a reason for action; for the psychoanalytic concept of "motive" is taken to imply "that the direction of the motive force is determined by its object." "Displaceability" is introduced to account for the fact that if one goal is unattainable for some reason (perhaps a reason of conscience, for example), substitute objects may be pursued.

Rapaport makes it plain that this definition of motive is intimately connected with the economic aspect of psychoanalytic theory, that is, Freud's concept of psychic energy. Defining motives as intrapsychic forces entails a definition in terms of energy: "Like all force concepts it involves a concept of energy."[85] Defining "appetitiveness" in the four ways indicated also is formulated in economic terms. Thus, "peremptoriness" ultimately turns out to refer, not to the urgency experienced by the subject, but to the accumulation of drive energies seeking discharge; " 'cyclic character' is conceptualized in terms of the accumulation and discharge of the energies of the motive force";[86] "selectiveness," which is not in itself defined in terms of energy, nonetheless implies that the objects that are one's motives, "are the specific necessary conditions for the discharge of the energies of the motivation in question";[87] and displaceability, although again not defined in terms of energy, is nonetheless accounted for in terms of an ability to discharge the accumulated drive energy through substitute gratifications.

Throughout Rapaport reminds us that the energies in terms of which motive is defined are not to be thought of as physiological processes of any kind:

> We must keep in mind that in dealing with the instinctual drives and the energy they expend in their work, we are not speaking about the muscular or other physiological energy expended in the course of executing the behavior, but rather about the psychological energy expended in the initiation, regulation, and termination of behavior—the physiological, biochemical, biophysical, or neurophysiological substrate of which we know, so far, nothing, or at best have but the vaguest conjectures.[88]

Although Rapaport hoped for the same physiological correlation that Freud envisioned, these concepts and the motive concept they define are to be judged as psychological terms whose value must be assessed independently of any correlation that may or may not exist with physiological terms.

Rapaport's elaborate definition of motive should be seen as part of his attempt to restate the most mechanistic of Freud's metapsychological viewpoints, namely, the dynamic (instincts) and the economic (psychic energy) viewpoints. Motive, so defined, becomes an intermediate-level theoretical term in a general theory of human behavior. Because for such theoretical terms Rapaport claims Humpty Dumpty's supposed ability to "make a word mean what we want it to mean," it may seem that this theoretical conception of motivation is not reductionist in character; for it need have little to do with motive in its ordinary sense (reason for action). Yet Rapaport's task *is* reductive insofar as he wants to claim that many reasons, though not themselves instinctual drives, are nonetheless really "highly neutralized derivatives of instinctual drives."[89] Altruistic reasons, for example, are reduced in this view to a kind of defense against an aggressive instinctual drive. Defenses in general are conceptualized in terms of psychic energy:

> When an instinctual drive reaches threshold intensity and the drive object is absent, and therefore no consummatory action can take place, a change in threshold is assumed to occur. This change is conceptualized as a heightening of threshold by means of a super-imposed collection barrier termed "anti-cathexis." When such anti-cathexes structuralize, we speak of them as defenses.[90]

There are two appropriate responses to this attempted reduction of beliefs and desires to patterns in the distribution of psychic energy. The first is to question the validity of the entire theoretical apparatus that Rapaport has by and large inherited from Freud[91] and later Freudians,[92] as well as from non-Freudian drive theorists. Critics both inside and outside of psychoanalysis have quite rightly questioned whether the idea of a "psychic energy cathecting" mental representatives and the like makes any sense at all.[93] Because of the current lack of clarity as to the criteria of adequacy for scientific theories, this is a difficult question to answer definitively. If this aspect of psychoanalytic theory is as vacuous as it seems, then of course there can be no reduction of reasons to psychic energy, and so on, for there would be nothing to reduce them to.

In any case, the other response is to doubt whether beliefs and desires could be identified with patterns of psychic energy (assuming for purposes of argument that talk of such energy makes any sense at all). For what Rapaport has tried to do is simply *stipulate* an equivalence that can only be *discovered*. In his effort to build a bridge between mechanistic notions (of energy, force, and instinctual drives) and ordinary reasons, Rapaport has warped each side of his proposed equivalence (that reasons are drive derivatives) for no reason other than to assert that such an equivalence exists.

With regard to one side of the alleged equivalence, the ordinary notion of reasons or motives, it should be apparent that the concept of reasons is being excruciatingly tortured in the usage Rapaport proposes. His "appetitiveness" stands the concept on its head. The notion that motives are peremptory, that is, that they make us do things we cannot help doing, is just the opposite of what we would ordinarily say. As set forth earlier, we cite motives only for human actions, that is, only for *voluntary* behavior of an intelligent agent. Since Richard Peters made this same point in his monograph about motivation (urging that "motive" be limited to situations in which an agent actively does something), Rapaport attempts to justify this particular departure from ordinary usage:

> The justification of this definition [Rapaport's] lies in the observation that the same motives (e.g., instinctual drives) are experienced subjectively at various times by the same person as actively willed (a state of affairs conceptualized by the term "ego-syntonic instinctual impulses"), and at times as passively suffered (a state of affairs conceptualized by the term "ego-dystonic instinctual impulse"). Peters is factually incorrect when he identifies the passively suffered as pathological.[94]

In assessing the reducibility of ordinary reasons to theoretical notions of instinctual drives it is hardly helpful to be told that one kind of reason — namely, an instinctual drive — has all the characteristics of an instinctual drive. Rapaport, however, seems untroubled by this framing of his definition of motive to fit his theoretical notion of an instinctual drive, for he admits that "this definition (of 'motive') is modeled on the defining characteristics of instinctual drives."[95]

Rapaport is equally willing to gerrymander the other side of his proposed reduction, that is, his definition of instinctual drive, so as to make it a kind of reason. Of the four defining characteristics of an instinctual drive (pressure, aim, object, source), Rapaport seizes on object as the concept making possible the bridge between reasons and energy. It is because instincts take objects that they are eligible to be motives or the source of motives:

> Even though the behaviors determined by instinctual drives are as a rule experienced as peremptory and compulsory, the instinctual drives are nevertheless causes of a motivational, purposive character, by virtue of the fact that their definition includes the object as a defining characteristic, the presence of which is the condition for their effectiveness . . . Peters' argument that the conception of motivation should be limited to "reasons," that is, to the "rule-following model," and that the causal motivational conceptions are logically fallacious, overlooks the fact that the crucial defining characteristic of the "rule-following model" is, on his own showing, purposive directionality, and that this is an integral characteristic of some causes, e.g., instinctual drives, also.[96]

What Rapaport has attempted to do here is to lump one salient characteristic of mental states—they take objects—with the mechanistic notion of energy discharges. For instincts are by and large defined, for Freud as well as for Rapaport, in terms of their tendency to discharge accumulated drive energies. The ideas of pressure, aim, and source are all part of this mechanistic conception of instinct. Rapaport seeks to lump objects with this mechanistic conceptualization by saying that "the direction of instinctual drive discharge is not unequivocally determined, but rather is contingent on the presence of the instinctual drive object." Yet to say this is to adjust his theory just so the equivalence between reason and energy formulations will hold. This is "reduction" by tautology, with *both* sides of the proposed reduction open for gerrymandering redefinition.

As a viable reduction of ordinary reasons to the mechanistic notions of energy and drive, this neobehaviorist kind of psychoanalytic theory fails dramatically. If the economic and dynamic metapsychologies explain behavior at all, which seems quite doubtful, they at least do not explain it in the way that reasons explain behavior. This difference in kinds of explanation becomes important later when we discuss the relation of responsibility to the unconscious. For now it is enough to see that reason-giving explanations are distinct from, and have not been shown to be reducible to, this kind of mechanistic explanation of human behavior.

2 The Legal View of Persons

Persons in Law, Morals, and Metaphysics

"PERSON," LOCKE TELLS US, "is a forensic term."[1] It is a term employed throughout the law in the assignment of legal rights and liabilities. The burdens of this chapter are, first, to ascertain whether the law has any systematic use of the concept such that some consistent theory of the person can be divined in such use, and second, to describe the most salient features of that legal theory of the person (assuming that some such theory exists).

Before proceeding to examine directly the legal contexts in which the concept of a person is employed, we must pause to ask some more general questions about legal concepts and what it is to seek their meaning. Prima facie, there are two quite distinct sorts of things one might advert to in "giving the meaning" of a legal concept such as "person": (1) One might seek to describe the set of *facts* under which the legal concept is correctly applied, or (2) one might seek to describe the set of *legal consequences* that attach to the authoritative use of that concept by judges.

Consider the concept of ownership. If asked to give the meaning of the two-place predicate, "X owns y," one might describe the facts under which a person X could correctly be said to own some thing y, facts such as that X received y as a gift from his uncle, that X purchased y, that X occupied y for a certain period, and the like. Alternatively, one might mention the kind of legal consequences that are supposed to flow from it being authoritatively pronounced of X, that he owns y. Such legal consequences include the fact that X has the power to dispose of y by gift, sale, or devise; that X can be taxed on y; that X may enjoin interference by others in the use and enjoyment of y; and so forth.

The reason for this Janus-faced aspect of legal concepts lies in what Hohfeld called their "dispositive" function.[2] Legal concepts such as ownership, malice, intention, or person are used both to describe in legal terms the facts in particular situations and to "dispose" of the issues in

The Legal View of Persons

cases by prescribing what results judges should bring about in the application of those concepts. Dispositive legal concepts form the "conceptual cement" that connects judges' factual findings to their legal remedies.

It is sometimes thought that this dual function of legal concepts renders them essentially ambiguous. Yet ambiguity is a semantic category having to do with two senses of a word.[3] "Entertain," for example, is ambiguous in that it can mean to think about or consider a question, or it can mean to behave in a hospitable and amusing manner. The two functions served by legal concepts constitute not a semantic distinction, but rather a distinction of *use*. Judges perform two distinct speech acts when they use a dispositive legal concept such as intention or ownership in legal proceedings. Their "assertorial" speech act is to describe the facts before them, while their "prescriptive" speech act is to prescribe that certain legal consequences should attach.[4]

These same dual functions are to be found in our use of language to express moral judgments. To use a moral term, such as person or intention, is often both to *describe* an entity or a state of affairs as being of a certain kind, and to *prescribe* that moral guilt or blame should attach to the entity or event so described.[5] The difference between moral and legal usages is that the consequences prescribed are not fixed by conventional rules of such detail as are the legal consequences attached to dispositive legal concepts. The "pragmatics," if you like, of moral utterances is not as conventional as the pragmatics of authoritative legal utterances.

There have been movements in both law and in ethical philosophy in this century that have sought to emphasize the prescriptive function of ethical or legal utterances to the exclusion of the descriptive function. In law this movement has had quite diverse roots. One can see such a position, for example, in H. L. A. Hart's ascriptivist theory of action.[6] According to this theory, one first decides whether responsibility is to be ascribed to some person for some harm, and only then does one decide whether the bodily motion causing the harm was an action performed by that person. If one wishes to ascribe responsibility, the behavior will be described as an action; if one wishes to say the person is not responsible, the behavior will be called an accident, in the sense of nonaction.

Hart's kind of argument—that is, because one is *ascribing* responsibility one cannot be *describing* some factual state of affairs with a concept such as action—has been made for each of the conditions employed to ascribe responsibility. George Fletcher, for example, notes that "the term 'criminal intent' may mean the intent to act under circumstances that make it just to treat the actor as a criminal."[7] John Dewey argued that motives are characterizations of conduct that are merely "a refinement of the ordinary reactions of praise and blame," so that motive words, such as greed, "simply [mean] the quality of [an] act as socially observed and disapproved."[8]

Judge Andrews, in dissent in *Palsgraf v. Long Island Railroad Co.*,[9] speaking no doubt as an accurate representation of the thoughts of many contemporary lawyers, urged that the requirement of proximate cause "is all a question of expediency [and of] practical politics: What we do mean by the word 'proximate' is that because of convenience, of public policy, of a rough sense of justice, the law arbitrarily declines to trace a series of events beyond a certain point."[10] Stanley Ingber has recently analyzed the excuse of duress as first consisting of the moral judgment that one is not responsible, and only then is the judgment made that the behavior in question was "involuntary."[11] Thomas Szasz and his legal followers are constantly contending that phrases such as mental illness have no descriptive meaning; such labels are merely after-the-fact labels applied to persons after deciding for one reason or another to degrade them as persons.[12]

Perhaps the most dominant strain of this kind of thinking in law has been the loose assemblage of persons known as American Legal Realists.[13] For the Legal Realists held that in applying a legal term one must look to the legal *consequences* being prescribed by its authoritative use by a judge, and further, that it was an illusion to think that such legal terms had a *meaning* that determined their correct use apart from such consequences. This general view came to be known as "functionalism"[14] (although it has very little to do with the functional approach in social science discussed in the preceding chapter).

Ethical philosophy has also had its share of theorists who urged that ethical utterances were used either to express the speaker's emotions or to prescribe what one ought or ought not to do.[15] Many of these "emotivist" and "prescriptivist" theorists in ethics urged that because such expressive or prescriptive functions were served by moral uses of language, descriptive functions could not also be served.

If one adopted such a position about the legal or moral usages of the word person, one would urge that *anything* could be called a person—it would simply depend on whether one wished to attach the legal or moral consequences to that entity of being so labeled. Consider, for example, the debate about whether corporations (as entities distinct from their shareholders, directors, and officers) are moral or legal persons. One adopting the functionalist analysis of legal concepts of American Legal Realism will collapse the question of whether corporations *are* moral persons into the question of whether they *should be called* moral persons in light of the consequences attached to so labeling them. Christopher Stone, for example, argues that the question of whether

> it is *intelligible* to blame the corporation draws on considerations that it is *useful* to speak in that manner. The validity of this claim, in turn, depends on what one supposes to be the function of moral discourse. If one argues that it is the function of moral discourse to educate about

what society considers right and wrong conduct (as opposed, for example, to describing non-natural moral qualities, as G. E. Moore claimed), then it makes perfectly good sense to speak of the company—the corporate entity—as blameworthy, if doing so can be grounded in the advancement of societal goals.[16]

Similarly in law, if one wishes to know whether a corporation is a legal person, one will inquire into "the likely effect of holding the corporate body legally accountable. One wants to know how making the corporation the law's quarry will affect those both 'outside' the corporation and those who labor 'within,' in terms of their perceptions (most importantly their self-perceptions) and their behavior."[17] Like any good functionalist, Stone relegates the descriptive question of whether corporations are legal persons, and thus can intelligibly be held legally accountable as persons, to the scrap heap of intellectual history and (pejoratively) academic pursuits: "The intelligibility of ascribing wrongdoing to the corporate body, once so lively an issue in law, is today mainly of historical and perhaps some lingering theoretical interest."[18]

An essential presupposition of the analysis of this chapter is that the emotivist-prescriptivist-ascriptivist-functionalist-Legal Realist analyses of moral and legal concepts are wrongheaded. Since I have presented extended arguments against each of these traditions elsewhere,[19] I will not recapitulate that discussion in any detail. My own view is that the legal and moral questions of whether some entity is or is not a person, whether that person performed an action, whether intentionally or with a certain motive, whether that act proximately caused harm, whether the actor acted under threats of another amounting to duress, and whether the actor is mentally ill are all factual questions. The concepts employed in discussing all such questions are not empty labels for a moral or legal conclusion reached on other grounds, or on no grounds at all; they are concepts having a descriptive and explanatory function, no matter what other expressive, prescriptive, or ascriptive functions they may serve in contexts such as those of responsibility assessment. It accordingly makes sense to seek the meaning of persons and its related terms (action, intention, and the like) in terms of the facts that must be true if such concepts are to be correctly employed.

I shall proceed in the following way. Because the legal consequences of calling some entity a person are different in different contexts, and because the descriptive significance of the concept *might* vary with these different consequences (I shall argue that it does not), I distinguish two very general legal consequences of calling an entity a legal person. First, legal persons are the appropriate subjects to be held legally responsible for either bringing about some harm, or at least trying to do so. Second, legal persons are the holders of legal rights, such as the rights to liberty, property, and equality.

Because I reject the Legal Realist et al. tradition, the analysis of the legal views of persons does not stop at drawing out these two legal consequences of personhood. It is not an adequate analysis of "person" in law simply to point out that a legal person is an entity such that it can be held responsible, or can hold rights. Rather, we need to ask what factual state of affairs must be true of any entity if it is to be correctly described as a legal person.

Within each of the two legal contexts I have distinguished I shall make a second major assumption. This is that the legal concept of a person does not differ from the moral concept of a person, despite the differing consequences of calling an entity a person in moral versus legal utterances. The defense of this assumption lies in a view of the relationship between law and morals. The content of much of our law is the same as the content of much of our morality. The relationship is thus one of (an at least) contingent identity between law and morality. Legal rights to property, to liberty, or to equality depend on moral rights to those things; legal liability to punishment or damages depends on moral responsibility. It is because legal rights and liabilities in each of these areas of law depend upon there being corresponding moral rights and moral responsibilities that the legal concept of a person can be said to be the same as the moral concept. Because the law is built upon morality in this way it is plausible to suppose that the law's crucial concepts, such as that of personhood, action, and intention, are also built upon the corresponding moral concepts. In this view, an entity is legally a person only if it is morally a person.

This fusion of law and morality is compatible with many psychiatrists' view of law and particularly of criminal law. They are quite happy to identify law with morality, because, given their skepticism about ethics, it makes it easier to contrast the law with their own "more scientific" approach. Legal theorists, however, may find the asserted law/morals connection somewhat more problematic. It takes considerable attention to the details of contract law, for example, to show that its doctrines are built upon the moral practices of promise keeping;[20] or that tort law is built either upon some utilitarian notions of efficient resource allocation or upon some corrective justice views, or upon some accommodations between these competing moral theories;[21] or that property law assigns rights on the basis of either utilitarian or natural (moral) rights theories;[22] or that criminal law doctrines are simply legal restatements of some moral theory of responsibility, either utilitarian or retributivist.[23] Although all of this is indeed what I think to be correct, the detailed examination required to establish these or like claims about other areas of law is of course not to be undertaken here. The literature cited in the notes makes a strong case for the view that our law is at least contingently connected to our morals.

What can be done here is to render this law/morals connection more

The Legal View of Persons

plausible by saying what it is not: It is not a natural law theory (or at least it need not be). The connection between law and morals asserted here is only a contingent one: The laws of our legal system turn out to be based on certain moral theories. Such connection to morality is not *necessary* for our laws to be law, as a natural law theory would assert. We *could have* laws that assign rights and liabilities in ways that have little resemblance to moral theory, and they would still be laws. As it happens, however, our laws do reflect underlying moral theories. It is because they do that it is plausible to suppose that the legal concepts in terms of which legal doctrines are framed depend upon the moral concepts employed in those underlying moral theories.

If one makes this second assumption (of the dependence of the legal concept of a person upon the moral concept of a person), then the task of this chapter is to articulate what the moral concept of a person comes to. The thesis defended throughout the remainder of this chapter is that an entity is a person in moral theory or legal doctrine only if it is rational and autonomous in the sense employed in the previous chapter, viz., only if it is a practical reasoner. To make out this thesis in each of the two contexts examined will require an analysis of the various theories and concepts in terms of which responsibilities or rights are ascribed. Because responsibility is more the locus of our concerns in later chapters, I will devote considerably more detailed attention to that context than to the ascription of rights. The payoff of such more detailed attention, apart from bringing out the view of persons implicit in it, will be to set the stage for later psychiatric claims about diminished or extended responsibility.

Persons as the Subjects of Legal and Moral Responsibility

THE CONCEPT OF RESPONSIBILITY

The following passage from H. L. A. Hart is useful in illuminating the nuances in the use of the word "responsible":

> As captain of the ship, X was [1] responsible for the safety of his passengers and crew. But on his last voyage he got drunk every night and was [2] responsible for the loss of the ship with all aboard. It was rumored that he was insane, but the doctors considered that he was [3] responsible for his actions. Throughout the voyage he behaved quite irresponsibly and various incidents in his career showed that he was not a [4] responsible person. He always maintained that the exceptional winter storms were [5] responsible for the loss of the ship, but in the legal proceedings against him he was found [6] criminally responsible for his negligent conduct, and in separate civil proceedings he was

held [7] legally responsible for the loss of life and property. He is still alive and he is [8] morally responsible for the deaths of many women and children.[24]

The first distinction to be drawn among these uses of responsible is one dependent on time. The second, fifth, sixth, seventh, and eighth uses of the word in the passage all share a common feature: The subject is said to be responsible *for* some event in the past. This can be called *retrospective responsibility*. In contrast, the first usage looks to the future and specifies what task was the captain's responsibility. This can be called *prospective responsibility*. The third and fourth uses of the word are timeless in that they do not assert that the actor is responsible for any particular action, past or future. Rather, the third asserts that he is the kind of person who is accountable, in general, for his actions, and the fourth asserts that he is not the kind of person who regularly meets his obligations.

In this section we are concerned with the conditions under which retrospective responsibility is ascribed to individuals in both civil and criminal law. The other senses of responsible have a role to play, but in this inquiry their role is a subordinate one, as will emerge in the ensuing discussion.

One can begin to systematize the conditions under which law and morality ascribe retrospective responsibility by paying some attention to the different uses of the retrospective sense of the word in the foregoing passage. Following Hart's suggestions, we can parse the retrospective sense of the word into four subcategories: (1) causal responsibility; (2) answerability; (3) culpability; and (4) liability.

Hart's fifth use of responsible asserts that there is a causal connection between the storm and the loss of the ship. Since storms are neither moral agents nor legal persons, the most that can be meant by saying that the storm was responsible for the loss of the ship is that the storm caused the loss. If one said that a person was responsible for some harm in this minimal sense, one would be claiming at the least that the person's body was causally implicated in the production of that harm.

One can fairly construe Hart's second use of the word as asserting more than this about the sea captain. Because his action of drinking was negligent, Hart's second use of responsible implies that the sea captain is *answerable* for the harm he has caused; the captain is answerable in the sense of being prima facie culpable in causing it. To be answerable in this sense requires, first, that the captain have performed some action or omission, and second, that he do so with a culpable state of mind. Because of this concurrence of act, mental and causation, the captain is prima facie to blame for what happened.

Hart's eighth use of the word responsible asserts that the ship's captain was not only prima facie, but also actually culpable in causing the harm. Not only did his actions and culpable mental state cause the harm, but he also caused the harm with none of the justifications or excuses that might have rebutted his prima facie culpability. He was, for example, not compelled to act as he did.

Hart's sixth and seventh uses of responsible both attribute legal liability to the sea captain: the sixth, liability to criminal punishment, and the seventh, liability to a tort judgment requiring that he pay damages. To these should be added another kind of liability, namely, the liability the sea captain may also have to moral sanctions, such as public shaming. This we might call being blameworthy. In all three cases, responsible is used to mean that under the justifications for imposing sanctions, the sea captain is liable to having certain harms inflicted on him.

The nonretrospective senses of the word responsible also have a role to play in completing this taxonomy of the conditions under which retrospective responsibility is ascribed. Hart's third use of the word uses responsible as a synonym for accountable. A presupposition of holding someone culpable or liable is that the person be an accountable agent. Young infants, the very seriously insane, and animals are examples of nonaccountable agents.

Finally, Hart's first use of the word to indicate prospective responsibility illustrates the need of another condition in ascribing fault: that there be a legal or moral *duty*, or obligation. In Hart's example the ship captain's obligation to look after the passengers, crew, and ship arises from his having undertaken to do just this when he accepted the position of ship captain. Such duties or obligations may arise in other ways as well, as illustrated by the obligations we have not to violate others' rights to bodily integrity without justification. In any case, some obligation or duty (moral or legal) must be violated by an actor before he may be held morally or legally liable.

With a bit of rearrangement, these senses of responsibility, and the conditions under which each kind of responsibility may be ascribed to an entity, may be represented on an increasing scale of retrospective responsibility:

Sense of "responsible":	*Conditions of ascription:*
1. Causally responsible	Causation
2. Prospective responsibility	Moral or legal duty
3. Responsible-accountable	Accountable agent
4. Responsible-answerable	Action and mental state
5. Responsible-culpable	No justification or excuse
6. Responsible-liable	Justification for imposition of sanctions met

The thesis implicit in this ordering of the senses of responsibility, and the conditions for each, is that we hold people retrospectively responsible in law or morals only if they are accountable agents who negligently or intentionally, and without justification or excuse, perform actions that cause some state of affairs they were obligated not to bring about. This is both a descriptive thesis, about the conditions we in fact employ in ascribing retrospective responsibility in law or morals, and a normative thesis about the conditions we ought to employ in ascribing such responsibility.

I shall shortly proceed to defend these theses by an examination of each of the conditions, and also seek to show how each of these conditions presupposes the notion of persons as practical reasoners. Before doing so, however, three items need to be cleared up about responsibility. The first is to eliminate any purported gulf between moral culpability and legal liability. This elimination is in two steps, corresponding to the two assumptions made in the previous section. Those two assumptions were, first, that the consequences of uttering a word such as responsible should not be regarded as a separate sense of the word. One of the consequences of agents' being morally culpable for causing some harm is that they are liable to moral blame for it. The moral liability is but the consequence of the moral culpability and should not be separated from it.[25] The second assumption was that moral liability is at least a (contingently) necessary condition of legal liability. Our criminal law, and to a large extent our law of torts, is such that one is liable to punitive or damage sanctions only if one is morally blameworthy.

The implication of both assumptions together is that moral culpability is the touchstone of legal liability. Because of this, I shall discuss both legal doctrines and moral principles indiscriminately as I attempt to divine the concept of a person implicit in the conditions under which fault is ascribed.

The second item to be cleared up has to do with the *objects* for which one might be held responsible. The retrospective responsibility spoken of herein is responsibility *for* a particular state of affairs being brought about. Distinct from such object is the responsibility sometimes ascribed to people for being the way they are, that is, for their character, including their mental states. One might say that people are retrospectively responsible for their character and are prospectively responsible for doing something about the bad aspects of their character.[26] Such responsibility is distinct from that ascribed to actors for bringing about some harm.

The third item to be cleared up has to do with the factual nature of one's responsibility judgments. Whether one is responsible for some harm depends upon certain factual judgments about one's actions, intentions, causation and the like being true. The responsibility spoken of is *real* moral responsibility. This is to be distinguished from the *feelings* of responsibility one may have on various occasions. One may *feel* that another is responsible for some harm simply because, as Nietzsche pointed out long ago, one resents having been harmed by that person.[27] One may feel such resentment even if the harm was done nonculpably and in such a way that the actor is not really responsible. Similarly, one may feel guilty for harm one has caused when one was not really responsible; nonculpably caused harm gives rise to such guilt feelings quite often. Indeed, one may feel such guilt even if one has not even caused the harm about which one feels guilty, as in survivor's guilt.[28] Although the psychology of resentment and guilt is a fascinating subject, it is distinct from the inquiry addressed in this section. Real moral responsibility is determined by those conditions that make it morally just to ascribe responsibility to oneself or others. It is to those conditions that I now turn.

THE CONDITIONS FOR ASCRIBING RESPONSIBILITY

Causation

The Role of Causation in Ascribing Retrospective Responsibility: Of all the concepts in terms of which we ascribe responsibility, causation is doubtless the least likely candidate for being a hidden repository of the idea of a person as a practical reasoner. Before assessing the degree to which this is true, more needs to be said about the role of causation itself in ascribing retrospective responsibility.

There are two extremes to be avoided here. One is the view that causation of some harm is alone sufficient for liability to pay for it, or to be punished for it. If such a view were correct, then it would indeed be difficult to make out any strong presupposition of a person as a practical reasoner in this area of the law (because, with the exceptions to be noted, causation is largely independent of this view of a person). Such a view might be thought to be supported by the undeniable existence of strict liability rules in criminal law and torts.

The other extreme is to think that causation is not necessary for responsibility, that culpability has nothing to do with the fortuity of whether some harm was caused or not. The substitute for causation, in this view, is intention or other mental state. Such a view of legal liability might be supported by the existence of criminal liability for attempting to bring about some harm, for conspiring to bring it about, or for aiding another in bringing it about (when that aid does not in fact causally contribute to the harm). Further support might be found in the dignitary torts, where actual harm being caused is not an element of the cause of action. In all such cases mental state alone might seem sufficient.

Strictly speaking, neither of these extreme views can be made out even in the area of law most favorable to them. A mental element is built into all strict liability rules because of their requirement that the actor at least have performed a voluntary action; a causal requirement is built into the notion of attempts, complicity, and perhaps even conspiracy because of their use of "causally complex" verbs of action, such as attempt or aid.

In any case, even if suitably softened, these extreme views about the role of causation are not correct. The central case of culpability is one in which an actor both causes harm and does so intentionally (or with some other culpable mental state). Strict liability statutes are abhorrent in criminal law and rarely do severe sanctions attach for simply causing harm. Attempt liability, accomplice liability, conspiracy law, and the law of dignitary torts are by comparison quite well established, but should still be seen as exceptional in comparison to the more standard cases of tort or criminal liability. One can perhaps perceive in such exceptional areas a genuine alternative to the standard case of culpability. If so, this alternative theory of culpability is quite compatible with the central thesis of this chapter. For such a theory of culpability, emphasizing as it does intention at the expense of causation, rather clearly presupposes the view of a person as a practical reasoner, as the subsequent discussion of the concept of intention will show. I accordingly turn to causation itself, where the connection to practical reason is much less apparent.

Lawyers commonly divide the idea of causation into two parts, one called cause-in-fact or factual cause and the other called proximate or legal cause. The first is thought to be the scientific question of whether, for example, cigarette smoking causes cancer or is only an accidentally present condition that happens to precede cancer regularly. The second is thought to be a less scientific question about whether the harm is sufficiently proximate to the defendant's act that he ought to be held liable for it. Although the matter is debated, I shall accept this traditional division of causal questions and discuss each separately.

Causation in Fact: The standard account of cause-in-fact in both law and the philosophy of science goes something like this. First, events or states are causes of other events or states; objects are not. When we speak of an object, such as a ship, as having caused harm, this is only an ellipsis for a more accurate formulation in terms of an event, such as the ship's moving, being the cause of the harm. Second, following David Hume, one event is the cause of another only if a regular connection is observed to hold between two *classes* of events of which the cause and the effect are each instances. This is the notion that causation involves general laws, namely, the laws that "cover" each of the two classes of events and assert that, if an event of the first class occurs, then an event of the second class also occurs. Third, not any old law will do as the covering law making possible a causal explanation. Rather (departing from Hume), one must distinguish between connections that *accidentally* hold and those that *necessarily* hold. In philosophy this is often put by saying that the laws connecting classes of

The Legal View of Persons

events must support a "counterfactual conditional," that is, a statement about what *would* have happened if, contrary to fact, the first event had not occurred. In law this is described as the sine qua non test: "But for" the ship's moving, for example, would there have been a collision? If the answer is yes, then there can be no causal connection between the first event and the second, for a cause must at least be a necessary condition of the harm it produces.

There are many problems with this conception of causation, forming a large literature in both philosophy and law; but then there are serious problems with the substitutes usually proposed as well. Of interest here are the problems the standard account of cause-in-fact faces in accommodating itself to the idea of a *person* causing harm. As stated, the standard account of causation makes no presuppositions about practical reasoning; I shall argue, however, that once this account of causation is modified to take into account a *person* causing some state of affairs, practical reasoning becomes involved.

Suppose some actor performs the act of moving his finger. Suppose further that his finger is on the trigger of a loaded gun that is directed at another person. Suppose further that X's moving his finger *causes* Y's death in a way that is not hard to imagine. This causal relation between the act event of X's moving his finger, and Y's death, presents no special problems for the standard account of causation; if that account is generally adequate, it is adequate here.

The standard account has more problems when we talk, not of *X's act* as a cause, but of *X himself* as a cause, as in: "X caused his fingers to move." There is no simpler, or more basic, act that X did in order to move his fingers. One cannot, accordingly, paraphrase away talk of X, the person, as a cause, to talk of some act event of X's being the cause. The causal agency of X seems to be primitive in the sense that it is irreducible to any notion of event causation. If the agency of X in bringing about the movement of his fingers is indeed a causal relation between X and his act of moving the fingers, then the standard account of causation in terms of events will have to be modified or abandoned for personal causation.

There are, to be sure, famous traditions in both law and philosophy that hold that one *can* reduce personal agency to event causation. These will be examined (and rejected) in the section on the concept of action. For now, it should be noted that if such reductions succeeded, practical reason would immediately be implicated in causation by persons. This is because such states or events as are proposed to be the causes of simple acts like moving one's fingers are just the states of belief and desire that are the essence of practical reasoning.

The more interesting question is thus not the question of reduction, but rather the question of whether we ever need to talk of a person as a *cause* of his own simple acts. Donald Davidson, for example, has argued that although personal agency is irreducible to event causation, such agency is not a causal notion at all.[29] If Davidson is correct, then the standard account of causation would not have to accommodate any notion of a person-as-cause and, being adequate without any such notion, would not presuppose practical reason in any sense.

We often paraphrase "X moved his fingers" to seemingly causal expressions such as, "X caused his fingers to move" or "X made his fingers move," or even "X brought it about that his fingers moved." Conceding as much, Davidson nonetheless argues that "the concept of *cause* seems to play no role" here[30] because it is as mysterious as that it was supposed to explain, personal agency: Attempting to explain irreducible personal agency by positing a special and equally irreducible causal notion is for Davidson a hopelessly vacuous enterprise.

What Davidson is arguing against is a notion of causation introduced by Richard Taylor, among others.[31] Taylor argued that "the relation between a certain kind of object—namely, a man—and certain events—namely, the voluntary motions of his body—which we sometimes still express by saying that he is 'the cause' of those motions, is . . . a basic, clear, and unanalyzable concept."[32] This basic concept, Taylor further argued, we have extended beyond its paradigmatic application (to persons and their simple acts) to other areas when we talk of causation. Taylor purported to see in all this a second and distinct *general* conception of causation quite different from the standard account. Taylor's anthropomorphic conception of causation springs from Locke's notion of objects having causal powers to make things happen (which ought not to be surprising in light of its being modeled on a person making his limbs move). Such a conception of cause, spelled out as Taylor does, entails a rejection of the standard Humean account of cause in terms of uniformity of sequence, laws, and necessary conditions.

It takes us too far afield to pursue these two competing conceptions of cause-in-fact. One would want to examine in detail the "hard cases" for the standard account of causation. In law these include: (1) the overdetermination, concurrent cause cases, in which two events are each sufficient for a particular harm at a particular time; since in such cases neither event was *necessary* yet we plainly want to say that each *caused* the harm, some non-Humean account of "cause" seems to be required; (2) the problems of coincidence, such as in the case of the motorist who speeds for ten minutes in the middle of Kansas and who ten hours later arrives at just that spot in the Colorado forest where a tree falls on him. Here, one may want to say that the speeding is not a cause-in-fact of the harm, yet it is an event but for which the harm would not have occurred (and thus should be a cause on the standard account); and (3) the problem of omissions, which on the standard account should be but-for causes; however, one may be reluctant to characterize omissions as even *a* cause of some harm since *everyone's* failure in some regard is equally such a cause.

If these and other causal puzzles convince one that the standard account is not right and that Taylor's kind of anthropomorphic conception of cause runs through our law, morals, and everyday thought, then Davidson's charge of triviality cannot be made out. For then, characterizing the relation between a person and his simple acts in terms of a special concept of causation, would not be the ad hoc positing of a causal relation as mysterious as that it was supposed to explain. Rather, such causal relation would be as legitimate a conception as its competitor, the Humean, or standard, conception of causation.

This not being an issue we can solve here, I shall leave it. To the extent that we have such an anthropomorphic conception of cause, and to the extent that it is the best characterization of the relation between a person and his simple actions, then causation itself presupposes the idea of practical reason. One can see the presupposition of practical reason here only by analyzing the concept of an action, and so I shall defer further discussion of this last point until we reach that concept.

Proximate Cause: One of the often-voiced objections to the Humean account of causation is that it is so overinclusive of what can be a cause-in-fact that it makes necessary some kind of second causal notion that can eliminate most but-for factors as causes. Let us nonetheless assume for purposes of this discussion the correctness of the Humean account of cause-in-fact and examine this second causal test.

One can see such a second causal test at work in the selectivity exercised by historians as they causally explain various events in history. Fortunately for the readability of historical narratives, historians do not explain each event by listing all the factors necessary for its production. Rather, most but-for causes are *not* mentioned when they explain what caused World War I, for example.

The secondary tests historians use in making such selections are a matter of some debate.[33] Some such test, however, is employed. The analogous test in law is called the proximate cause test. In torts, contract, and criminal law there are two dominant versions of such a test, the foreseeability version and the direct cause version. Each version presupposes the idea of a person as a practical reasoner, although since each is a bit different I shall discuss them separately.

The foreseeability version of proximate causation allows that an actor is liable only if the harm that occurred was a type of event that was foreseeable to him at the time he acted. Whether such a type of harm is foreseeable depends on whether the average person of reasonable foresight *would have* foreseen a harm of that type resulting from his actions. If the average reasonable person would have foreseen such type of harm occurring, then the defendant who did not in fact foresee it, should have, and can be held fairly blamable for it.

What is presupposed in this test is not that the defendant on this occasion actually engaged in a set of practical inferences that included some description of the type of harm that occurred as the object of one of his beliefs. It is rather that the defendant has the *capacity* to engage in such inferences even though on this occasion he did not. It is only because the defendant is in fact enough like that ideal of a rational, practical inference drawer—the average, reasonable person—that he can fairly be held liable for harms that he in fact did not foresee. The only agents to whom such a test can fairly apply are agents who are in general pretty good practical reasoners.[34]

The direct cause version of proximate cause is a bit more elaborate. A direct cause of harm is (a) any cause-in-fact of that harm for which (b) there is no "intervening" or "superseding" cause. Obviously what is needed to make sense of this definition of direct cause is to give sense to the idea of an intervening or superseding cause. By far the most sophisticated articulation of this last notion remains Hart and Honore's impressive *Causation in the Law*.[35]

Hart and Honore attempt to get at the idea of an intervening cause (and thus at the idea of proximate causation itself) by first proposing an ingenious detour. Historians and all of us in daily life, they tell us, discriminate among all those conditions necessary for the production of some event. A few such conditions are called "cause" whereas most are "mere conditions." The criteria implicit in this selection are two, according to Hart and Honore. First, abnormal events are preferred to normal ones. One does not cite the presence of timber on English soil to explain the defeat of the Spanish Armada any more than one cites the presence of oxygen to explain a house fire, although each may have been necessary for the respective events to have occurred. Second, voluntary human action is preferred over natural events and involuntary human action. Drake's decision to penetrate the Spanish bird formation of ships will be cited to explain the Armada's defeat over the constricted channel in which the battle took place, although each was a factor necessary for the defeat of the Armada.

Historians use such criteria, Hart and Honore assert, because they, like all of us, have been raised in a culture in which these criteria are employed in making causal discriminations in daily life. Even when moral responsibility is not at stake, we all will explain, for example, train wrecks by citing abnormal factors (bent rails over inertia of the train at normal speed) or fires by voluntary acts (thrown matches over normal light winds).

The Legal View of Persons

The ingenious aspect of Hart and Honore's argument is that it utilizes these criteria (of which among a host of equally necessary conditions was *the* cause or "the most important" cause of some event) as a *limit* beyond which consequences will not be traced. That is, as we are charting the chain of consequences any human action causes in fact, when we come to the intervention of an abnormal event or *another* voluntary action, we trace consequences no further. A waiter who sets a table with knives does not cause the death of some victim who dies because a third party picks up one of the knives and stabs the victim with it. The waiter's table setting is not the cause because B's fully voluntary action intervened between A's act and the harm. As judges often put the matter, A's action was a mere condition whereas B's action was the cause.

Hence, this concept of direct causation is thought to be drawn from the conditions under which we explain the world in daily life. In assigning moral responsibility, we incorporate those criteria in terms of which we more generally assign causal responsibility to persons and natural objects.

The link to practical reason in this version of proximate causation lies in the two criteria proposed for intervening causes. With regard to the idea of a "fully voluntary human action" that breaks the causal chain, in most cases such an action, as analyzed by Hart and Honore, turns out to be an intentional action. Since both action and intention are themselves explicated in terms of the idea of practical reason, as I shall discuss shortly, so is this criterion of an intervening cause.

The other criterion of intervening cause that Hart and Honore propose has to do with abnormal natural events. If the defendant strikes the victim and knocks him out, and a tree falls on just the spot where the victim lies unconscious, the defendant did not cause the death even though but for his hitting the victim the latter would not have died; this is because the tree's falling was an intervening cause. In such cases, Hart and Honore tell us, we have an abnormal conjunction of events amounting to a coincidence.

Practical reasoning is presupposed even in this version of intervening cause because of the hidden role of intention in all of this: If the defendant foresaw the tree's falling, and used this natural event, unlikely as it was, to accomplish the intended death of the victim, then the tree's falling does not constitute an intervening cause.[36] Such a means/end calculation is the essence of practical reasoning.

Duty

"Duty" has come to be something of a technical term in tort law, where it picks out an element of the negligence cause of action. So used, it deals with issues such as the question of whether landowners need to look out for trespassers and whether providers of goods or services who are not in "privity of contract" with consumers may nonetheless be held liable for injuries to such customers. The high water mark of duty in torts is the more general notion defended by Cardozo in *Palsgraf v. Long Island Railroad Co.*[37] wherein Cardozo used the concept as a means of limiting recovery to those persons who were in the class of persons foreseeably injured by a defendant's activities (and to whom, thus, the defendant "owed a duty").

Such tort law usages of duty are a special case of the broader usage I intend, which is more akin to Hohfeld's usage of the term. This is to use it to name obligations created by any type of law — tort, criminal, contract, or whatever. Moreover, because of the earlier assumption of the connection between legal and moral concepts, duty not only will name a legal obligation, but it will also be the case that there is an underlying moral obligation as well.

The source of legal obligations is no simple matter to spell out. A legal positivist will argue that legal obligations are created by standards that are legally valid because they have been promulgated in accordance with some value-free test for law. A natural lawyer will argue that legal obligations can come into being only if the standards creating such obligations: (a) are promulgated in a way that meets certain moral requirements "internal" to the law;[38] or (b) are in content congruent with the content of contemporary moral norms;[39] or (c) are standards whose content forms part of the best moral theory one can articulate of both "background" and "institutional" morality;[40] or (d) are standards whose content is morally right.[41]

The rather strong assumption made earlier, that is, that there is a contingent connection between moral principles and concepts and legal principles and concepts, does not commit us one way or the other in this legal positivism/natural law debate. Although my own position is the natural law position, and closer to the last than to the others, defending such a position is the subject of another book. Let us therefore focus on one aspect of the source of legal obligations on which most legal positivists and natural lawyers would agree. This is Fuller's idea that a set of standards must conform to some "internal morality of the law" in order to be the kind of standards that are capable of creating legal obligations.

By the internal morality of law Fuller had eight principles in mind.

1. The standards must be general in that they are capable of being applied to more than one person or situation; they must apply to *types* of situations and persons.
2. The standard must be publicly promulgated, so that all bound by it can read it.
3. The standard should be prospective in application and not

The Legal View of Persons

   made retroactive to actions that were done before the standard was promulgated.
4. The standard should be sufficiently free of vagueness that it can be understood.
5. The standards should be sufficiently unambiguous in what they require that they can be understood.
6. The standards should not require acts that cannot possibly be done.
7. The standards should be consistently applied.
8. Such standards should not be ignored by those who authoritatively apply them.

As Fuller recognizes, various of these principles find expression in certain legal doctrines, particularly in those areas of law where responsibility is ascribed. These doctrines include the void-for-vagueness doctrine, the ban in many states on court-created crimes, the constitutional ban on retroactive reinterpretation of criminal statutes, the rule of strict construction sometimes applied in criminal law, the constitutional ban on ex post facto laws, and the publication requirements for statutes.

There is a common thread to all of these doctrines and Fuller's principles that underlie them: Citizens are capable of adjusting their behavior to legal standards if they are given the chance to do so. These eight principles are no more than the conditions necessary for the exercise of that human capacity. Only if there are general standards that do not require the impossible can citizens use these standards as the major premises of their practical syllogisms. Similarly, only if they know what those standards are—which they can only if they are promulgated beforehand and publicly available—can they use such standards as the major premise in their practical reasoning about what they should do. It is also true that they can reason from such standards to the action that will satisfy them, only if the standards themselves are clear enough that they can see how they apply to their situation. Standards that are vague, ambiguous, inconsistently applied, or ignored by officials do not allow citizens to do this.

The short of it is that the "rule of law" virtues that Fuller lists are virtues for law only because the persons to whom laws are addressed are practical reasoners capable of forming belief/desire sets around such laws, and then acting accordingly. If persons were not like this, these characteristics of laws would not be prerequisites of legal obligation, and thus of legal liability, because they would have no point. Fuller himself was clear about this. The internal morality of the law, he argued, "cannot be neutral in its view of man himself. To embark on the enterprise of subjecting human conduct to the governance of rules involves of necessity a commitment to the view that man is, or can become, a responsible agent, capable of understanding and following rules."[42] We might add, as Fuller did not, that the capacity to understand and follow rules is but an aspect of the capacity to reason practically.

Accountability

Any system of moral or legal standards has implicitly within it an idea about the audience to whom such standards are addressed. One sort of boundary condition with which we need not concern ourselves is *territorial* limits on the reach of any state's laws. More pertinent to our concerns is the kind of limit Kant envisioned when he proclaimed that the general form of moral judgments was a categorical imperative *for all rational beings* (including, but not limited to, persons). This kind of limitation on the audience of a norm limits the entities that are obligated by the norm, by virtue of *what* they are rather than *where* they are.

There are many entities in this world (we need not posit Martians) capable of causing harm. Yet legal and moral injunctions such as, "Don't kill human beings," do not apply to most such entities. If such norms do not apply and do not obligate such entities, then they cannot be held responsible for causing death or other harm to persons.

Consider in this regard entities such as plants, stones, ships, earthworms, dogs, computerized robots, corpses, corporations, infants, and very crazy human beings. Culpability is not attributable to any of these entities and, as a result, they are not legally liable whenever culpability is prerequisite of liability. These entities (with the possible exception of corporations) are by and large not the addressees of our moral and legal norms. Only *persons* are such addressees and these entities are either not persons at all, or are at least entities whose personhood is in question.

One necessary condition of personhood all such entities lack is rationality and autonomy, defined as the ability to perform actions in response to valid practical inferences. Such entities are not, or are not fully, practical reasoners. They are accordingly not the kind of moral agent obligated by moral norms; they thus cannot fairly be held responsible for the breach of such norms. It is only persons like us – practical reasoners – who are obligated by moral norms and thus have the capacity to be responsible (culpable) when we breach them.

One can see this link of practical reason and culpability/liability in those areas where the law has on occasion blamed these nonpersonal entities. Animals at one time were punished for causing harm – not just destroyed or conditioned to be nondangerous, as we might do if they present a danger, but *punished* for having culpably caused a harm. In the opening chapter of *The Common Law,* Holmes gives numerous examples of ancient legal systems punishing dogs, oxen, tigers, or horses if they caused

The Legal View of Persons

harm.[43] Holmes argued that it was a refinement of these punitive practices of blaming animals first to allow their surrender, and then to allow their owners to pay damages rather than to forfeit the offending beast. The right of surrender did not evolve as a limitation on the liability of an animal's owners, but rather, as a remnant of the more primitive liability of the animal itself.

Even more primitive are the practices of punishing inanimate things. In both primitive and early English law the tree that fell on a person, or from which someone fell, was chopped to bits. The club or other instrument with which one person killed another was an "accursed thing" on its own, in Blackstone's language, and was forfeited as "deodand."[44]

Holmes's general thesis about all of this was that all punishment was rooted in a passion for revenge. But, he asked, how could inanimate objects and animals be punished in these ways if the object was to seek revenge? Holmes thought that the answer was to be found "in the personification of inanimate nature common to savages and children ... without such a personification, anger towards lifeless things would have been transitory, at most."[45] What Holmes meant by the personification of the natural world is what is often called "primitive animism," that anthropomorphic view of the world that attributes all that happens to intelligent design. It is the view that stones, plants, animals, and human instruments such as ships all have their own (nonfunctional) purposes for which they act, their own belief/desire sets the contents of which form valid practical syllogisms. What we learn from the coupling of such primitive practices of blaming and the animistic view of nature is that practical reasoning (personification) and the attribution of responsibility go hand in hand. Without the primitive belief in the capacity for practical reasoning in stones, plants, and animals, the attribution of responsibility disappears.

A much more contemporary example of this presupposition of practical reasoning capacities by accountability is to be found in the very current debate about the moral status of corporations. Can one meaningfully attribute moral blame and culpability to, say, Ford Motor Company for its failure to recall automobiles that had dangerously located fuel tanks? To even see what this debate is about, one must put aside instrumental calculations about what educative or other benefits may be achieved by *saying* that Ford is culpable.[46] One must also put aside the culpability of Ford's officers, shareholders, directors, or employees—*they* as persons may of course be culpable on their own. Stripped to its essentials, the interesting question is whether a nonhuman thing, a corporation, possesses sufficient attributes of personhood that *it* is a moral agent fairly blamable for *its* actions.

It is not my purpose to answer this question, but only to show that those who would argue that corporations are or are not themselves accountable as persons do so in terms of the nonreducible practical reasoning that they argue can be attributed to such entities. John Ladd, for example, argues against corporate accountability on the grounds that "organizations are like machines, and it would be a category-mistake to expect a machine to comply with the principles of morality."[47] The category mistake for Ladd is the attribution of rationality to organizations. Peter French, on the other hand, argues that corporations are moral persons because "there is sense in saying that corporations and not just people who work in them, have reasons for what they do."[48] Proponents of corporate accountability, such as French, acknowledge that they must make sense of the idea that a corporation can form a desire and act on it in light of a belief. One might try to do this by showing that a corporation is structured in such a way that no human being within it makes the disputed decision or forms the culpable desire; such decisions may be thought to be made incrementally by employees so that the culpable practical inference emerges only at the level of *corporate* action and decision. In any case, that some such argument is necessary to any contention that corporations are moral agents evidences the crucial role practical reasoning abilities have in such status.

The tie of practical reason to the personhood required for accountability may also be seen in the uniform unwillingness of our culture to attribute responsibility to two other classes of entities, very young children and very crazy adults. Although such entities are clearly human beings (in the sense of being members of that species), and although such human beings have the potential to become persons, both are entities that are not fully persons and thus are not the addressees of moral norms.

With regard to children, the common law settled into its present form by the time of Lord Coke: A child under the age of 7 was (and is) conclusively presumed to be incapable of being criminally culpable, and children between the ages of 7 and 14 were presumed to be similarly incapable, but the presumption was one that could be rebutted on a proper showing by the prosecution.[49] The rationale the common law adopted in the early fourteenth century as to why a child under 7 lacked capacity, was "because he knoweth not of good and evil."[50] Similarly, to show that a child between the ages of 7 and 14 had the capacity prerequisite to culpability, the prosecutor was obliged to show that the child knew the difference between good and evil.[51]

There is something important lurking in these archaic-sounding phrases that has often been overlooked after this language was altered and then frozen in its altered form into the long-dominant insanity test of English and American law. The language of knowing good and evil apparently originated in the Bible, where, in Genesis, God likens humans to God once they have come to know of good and evil.[52] Such godlike knowledge the common law adopted as the mark of maturity of a child, the kind of maturity that gave the child the status of being an adult accountable for its actions.

The confusing gloss often put on such language is to treat it as specifying a kind of *excuse* for children, as if they got a kind of special mistake of law or "mistake of morals" defense. Young children are not held to lack the capacity to be accountable because they lack knowledge of the moral or legal norm they violate. Often they have such knowledge, and in any case, mistakes of law or morality do not generally excuse. The "knowledge of right and wrong" language marks a *general* capacity, a status, that young children are thought to lack: They are not yet sufficiently rational that they can reason about moral or legal norms and adjust their behavior to them. In a phrase, they are not yet good practical reasoners. They are thus not enough like us in one of our essential attributes, our rationality, to be fully *persons* who are accountable. It is only when we begin to see a child's actions as regularly flowing from valid practical inferences that we accord it the status of a person and a moral agent.

The same sort of confusion exists as to why we do not hold insane human beings accountable for the harm they may cause. The dominant theory of insanity is that it is a kind of excuse attached to particular actions of an insane human being. What kind of excuse is a matter of some debate, the three leading candidates being the excuses of ignorance, compulsion, or "lack of free will."

I shall examine these conceptions of legal insanity in Chapter 6 and reject them as being unfaithful to our actual practices in attributing legal and moral responsibility to the mentally ill. If we can anticipate the result of that discussion and put aside these excuse theories of legal insanity, we can see the alternative idea: Very crazy human beings are not enough like us in one of our essential attributes, rationality, to be considered persons to whom moral and legal norms are addressed. Crazy people are "excused" from responsibility for the harm they cause for the same reason that young children, animals, stones, and perhaps corporations are excused: None of them has the *status* of being a person, the only kind of entity obligated by moral and legal norms.

Working out more precisely the senses of rationality and their tie to responsibility will be one of the central tasks of Chapter 6. One can at least make plausible here this conception of legal insanity by examining very briefly the historical tendency to analogize the mentally ill to other defective practical reasoners, children and animals.

Insanity in some form was recognized in most ancient systems of law, which likened the insane to the young. Ancient Moslem law applied punishment only to "individuals who have attained their majority," and "who are in full possession of their faculties."[53] This analogy of the insane to children exists as well in ancient Hebraic law, which recognized that deaf-mutes, idiots, and minors were not responsible for their actions.[54] Roman law, at least during the latter period of the Empire, also relieved the mentally ill of responsibility for wrongful actions, again drawing the analogy of insane persons explicitly to children.[55]

Two analogies dominate the earliest ideas about the insanity defense in Anglo-American law. The first of these is again the analogy to children. Sir Matthew Hale, Chief Justice of the Court of the King's Bench, in his *Select Pleas of the Crown,* expressed the view that the best measure of legal insanity was whether or not the accused "hath yet ordinarily as great understanding as ordinarily a child of 14 years hath."[56] This *explicit* analogy to the responsibility of children was *implicit* in a much earlier development in Anglo-American law, the good and evil test, which was later to influence the M'Naghten test of insanity in the nineteenth century. It was this explicit analogy to the conditions under which children could be regarded as responsible agents that was behind the infusion of this language into a definition of legal insanity.[57]

The second famous analogy of early Anglo-American law was to animals. As early as the thirteenth century, Bracton, in *De Legibus et Consuetudinibus Angliae,* the earliest comprehensive treatise on English law, thought that the insane were "not greatly removed from beasts for they lack reasoning."[58] Lord Coke, in Beverly's case in 1603, quoted what he took to be Bracton's analogy with approval.[59] It was in Arnold's case, however, in the early eighteenth century, that the analogy to animals became well entrenched in English law. Justice Tracy, presiding at the trial of Edward Arnold, said that in order to avail himself of the defense of insanity, "a man must be totally deprived of his understanding and memory, so as not to know what he is doing, no more than an infant, a brute, or a wild beast."[60]

In all of these instances an entity is an accountable agent only to the degree to which it possesses one of the defining characteristics of personhood, namely, rationality. Some entities, such as plants, stones, and corpses, do not possess this attribute of personhood at all. Others, such as the insane, the young, and the higher animals, exhibit some practical reasoning capacities, although less than is required for personhood. With regard to still other entities, such as corporations and sophisticated computers, we are uncertain about whether they are fully rational agents or even rational agents at all. About these last two kinds of entities the law has certainly wavered as to where to draw the line separating persons from nonpersons. About what the line is, however, there has been no such wavering. In such line drawing, perhaps more clearly than anywhere else, the law has revealed its hidden image of a person: A person is a rational being, a being who acts for intelligible ends in light of rational beliefs.

The Legal View of Persons

Action and Mental State

Acting: In law no less than in morals, the idea of human action lies at the heart of ascriptions of responsibility. One is responsible only for those consequences that are caused by one's actions, and not for those things in which one's body, but not the acting self, is causally implicated. One is responsible if one hits another with a stick, but is not responsible if one's arm-with-stick is caused by wind to strike another. On what basis do we distinguish those bodily motions that are actions from those that are not? Our immediate motive in asking this question is to assess the role of practical reason in this fundamental legal and moral category. Later, in Chapter 9, we will rely on this analysis in answering one of the basic questions concerning the impact of unconscious mental states on responsibility, namely, whether the discovery of unconscious mental states can show that what one took to be accidents are truly actions.

A more problematic and more complicated example will further the analysis. Consider the case of Rosa:

> Everyone has an anecdote to tell about the first time he drove a car. But no one can top the story of Rosa Carolle.
>
> Rosa, 19, was going to get her first driving lesson from Hector Cervantes, a young man she had dated a couple of times.
>
> Hector drove her to the Harrison High School parking lot on the Southwest side. After a few minutes, though, something went wrong with the car. Hector couldn't get it into gear.
>
> Hector doesn't know much about mechanical things, but he has a friend who does. So he told Rosa to wait and he would return with his friend.
>
> While waiting, Rosa decided to listen to the radio. So she started the engine. Then — and Rosa isn't sure how it happened — the car got into reverse and began moving.
>
> At that moment a squad car was going by and the policemen noticed the car in the parking lot. Since it was evening, they decided to check the car out. They pulled into the lot and got out.
>
> Rosa, meanwhile, was in a state of confusion. The car was moving and she wanted to stop it. But her foot hit the gas pedal instead of the brakes. At the same time she was frantically trying to get the car out of gear.
>
> Lurch. The car slammed into the school building wall.
>
> Lurch again. It rammed a fence.
>
> Another lurch and it was flying across the lot and whacked the open squad car door, which in turn whacked Patrolman Grecencio Gonzales. With a car roaring wildly around the parking lot, the policemen understandably believed somebody was out to run them over.

So Gonzales took out his pistol and shot at the car.

This did little to calm Rosa, who had not yet figured out how to make the vehicle stop. So the car continued to carom around and across the parking lot, from building to fence to building, while the policemen tried to get out of its way.

Finally, Patrolman John Bria ended the driving lesson by shooting out a front tire.

Rosa, looking more than a little shaken, stepped out. The policemen, who were also shaken, announced that she was under arrest.[61]

If it is both a moral and a legal offense for one to drive in a manner dangerous to others, did Rosa perform the action of *driving?*

To answer this question requires that it first be divided into two distinct questions, often unfortunately conflated both in the older philosophy of action and in the criminal law's supposedly univocal requirement of an *actus reus*: (1) Did Rosa perform any action at all? And (2) if so, *what* action(s) did she perform? (And, more practically in the context of assessing her responsibility, is included in the proper descriptions of her actions one called driving?) Each question corresponds to a distinct inquiry in the philosophy of action: the first, to an analysis of the idea of a simple or basic action; the second, to an analysis of the ways in which complex action descriptions are built from simple ones. I shall pursue each in turn.

Basic Actions: A basic or simple action is an action one performs by doing no other action.[62] One opens a door by pushing against it; one pushes against it by moving one's arm; but by what further act does one move one's arm? Simple motions of the body that a person brings about are basic acts because we do not do anything else in order to do them.

Arthur Danto has argued persuasively that the concept of a human action depends on there being a concept of a basic action. It is only because there is an act not done by the performance of some further act (a basic act) that one has any place at which to stop in the search for ever simpler descriptions of any action. Otherwise one would redescribe X's raising his arm as "X flexed his deltoids," or perhaps, "X sent a nerve impulse to his deltoids." Yet none of these is a basic action X performs.[63] X did not raise his arm by flexing his deltoids, nor did he do the latter *by* sending a nerve impulse. It is true that these events occurred when X raised his arm, yet X caused these events to occur by raising his arm, not vice versa. If X is an average person, he does not know how to send a nerve impulse and may not know which muscles to stimulate, except by doing that which he does know how to do, namely, raise his arm.

If there were no such natural beginnings of actions as basic actions, then the infinite regress objection often advanced against volitions would apply here as well: If every time actor X does action A, he must first do action B,

The Legal View of Persons

and to do B, he must do C, and so forth, one could never *do* anything. Since people do perform all sorts of actions, there must be basic actions.

One wants to isolate such simple acts, not because they figure often in legal or moral norms, but because they properly focus the first question: What is the difference between the (simple) *action* of raising one's arm, and the mere *movement* of the body described by saying that the arm went up? One is morally responsible for raising one's arm (and, if other conditions are met, also responsible for all the further, complex actions one may thereby perform that *are* prohibited by legal or moral norms, such as killing another with a knife); one is not responsible if one's arm only went up but was not raised. It is necessary to focus on simple actions in order to avoid the errors of some philosophers who have mistaken certain features of complex actions as the hallmark of action itself.

The question to which we here seek an answer is Wittgenstein's famous question: "What is left over if I subtract the fact that my arm goes up from the fact that I raise my arm?"[64] Seemingly "something" is left over, as is shown by the relationship between the following statements:

1. X raised his arm.
2. X's arm went up.

(1) implies (2), but (2) does not imply (1). X's arm may go up because, for example, the wind blows it, someone grabs it, or a reflex occurs. Hence (1) and (2) are not equivalent statements. To say that X raised his arm is to say *more* than that certain motions of his body took place.

This is demonstrably not true for the "actions" of inanimate objects.[65] Suppose the following is said of some water that was partly elevated in a U-shaped tube.

3. The water sought its own level.

Although the grammatically active mood might suggest that the water performed some action in the same sense that X performed some action in (1), this is not the case. Compare (3) with the following statement:

4. The water fell to a constant level.

Not only does (3) imply (4), but (4) also implies (3). The statements are equivalent; the actions of inanimate objects, such as water, do not share some crucial features of *human* action. Action language applied to inanimate objects is but a metaphorical way of describing the motions of those objects. In principal, all such metaphor could be eliminated, and any talk of water performing *actions* could be reduced to talk of the motions of that water. Thus, one should be a simple behaviorist with regard to the actions of inanimate objects, but no simple behaviorism will do as an account of *human* action. The language used to describe human action presupposes that more than some motion of a person's body took place in the world.

This contrast between the actions of inanimate objects and the actions of persons is important beyond its usefulness in clarifying what is the right question to be asked about human actions. In addition, this contrast is important as a reminder that one does ascribe actions to objects other than persons, that one does talk of objects that are not persons causing things to happen, and that one does invoke agencies that are not *personal* agencies.

It is important to keep this fact in mind when confronted with claims such as those examined later, viz., that what one takes to be accidents are really actions one performs. There is a sense in which such claims will obviously (if trivially) be true, namely, a sense relying on the concept of action applicable to inanimate objects. Suppose, for example, one is told that X's hitting Y, nominally an accident because X stumbled and hit Y as he fell, was really an action X performed. If "X" is taken to refer to the physical body of X, then it is true that X performed the action of hitting Y because there is a hitting that one can ascribe to the agency of *some body*. Such a hitting will be X's action in the same sense that the hitting of one billiard ball by another is an action of the ball in motion. So construed, such a claim says nothing about whether X, *the person*, performed a human action in hitting Y. Since in law and morals it is *persons* performing actions with which we are concerned, we may put aside the behaviorist sense of action, which reduces it without remainder to bodily motions.

Legal theorists may appear to ignore any distinction between human actions and mere bodily movements, for often the two are equated. The American Law Institute's Model Penal Code, for example, defines act or action as meaning "a bodily movement."[66] Much earlier, O. W. Holmes argued that an action was "a willed muscular movement, and nothing else."[67] Yet these lawyerly usages do not obliterate the important distinction between actions persons perform and bodily movements that are not actions because the person whose body was involved did not perform them. For lawyers reintroduce exactly the distinction between action and bodily movement with notions of volition, will, or voluntariness. The Model Penal Code, for example, states that a person cannot be held responsible "unless his liability is based on conduct which includes a *voluntary* act."[68] Voluntariness is then itself defined in terms of "the effort or determination of the actor, either conscious or habitual."[69] This last phrase is no more than an attempt to answer Wittgenstein's question about what is left over when we subtract an arm going up from an arm being raised:

The Legal View of Persons

The will of the actor is left over. This may not be a very helpful answer, but the only point here is to see that it is an answer to the same question that concerns philosophers when they ask, What is the difference between an action and a mere bodily movement?

The answer to this question that is most congenial to the thesis of this chapter has many adherents in both legal theory and philosophy. In general form the theory asserts that a bodily movement will be an action if it is caused by some mental state of desire, intention, or volition. John Stuart Mill succinctly stated an early version of this theory as follows:

> Now what is an action? Not one thing, but a series of two things: the state of mind called a volition, followed by an effect. The volition or intention to produce the effect, is one thing; the effect produced in consequence of the intention, is another thing. The two together constitute the action. I form the purpose of instantly moving my arm; that is a state of my mind: my arm (not being tied or paralytic) moves in obedience to my purpose; that it is a physical fact, consequent on a state of mind. The intention followed by the fact . . . is called the action of moving my arm.[70]

This causal theory of action is echoed in legal theory by John Austin in his *Lectures on Jurisprudence*,[71] and more recently by J. L. Mackie.[72] Mackie shifts the Mill–Austin theory slightly to take into account an objection H. L. A. Hart once voiced.[73] Hart's objection was that we do not desire to move our muscles or our arm, even when our arm's moving is an action by us; we normally desire to do more complicated sorts of things to which the arm's moving is but a means. A causal theorist can take this into account, Mackie tells us, by retaining the causation-by-desire requirement but rejecting any notion that an actor must desire *to move his arm* in order for that arm movement to have been an action. It is enough that such movements, "though not themselves desired, . . . were such as would normally fulfill the desire that brought them about and that they came about because they were so associated with its fulfillment."[74]

The modified causal theory Mackie articulates is the modern version of the causal theory of action according to which movement is an action if and only if it is caused by a belief/desire set whose contents form a valid practical syllogism. Although Mackie seems to believe that it is the causation by a *desire* that makes movement an action, as Alvin Goldman (a leading exponent of this theory of action) has shown, *both* a belief and a desire must cause the movement. Further, such belief and such desire must be related to one another and to the action they cause in the manner earlier described for reason-giving explanations.[75]

If the Mill-Austin-Mackie-Goldman theory of action were correct, then the connection between the concept of an action and reason-giving explanations would be direct: The second would be a necessary and sufficient condition for the first. The problem that appears insurmountable for any version of the causal theory stems from what are called "deviant causal chains."[76] Suppose someone like Rosa is behind the wheel of a car and sees her hated enemy step before her. Suppose further that she forms the desire to run over her enemy and believes that if she pushes down with her foot from the brake to the accelerator, she will run over her enemy. Suppose further that her foot moves from the brake pedal to the accelerator, and that this movement was caused by her desire and by her belief. Is the causal role of this belief/desire set enough to say that Rosa *acted* in moving her foot? Before one says yes too readily, consider the following elaboration: Rosa's beliefs and desires got her so excited in anticipation of finally being in a position to kill her enemy that her foot slipped off the brake to the accelerator. Our intuitions are plain in such a case that Rosa's foot movement is *not* an action, despite the causal role of her belief/desire set. If this is so, then our idea of what an action is is not captured by the causal theory even in its most sophisticated modern form.

The common way to try to repair this kind of example is by adding "the requirement that action-plans not merely *cause* basic acts, but that they cause the basic acts '*in a certain characteristic way.*' "[77] Goldman tells us that "we are aware, intuitively, of a characteristic manner in which desires and beliefs flow into intentional acts."[78] The problem with this response is the ad hoc, gerrymandered notion of causation on which it must rely. No independent characterization is given of the kind of causal relation that will do here, except by saying, "the kind of causation involved in *acting*." Causation that is merely synonymous with acting will not, of course, do in analyzing action.[79]

That one cannot make out the causal theory of action in no way contradicts the Lockean notion that persons have causal powers, as discussed earlier. That analysis left open whether such causal power was truly a causal notion, or whether it was not better conceptualized in terms of some noncausal notion of personal agency. The Mill-Austin-Mackie-Goldman causal theory attempts to eliminate either of these alternatives — the causal power of a person or personal agency — in favor of the Humean notion of event or state causation. Yet the causal theory fails precisely because it leaves out the central ideal of human action captured by the ideas of personal agency or causal power, namely, the notion of a *person* bringing about some new state of affairs.

Unfortunately, this causal power/personal agency account of human action does not say very much. It is about as helpful as Aristotle's idea that an action is where the moving principle is inside the person. What is needed is some further indication of what it is that allows us to distinguish patterns of movements that are to be attributed to personal agency from those that are not. Attention to the kinds of movements not thought to be

The Legal View of Persons

actions, both in law and in everyday life, may help to isolate such further indicators.

Imagine three different ways in which the arm of some person may move upward:

1. X's arm is blown upward by the wind.
2. X's arm rises because of a reflex reaction to some stimulus operating through his central nervous system.
3. X is asleep and his arm goes up.

Although the behavior in each of these cases might be identical when considered as the motion of a physical body, each is distinguishable from each other and from an action by X of raising his arm. In the first example, a known external force raises X's arm; X's muscles are not even involved. Thus, this is an easy case in which the arm movement is not an action by X. In the second example, it is X's muscles that cause his arm to rise, but X, the person, is not causally responsible for his arm going up. It is therefore not his action. The third example is the most difficult case. Cases of sleepwalking, posthypnotic acts, and similar behavior are often sufficiently complicated that they appear to be intelligently directed actions. In such cases one is loath not to attribute these acts to *some* agency, but if not to X, then to whom? It is as if one is prepared to say that sleepwalking is an action, but not of X, even though it is performed by his body.

Criminal law and the law of torts have consistently held that sleepwalking, posthypnotic and similar acts are examples of nonaction. Case law,[80] model codes,[81] and commentary[82] uniformly classify unconsciously directed behavior, or behavior engaged in while unconscious, as nonaction. Although I shall ultimately conclude that the law is correct in this regard, it is necessary to examine the conceptual issue prior to the moral and legal issues due to the importance of the conceptual issue to later analysis.

There seems to be an important relationship between the concept of a basic act and the knowledge of the acting subject.[83] What a person can do as a basic act is limited by what that person *knows* he can do as a basic act. For example, the complicated muscle flexings necessary to raise one's arm are not basic actions because the actor does not know how to move them in just the way that will raise his arm. The act of raising one's arm is a basic act, however, because the actor knows he can raise his arm and because he knows when he is exercising that power.[84]

This relationship between action and knowledge provides a kind of epistemic indicator of action: An actor's bodily movement is a basic action only if he knows that he can perform that movement as an action and knows that he is doing so on that particular occasion. This epistemic account of action may gain further plausibility when "mental acts" are considered. A person performs the mental act of calling to mind some memory if, and only if, he knows he is doing so. This is not to say that thoughts that are not mental acts were uncaused, but only that bringing them forth was not something *he* did. What else could distinguish mental acts from mental happenings *but* that person's knowledge of doing the act in question? Hence, the correctness of Wittgenstein's answer to his own question: Human actions are marked by the absence of surprise.[85]

The law's treatment of nonconsciously directed behavior as nonaction is, at least prima facie,[86] in line with this epistemic criterion of an action. In cases where the actor is unconscious, the person is not awake to possess the requisite knowledge (in the sense of awareness) that would make the movements of his body an action attributable to him. In cases where the actor is conscious, such as in cases of posthypnotic suggestion, the actor, although awake, does not know that he is raising his arm. He doubtlessly does know that his arm is going up, just as he would know during an epileptic seizure that his limbs were moving, but in neither of these cases does he know that he is exercising his power to move his limbs.

The tie of action to practical reasoning is much less direct on this epistemic account of action than it would be if the causal theory were true. It is possible, in the account just concluded, that a person: (1) performs a basic action even though not caused to do so by a belief/desire set, and (2) does not perform a basic action despite having certain bodily movements caused by a belief/desire set. Causation by belief/desire sets is neither a necessary nor a sufficient condition for there to be a basic action. Despite this, there remains the stubborn intuition, expressed by Richard Peters but shared by many, that "the paradigm case of a human action is when something is done in order to bring about an end."[87]

One wants to separate two aspects of this intuition to see what it comes to. The first aspect has to do with the contingent connection that does exist between basic actions and reasons: Although not strictly necessary to there being a basic action, it is almost always the case that basic acts are done for reasons. No one we know just moves his limbs on a regular basis for no reason. Not even in existential fiction does one find *actes gratuits* that are *basic* acts. Mersault, in Camus's *Stranger,* does not just move his fingers but does so in order to pull the trigger, and perhaps, to kill. Similarly, Gide's Lafcadio, of *Lafcadio's Adventures,* does not just raise his foot for no reason; he does so to push the old man out of the train. Although our personal agency, or will, could be exercised over our bodies without our forming any desires, it is very rare that such basic acts take place.

The second aspect of Peters's intuition has to do with the limited domain of reason-giving explanations earlier noted: Reasons only explain actions. A reason-giving explanation can be true only if what it explains is an action. This is a noncontingent connection between reasons and action: Reason-giving explanations presuppose, or imply, action. This presupposition of actions by reasons does *not* mean that causation by a belief/desire set is a sufficient condition for there to be an action; it means that built into the idea of reasons is the concept of action.

Because of this, there is, to be sure, a trivial sense in which to act for reasons is a sufficient condition of action: If one acted for reasons, necessarily one acted. This, however, does not allow one to use reasons as a criterion of action, any more than the trivial truth that if a thing is a red ball, it is a ball, allows one to use redness as one's criterion of "ball."

The relation of basic action to reason-giving explanations is thus not a simple one. We cannot reduce basic actions to causation by rationalizing belief/desire sets, as the causal theory attempts to do. Still, the idea of a basic act — an exercise of personal agency over our bodies — is a necessary part of the idea of practical reasoning. It is also true that basic acts are contingently connected to reasons by virtue of their not being done (for all practical purposes) except as means to some other ends.

Complex Action Descriptions: Suppose we conclude that the arm we see rising before us is an instance of some action. We conclude, that is, that it is the result of a personal agent's making his arm go up. We cannot yet conclude *what* action it is we have witnessed, even though we know that it is *some* action. To know *what* action it is depends on a host of considerations different than simply knowing that an agent was causally responsible for the arm's going up.

We often are performing many other actions when we perform the simple action of raising our arm. We may, for example, be opening a window, if a *consequence* of raising our arm is such that a window opens; voting, if the *conventions* are such that in these *circumstances* the hand will be counted as a vote; signaling to another, if our *intent* is to signal. Depending on what else is presupposed by the complex description beyond the performance of a simple action, we may say that some actions are causally complex, conventionally complex, circumstantially complex, and/or intentionally complex.[88] A description is causally complex if it presupposes not only that some basic action was performed, but also that a certain state of affairs was brought about by that basic action. "A killed B" is a causally complex description, because in addition to whatever basic action was the means of B's death, it had to cause B's death for A to have killed B. Similar analyses apply to rules presupposed by conventionally complex descriptions, circumstances or intentions presupposed in circumstantially or intentionally complex descriptions.

For any action one may build up a chain of such descriptions, beginning with a basic action and incorporating some further consequences, conventions, and so on, to build further and more complex descriptions. For example:

1. A raised his arm
2. A opened the window
3. A signaled a warning to his comrades
4. A chilled the room

These could be actions A performed, depending on the consequences of raising his arm (for 2 and 4) and on his intentions (for 3).

Returning to Rosa for a moment will illustrate the ways in which practical reasoning is related to certain complex action descriptions. Before we ask whether Rosa *intentionally* drove the car, we might ask whether she *drove* it at all, intentionally or unintentionally. Indeed, in the law, where driving offenses are typically framed without a *mens rea* requirement, this inquiry would be forced upon us. Even if we stipulate that she performed the basic actions of pushing her foot down on the accelerator and turning the steering wheel, would we say that she was driving?

Richard Peters once urged that "general standards or rules are implicit in the concept of an action."[89] As a general statement about actions, this is false. It is, however, an accurate statement about conventionally complex actions such as driving. "Driving" is like "castling a king" in that both action verbs are truly predicable of a person only if he is engaged in a bit of practical reasoning. One can be said to be castling one's king, not just because one physically moves the chess pieces in such a way that the king is castled; in addition, one has to know the rules of chess and be following them in order to be said to be castling one's king. Similarly, it might be urged that one has to know how to drive (the practical and legal rules of driving) in order to be said to be driving. A. I. Melden, for example, asks us to

> consider the enormously complex set of practices acquired by those driving their automobiles through traffic, responding to a variety of cues – the condition of the road surface, the sound of the motor, the presence of pedestrians and vehicles blocking the way, the signals of other motorists, the road signs, the traffic lights, and the instructions of the traffic police. In this complex set of practices we may recognize the observance of rules.[90]

Rosa, in such a view, was not driving because included in the practical syllogisms that governed her basic acts of foot pushing and arm movements were none that made reference to the rules of driving.

A similar presupposition of practical reasoning is to be found in intentionally complex act descriptions. As G. E. M. Anscombe once noted, "A great many of our descriptions of events effected by human beings are *formally* descriptions of executed intentions."[91] If one performs the action of *concealing* a gun, for example, one necessarily intended to conceal it. If intentions are closely tied to practical reason, then so must be this class of actions. It is the burden of the next section to show the close tie that exists between practical reasoning and intentionality.

Mental State: It is the hallmark of civilized legal systems that a person act with a culpable mental state, or *mens rea,* before being held liable to legal sanctions. Moral culpability, too, is ascribed only to those with a "guilty mind." I shall deal with three such mental states: those involved in intentional action, in action for a further intention, and with that substitute for a mental state involved in acting negligently.

Intentional Action: G. E. M. Anscombe helpfully distinguished three usages of the word "intention": We speak of an action being *intentional,* of an action being done with some *further intention* in mind, and of an actor *intending* to do some action in the future.[92] The usage most generally pertinent to assessing responsibility is the first, using "intentional" as an adjective or adverb ("intentionally"). In criminal law this is often called "general intent"; in morals, it marks the fundamental distinction we all learned as children, between things done "on purpose" and those that are not.

By what criterion is an action intentional? Suppose that actor X, in performing the basic action of raising his arm, caused the window to open, which in turn caused the room to become chilled. When can it be said that X's chilling of the room was intentional? The first thing to notice is that it is not enough to conclude that X performed a basic action nor even that X performed the complex action of chilling the room. To have *intentionally* chilled the room requires that something else be the case beyond the fact that X performed that action.

For basic actions it is important to see that this is not the case. A bodily movement will be a basic action if and only if it is intentional. Bentham saw this quite clearly: "If the act be not intentional in the first stage [what we would call a basic act], it is no act of yours."[93] This is the grain of truth to the otherwise false claim that every action is intentional if it is an action at all.

Because of this link of intentional to basic action one might well expect some parallels to exist between theories of action and theories of intention. This is indeed the case. Those who urge that causation by belief/desire sets is the criterion of when a bodily movement is a basic action are logically committed to a like theory of when a basic act is intentional.[94] More generally, the causal theory of intention is that for any action (basic or complex) to be intentional, it must be caused by a belief/desire set the contents of which form a valid practical syllogism.

The causal theory fares no better as a theory of intention than it does as a theory of action: (1) Causation by such belief/desire sets is not necessary, for people often act intentionally for no further reasons, and (2) causation by such belief/desire sets is not sufficient, for counterexamples with deviant causal chains are easy to imagine. Accordingly, if there is a connection of practical reasoning to intentionality, it is not as direct a connection as this.

One can get at a more plausible account of intentional that also links the concept to that of practical reasoning in the following way. Suppose that X's reason for opening the window was to signal his comrades but that he also knew his action would result in chilling the room. Both philosophers and lawyers have long been split as to whether or not X's chilling the room under these circumstances can properly be described as intentional.

Clearly, the *further intention* with which the action of opening the window was done was not to chill the room but rather to signal a warning. Similarly, if X were asked what he *intended* to do prior to raising his arm, he would probably *not* list chilling the room as something he intended to do. To the extent that the common usage of further intention and intend governs the usage of intentional, these considerations suggest that mere knowledge of a consequence resulting from a given action is not enough. For X's chilling the room to have been intentional, this view requires that the consequence has been one of X's reasons for opening the window. This analysis is sometimes called the purposive theory of intention.[95]

The purposive theory has a quite direct link to the idea of practical reason, for in this theory, an action is intentional only if bringing about the state of affairs the action describes was part of the actor's chain of reasons for acting. This differs from the causal theory earlier rejected in that no *further* desire/belief set need cause the action of chilling the room for that action to be intentional. It is enough on the purposive theory that the desire to chill the room, together with the belief that opening the window would chill the room, was X's reason for opening the window.

The other competing theory of intention stems from Bentham, who held that knowledge alone was sufficient for intentionality.[96] In the example given, Bentham would say that X, who only knew that his opening the window would chill the room but did not have that consequence as his reason for opening the window, *obliquely* intended to chill the room. If X not only knew that his opening the window would chill the room but had that consequence as his purpose, Bentham would say that X *directly* intended to chill the room. Bentham's theory of intention is thus more inclusive than the purposive theory, for Bentham allows either knowledge or purpose to suffice for intentionality.

One can muster some support for Bentham's theory in our ordinary

The Legal View of Persons

usage. X's chilling the room would probably not be called *unintentional* if he knew that it was certain to occur as a result of his opening the window. To call it unintentional would suggest, as H. L. A. Hart once pointed out,[97] that X opened the window in ignorance of the fact that it would chill the room, under the mistaken belief that it would not chill the room, or perhaps that the room's becoming chilled was inadvertent. Since X's knowledge of chilling the room is inconsistent with the existence of any of these three excuses, "unintentional" is not properly applied to the action. If one believes that intentional and unintentional are contradictories and not merely contraries of one another,[98] it follows that X's chilling the room was intentional so long as X knew that was what he was doing, even if that consequence was not a reason for his opening the window.

It would seem that the only convincing conclusion of the considerable ordinary language analysis that has been applied to this problem is that one's linguistic intuitions do not resolve the problem. Intentional, like many other words, is intensionally vague; that is, it is vague with respect to its sense or criteria (its intension).[99] That being true, one should simply stipulate a definition of intentional that best marks the significant moral distinction between those who act with the most culpable mental state and those who act with a markedly lesser culpability.

Although this point has been argued to the contrary by other commentators,[100] I shall again follow the law of torts[101] and crimes[102] in adopting Bentham's more inclusive definition of intentional as those actions done by an actor who knows he is performing them. Such a definition is based on the moral notion that one who does an act knowing it will lead to some bad result is equally as culpable as the person who performs that act having the bad result as his purpose.

This more inclusive definition of intentional parallels the epistemic account given earlier of basic actions, for in both cases it is the knowledge of the acting subject that makes his movement a basic action or an intentional complex action. Although knowledge is a criterion of both basic action and intention, for any given instance of complex action the knowledge required will of course be different. A killing will be X's *action* if the victim's death follows as a consequence of some basic action performed by X, the performance of which X had knowledge; but a killing will be X's *intentional* action only if death follows as a consequence of some basic action by X *and* X knew that it would so follow.[103]

Because intention, like basic action, relies on the knowledge of the acting subject, the ties of intentionality to practical reasoning will also be the same. First, it is often (although not as often) true that intentional actions are performed for further reasons. Second, the idea of intentionality is built into reason-giving accounts as solidly as is the idea of a basic action. If X performed some complex action for certain reasons, necessarily that complex action was performed intentionally. If X chilled the room in order to offend his guests, necessarily his chilling of the room was an intentional action by him.

This is the limited truth in Anscombe's claim that an action is intentional when reason-giving accounts are appropriate for it.[104] Such accounts are appropriate *only* for intentional actions. The problem for Anscombe lies in her attempt to make this into a *criterion* for intentionality, which it cannot be without a vicious circularity: The appropriateness of reason-giving explanations cannot be an informative criterion of intentionality when those very explanations presuppose intentionality.

What one can say is this, and it is important: The three ideas of a basic act, of intentionality, and of reason-giving explanations are all importantly linked to each other. To use any one of them to describe or explain some bodily movement of a person is to presuppose the applicability of the other two. The three together form the basic vocabulary in terms of which we understand and evaluate ourselves as persons.

Acting Intentionally for a Proscribed Further Intention: As discussed in connection with causation, a plausible case can be made that *trying* or intending to cause some harm is equally culpable with causing it intentionally. Criminal law recognizes such noncausal culpability in three different theories. The first is attempt liability, wherein one is held liable for coming close enough to causing a harm that one can be said to have attempted it. The second is conspiracy liability, where one may be liable for intending to commit a crime so long as that intent is communicated to another in the form of an "agreeing." The third is accomplice liability, whereby one can be held liable for acts that do not in fact causally contribute to a harm so long as those acts were intended by the accomplice to help cause it.

Common to all of these theories, and to the moral theory that underlies them, is that an intention to do something bad, when acted upon, is sufficient for serious culpability. Although one might debate the merits of this idea (in terms of whether there is not such a thing as "moral luck" in not causing a harm that one tried to cause), the main point here is to examine the nature of the intention, the touchstone of culpability here.

Of the three ordinary usages of intention earlier distinguished, it is the second, further intention, that is relevant here. If one wants to know whether X, when he shot Y, was trying to kill him, then the inquiry is not into whether X *intentionally* shot at Y. Rather, what one needs to know is whether X shot at Y with the *further intention* of killing him. Only if X had this further intention could X be said to have tried or attempted to have killed Y.

Further, on this usage of intention, the ambiguity earlier noted for intentional (between purpose and knowledge) disappears. For if one's question is not whether X shot Y intentionally, but rather, whether the further intention with which X shot was to kill Y, it is clear that knowledge will not suffice. X shot with the further intention of killing Y only if killing Y was the purpose or reason for which X shot. If X shot at Y for some other reason, but knowing to a substantial certainty that he would kill him (but miraculously he fails), then X did not shoot with the further intention of killing Y.

In both of these respects the law follows ordinary usage quite closely. All three kinds of crimes—attempt, conspiracy, and complicity—are said to be specific intent crimes. What the latter phrase means in these contexts is exactly what is meant in ordinary speech by the idea of further intent. As LaFave and Scott describe the phrase: "The most common usage of 'specific intent' is to designate a special mental element which is required above and beyond any mental state required with respect to the *actus reus* of the crime."[105] The act involved in the hypothetical situation was X shooting at Y. Specific intent is the further intention to kill, which one must have beyond the intention to shoot (which was the act done) if one is to be guilty of attempted murder.

In addition, specific intent in law, just as further intent in ordinary speech, carries with it the requirement that the forbidden consequence be one's purpose in acting. Shooting at Y, with knowledge to a substantial certainty he will die, but not having Y's death as the reason for which one shot, will suffice no more as specific intent than as further intent.

The theory of culpability/liability based on intention rather than causation uses a clear and unambiguous notion of further or specific intention. The connection of this notion to reason-giving explanations should also be clear: The further or specific intention with which an action was done is just the reason for which it was done. These phrases are simply different names for belief/desire sets whose contents form valid practical syllogisms. Persons must have actually engaged in a certain instance of practical reasoning to possess the culpable *mens rea* described as "specific intent."

Acting Negligently: Negligence in both law and morals will suffice for culpability/liability for causing a harm. The degree of culpability is less than if the actor either had the harm as his reason for acting, or if he at least knew that the harm would result from his actions. Such lesser culpability for negligence is reflected in the concept's differential importance in criminal law and in torts: It is a central concept in torts but of secondary importance in criminal law, where intention is central. The fault required to make one liable to compensate is less than the fault required to make one liable to punishment, and thus negligence has its much more central role to play in tort law than in criminal law.

The lesser culpability attached to negligence stems from the fact that it is not a state of mind, unlike intention. To act negligently is not to possess some state of mind of carelessness or inadvertence, nor is it even to *lack* some state of mind. To act negligently is to fail to measure up to a standard of behavior we expect of all persons. This is one of the meanings of the often expressed notion that negligence is an *objective*, not a subjective, standard of liability.

The concept of negligence itself was classically defined by Learned Hand in his opinion in *United States v. Carroll Towing Co.*[106] Hand's definition makes any actions negligent if the seriousness of the harm resulting from the action, discounted by its improbability at the time of acting, outweighs the cost of the precautions the actor could have taken to prevent the harm. Negligence, in short, is the failure to make, or to make badly, a cost/benefit calculation about the desirability of an action. If the costs of not doing the action (including not only Hand's costs of prevention but also the costs of forgoing any benefits that might have accrued from the action) outweigh the benefit that is the harm's prevention, then the action is not negligent if performed. If such costs of not acting are outweighed by the benefit (prevention of the harm) of not acting, then the action is negligent if performed.

There is nothing in the objective concept of negligence as so far stated that says anything about the nature of persons as practical reasoners. The cost/benefit definition of negligence is simply a utilitarian mode of thinking that tells us what, according to utilitarianism, are good actions because they maximize good states of affairs. One could use such a concept to decide upon the proper behavior of a wide variety of beings, and then *condition* them (à la Skinner) or *rewire* them (via a knowledge of neurophysiology we do not yet possess) into behaving in that way.

The presupposition of persons as practical reasoners comes from the use to which the concept of negligence is put in the criminal and tort rules employing it. Two different uses are relevant here. The first is the use of such rules to guide behavior (the deterrence theories of tort and criminal law). There is a well-known tendency of our negligence law not to frame specific rules of negligence, but to leave it to individual actors and the juries that judge them to decide whether some particular action was or was not negligent.[107] Our law of torts and crimes is here built on the assumption that the general negligence standard itself—Hand's cost/benefit formula—will be action guiding; this can be true only if people can and do reason in this way. Although one might condition horses and dogs as well as persons to stop, look, and listen each and every time they come up to cross a railroad track, such programs would be much less likely to succeed with such a wide range of beings when the only directive was, "don't be negligent." To guide behavior with the latter directive presupposes that the directive's intended audience can calculate costs and benefits themselves, that is, that they can reason practically.

The Legal View of Persons

The second use of the negligence standard is to parcel out legal liability only to those who are culpable (a retributivist or mixed theory of criminal law and the corrective justice theory of torts). Because "negligence" does not name a state of mind, some legal theorists have found it difficult to understand how merely negligent behavior could be culpable. The answer to this is hinted at in the law's *personifying* Hand's calculus of risk into that ideally rational being who gets it right more often than do most defendants, the "average reasonable person."

The average reasonable person may strike one on first acquaintance as a redundant, unnecessarily anthropomorphic conceptualization of a negligence standard better stated by Hand's formula. Why take a clear standard in terms of cost/benefit calculations and transform it into a standard calling for people to behave as would the average reasonable person (who, of course, is no real person but rather an idealization who calculates just as Hand would wish him to calculate)? The answer lies in the function the anthropomorphic way of putting it serves: It makes explicit the connection of negligence to culpability only implicit in Hand's kind of formula. A biography of the average reasonable person reveals that he embodies those qualities of character that we think persons should possess, and those capacities of mind that we think all persons do possess. The average reasonable person is benevolently motivated – he counts all persons' interests as equal to his own; he is thus neither unduly selfish nor unrealistically altruistic. In addition, he knows the true worth of things and is able to compare the value of a life with the dollars and cents cost of altering the design, say, of an automobile. He is also capable of calculating what actions are likely to lead to what results and even to assign relative probabilities to each. He is, in other words, a preeminent practical reasoner, finding the morally and legally correct major premises (in terms of costs and benefits) for his practical syllogisms, and forming the accurate means/end beliefs (in terms of probabilities) for his minor premises. Conceptualizing the negligence standard in terms of such a person makes explicit the assumptions we must make about people if their failure to make the right cost/benefit calculation is to make them culpable: It is because people have the capacity to reason in this way that they can be said to be culpable when they do not do so.

"What is crucial," H. L. A. Hart states in his analysis of the culpability to be found in negligent action, "is that those whom we punish should have had, when they acted, the normal capacities, physical and mental, for doing what the law requires ... and a fair opportunity for exercising those capacities."[108] In cases where the action is negligently but not intentionally done, Hart adds, "At least we may say 'he could have thought about what he was doing' with just as much rational confidence as one can say of any intentional wrongdoing, 'he could have done otherwise.'"[109] Just as the culpability of choice (for intentional wrongdoing) presupposes a kind of being who makes choices, so the culpability of unexercised capacity presupposes a kind of being who has that capacity. The kind of being presupposed in each case is a person who reasons practically.

One can see this presupposition of what people are like most clearly at work when some defendants in fact do not have the capacities negligence law supposes them to have. If there is a demonstrable category of beings who do not have the capacity to know the good and calculate what actions tend toward its achievement, then those beings are not culpable and should not be liable. The mentally retarded and the young are two such well-established categories. One cannot judge them in comparison to what the average reasonable person would do because they do not have the capacities to be the kind of being on whom the law is based; they are not fully persons who reason practically.[110]

Justification and Excuse

The last condition that must be met before one is culpable is that the action be done without either of those kinds of responsibility-diminishing factors we call justifications or excuses. The distinction between a justification and an excuse is an important one. This difference is usually put as a difference in how we regard the actor and the act if a claim of justification or of excuse is made. George Fletcher, for example, so distinguishes the two:

> Claims of justification concede that the definition of the offense is satisfied, but challenge whether the act is wrongful; claims of excuse concede that the act is wrongful, but seek to avoid the attribution of the act to the actor. A justification speaks to the rightness of the act; an excuse, to whether the actor is accountable for a concededly wrongful act.[111]

There is nothing wrong with this as far as it goes. The moral and legal consequences attached to justifications are different from those attached to excuses. Still, what one would like to know is what the difference is between the two modes of mitigation that justifies these different consequences being attached to each.

A justification has to do with certain circumstances in which a normally wrongful act was done. Such justifying circumstances make the act not wrong as performed on this occasion. An excuse has less to do with the act or its circumstances than with the actor's state of mind. Actors may be excused if their state of mind is innocent even though their acts are wrong (even when considered in light of all circumstances).

Justifications such as self-defense, defense of others, defense of property, or balance of evils need not detain us since they present no new problems.

The Legal View of Persons

Such justifications simply form more complete descriptions of what actions are bad or illegal. The legal or moral injunction, "Do not kill," for example, is more completely and thus more accurately phrased as, "Do not kill except in self-defense." Such more complete norms presuppose the same kind of audience as do legal and moral norms generally, namely, an audience composed of beings who reason practically and thus can take such norms into account in planning their behavior.

Of more interest to the concerns of this and later chapters are the excuses. In his discussion of when behavior is voluntary, Aristotle divided excuses into two kinds, those of ignorance and those of compulsion.[112] This is still a pretty good division of legal and moral excuses, and I shall adopt it in discussing each in turn.

There are three excuses having to do with the knowledge of the actor: ignorance proper, mistake, and inadvertence. The difference between the first two can be seen by introducing a distinction from modal logic, the distinction between internal and external negation. If I say of some person, X, that he believes some proposition, p, there are two ways in which negation can enter into the overall statement that X believes that p. First, it is not the case that X believes that p. Second, X believes not-p. The first is known as external negation, because what is negated is external to the proposition that X believes; the second is known as internal negation because what is negated is the proposition that X believes.[113]

If p is some true proposition about some matter of fact, then external negation represents that there is *ignorance,* or no belief, about that matter of fact, whereas internal negation represents that there is a belief about that matter of fact, but it is a *mistaken* belief. Let p, for example, represent the truth, "There is marijuana in the car." One who is ignorant of that fact has no belief that there is marijuana in the car. One who is mistaken believes that there is no marijuana in the car.

Inadvertence is a special case of mistake or ignorance dealing with the consequences of actions rather than with their circumstances. If one shoots a donkey by aiming at a tree but missing, one kills a donkey inadvertently and thus unintentionally. All this means is that one either believed that the bullet would not hit the donkey (mistake), or that the thought that it would hit the donkey did not cross one's mind (ignorance). Because of this, inadvertence will not require separate discussion.

It is commonly said that both mistake and ignorance are merely the contradictories of general intent (or knowledge), and thus that they are not truly excuses.[114] To understand the extent to which this is true is to understand the relation between practical reasoning and these excuses.

Reexamination of the distinction between internal and external negation should allow one to see that only ignorance is the contradictory of knowledge. Only when one conjoins the statement, "X believes that there was marijuana in the car," to the externally negated statement. "It is not the case that X believes that there was marijuana in the car" does one obtain a contradiction.[115] A statement that X made a mistake – "X believed there was no marijuana in the car" – is not the contradictory of the statement that X had knowledge of marijuana being in the car.[116]

Ignorance, being simply the contradictory of knowledge, is related to practical reasoning in the same ways as knowledge itself. The connection between mistake and practical reasoning is slightly less direct. Mistakes excuse because of a hidden presupposition of rationality we make about persons: Persons by and large have consistent beliefs. If we assume that X, for example, has consistent beliefs, then we can rule out the possibility that X believes both that there is marijuana in the car and that there is no marijuana in the car. If we can rule out this possibility, and if X has the mistaken belief supposed – that there was no marijuana in the car – then as a matter of elementary logic we can deduce that X did not have the guilty knowledge (that there was marijuana in the car) and thus should be excused.[117]

Occasionally this hidden presupposition of rationality is not made, as in the Model Penal Code's definition of willful blindness. According to the Code, a defendant who knows that there is a high probability that there is marijuana in his car is guilty of knowing possession of marijuana, unless it is *also* the case that the defendant (mistakenly) believes that there is no marijuana in the car.[118] What the Code here envisions is that there are some people who believe both that (to a high probability at least) there is marijuana in their car and that there is not. Mistake in such a case becomes problematic as an excuse, because in some sense the actor did have the culpable knowledge even if he was "of two minds" about it.

Such cases, however, are the exception. Most of the time we are able to assume consistency in the beliefs of most persons. This presupposition behind mistakes as an excuse is a presupposition about the kind of beings persons are: They are rational beings whose practical reasonings proceed from (usually) consistent minor premises.

The excuses sounding in compulsion rather than ignorance require more extended treatment. Following categories traditional in criminal law, consider four nominally different kinds of cases:

1. An individual, W, robs a bank, but only because other bank robbers hold a gun at his head telling him they will kill him unless he aids in the bank robbery.
2. An individual is hanging onto a plank large enough to support only one person. Another, X, who would otherwise drown, ousts the first, who then drowns.
3. An individual, Y, becomes extremely upset upon learning that

The Legal View of Persons

his wife has just been raped by another. His anger leads him to find the other and shoot him "in a fit of passion."
4. A drug addict, Z, is trying to kick his heroin habit. Yielding to his craving for the drug, he purchases and uses some heroin in violation of the narcotics laws.

Each of these fits a different category of legal excuse. W was coerced to rob the bank by the threat of another (duress). X was coerced by nonhuman, but still external, circumstances; he himself would drown unless he caused another to drown (necessity). Y was not coerced by any external circumstances, human or nonhuman; rather, Y's action was caused by the extreme passion of the moment. His legal defense would be one of provocation. Z also was not coerced by any external circumstance; his use of the drug was caused by his craving for it. His defense would be one of addiction.

Despite these differing legal categorizations, each of these is an instance of compulsion. Common to all such cases is the fact that the actor has made a "hard choice." The factors that made the choice hard differ in each case. External threats, external but natural necessity, internal emotional turmoil, or passionate cravings are different from one another, yet all make a choice difficult. Each at least mitigates the actor's responsibility because of the difficulty of refraining from doing what he ought not to do.

The excuse of compulsion differs from the excuse of ignorance and mistake in the relation of compulsion to the intentionality of the action. W, X, Y, and Z each performed the *actions* of robbing, killing, or drug taking; moreover, each did so *intentionally*. That they were each compelled to do what they did in no way affects the intentional quality of their actions. This distinction is often obscured because of an ambiguity in the word "involuntary." From Aristotle's writings[119] to Fletcher's recent treatise on criminal law,[120] examples of no action or no intentional action are juxtaposed with examples of duress, both being called involuntary. That the word is often employed, both in law and in ordinary speech, to describe all such examples, does not mean that they are the same. There is an important difference between grabbing a person's arm and hitting a third person with it, and telling him to hit another under a threat of being shot. In the first case there is no action, whereas the second is a case of intentionally hitting another, albeit under duress.

The connection between compulsion and practical reasoning will accordingly be different from the connection between ignorance/mistake and practical reasoning. Compulsion is an excuse because, in various forms, it is an impediment to practical reasoning. There seem to be two quite different ways in which compulsions "get in the way" of practical reasoning.[121]

First, one may view compulsions as constraints on the actor's choice that are not part of his character. Compulsion viewed in this way is essentially a feature of the actor's situation that significantly limits the alternative courses of action that he may choose.[122] It is a restriction on the freedom of his decisions imposed by something other than his own character. This restriction may take the form of very bad consequences attached to some alternative course of action. This is most often coercion by others, but it may also be the compulsion of natural circumstances, such as in X's drowning another. Significantly, one can make mistakes about these circumstances and yet be compelled; it is the actor's beliefs about such constraints that make his choices hard and not the actual facts of the matter. Cases of compulsion may thus be made out where one would not have ordinarily expected them, if one can discover that the actor had some beliefs about being constrained of which one (and perhaps the actor) was not aware.

One must stipulate that the actor's character is not a constraint that makes an action compelled, at least that part of his character one would call his "evaluational system."[123] One might otherwise think that an actor's characteristic evaluations constrain his choices in the way in which a gun at his head would. One's character does not constrain one in this way; rather, characters are themselves constructs created by generalizing about what one does when one's choices are unconstrained.

Viewing compulsion as essentially uncharacteristic constraints on choice gives it an obvious connection with acting for reasons. The feature of the actor's situation that compels him also necessarily provides him with a reason for acting. Indeed, if his reason for some action is not supplied by the compelling circumstance, then he was not compelled. For example, when a person with a gun at his head robs a bank, he obviously has a constraint upon his alternatives. The idea of there being "constraints upon his alternatives" presupposes that he has something he wants to do, namely, stay alive. Without this motive the person would not be able to say that his alternative courses of action were constrained, for the constraint is relative to some end he wishes to pursue. What is constrained is the means to something that he wants very much. Thus, when a person acts to obtain that thing in the only way left open to him, that act is necessarily motivated by reasons; compelled action of this first sort is action for certain reasons.

This view of compulsion works for the first two cases of compulsion, W and X. It does not do so well, however, for the kind of compulsion involved in provocation or addiction. In the case of killings done in states of extreme passion, there is nothing one wants a great deal, the means to which are constrained, other than to kill. One cannot, as in the earlier examples, point to some acceptable motive, such as survival, the means to the satisfaction of which are artificially constrained. Indeed, in such cases,

The Legal View of Persons

the act of killing, although intentional, need not be done for reasons at all; the passionate emotional state may simply cause the agent to kill. Further, such impassioned emotional states may be "in character" for the actor, if he is an emotional type, and yet his action be compelled.[124] How this is possible no doubt requires some spelling out, which will also elucidate the second sense in which compelled choices may be hard.

The use of emotion words in language is a slippery business. One can use them simply as a way of talking about a person's reason for acting. When someone's failure to show up at an engagement is said to be because he was *afraid* he would be asked about his past, it is likely meant that the actor stayed away because he did not want to be asked about his past and believed that if he came he would be. Alternatively, emotion words can be used in purely causal explanations of human action. If someone's rapid conversation during an electricity failure is explained as being caused by fear of the dark, the fear is not his reason for speaking rapidly, but rather, his speaking rapidly is caused by his fear.[125]

"Desire" can be used in both of these ways as well. Its use as part of a reason for action should require no further attention at this point. Desire in the sense of "passionately wish" or "crave" can also be used in a mental cause explanation of action. An example of the latter usage is provided by *An American Tragedy*. In Dreiser's novel Clyde may properly be said to have craved the company of the socially elite Sondra. Indeed, much of Dreiser's social commentary in the novel about the causes of Clyde's craving depends upon the fact that Clyde desired to be with Sondra in this sense. Such cravings may cause actions, and yet not be the reason for which the actor acted. Clyde may have struck Roberta because he desired to be with Sondra; yet he did not strike Roberta *in order* to be with Sondra, or at least the "because" need not be so construed.

The distinction that the foregoing examples are intended to bring out is between emotions that are part of reasons for actions and emotions that explain actions in a purely causal way. The distinction does *not* preclude an actor from both craving something passionately and acting with the object of that craving as his reason for acting. The distinction only shows how this species of compelled action need not be, but may be, an action done for reasons. Whether one acted with the object of the passionately felt emotion as one's reason is not determinative of whether one was compelled by one's emotions.

Such choices, made under the influence of powerful emotions, are hard choices. Cravings, passionate desires, and emotions can produce strong inducements to act that are difficult to resist. Society recognizes this by excusing or partly excusing those who perform bad acts because of their emotions. This may be done even though such desires or emotions are in character for the actor. Those who are more prone to losing their temper, being very fearful, or craving high social position are still not as culpable as those who perform equally bad acts while not under the influence of such emotions.

There is a weak sense in which both kinds of compulsion presuppose practical reasoning abilities in persons: the first, by allowing an excuse only to those who act for certain good (or at least understandable) reasons, such as saving their own life; and the second, by allowing an excuse to those who *intentionally* act in a way that violates law or morality even if the reason for which they act is not a good one. In such cases it is only persons who reason practically who *can* be compelled, because only persons act for reasons and act intentionally. The ultimate rationale for both kinds of compulsion, however, reveals a much stronger presupposition of persons as practical reasoners. People are excused when compelled because their opportunity to reason practically from acceptable norms is disturbed. In quite different ways the abilities of W, X, Y, and Z to use legal or moral norms as the major premises of their practical syllogisms are disturbed. The strong presupposition is that persons *in general* are sufficiently able to engage in such reasoning that when external circumstances or even someone's own appetitive makeup makes it harder *for him,* he can be excused. If the world were a much harder place to survive in than it is, or if we were much more childlike in our susceptibility to being disturbed in our reasoning by the passions of the moment, we would have either no excuse of compulsion or one so broad as to swallow up responsibility. That we have the limited excuse we do reflects our view of persons as relatively sturdy practical reasoners despite the inevitable vicissitudes of life.

Persons as the Holders of Legal and Moral Rights

If many lawyers were called upon to give a definition of "legal person" they would give a simple functional definition in terms of an entity being the holder of legal rights. Peter French nicely describes this tradition:

> Following many writers on jurisprudence, a juristic person may be defined as any entity that is a subject of a right. There are good etymological grounds for such an inclusive neutral definition. The Latin *"persona"* originally referred to *dramatis personae*, and in Roman law the term was adopted to refer to anything that could act on either side of a legal dispute ... In effect, in Roman legal tradition persons are creations, artifacts, of the law itself, i.e., of the legislature that enacts the law, and are not considered to have, or only have incidentally, existence of any kind outside of the legal sphere. The law, on the Roman interpretation, is systematically ignorant of the biological status of its subjects.[126]

The Legal View of Persons

Because of our earlier assumption that the *legal consequences* of being a person do not adequately explicate the concept, we should reject this functionalist, or "Roman interpretation," of legal personhood. What we seek in this section is the metaphysical notion of a person that the law implicitly employs when it ascribes rights to persons. My thesis is that the law's metaphysical views about what sort of being can hold legal rights is the same as its views about the sorts of beings who can be held responsible. In each case, rights and responsibilities are ascribed only to those practically reasoning agents we call persons.

I shall also again assume that we need not differentiate between legal rights and moral rights. Because of the contingent connection between law and morals noted earlier, there is good reason to believe that legal rights of property, liberty, or equality are grounded in the corresponding moral rights. Accordingly, the person who can hold moral and legal rights should be the same, that is, have the same metaphysical attributes.

RIGHTS, DUTIES, AND PERSONS

The concept of a right itself is doubtlessly one about which much can be said. Since the concept does not figure in the discussion in subsequent chapters nearly to the extent as does the concept of responsibility, I shall devote less attention to it and to the conditions of its ascription. One aspect of the concept of a right that is here important is the relationship between rights and obligations. It is often said that rights of one person presuppose duties of others, and vice versa. It might, accordingly, be thought that the concept of a person presupposed by the obligations discussed in the previous section must be the same as the concept of a person presupposed by the idea of rights. This does not have to be so, however, for several reasons. First, this doctrine about "correlative" rights and duties is not everywhere true. There may be duties where there are no rights and rights where there are no duties. An example of the first is the duty we have not to harm animals without justification. An example of the second is the rights of an economic nature that we are sometimes said to have, such as the right to minimally adequate housing. Second, it is possible (even if it is unlikely) that the person who holds the right can be a different kind of entity than the person who has the correlative duty. Those who talk of "animal rights" typically ascribe rights and duties in this asymmetrical way (animals having rights but no obligations). Third, and most fundamentally, there is an important attribute of "rights talk" that reduction to "duty talk" does not preserve. This is the notion that rights are by their nature exercisable or not at their holders' option. There is built into the notion of rights the idea that their holder has the choice to stand on them, or to waive them.

Bentham in discussing legal rights was one of those who would reduce rights talk to duty talk. According to Bentham, "To know how to expound a right carry your eye to the act which in the circumstances in question would be a violation of that right; *the law creates the right by forbidding that act.*"[127] Such reductions ignore any difference between saying "X has a right that Y do action A," and saying, "Y has a duty to X to do action A." Left out of such reductions is, as H. L. A. Hart observed, "the special position of one who has a right ... as to whether the corresponding duty shall be performed or not." For, Hart continues, "it is characteristic of those laws that confer rights (as distinguished from those that only impose obligations) that the obligation to perform the corresponding duty is made by law to depend on the choice of the individual who is said to have the right."[128]

To test whether Hart or Bentham is correct, consider the use of the concept of rights by those who would justify various paternalistic state interventions. Suppose one spoke of a "right to treatment" possessed by all those involuntarily committed to a mental institution, and meant by this not only that patients should have adequate *opportunities* for treatment but also that such patients should *have to* exploit such opportunities. Or consider the "right to punishment" locution of those whose intuition is that punishment is inflicted in order to make the criminal a better person: By such a right to punishment is meant not only the opportunity to be punished but also that one must be punished in order to become better. In each case rights talk is misleading. Such talk makes it sound purely beneficial to the patients or prisoners because it affords them an opportunity they can take advantage of or not; in fact, patients and prisoners have no such choice, and "rights" is an inappropriate description of their *obligations* under paternalistic regimes. To have a right and yet have no choice over its exercise seems contrary to the established sense of the word.

If having a right implies (as S. I. Benn puts it), "neither what a man must or what he ought to do, but what he may do if he chooses,"[129] then built into the concept of a right is an image of its holder as one who *chooses*. The idea of choice, in turn, implicates rights holders as beings who act for reasons in exercising their choice of whether to enforce their rights. They may make their choices based on prudential reasons, or they may have certain moral reasons favoring either a right's waiver or its exercise. The only point of importance here is that rights are meaningfully ascribed only to those who reason practically and are thus capable of choice.

There are two aspects to this presupposition of practical reason in rights holders that should be separated, paralleling our separate discussion of duty and accountability in the discussion of responsibility. The first is the degree to which right-creating norms should be knowable to the citizens whose rights they are. The aforementioned eight virtues Fuller thought to be the inner morality of law, are virtues for right-creating as well as obligation-creating norms. Generality, publicity, clarity, nonretroactivity, and the like allow rights holders to take such norms into account in planning their behavior. There is thus the same image of human beings here as Fuller describes with obligation-creating norms, namely, that persons are beings sufficiently rational that they can take such norms into account in choosing to act in accordance with the powers or obligations they create for them.

Second, rights, like obligations, apply only to accountable agents. Agents who cannot *rationally* choose to exercise a set of rights are not the holders of moral or legal rights. Plants, dogs, earthworms, stones, corpses, very young infants, and very crazy adults all either hold no rights, or suffer very serious disabilities in the set of rights they are accorded. They suffer such lack of rights or such disabilities because they lack the capacities of intelligent choice that is presupposed by the ascription of rights.

Consider, for example, the much-debated matter of animal rights. Animal rights is simply an unhelpful way of talking about the *duties* persons have to animals, such as the duty not to torture them. Although animals can be both the objects of a person's duties and perhaps even an independent source of *interests* that the law can take into account, talk of animal *rights* makes little sense because animals lack the capacity of intelligent exercise of those rights. The same applies to plants, stones, and other objects in the environment. Although one might consider such objects as having *interests,* to say they have rights is unnecessarily anthropomorphic.

Consider, analogously, fetuses. These may be legitimate sources of interests for the law to protect in various ways, such as the prohibition against intentional assaults by others or even by taking such interests into account in considering the mother's right to an abortion. Treating fetuses as interests to be protected, and imposing obligations on persons accordingly, does not require that fetuses have rights.

The severe limitations on the rights of children and the insane highlight perhaps better than any other examples how having rights presupposes the capacity for rational choice. The young, the retarded, and the insane are disabled from the rights to make wills, deeds, contracts, to manage their own property, to refuse certain treatments, to marry or divorce, to be granted custody of children, or to have abortions on demand. Only beings that can make rational choices about these matters have such rights. Only entities, in other words, who can reason practically with sufficient skill that they can choose intelligently whether and how to exercise such rights, have such rights to begin with. To be sure, infants and the insane do not lack all legal and moral rights. But that is because such beings have both *some* practical reasoning abilities and, more importantly, the potential for that more complete reasoning capacity that is distinctive of persons.

Aside from this very general presupposition of a person as a practical reasoner inherent in the general concept of a right, the *particular* rights persons have also presuppose this concept of a person. I shall distinguish two kinds of rights and discuss each in turn: (1) the rights persons have "qua persons," and (2) the rights persons have because they have earned them. Built into each of these kinds of rights are ideas of what persons are.

There is obviously some disagreement about what moral or legal rights persons have. Any claims about the presuppositions of personhood implicit in various rights people have will be hostage to people actually having those rights. I have chosen to discuss four rights persons have that are hopefully not too controversial. I discuss the rights to liberty and to equality, as well as property rights and contract rights.

The way in which some concept of a person is presupposed for each of these rights is not only different from the presupposition of personhood in the concept of a right itself (see the preceding discussion); the presupposition of personhood is also different for the first pair of rights than for the second. Some rights are rights persons have *just because they are persons*. These are often called natural, human, or basic rights. I shall call them personal rights; liberty and equality I take to be two such rights. What one wants to know here is what minimal attributes an entity must have to have this kind of right. Other rights certain persons have because they have earned them by their actions. I shall call these desert rights, of which I take property rights and contract rights to be two species. What one wants to know here is what sort of being a person must be to have earned such rights.

THE RIGHTS TO LIBERTY AND EQUALITY

Each person, simply because he or she is a person, has a right to liberty and to equal treatment. A great deal can be (and has been) said about these rights. Sufficient for our purposes is to distinguish formal equality from egalitarianism, and formal liberty or freedom from libertarianism.[130] The formal principles of equality and liberty do not by themselves say very much. The formal principle of equality is that some justification is required to treat people in unequal ways or with unequal respect. The formal principle of liberty is that some justification is necessary for a state to restrain by law a person's freedom to act. Egalitarianism goes beyond the formal principle of equality to assert that certain purported justifications of unequal treatment or respect are unacceptable, such as those based on race. Libertarianism goes beyond the formal principle of liberty to assert that the imposition of certain purported justifications of legal restraints on individuals is unacceptable, such as those imposed on competent adults "for their own good."

The Legal View of Persons

The formal right to equal treatment or respect can accordingly be said to be no more than a kind of prima facie right to such treatment, a right good only in the absence of adequate justifications for differences in treatment because of morally relevant differences between people. The more substantive right to equality of egalitarianism is the right of all persons to receive certain kinds of benefits in equal shares, such right being premised on the ground that for such benefits there are no morally relevant differences that could justify different treatments. The formal right to liberty, analogously, can be thought of as no more than a kind of prima facie right to be free from legal restraint, good only in the absence of some justification for the restraint; the more substantive right to liberty may be thought of as the right to do certain sorts of things or be free of certain sorts of legal restraint, such as paternalistic state interference. The question for us is, What is it about persons qua persons that at least makes it plausible to suppose that they have either the formal or the more robust rights to equality and liberty?

The very conception of there being personal rights—rights persons have just because they are persons—presupposes that the differences between individual people can be stripped away to reveal some essence of personhood. A very traditional answer, and one I adopt, is that it is human beings' autonomy and rationality that ground their rights to liberty and equality and without which they would have no such rights.

Rationality and autonomy have, of course, been proposed as the morally relevant aspect of human beings by moral philosophers as different as Aristotle, Kant, and Rawls. What I have in mind for these sometimes slippery words is a meaning tied to the idea of practical reasoning. By autonomy I mean the capacity to perform human actions in the sense discussed earlier, viz., the irreducible causal agency persons but not other objects possess. By rationality I mean both the capacity to act for reasons of some kind (the "minimal rationality" of Chapter 1) and the capacity to act for desires that are themselves intelligible and beliefs that are themselves rational (the "full rationality" of Chapter 1). The thesis, in short, is that the rights to liberty and equality are personal rights because all and only persons possess the capacity to act for reasons, that is, to reason practically.

Such presuppositions of practical reasoning capacities in the holders of personal rights can be seen most easily in the right to liberty. With regard to the formal right of liberty, it is, as S. I. Benn has said,

> part at least of what is meant by saying that someone is a moral person. For if one denied a man this right, it would be open to others to use him, like their beasts and their tools, for their own purposes and as they choose, without being called upon to show by what right they

did so . . . To recognize a man as a moral person is thus to recognize that he has interests and not merely functions and thus to concede at least this minimal right.[131]

The reason we recognize that persons are "ends and not merely means" is because we all, if we are persons at all, have our own purposes, goals, and life plans. Strip away such "prospective purposive agency,"[132] and the rationale for a minimal (or formal) right to liberty would not exist. Such right makes sense only for agents who have the capacity to act for reasons.

Moreover, a more substantive right to liberty, such as that defended by Mill in his famous essay against paternalism,[133] also is grounded in the rational capacities of persons. More specifically, Mill's antipaternalistic principle of liberty is partly supported by the notion that persons are good practical reasoners, that is, that they by and large know the good and their own self-interest and can calculate what actions tend toward their achievement. Without such capacity, as in the young and the insane, even Mill would concede that there could be no freedom from paternalistic state interference.

The right to equality is similarly grounded in a view of persons as agents with their own projects. The formal principle of equality, like the formal principle of liberty, is intimately connected with our ideas of a person. One can see this by recognizing what the formal principle of equality is not: It is not simply the principle of universalizability. It is true that to think (in terms of general categories) we must judge like cases alike. This much is presupposed by using general predicates, such as "red"; to say X is red is to be committed to saying Y is red, if X and Y differ in no relevant respect.[134] Our use of general predicates presupposes that we will universalize our application of them to all (qualitatively) identical objects. It requires a separate step, however, to say that *persons* are sufficiently alike that, prima facie, they are to be treated alike. There is nothing in a principle of universalizability that prevents universalizing over other categories, such as left-handed people, Jews, or all sentient creatures.

The formal principle of equality can be arrived at only by some independent judgment that *persons* are presumptively the relevant category over which one should universalize in treating like cases alike. If one believes that there is a right to formal equality, it can only be because of some idea of what it is that *persons* share that is morally relevant. Again, the idea of a person that seems relevant is the idea of a being who can *use* whatever benefits, opportunities, or entitlements are being distributed. It is beings who can reason practically that can make such use of such goods.

The more substantive rights to equality of egalitarianism are premised on the rejection of certain distinctions among persons as being morally justifiable. Distinctions based on race or sex are morally odious distinctions among beings all of whom are fully persons. Distinctions based on

The Legal View of Persons

maturity or sanity are not suspect for such egalitarian ideals, because the latter, but not the former, attack the presupposition of what persons are like for equality between them to be appropriate: Persons must be autonomous and rational agents.

There is, to be sure, an entirely alternative way in which one might seek to show how the concept of basic rights such as equality and liberty is connected to the concept of a person. A. I. Melden, in his recent *Rights and Persons*, takes such a tack:

> It is not . . . by reference to some attribute that constitutes the essence of human beings, to their rationality, autonomy, uniqueness or to the actual or potential realization of value in the experience of individuals—matters that pertain to their endowments merely as individuals—that it is possible to comprehend how it is that each person has that moral status as the possessor of human rights.[135]

Melden urges us to attend to persons, "not in some never-never ideal land in which all of the differences between persons . . . have been erased, but [to] persons as we actually find them in the actual circumstances here on earth."[136] The circumstance that Melden finds relevant is the interaction between persons as they participate in an "enormously complicated and moral form of human life."[137]

If Melden's kind of thesis could be made out, the concept of a person presupposed by talk of natural or human rights would be different. Yet what Melden's Wittgensteinian patter about a "form of life" itself presupposes is that individual human beings *communicate* with one another (i.e., form reflexive intentions); "have interests in the pursuit of which they seek to achieve a variety of goods for themselves and for others," as Melden himself notices;[138] and pursue intelligible desires, including altruistic and cooperative desires—in short, that human beings are those practically reasoning agents we call persons.

PROPERTY AND CONTRACT RIGHTS

Property rights and contract rights are representative of the rights that people have because of what they as individuals *have done* to deserve such rights, as opposed to the rights they have simply because they are persons. The rights we discuss here are not the rights to hold property or to contract; *these* are arguably personal rights, or derivable from some personal right, such as the right to liberty. Rather, the rights in question are those rights particular people have with regard to certain other people's performance (contract) or with regard to particular things (property). Legally and morally there are certain conditions under which people acquire such rights, and what we wish to examine is the concept of a person implicit in such conditions.

Property rights to newly found or created goods (as opposed to goods transferred from a prior owner) are allocated by our law under one of two normative theories. The first is the economic notion that property entitlements should be allocated in a manner that best mimics a market in which there are no transaction costs. To what point, this theory asks, would people trade and trade no further, with regard to something, if they had perfect information and it cost them nothing to transact? Wherever the property rights would end up is where they should by law be allocated, according to this theory.[139]

Such a mode of allocating property rights makes sense only in light of some view about persons. Hypothetical market behavior in a costless market is normatively relevant because of what such behavior is thought to show about what persons prefer: If people trade one thing for another, they prefer the second to the first; if one person pays more for a thing than another person is willing to, the first must want that thing more than the second. If one's social theory is utilitarian, so that maximizing the net sum of satisfied preferences is a desideratum to be sought, then property rights should be allocated to mimic the costless market. Built into this complex of ideas is a view that persons know what they (most) want and can reason effectively about the means necessary to get what they want. That persons are rational in this sense is presupposed by any economic regime of allocating property rights.

The other normative theory under which property rights are allocated by our law is the natural rights theory that runs from Locke through Nozick and Epstein.[140] Each person, Locke proclaimed, has "within himself the great foundation of property." This was because each is "master of himself and proprietor of his own person and the actions or labor of it."[141] What Locke meant is that we are all entitled to the fruits of our own labor because that labor was ours to start with.

Such Lockean notions run through diverse areas of our property law. One who just takes possession of a wild animal, or kills it, has a property right to it that cannot be appropriated by another; one who collects abandoned manure into little heaps also acquires a property right to it, as does one who improves shells by making them into buttons; one who simply takes possession of land or chattles has a property right good against all save the true owner, and even good against the latter if possession continues for a long enough period of time; the person who first uses flowing water has the property right of a "prior appropriator" under the water law of the western states; first by common law and now by statute, one person cannot appropriate the creative efforts of another in writing a book, a play, music, and so on, nor can one appropriate the labor of another by copying the news he has gathered or the picture or name that he has built into an asset. In each of these areas our law is Lockean in its allocation of

The Legal View of Persons

rights to those who first mix their labor with a thing or even (as in the case of copyright) create that thing to start with.

The persons who figure in this moral and legal theory are the beings who are masters of themselves, that is, beings who have the causal powers of persons over their own bodies. They are, in other words, the beings who can perform basic actions. Moreover, to labor is not just to act in a nonplayful way. It is the unfairness of one person's appropriating the *labor* of another in the sense of depriving the other of something he could use, and giving to oneself something one can use, that gives Locke's theory of acquisition of property rights the persuasive power it does possess. Thus, to *labor,* as Locke is using the term, is to act in such a way as to bring forth something of use to oneself or to others. In this sense, to labor is not only to perform some basic acts with one's body, but also to do so with a result in mind. Locke's laborers are persons with causal powers over their bodies and the capacity to exercise them so as to produce things they want. Such laborers are the practical reasoning persons we have encountered throughout this chapter. They are the persons who can exercise will and reason over all things, including their bodies, in order to get what they want. Basic to Locke and to the property law doctrines reflecting his influence is this view of persons as having causal powers and the reason with which to exercise them. It is only because all persons have such powers that it is unfair to deprive those who have exercised them of their reward — their property right — and to give it to others who have not exercised their own distinctively human capacity.

Our idea of a contract right also reflects this view of a person. The right to contract (in general) of course reflects a view of persons as rational masters of their fate, being one strain of the more general right to liberty. But the more particular conditions under which particular contract rights are created in certain people also reflect this view of human beings.

If the conditions under which contract rights are ascribed were as much the subject of our concern in later chapters as are the conditions under which responsibility is ascribed, we could easily devote as much detailed attention to them. For the ascription of contract rights is justified in law and morals under much the same conditions as those under which responsibility is ascribed. The norms creating contract rights apply only to accountable agents, so that the young and the insane are disabled from possessing such rights. The analogues of the *actus reus* and *mens rea* conditions of responsibility ascription are to be found in the idea of a communicated promise around which two or more persons form reflexive intentions (or, in the language of contract law, in the ideas of offer and acceptance). There must be both an *act* of communication and an *intention* of the kind found in standard theories of communication (whereby a speaker intends that the audience themselves form certain intentions).[142]

There are, in addition, the same two kinds of excuses, which vitiate any prima facie contract rights.[143] The ignorance excuses consist of the doctrine of ignorance or mistake with regard either to present circumstances or to the future (this latter kind of mistake or ignorance excuse is in law called "impossibility of performance" or "frustration of purpose"). The compulsion excuses consist of duress, a kind of natural necessity by virtue of economic hardship, and procedural unconscionability. All such excuses may seem to defeat or "defease" the prima facie contract right the recipient of a promise otherwise would have.

Given the similarity of the conditions under which contract rights and responsibilities for causing harms are ascribed, it is to be expected that the concept of a person presupposed by each is very much the same. The concepts of action, intention, accountability, and excuse all presuppose the same image of persons here as they did before, as beings with causal agency and practical reason. Indeed, contract rights presuppose two such people, for a promisor not only (usually) intends to perform a certain action in the future, but also intends that the promisee form an intention around the promisor's promise. Moral promises, legal contracts, and the moral and legal rights they generate make sense only between beings who are capable of acting with such intentions. Here, as clearly as anywhere else, the law's view of a person as a practically reasoning agent comes to the fore.

The Legal View of Persons

In the ascription of both responsibility and rights the legal view of persons is of autonomous and rational agents. Most fundamentally, autonomy and rationality are to be understood by the concepts of acting, and of acting for reasons, explicated in this chapter and the preceding chapter. *The* kind of explanation of human behavior relevant to law is that in terms of the concepts of action, intentions, and reasons. The law is thus not neutral between the various ways in which human behavior might be described and explained. It, like morality, is built around the commonsense psychology captured by the notion of acting for reasons.

That such a view of persons is embedded in our law and morality is the main point of this chapter. One may have noticed, however, that somewhat more particular ideas about what persons are like are embedded in various aspects of the law discussed earlier. Aside from viewing persons as those practically reasoning beings for whom action descriptions and reason-giving explanations are appropriate, other presuppositions about persons can also be discerned in the doctrines just examined. Each of these more particular presuppositions about persons has to do with either rationality or autonomy, each of which I shall discuss.

The Legal View of Persons

RATIONALITY

To say that an agent acts for reasons is already to say that an agent is rational in the fundamental sense explored in Chapter 1. That is, to act for reasons is to act on a belief/desire set the contents of which form a valid practical syllogism. Also mentioned in Chapter 1, however, were two additional constraints we impose on each of the two premises of a practical syllogism in order to say that an action done because of it is fully rational: The end must be an intelligible end to seek, and the belief about the action being a means to the fulfillment of that end must itself be a rational belief. It is now time to delineate somewhat more precisely what constraints might be imposed on each of the premises of a practical syllogism in order to say that it fully rationalizes an action. For some of these constraints on what can be considered rational behavior are presupposed by at least some of the legal doctrines we have examined. Each of these stronger senses of rationality, in other words, names attributes the law, in places at least, supposes persons to possess. Because there is some difference in the way in which each constraint applies to desires as opposed to beliefs, I address each separately below.

The Rationality of Desire

Intelligibility: The weakest constraint that might be placed on the desires or moral beliefs eligible to serve as the major premises in practical reasoning is the constraint mentioned in Chapter 1. This is the idea that in order to rationalize an action a reason-giving explanation must utilize an end that is intelligible as something a person could want. Some consequences of human action seem too remote from any human concern to count as intelligible ends of action. Soaking one's elbow in the mud all day for no further reason,[144] or carrying all of one's green books to the roof for no reason other than having them on the roof,[145] may be examples of such unintelligible ends. Intelligibility is not much of a constraint, because the limits of our empathetic understanding are quite broad once we make the effort to be nonparochial in our understanding of others. Still, it may rule out some of the most bizarre desires of Martians (or perhaps very crazy human beings) as being the kinds of ends that can rationalize an action and thus serve one of the two functions of reason-giving explanations.

The law everywhere assumes that its subjects—persons—not only act for reasons, but also that the reasons are intelligible ones. One can perhaps see this legal presupposition most clearly in the law of evidence. It is generally true that proof that an accused had a motive for committing a crime is relevant circumstantial evidence tending to show that he indeed did commit the crime; it is also generally true that proof that the accused had no motive to have committed the crime is relevant as tending to show that he did not commit the crime.[146] Central to the idea of "having a motive" to do some act is the idea of a person standing to gain an intelligible advantage from that act. The law here assumes that persons act only for such intelligible advantages. Only in light of this assumption can the presence or absence of such motives give rise to the respective inferences about whether the accused did some particular act or not.

More generally, intelligibility of desires is a basic feature of reason-giving explanations; it is only because the ends cited in reason-giving explanations are intelligible that such explanations can serve their rationalizing function. Wherever the law presupposes that agents act on valid practical syllogisms, it also assumes that the major premises of those syllogisms contain an object of a desire or moral belief that is an intelligible end on which a person could act.

Consistency: A stronger constraint on the desires eligible to fully rationalize an action is the requirement of consistency. To be rational in this sense a desire or a moral belief must have a propositional object that is not the contradictory of the propositional object of some other desire or moral belief of the agent. Rationality in this sense is logical consistency in the objects of one's desires.

Rationality in this sense does not demand that one be free of conflicting desires in particular situations. Such freedom would only be possible if one had a very impoverished list of wants. Given the scarcity of time and material resources, we all experience the conflicting demands of our desires as we choose various courses of action. Rather, the conflict relevant here is one where the desires *necessarily* conflict because their propositional objects are contradictories of one another. To desire to help people and to desire not to help people would be the kind of conflict labeled irrational, in this sense of rationality; to desire to help someone in need yet also to desire to get to one's own work is not the kind of necessary conflict that can be termed irrational in this sense.

Rationality in the sense here explored does not even demand that one be *completely* free of conflict between desires whose propositional objects are contradictories of one another. A person should be considered rational in this sense if there is an answer to the question of what he *most* wants when faced with conflicts of this kind. So long as he is able to merge his component desires into an overall intention, or want, on which he can act, he should be considered rational in the sense of *acting* on a consistent set of desires.

The law almost everywhere supposes that persons are rational in this sense as well. One sees this in the centrality of intention in the ascription of both responsibility and desert rights. If the law did not assume consis-

The Legal View of Persons

tency in desires, then the many criminal and contract law doctrines turning on the intentions of the parties would make little sense because they would be radically indeterminate: A person's intention to rob a bank or form a contract could not be sufficient to satisfy the *mens rea* requirements of attempted bank robbery or the making of a contract offer, because it might also be the case (if persons were not rational in this sense of consistent) that the person intended not to do these things. The law must thus generally assume that persons, whatever their initial conflicts of desires might be, are able to resolve them into overall wants and intentions.

Transitivity: Having transitively ordered preferences is not the same as having preferences whose propositional objects are free of contradiction.[147] Assuming that the desires of a person are transitively ordered is a stronger assumption than merely assuming that the desires of a person are consistent (free of contradiction). Accordingly, it is a stronger presupposition about persons to say not only that they have intelligible desires whose contents are not inconsistent with one another, but also that those desires have a transitive ordering that might be called a preference order.

It is the heart of "economic rationality" to assume that the desires of a person are transitively ordered. Only with such an assumption can one take "the point to which people will trade and trade no further" as having any normative relevance because it is indicative of maximum satisfaction of preferences. To the extent the law allocates entitlements by any scheme of mimicking the outcomes a costless market would achieve, it too supposes that persons are rational in this distinct and stronger economist's sense.

Consistency and Transitivity over Time: The law to some extent also assumes that the desires of persons are consistent and transitively ordered, not just at any given time, but also *over* time. In a phrase, the law assumes that a person has a character structure. The idea of binding a future self by a promise made now assumes some continuity of self over time, as does the idea of punishing someone now for what *he* (the same person) did in the past (particularly if we punish him now for the dangerous propensities his past act manifested). Giving a person property rights continuing over time contains this same presupposition of continued character through time. Character consists in part in the set of desires that people maintain over time. That persons exhibit some degree of stability in this regard is another of the law's stronger presuppositions of rationality.

Correctness: To some it no doubt sounds odd to speak of the correctness of desires. Alternative phrasings, in terms of the rightness of desires or the truth of moral beliefs, probably do not, to such ears, sound any more intelligible. For all such attributes of desires or moral beliefs assume that there can be objective values, an idea that moral skeptics have difficulty in crediting. Nonetheless, a well-established sense of rationality is built on just such notions. To act rationally, in this sense, is to act on a desire that is correct, or on a moral belief that is true. There are correct ends to be sought by any rational being, in such a view, and to be rational is to desire their achievement.[148]

The legal doctrines assigning rights and responsibilities do not generally presuppose that persons are rational in this strongest sense. In some instances, however, the law does presuppose that persons have the *capacity* to form correct desires. In such cases, the law does not presuppose that persons actually *have* such desires, that is, that each of us actually possesses the correct set of values; it presupposes only that we have the capacity to be rational, that is, the capacity to form the correct desires and true moral beliefs. One sees this limited presupposition of the rationality of correct desires in the negligence concept, where the reasonable person has to weigh competing values *and get it right*. A similar presupposition stands behind that most general of justifications in criminal law, the balance-of-evils justification, wherein one is not culpable for causing some harm if one correctly compares the evil that is done by the act to the evil that would follow if the act were *not* done.[149] In each case it is only if persons are in general capable of being rational in this noninstrumental sense—of knowing what is right or good—that individuals who fail to exercise such a capacity can fairly be held responsible. Likewise, in according all persons, just because they are persons, a right to liberty, our law presupposes that persons in general are rational in the sense of having the capacity to use their liberty to find the good.

In its occasional presupposition of rationality in this strong sense the law does not adopt some motivational theory about the ends persons in fact seek or think they ought to seek. It is not like economics, which implicitly posits people as creatures of selfish ends, or like other theories positing that persons only (really) seek pleasure, the avoidance of pain, sex, or power. Even where the law does presuppose a view of persons as beings who have the capacity to know the good, it does not presuppose any particular theory about what sorts of ends actually motivate persons. It does not, in short, have anything like an instinct theory.

The Rationality of Beliefs

The five stronger constraints that we may mean by rationality when applied to desires have their parallels in the constraints one might also impose on beliefs when we characterize them as rational. As before, some of these constraints on the minor premise of practical reasoning are not only legitimate senses of rationality, but are also characteristics the law in some places supposes persons to have.

Intelligibility: Intelligibility applied to beliefs is a matter of inconsistency or incoherence with popularly held beliefs of a society. Those beliefs that are wildly at odds with enough widely shared beliefs will be regarded as unintelligible. A belief that the earth is flat, held by someone raised in our society, is an unintelligible belief because it too flagrantly contradicts general factual beliefs that are widely shared.

As before, the clearest place in which the law reveals its presuppositions that persons hold beliefs not wildly inconsistent with shared beliefs is in the law of evidence. One ascertains possible motives for a crime as much in light of intelligible beliefs as in light of intelligible ends. More generally, full empathetic understanding is possible only if the actor acts on familiar beliefs as well as for familiar ends. An action will be fully rationalized only if the means/end belief does not leave us wondering, How could that person believe that? If this is so, then the law generally presupposes that the minor premises of its subject's practical reasonings are intelligible no less than are the major premises; for wherever reason-giving explanations are appropriate in the law, so will be one of the features of that form of explanation, its ability to rationalize an action.

Consistency: In some places the law also presupposes that an actor's factual beliefs are relatively consistent with one another. (As with desires, consistency of belief means freedom from contradiction in the propositional objects of belief.) As we saw earlier, mistakes excuse from responsibility or vitiate a contract only when they negate the possibility that a harm or an agreement of a certain sort was *intended,* and they can do this only on the supposition that generally, persons do not both believe a proposition and believe its contradictory. It is this hidden premise of consistency that allows one to infer the absence of knowledge of some proposition (i.e., the absence of intentionality) from the (mistaken) belief in the negation of that proposition. In terms of our earlier example: Only on a premise that an actor's beliefs are consistent can we infer that he did not know there was marijuana in the car from his belief that there was no marijuana in the car.

Coherence. Just as transitivity of preferences is distinct from consistency of preferences, so coherence of factual beliefs differs from consistency of such beliefs. Coherence is a stronger notion than mere freedom from contradiction, although it is no small matter to specify just what the relation must be between the objects of belief before one says that they cohere with one another. Mutual entailment of propositions seems much too strong a notion; having *some* entailment relations with some other beliefs is better, although it is pretty vague. However coherence theorists in epistemology resolve these matters,[150] one sense of judging a belief to be rational is that it implies or is implied by (coheres) with other things one believes.

The clearest presupposition of rational belief (in this sense of coherence with other beliefs) by the law is in some applications of the concept of negligence. Persons are often held negligent in both criminal law and tort for what they did not know but should have known. They are held responsible, in other words, for a failure to infer one belief from some other beliefs they did possess. A person who knows, for example, the general truths about spontaneous combustion may be held negligent if he fails to use such general beliefs as the basis for the inference that the wet hay drying on his land may ignite and that the conflagration may spread to his neighbor's house. Such failure to draw the correct inference in particular instances is only fairly blamable in beings who in general have the capacity to draw such inferences, only, that is, in beings who can cohere their beliefs into a system of beliefs making such inferences possible. By using negligence to cover such failures at inference drawing the law supposes persons to be such rational beings.

Consistency and Coherence over Time. Character is constituted by a consistency and coherence in one's factual beliefs no less than by one maintaining such consistency and coherence in one's preferences and moral beliefs. Inasmuch as the law supposes persons to have continuity over time (character), it supposes that persons have some consistency and coherence of their factual beliefs over time too. How much consistency and coherence is required has no clearer answer than to say that it is whatever amount we require in order to say of an individual that he is the same person now as he was some time ago.

Truth. As with desires, the strongest sense in which we say that a belief is rational is the sense that includes as rational all and only beliefs that would be accepted by an ideally rational agent with all possible information — *true* beliefs, in other words. As with desires, the law nowhere supposes persons to have all and only true beliefs. Everyone obviously has some false factual beliefs, no less than he has some bad moral beliefs and some incorrect desires. In its use of the negligence concept, however, the law does suppose persons generally to have the capacity to form true beliefs. It is only because persons can form true beliefs that they can fairly be held responsible for basing their actions on false beliefs. Persons are in effect held responsible for forming false beliefs whenever their negligence consists in miscalculations of the likelihood of good or bad consequences following upon their actions, as opposed to mistaken evaluations as to the goodness or badness of those consequences.

The Legal View of Persons

Rationality and the Emotions

There is no doubt a rationality *of* the emotions. It would be an interesting matter to explore the senses in which one might say of emotions, as of desires and beliefs, that:

1. They can be more or less intelligible (here meaning the appropriateness of feelings to their causes and objects).[151]
2. They can be more or less consistent (freedom from logical contradiction of propositional objects does not seem to be the right notion of consistency here, as in the opposition of love and hate of the same object).
3. They form some kind of hierarchy of importance to the individual, some more valued or more trusted than others.
4. They are both hierarchically ordered and consistent over time, sufficiently to add "emotional makeup" as an ingredient in character.
5. They are the right or correct emotions to experience (tolerance, not prejudice, for example).[152]

The philosophy of the emotions is not nearly so extensive as has been the philosophy of belief and desire, so that these suggestions about the senses in which one might judge emotions to be rational are just that, suggestions. Fortunately for our inquiry here, it is not necessary to work out a notion of rational emotions. The rationality presupposed by the legal doctrines ascribing rights and responsibilities has little to do with the rationality of the emotions, however that notion were to be fleshed out. The rationality the law supposes persons to have is the rationality of will and reason, not that of the passions. By and large the rewards or the sanctions one deserves are parceled out on the basis of reasoned choices, not on the basis of appropriate, correct, or in some other sense rational feeling.

Here morality is no doubt a good deal more subtle than the law, for morally we do take into account the emotions with which persons act or that they feel after they act. Morally, if not legally, it matters to us whether a criminal suffers from remorse, guilt, or regret after his act; morally if not legally it matters to us whether a killing is accompanied by pity and empathy for the victim, or by indifference. One can perhaps detect a hint of such use of an idea of rational emotions in the "unofficial" version of the provocation defense to murder. To the extent that one takes the provocation formula to be a justification (or partial justification) of killing, then one is judging the passions aroused by the victim's provoking act as appropriate or even correct. If, for example, one were legally entitled to be enraged at seeing one's wife in the arms of another, and thus entitled to kill them both, then the law would be presupposing persons to have emotional makeups in line with these entitlements.

The official version of provocation, however, is that it is an excuse, not a justification. As courts often put it, provocation is a concession to human weakness. So conceived, provocation joins duress, necessity, and addiction in criminal law (and duress and procedural unconscionability in contract law) in viewing persons as basically reason-governed beings, but on occasion unhinged by their emotions. Emotions in such excuses are viewed as impediments to reasoning, irrational factors that prevent the actor from doing what his reason would otherwise tell him he should do. The rationality presupposed by these legal doctrines is not any rationality *of* the emotions, but rather, a rationality that can win out *against* emotions.

This last is a sense of rationality that should be added to the senses of rationality having to do with the form of the practical syllogism or with the contents of each of its premises. For in the doctrines of criminal law and contract law having to do with compulsion, we see another presupposition about persons: Persons are able to reason practically, and to act on the dictates of those practical reasonings, despite most (but not all) disturbances in their emotional life.

In each of these stronger senses of rationality the law in various places has an image of persons as rational. The fundamental sense of rationality presupposed throughout the law, however, is that defined by the ability to act on valid practical syllogisms.

AUTONOMY

The fundamental sense of autonomy the law attributes to persons is that explored throughout this chapter: Persons have that causal agency, or will, that allows them to perform basic actions with their bodies. Persons are, to paraphrase Locke, masters of their bodies and thus proprietors of their actions. As with rationality, one can discern other, stronger notions of autonomy attributed to persons in various parts of the law. A slightly stronger notion of autonomy is presupposed by thinking that persons not only can cause their bodies to move but also can cause many things to happen *by* moving their bodies. The factual assumption here is that the world is such that persons can, by their basic acts, change things. Slightly stronger yet: Persons are able to *intentionally* cause such further changes. Autonomy in this sense is the idea that persons have the causal powers to change the world, not just in some unforeseeable ways, but in conformity to what they want. The factual presupposition here is that people by and large do not want the impossible.

One can put these two stronger senses of autonomy together to assert

The Legal View of Persons

that the world and human wants are such that persons are not inherently frustrated in their actions. Whether persons have such autonomy is much more controversial than autonomy in the basic sense of causal agency. One kind of classical, tragic view, focusing on how the world is, would have us believe that gods or natural events ("fate") will intervene in just those ways that will frustrate our designs. Another, more modern view, focusing on people's godlike aspirations, would have us believe that we are "useless passions," beings who intrinsically yearn for the impossible. Either of these views would deny that persons are autonomous in the stronger sense (but not the basic sense of causal agency).

Despite the artistic appeal in the tragic or the Sartrean view of people, our law, morality, and commonsense psychology together presuppose some good measure of autonomy in this stronger sense. This is evidenced by the very vocabulary with which we describe the (complex) actions by persons in both statutes and everyday life: The causally complex ("killing") actions persons perform presuppose that persons cause events beyond bodily movements; the intentionally complex ("concealing") actions persons perform presuppose that persons successfully execute their intentions in action. Persons must have some measure of autonomy (in this stronger sense) for this way of conceptualizing what people do to make any sense.

Two much stronger notions of autonomy are often attributed to the law's view of persons. Both of these are often labeled with the phrase "free will." The first is the indeterministic view that persons are free of causation by other agents or events when they act. Free will, or autonomy in this mind-bogglingly strong sense of the word, means freedom from causation in one's actions. We shall have occasion in Chapter 10 to discuss this notion of autonomy, since it is one that psychiatrists have some fondness in attributing to the law's view of persons. In Chapter 10 I shall argue that autonomy in the sense of contracausal freedom is not an attribute the law supposes persons to have. Sufficient for present purposes is to note that this is a very different notion of autonomy than either of the kinds of autonomy discussed before. To conceive of autonomous agents as those who have sufficient causal powers over their bodies and other objects so as to achieve some of their wants is one thing; it is quite another to conceive of autonomous agents as those who are *uncaused* ("free") agents who nonetheless can themselves cause other things to happen—uncaused causers.

The second idea of autonomy sometimes expressed by the idea of free will has nothing to do with indeterminism. Rather, this idea of autonomy is one whereby a particular human capacity is posited. This is the capacity to form second-order desires with regard to oneself *and* to carry out such desires in remaking one's character. This is not an indeterminist's notion (or at least it need not be), because a believer in this kind of autonomy could admit that the possession of this capacity, and the conditions of its exercise, are fully determined. Autonomy in this sense only requires that the second-order desires one forms about one's own character be causally efficacious in achieving their object, namely, a remaking of the self. This is a straightforwardly causal hypothesis involving no indeterministic assumptions. The hypothesis is that certain belief/desire sets "win out" against other causal factors (such as emotional states, past conditioning, and present temptations) in forming who we are. This is the hypothesis that it is possible to be, somewhat at least, a self-made person, in the noneconomic sense of the phrase.

If there is a popular sense of autonomy, this self-creating sense of the word is probably it. There are very strong views about each person's autonomy in this sense, such as Heidegger's and Sartre's notions that a person is a subject for whom the question rises inescapably, what kind of being to become.[153] Such a question arises for persons just because they can remake themselves into whatever they want to be. Echoes of a more moderate view are to be found in Aristotle as well, who thought that because human beings have the capacity to shape their character they can fairly be held responsible for being the kind of persons they are.[154]

Some of this self-creating kind of autonomy is implicit in the legal view of persons in each of the two contexts discussed. Inner compulsion is not a broad-ranging excuse because the law assumes that persons have the capacity to stand back from their own cravings, to judge their worth, and thus not yield to those deemed unworthy. In the language made familiar in philosophy by Harry Frankfurt,[155] there are causally efficacious second-order desires that win out over cravings or other emotional states in determining how we act. The same assumption that persons have autonomy in this sense is to be found in the contract law doctrines allowing a limited invalidating condition for compelled promises.

More generally, it is arguable that to talk at all about what people *deserve* – either liability for bad acts or rewards for good acts – presupposes autonomy in this strong sense. In the context of responsibility, one might think that behind our practice of blaming for bad *acts* there is an assumption that bad acts generally manifest bad character, and that what we really blame is bad character. This we can do only if persons have the capacity to alter their character, that is, only if persons are autonomous. Analogously, in the context of ascribing desert rights, one might think that behind our practices of granting rights to those who have acted in certain ways is an assumption that such acts are deserving of reward only because they are attributable to a person's character and not to those accidents of fate (social position, genetic endowment) in which he had no hand. Only autonomous persons would ever deserve rights on such a view of our

The Legal View of Persons

practices of ascribing desert rights, for only persons who had a hand in forming their character could claim credit for it.

Such views about the ascription of responsibility and rights, if correct, would reveal a general presupposition in the law that persons are autonomous in this strong (self-determining) sense. Yet it is very doubtful that such views are correct. Legally and morally we ascribe responsibility to persons for actions "out of character" so long as the conditions discussed earlier (action, causation, *mens rea,* etc.) are met. Legally and morally we ascribe rights to persons for having invested their labor in a thing, even if the creative urges that led to the investment of that labor were not themselves in character (i.e., they were not the exclusive product of character-forming desires). An individual who intentionally kills another or who writes a novel is liable to punishment in the one case and entitled to certain rights in the other, no matter how out of character such acts may be. Accordingly, autonomy in this strong sense should not be seen as a general presupposition of our law as to what persons are like; it is a presupposition of some parts of our law, as in the law's notions of when someone is compelled. The truly general presuppositions of autonomy are those considered earlier: that persons are beings who can perform both basic and complex actions in order to achieve what they want.

What we shall next examine is where psychiatry appears to challenge this view of persons most dramatically. Before doing so, however, one last word needs to be said about the legal view of persons. It is easy to parody the view of persons as autonomous and rational agents by showing that it leaves out much of what we know to be true. One such parody is A. P. Herbert's portrait of tort law's reasonable man:

> He is one who invariably looks where he is going, and is careful to examine the immediate foreground before he executes a leap or a bound; who neither star-gazes nor is lost in meditation when approaching trapdoors or the margin of a dock; who records in every case upon the counterfoils of cheques such ample details as are desirable, scrupulously substitutes the word "order" for the word "Bearer," crosses the instrument "a/c Payee only," and registers the package in which it is dispatched; who never mounts a moving omnibus and does not alight from any car while the train is in motion; who investigates exhaustively the bona fides of every mendicant before distributing alms, and will inform himself of the history and habits of a dog before administering a caress; who believes no gossip, nor repeats it, without firm basis for believing it to be true... Devoid, in short, of any human weakness, with not one single saving vice, sans prejudice, procrastination, ill-nature, avarice, and absence of mind, as careful for his own safety as he is for that of others, this excellent but odious creature stands like a monument in our Courts of Justice... The Reasonable

> Man is always thinking of others; prudence is his guide, and "Safety First," if I may borrow a contemporary catchword, is his rule of life. All solid virtues are his, save only that peculiar quality by which the affection of other men is won.[156]

Such parodies are not *challenges* to the legal view of persons because they only show such a view to be incomplete. Many of the most valued attributes of the particular persons each of us care about have nothing to do with autonomy and rationality, in either their fundamental or the more extended senses just discussed. The very abstract view of persons in terms of autonomy and rationality is of course radically incomplete as a picture of any person we know. In particular, left out is the life of the emotions where, if anywhere, the "affection of other men" is gained. Yet the radical incompleteness of the law's view of a person is no argument that it is *wrong*. As far as it goes, the law's view of persons could be quite correct even if radically incomplete. It takes a view of mind quite different from that of commonsense psychology to challenge the law's own view of persons, rooted as the law's view of mind is in *part* of that commonsense psychology. One such more serious challenge is that of psychiatry, to which we now should turn.

3 The Challenge of Psychiatry

FORTUNATELY IT IS NOT necessary to attempt to extract from psychiatry some general theory of the person with which to compare the legal view. Given the divergent theories prevalent among psychiatrists, extracting any general view would be extremely difficult. The burden of this chapter is much more modest. It is to isolate those aspects of a psychiatric view of persons most challenging to the legal view of persons. These aspects of psychiatric theory do not themselves cohere into a theory of the person, nor do all psychiatrists adhere to them. They are simply those features to which a substantial body of psychiatric opinion would subscribe, and which, if true, most challenge the legal presuppositions of what persons are like.

There are three main challenges to the legal view of persons coming from psychiatry. The first is a kind of conceptual imperialism whereby the medical notions of health and illness are urged as substitutes for the ethical notions of goodness and badness. These are the familiar views that identify mental health as human flourishing or that identify any form of social deviance as mental illness. Such views, if accepted, would make meaningless the law's attempt to separate the sick from the bad. For in such views no one is really bad except in the sense that one is sick or ill. According to such views the law's division of human beings into accountable or nonaccountable agents makes little sense; given the merger of badness into sickness, *all* human beings are not accountable for the bad results they may cause. Attacked in such a case is the law's idea that persons are beings who have passed some threshold of rationality such that they can fairly be ascribed responsibilities and rights.

The second challenge stems from the idea that Freud made almost definitive of twentieth-century psychiatry, that of the unconscious. "All of the categories which we employ to describe conscious mental acts, such as ideas, purposes, resolutions and so forth," Freud wrote, could be applied to describe the *unconscious* mental life.[1] "Indeed, of many of these latent states we have to assert that the only point in which they differ from states which are conscious is just in the lack of consciousness of them."[2] This idea, of there being a kind of shadow mind, the existence and contents of which are unknown to its possessor, could have several radical impacts on the legal view of persons, depending upon how the unconscious is conceived. These differing impacts, and the differing conceptions of the unconscious behind them, I shall summarize later in this chapter and deal with in detail in subsequent chapters.

The third challenge to the legal view of persons comes from the temptation, not only of psychiatrists but others as well, to fractionate the person into smaller selves. An animistic conception of the unconscious—as a kind of second autonomous and rational self—is one strand of this kind of subdividing of persons. But there are other strands as well. Whenever a theory attributes causal agency and practical reasoning to subpersonal entities, be they called ego, id, censors, the past, ancestors, roles, other people, or System Ucs, one presents the same challenge to the legal view of persons. The challenge is to the legal assumption that one, but only one, rational agent with causal powers resides "in" any human being.

The main task of this chapter is to flesh out these three challenges to the law. This I will seek to do for each of these three challenges, first, by elaborating on the psychiatric views themselves, and second, by attempting to articulate how such psychiatric views in fact challenge the legal view of persons.

The Human Being as the Universally Sick Animal

THE EXTENDED VIEW OF MADNESS OF PSYCHIATRY AND NATURALISTIC ETHICS

When Bernstein and Sondheim have one of the young hoodlums in *West Side Story* proclaim that he has a social disease, they parody a dominant theme of a substantial body of twentieth-century psychiatric opinion: that to engage in morally bad behavior is to be mentally ill. Before drawing out the legal consequences of such a claim if it were true, I shall attempt to make the claim itself somewhat clearer.

Very generally, there are three conceptually distinct routes by which psychiatrists come to the view that to act badly is to evidence illness. It is useful to separate them, even if they are often intertwined in psychiatric thought.[3] The first route depends on the deterministic assumption that all behavior is caused. On such an assumption we are all "patients" in the ancient sense of the word, viz., passive with respect to our own behavior. If to be ill is to deviate from some sort of norm, and to passively suffer such deviation rather than actively cause it, badness becomes one kind of illness.

The second route focuses on the obvious connection of sanity to rationality. The argument here is that since criminal behavior is ultimately irrational, the criminal must be crazy to engage in it. In one version of this view, bad behavior is inherently self-defeating and pathetic—irrational even from the narrow viewpoint of the criminal's self-interest.[4] A more theoretical version of this view posits a hidden irrationality that underlies all our apparent, or surface, rationality. This is the Freudian view that conceives of a "primary process" kind of thinking, which does not obey the ordinary laws of logic but which governs all our "secondary processes" of thinking. This last view is, of course, one kind of determinism, being differentiated from other kinds of determinism by the kinds of causes it mentions. In this view, the ultimately irrational nature of our motivations makes us all at least a little bit crazy.

Last, there is the route that does not rest on a supposed scientific discovery—that we are at bottom irrational—or upon some supposed scientific posit of determinism; rather, such a route is conceptual in character. The argument here is that if one examines the meaning of moral concepts such as good or bad, one will discover that they form but a misleading way of speaking about situations better discussed in the medical vocabulary of health and sickness. This last route represents a kind of conceptual imperialism, for it argues that the concepts of health and sickness can and should replace our ideas of good and bad. Such a claim has been called, aptly enough, the "psychiatric turn." As described by Christopher Boorse: "In this century a strong tendency has developed to debate social issues in psychiatric terms. Whether the topic is criminal responsibility, social deviance, feminism, or a host of others, claims about mental health are increasingly likely to be the focus of discussion. This growing preference for medicine over morals... might be called the *psychiatric turn*."[5] The psychiatric turn is a conceptual claim because it rests on claims about the meaning of medical concepts, the meaning of moral concepts, and the relationship between the two.

In Part II of this book I shall deal with this third kind of claim. What I shall attempt to show is that the extended view of illness such that all bad behavior is sick is unwarranted, even in psychiatry, but certainly in law and morals. The first two kinds of claims—those depending on determinism or on a hidden irrationality—are better dealt with in Part III, which is concerned with the unconscious. For the most interesting form of psychiatric determinism is that stemming from Freud and goes beyond the simple idea of determinism to a more uniquely psychiatric claim that our behavior is determined by mental states that show us to be irrational. Since such primary process ideas are part of what Freud meant by the unconscious, these claims are better dealt with as aspects of that kind of psychiatric challenge to law.

It is, accordingly, the conceptual route to the conclusion that badness is sickness that needs some elaboration here. Such elaboration must begin with the meanings of health and of its opposites — illness, disorder, sickness, and disease. In approaching the meaning of health and of its opposites it will help to recall an admonition of J. L. Austin:

> In general, it will pay us to take nothing for granted or as obvious about negations and opposites . . . . above all it will not do to assume that the "positive" word must be the one to wear the trousers; commonly enough the "negative" [looking] word marks the [positive] abnormality, while the "positive" word . . . merely serves to rule out the suggestion of that abnormality.[6]

In the present context what Austin's suggestion comes to is that it is not obvious whether it is health or illness that "wears the trousers." Health might be the main idea, and illness merely defined as "not health," or illness could be primary, and health defined as "not-ill."[7]

These two possibilities track into the two conceptual ways in which psychiatrists and others have sought to show that being bad is to be ill. The first conceives of health as the primary concept and identifies it with human flourishing, that is, with the good for humankind. Anything less than a complete fulfillment of this human potential is not health (i.e., illness). Such a view collapses all badness into an unhealthy failing to realize the human potential. The second possibility is to regard illness, sickness, and disease as the primary concepts and health as derivative. This approach accordingly seeks a general definition of illness directly. Badness becomes illness in this approach by showing that implicit within the judgments we make when we classify a condition as an illness are criteria sufficiently broad that they include bad behavior. I shall elaborate on each such view in turn.

Goodness as Mental Health

The idea that the good of a person should be conceptualized in the medical terminology of health is an ancient one. Plato, for example, held that justice and injustice "are in the soul what the healthful and the diseaseful are in the body."[8] More generally, Plato thought, "virtue . . . would be a kind of health and beauty and good condition of the soul, and vice would be disease, ugliness and weakness."[9] One need not be a Platonist, however, to be tempted by the "medicalization of morals." Any objectivist view of ethics may incline one toward a medical view of the good for people. Objectivists in ethics are led to medical conceptualizations because they believe there is a right way for people to be. Such an objectively correct state for human beings is easily conceived of as a kind of health, and anything less than such an ideal is seen as a kind of sickness of the soul (in modern terminology: a disease of the mind).

The Challenge of Psychiatry

Although a Platonist kind of objectivism in ethics could be the basis of modern psychiatry's extended views of health and illness,[10] the oddness of Platonist ontology has kept most medical professionals from grounding their extended view of health in his kind of objectivist ethics. Much more compatible with the empirical cast of mind of medical theoreticians is the naturalist tradition in ethics stemming from Aristotle. Aristotle's kind of ethics is called "teleological," because it holds that there is a valuable goal (a *telos*) toward which events or objects must contribute if they are to be judged good. The goal for human beings, Aristotle thought, was happiness. Happiness for Aristotle was both normatively *desirable,* and in fact desired by persons above all else: "Happiness . . . is something final and self-sufficient, and is the end of action."[11]

To say that happiness is good for humans is not, as Aristotle recognized, to say very much until "happiness" itself is fleshed out a bit. This Aristotle thought one could do by ascertaining the function of human beings, which was to be found in their rationality. Their function was to lead a certain kind of life, namely, a life in which the "activity of the soul . . . follows or implies a rational principle."[12] To be happy is to fulfill this natural human function. Happiness for Aristotle is an activity of soul, an exercise of that distinctive human capacity to reason.

Such a naturalist account of goodness invites the extension of the concept of health to name the ethical ideal of what people should be like. Aristotle himself likened the "student of politics" who would treat the soul to the doctor who treats the body:

> By human virtue we mean not that of the body but that of the soul; and happiness also we call an activity of soul. But if this is so, clearly the student of politics must know somehow the facts about soul, as the man who is to heal the eyes or the body as a whole must know about the eyes or the body.[13]

One must study the mind and its workings—including, Aristotle thought, its irrational part[14]—in order to know what virtue is for a human being.

Psychiatrists (having supplanted Aristotle's student of politics as the shapers of our psyche) have easily assimilated these Aristotelian ideas into their own view of people. Psychoanalysts in particular have sought to insert the Freudian view of human nature into Aristotle's naturalistic ethic. The result has been a kind of ethics of freedom, spontaneity, authenticity, self-actualization, self-realization, or self-fulfillment.

Representative of this last group is Erich Fromm's ethic of "productiveness." Fromm faithfully recapitulates Aristotle, in that he posits that there is a human nature such that people have an end given for them: "Man is not a blank sheet of paper on which culture can write its text; he is an entity charged with energy and structured in specific ways, which, while adapting itself, reacts in specific and ascertainable ways to external conditions."[15] Second, for Fromm as for Aristotle, happiness is the ultimate human goal.[16] Third, Fromm also follows Aristotle in holding that happiness is not to be identified as subjectively experienced pleasure, but rather as the exercise of those of our capacities or powers that are distinctively human: "All organisms have an inherent tendency to actualize their specific potentialities. *The aim of man's life,* therefore, is to be understood as *the unfolding of his powers according to the laws of his nature.*"[17] Fourth, the happiness of exercised powers (or realized human potential) is identified as psychic health. "Health and virtue are the same"[18] in this view. Such health includes the realization of our moral capacities, specifically including our capacity to respect other persons: "The respect for life, that of others as well as one's own, is . . . a condition of psychic health."[19] Fifth, and finally, anything less than health (in this sense of a flourishing of human potential) is illness, or unhappiness, which comes to the same thing. As Fromm puts it, a "man's failure to use and to spend what he has is the cause of sickness and unhappiness."[20]

Fromm's views should be seen as a part of the so-called third-force psychology. Although Fromm is perhaps most explicit in his paralleling of Aristotle's naturalist, eudemonic ethics, many psychiatric theorists have shared those views. Maslow and Mittelmann, for example, urged an eleven-part definition of "psychological health" or "normality," which included such things as a person's having "adequate life goals,"[21] a "fairly rounded development, versatility, interest in several activities" and a set of "morals . . . which are not too inflexible from the group's point of view."[22] Also included as healthy for Maslow and Mittelmann were an "adequate self-evaluation,"[23] "adequate spontaneity and emotionality,"[24] "adequate bodily desires,"[25] and "adequate self-knowledge."[26] Such a list should be seen as strictly parallel to Aristotle's taxonomy of the virtues in *The Nicomachean Ethics,* the main differences being what is considered virtuous and the explicitness with which virtue is reconceptualized as psychological health.

A like example is provided by Rollo May, who urged that "a person is healthy psychologically and emotionally to the extent that he can use all his capacities in day-to-day living."[27] Similar conceptualizations of health as realization of human nature may be found in the work of Kurt Goldstein, Karen Horney, and Carl Rogers.[28] What all such theorists share is Aristotle's naturalistic ethics according to which the human good is to be found in our realization or fulfillment of our essential nature.

Standing behind the expansive view of health of Fromm et al. is not only Aristotle but also Freud. As F. C. Redlich once observed, after Freud, "psychiatrists who followed his thinking began to abandon the island of nuclear psychiatric disease and thus were engulfed in the boundless seas of human problems."[29] The reasons for this were twofold. One is a Freudian's understandable normative commitment to the therapeutic goals of psychoanalysis. The natural temptation of a therapist is to define such therapeutic goals as "making the unconscious conscious" or "where id was there ego shall be" into standards of health.[30] To be totally healthy, in such a view, would be to be without an id or unconscious. By such a standard of health we are all somewhat sick. As Redlich puts it, "The concept of health thus becomes an ideal which is never completely reached."[31]

The second (although related) reason for Freud's influence toward a broadened ideal of mental health stems from psychoanalytic theory proper (as distinct from therapy). As I shall examine in Part IV, the bedrock of Freud's view of minds and persons is that we are all conflict ridden. We are all engaged in the maintenance of a precarious balance between opposing systems of desires, beliefs, and emotions. Such universal conflict, for Freudians, again meant that we are all sick:

> If it is reasonable to assume that such conflicts are universal, we are all sick in different degrees. Actually, the difference between anyone and a psychotic may lie in the way he handles his conflicts and in the appearance or lack of certain symptoms. If this is so, mental disease must inevitably be inferred from behavior. But, apart from extremes, there is no agreement on the types of behavior which it is reasonable to call "sick."[32]

Because of Freud's influence, the broad notion of "positive" mental health is subscribed to by many psychiatrists not usually classified as part of the third force in psychiatry. Hartmann's suggested identification of mental health with capacities for adjustment (adaptation) to reality,[33] for example, and Karl Menninger's similar definition ("the adjustment of human beings to the world and to each other with a maximum of effectiveness and happiness")[34] both illustrate such influence.

The upshot of the tradition stemming from Aristotle and Freud is that there is a well-legitimated conception of mental health so broad that it includes all that might otherwise be thought of in terms of "virtue" and "goodness." The famous definition of health in the Constitution of the World Health Organization indicates the breadth of this influence. Health is there defined as "a state of complete physical, mental and social well being and not merely the absence of disease or infirmity."[35]

We shall examine the impact such a medicalization of morals would have on the law if it were adopted once we have its companion (starting with the concept of illness rather than with the concept of health) before us. Before turning to that second psychiatric view, however, it may be worth defusing one kind of objection to the Aristotle-Fromm view of health. This is the broadside delivered by philosophers from Moore to Hare who accuse naturalists of having committed some fundamental howler called the "naturalistic fallacy."[36] According to such philosophers, one can dismiss the naturalist ethics of Freudians, Aristotelians, or anyone else by paying closer attention to the meaning of moral words such as good and bad, right and wrong. Such closer attention to the meaning of moral words is supposed to reveal that no natural state of affairs, such as health or happiness, could possibly be named by such moral words as "good." For moral words either describe *non*natural states of affairs, as Moore thought, or they describe nothing at all. In the latter view, their function is merely expressive or hortatory but not descriptive of anything, health included.

I have elsewhere argued against this view of ethics and defended an objectivist position about moral judgments.[37] What I have argued is that there is no *linguistic* or *logical* argument with which one can show that good cannot mean healthy or happy. One cannot thus dismiss out of hand naturalist views of psychiatrists, as if they were the product of an impoverished education in elementary philosophy. Although I shall argue in Chapter 5 that psychiatry is wrong in seeking to analyze virtue as mental health, that is a matter of detailed considerations about the lack of synonymy or equivalence between health and virtue; it is not a matter that can be settled by recourse to supposed categorical differences between descriptive and moral speech.

Deviance as Mental Disease

Many psychiatrists would be embarrassed to profess an objectivist view of ethics such as is so forthrightly stated by the likes of Erich Fromm. Such psychiatrists may feel that they can help people, but are unwilling to categorize the states that such people are helped to attain as being objectively correct for a human being. Some of these more ethically cautious psychiatrists nonetheless identify badness with illness.

One way to do this is the route long fashionable in sociological and anthropological approaches to mental illness, approaches that are now called "labeling theory." The merger of badness and illness by such an approach has three essential steps. First, it is asserted (or, more likely, assumed) that moral judgments such as "bad" are logically dependent upon there being some cultural norms that condemn the behavior being labeled bad. This view, known as ethical relativism, holds that there are no cross-culturally valid judgments of good or bad—indeed, such moral judgments are thought to be nonsense; the only moral judgments that make sense are those made relative to a society's norms about what it likes and what it dislikes.[38] Second, medical judgments of illness are viewed in the same way, as being convention-dependent judgments about behavior that a given society does not like. The third step of the argument is to deny that there is any significant difference between the disapproval norms presupposed by judgments of badness and the disapproval norms presupposed by judgments of illness. Judgments of mental illness, in such a view, are simply one form of moral disapproval that white-coated members of some societies happen to use.

Such a view found early expression in Ruth Benedict's now classic *Patterns of Culture,* in which she acknowledged the fact that in some societies, "some impulses are recognized as bad ways of dealing with the situation; some as good. The bad ones are said to lead to maladjustments and insanities, the good ones to adequate social functioning. It is clear, however, that the correlation does not lie between any one bad tendency and abnormality in any absolute sense."[39] Such a view finds considerable support among the many contemporary social scientists and psychiatrists who focus their efforts on the social consequences of labeling someone mentally ill. According to Tom Scheff, for example, it is only "the culture of the group [that] provides a vocabulary of terms for categorizing many norm violations."[40] "Criminal," "drunk," and "insane" are, Scheff tells us, all labels for behavior that deviates from the cultural norms in one way or another, the last being a kind of residual or catchall category for social deviants.

This sociological view of mental illness merges illness and badness together in terms of a larger category, social deviance. Such a merger is accomplished by focusing exclusively on the social consequences of being labeled bad or crazy, for both such labels do carry various social stigmas. But to focus on these social consequences of labeling is not to take seriously the task of seeking the *meaning* of "mental illness" and like terms. As we observed at the beginning of Chapter 2, if we wish to get at the meaning of a term or phrase such as person or mental illness, we cannot fasten onto the *consequences* of the use of such terms or phrases in certain contexts. We cannot accept the commonly given advice of Philip Roche that "lawyers and psychiatrists [should] agree to regard 'mental illness' and 'insanity' less as they are verbally defined and more as what we do to people to whom we attach such terms."[41] We need rather to ask under what conditions is an entity *truthfully* so labeled?

It may turn out, as Scheff and other labeling theorists appear to believe, that there are no coherently and consistently statable conditions under which a term or phrase is applied. In such cases, the term or phrase has no meaning even though consequences are attached to its use in certain contexts. That mental illness is such a phrase is a view that I shall examine in the next chapter and reject. Anticipating the results of that discussion, we should accordingly take seriously the task of articulating the meaning of mental illness. This is not done by identifying consequences of uttering "He is mentally ill" in certain contexts. To be satisfied that one has discovered the meaning of mental illness when one has discovered the consequences of applying the phrase would entail a like satisfaction with an analysis of "death": Death means to be the subject of others' grief and mourning, to have one's property given to others, and to be subject to burial.

I shall accordingly put aside the sociological merger of badness and sickness into "social deviance." More interesting as a challenge to the law's separation of the sick from the bad are the definitional efforts of those psychiatrists who do take seriously the idea that mental illness has some meaning apart from the social consequences of its use. Most of the latter kind of psychiatric theoreticians offer definitions of mental illness that only somewht erode the line between badness and sickness. I shall examine some of these more moderate definitional schemes in Chapter 5. More challenging to the legal view of persons are the more radical definitions that entirely collapse badness into sickness.

An example of the latter is Karl Menninger's lifelong effort to define mental illness so broadly as to make badness but a form of sickness. This has been one of Menninger's persistent themes, from his early thoughts[42] to his more recent (if inelegant) broadside against the law, *The Crime of Punishment*.[43] Menninger's most systematic views are to be found in *The Vital Balance: The Life Process in Mental Health and Illness*.[44] Menninger and his coauthors tell us that this "entire book is an extended definition—a definition of the new view of mental illness."[45] I shall accordingly adopt this book as the best representative of Menninger's extreme views of the merger of badness into sickness.

Menninger does not make it easy to say what the "new view" of mental illness comes to. At one point he tells us that "to define either health or illness is an almost impossible task."[46] That does not stop him from defining it, however: "We can define illness as being a certain state of existence which is uncomfortable to someone... The suffering may be in the afflicted person or in those around him or both, but a disturbance has occurred in the total economics of a personality."[47] Such language may make one think that it is *suffering* that is the essence of illness for Menninger. In fact, however, such suffering is but the experience of one who has a "*disturbance... in the total economics of a personality.*" It is the latter notion that is the essence of illness for Menninger.

Giving content to his idea of "disturbance" is Menninger's theory of normal human functioning. A person, for Menninger, as for other traditional Freudians, is to be conceptualized as a kind of homeostatic mechanism that maintains a "vital balance" between disturbing and controlling impulses. Relying on the mechanistic metapsychological viewpoints of Freud, this balance is conceived of in terms of instincts with psychological energies that must be discharged in one way or another. Mental health is to maintain the balance, and mental illness is a "shift in balance... with a lowering of the effective level of living."[48] To be mentally ill is thus not to lose entirely some balance between instinct and control; illness rather is to maintain the vital balance in an expensive and self-defeating way:

> It is this view of mental illness as personality dysfunction and living impairment which is presented in this book. It sees all patients not as individuals afflicted with certain diseases but as human beings obliged to make awkward and expensive maneuvers to maintain themselves, individuals who have become somewhat isolated from their fellows, harassed by faulty techniques of living, uncomfortable themselves, and often to others. Their reactions are intended to make the best of a bad situation and at the same time forestall a worse one—in other words, to insure survival even at the cost of suffering and social disaster.[49]

It should be apparent that to talk of "lowered effective levels of living" or "faulty techniques of living" as constituting imbalance and mental illness will generate a very broad concept of mental illness. It will not be as broad as one (such as Fromm's) that begins by defining health as an ethical ideal of what persons should be like, and illness as anything less than that; but Menninger's concept will be broad enough to capture all behavior we would think of as morally bad and criminal. Menninger arranges the conditions that his concept of mental illness would include along a continuum, with five "orders of dyscontrol." Sandwiched in between neurosis, the second order or dyscontrol, and psychosis, the fourth, is violent behavior.

The rationale for including violent behavior as an illness less severe than psychosis but more severe than neurosis is that such behavior is seen as sharing with traditional mental illnesses the character of "personality dysfunction." There has been, in other words, a disturbance in the economics (energy balance) of the total personality. Menninger seeks to characterize violent behavior as being a desperate mode of coping with aggressive instinctual drives. There has been in such cases "ego-rupture," by which Menninger means a "disruption of the ego functions of instinct-control."[50] Such rupture "permits some aggressive energy to be discharged [which] has the economic value of affording sufficient temporary relief from internal pressure for the healing-over of the ego's ruptured wall to occur."[51] All of this, Menninger tells us, allows us "to see clearly how the disorders of these patients [i.e., violent criminals] resemble . . . personality disorganizations of lesser and greater degree."[52] This gets us back to the hoodlum in *West Side Story* who mimics a social worker in proclaiming, "Hey, I got a social disease."

Menninger's view is extreme and doubtlessly does not represent any majority viewpoint among psychiatric theorists. Yet Menninger's view is useful just because of its polar nature: He trumpets clearly the challenge to law that is present but muted in more moderate psychiatric views about how mental illness should be conceptualized. The challenge to law, but also to more moderate psychiatrists, is to come up with some conceptualization of mental illness that does *not* collapse badness into sickness.

THE CHALLENGE TO LAW OF THE EXTENDED VIEW OF MADNESS

As the discussion just concluded makes clear, the challenge to law of the extended view of madness is to collapse all bad behavior into sick behavior. The route that takes the concept of illness to be primary does this directly: Illness, properly defined, includes criminal behavior. The route that takes health to be primary does this indirectly: Health is the ideally good; illness is a failure to achieve the good, which of course includes bad behavior.

In either case there is a kind of conceptual imperialism against the moral concepts that undergird the law. The route that takes health to be primary seeks to *reduce* moral terminology to medical terminology. The result is not so much an elimination of our customary moral vocabulary as a translation of it into the language of health and illness. The route that takes illness to be primary seeks to *replace* moral terminology with medical terminology. Here what is sought is not a translation of moral terms, but rather, their elimination as inapplicable to the behavior to which they have customarily been applied.[53] The medicalization of morals in the first case has as its consequence that people can indeed be characterized as being bad but only when badness is understood to entail sickness; in the second case, such medicalization of morals entails that people are not at fault (bad) for their apparently intentional actions, and they lack such moral fault just because they are properly conceptualized as being sick.

There is thus a special assumption to the route that takes illness to be primary that needs to be made explicit. This is the incompatibility of the medical judgment, "diseased," with the moral judgments, "bad" and "responsible" (and thus with legal judgments of liability to punishment). Implicit in much of the discussion of this area is the assumption that if a condition is properly labeled by doctors as a disease (illness, sickness, etc.), then the person having it is not responsible either for getting into that condition or for staying in it.

This assumption is a very common one among psychiatrists, sociologists, philosophers, and legal theorists, even if they do not share the extended view of madness discussed herein. Donald Klein, for example, assumes in his recently proposed definition of mental illness that "the attribution of illness both legitimizes the sick role and is a defense against criminal prosecutions, so that the definition of illness has a marked social impact."[54] Illness for Klein, as for many psychiatrists, precludes the negative moral judgments of bad and responsible. A similar assumption pervades much of the sociology of medicine, beginning with Talcott Parsons's explication of the sick role as implying exemption from normal responsibilities.[55] Many philosophical analyses of the ordinary meaning of illness have also shared this assumption that illness precludes responsibility.[56]

One can see such an assumption at work most dramatically in the examples of alcoholism and drug addiction. Many doctors in the 1950s and 1960s urged that drug addiction and alcoholism were diseases.[57] A corollary of this for many such doctors was the assumption that so classifying these conditions precluded responsibility for such "patients":

> As physicians, we say that alcoholism is a sickness... For forensic purposes alcoholism is not a sickness but a bad habit. If psychiatrists keep repeating that alcoholics are sick people, some day judges may begin to believe us. Then a person will be able to get away with murder by the simple process of fortifying himself with enough whiskey to allow him to commit the crime. Since by that time you will have classed alcoholism with pneumonia, you will be no more able to hold him responsible for murder than you would be able to hold responsible a man who commits an assault during the delirium of pneumonia. This would be the logical result of classifying alcoholism as a disease.[58]

The United States Supreme Court, a majority of whom indeed began to believe the psychiatrists that drug addiction and alcoholism were diseases, also came to share this assumption that as a "logical result" of the disease classification these conditions were incompatible with culpability and thus could not be constitutionally punishable. In 1962, the Court in *Robinson v. California* assumed for largely unstated reasons that any condition properly thought of as a disease could not be punished:

> It is unlikely that any State at this moment in history would attempt to make it a criminal offense for a person to be mentally ill, or a leper, or to be afflicted with a venereal disease; ... a law which made a criminal offense of such disease would doubtlessly be universally thought to be an infliction of cruel and unusual punishment... Even one day in prison would be a cruel and unusual punishment for the "crime" of having a common cold.[59]

It was not until *Powell v. Texas* in 1968 that four of the members of the Court made clear what it was about a condition being a disease that had to do with its punishability. In *Powell,* the dissenters found that the "core meaning" of the idea that alcoholism is a disease "is that alcoholism is caused and maintained by something other than the moral fault of the alcoholic, something that, to a greater or lesser extent depending upon the physiological or psychological makeup and history of the individual, cannot be controlled by him."[60]

The assumption that illness precludes moral responsibility highlights one of the most direct implications of an extended view of madness: No one is really responsible for hurting others. More generally, however, the medicalization of morals of either kind tends to foster a paternalistic attitude toward persons, with regard to their rights as well as their responsibilities. The paternalistic orientation about responsibility is a familiar theme in criminal law theory, wherein one speaks of reforming criminals ("the sick") for their own good rather than punishing them for their misdeeds.[61] Such criminal law theories are paternalistic in character because punishment (or "treatment") is not justified by the increased safety reformed criminals mean for all of us, but rather, by the better persons that reformed criminals will be if they are "cured." Less familiarly, such paternalism is also fostered about a person's rights. A reduction of morals to (or replacement by) medicine tends to encourage the attitude that persons who are less than ideal cannot be trusted to exercise their rights in a "healthy" way. Particularly eroded, of course, is any right to liberty.

This encouragement of paternalism by the medicalization of morals is not due to the objectivity of moral judgment that one version of the view accepts. One can think that there are right answers to questions of morals and yet think that one of those right answers is that persons should be accorded as much liberty as is compatible with a like liberty for others.[62] Rather, paternalistic social theory results from the erosion of the legal view of persons done by extended ideas of madness. It is because a person as a patient lacks the kinds of autonomy and rationality that the law supposes persons to have, that the extended view of madness generates the paternalistic social theory that it does. The task of Part II will be to assess whether the extended view of madness of modern psychiatry is in fact warranted in making this apparent challenge to the legal view of persons.

The Omnipresent Unconscious

THE MEANING OF "UNCONSCIOUS"

The second psychiatric conception that challenges the legal view of mind and persons is the idea that we are each possessed of an unconscious. Before assessing what kind of challenge this idea presents, we must have some understanding of what is meant by saying that persons have an unconscious. This I shall undertake in three steps: first, by examining "conscious" and "unconscious" as used in ordinary speech; second, by examining Freud's own nontheoretical use of these terms; and third, by analyzing the more theory-laden meaning such terms are given in the body of Freudian theory.

Conscious/Unconscious in Ordinary Speech

To begin with, conscious can refer to a state of an individual. One can be said to be conscious if one awakens from a coma and unconscious if one is knocked out by a blow to the head. In this usage one is not conscious *of* anything; one is simply conscious. Since conscious in this first usage is not used to modify things like wishes, motives, or emotions, but only persons in toto, the more pertinent usage for our purposes is that of being conscious *of* something. This is particularly true since we wish to use the ordinary sense of the word as our springboard into the Freudian usage; Freud's term in German, *bewusst,* does not have this first meaning, but *only* means to be aware of something.

One may be conscious *of* the discomfort of a tight shoe, of being nauseous, of desiring apple pie, of imagining a yellow ball, of what one is doing and why one is doing it, of the fact that the cost of living is rising, or of a host of other and quite disparate things. What does it mean to be conscious *of* such things? One answer, which we shall call the "stream of consciousness" answer, is that "being conscious" means, first, that some datable mental process is occurring that we experience, and second, that our attention is directed upon that mental experience. Thus, in the foregoing examples, to be conscious of each of these things is, respectively, to experience a throb of pain in the foot, a feeling of nauseousness, an urge or uncomfortableness in longing for apple pie, a picturing "in the mind's eye" of a yellow ball, a deliberation of what one ought to do and for what reasons, the silent saying to oneself that the cost of living is rising, and it is to have one's attention focused on these things. Being conscious of one's pains, feelings, desires, imaginings, motives, emotions, and perceptions in this sense means that some such activity was occurring in the "inner phenomenology" of the conscious subject.

That the stream of consciousness account is not the only sense of "conscious of" that we employ in ordinary speech can perhaps best be brought out by an examination of the example of being conscious of the fact that the cost of living is rising. From being conscious of that fact it does not follow that I necessarily told myself some story to that effect. I could have learned it by reading it in the newspaper or even having a recording of some statement to that effect playing at my bedside one night while I was asleep; in neither case is my being conscious of it dependent on my having experienced some conscious process of silent soliloquy. Being conscious of such a fact means that one has achieved something, a state of knowledge: One *knows* that the cost of living is on the rise. Being conscious of some fact about the external world is simply knowing it to be true. And the clearest case of knowing that some proposition is true is given by the ability, if asked, to state what it is one knows. The most straightforward way in which one tests whether another knows that the atomic weight of helium is 4 is not to seek out evidence of the occurrence of some conscious process at some time (presumably a learning experience), but rather to ask the subject what the atomic weight of helium is. If he can state that fact, then he knows it; if he cannot state it, that is some evidence that he does not know it (although he may once have known it and forgotten it).

Hence, to be conscious of the fact that the cost of living is rising may mean that if asked one could so state. Being conscious in this dispositional sense does not require that one have experienced anything or have one's attention directed in one way rather than another. Rather, synonymously with one sense of "knowing," it means only that the subject has the ability to state that of which he is conscious.[63]

One also has the ability to describe one's pains, feelings, desires, emotions, imaginings, and perceptions, and so on. If one is conscious of such "internal" facts in the dispositional sense of conscious of, this also means that one can state what they are. If one is conscious of them in this sense, one necessarily knows what they are. But *how* one knows that one is in pain, feels nauseous, hates another, is imagining something, or desires apple pie is different from the way in which one knows some fact about the external world such as that the cost of living is rising. We seem to know these former things immediately, noninferentially, without resort to observation, experiment, or evidence, whereas one can only know facts in the external world (including *other people's* mental states) by such observation and experiment, and on the basis of the available evidence. One must make inferences from the evidence, whereas in the case of our own pains and the like, if we know we have them we seem to possess such knowledge without inference or observation. This is the famous "privileged access" we seem to have to the contents of our own minds that we do not have to other aspects of the world.

This special way of knowing our own feelings and sensations seems to be involved in the meaning of conscious of. To be conscious of such things means not just to know what they are, but to know it in this special direct or nonobservational way. One cannot, for this reason, be said to be conscious of someone else's pains. I may know that you are in pain, yet I am not conscious of it—only you can be said to be conscious of it. At most, all I can say is that I am conscious *of the fact that* you are in pain, which is equivalent to saying only that I know that to be the case.

Recall our earlier example of being conscious of the fact that the cost of living is rising. Can we say "He is conscious of the cost of living rising"? He can be conscious of that fact (he knows it), but can he be conscious *of it?* We have, I think, a hard time imagining what it would be like to be conscious of the cost of living rising. We have less difficulty imagining being conscious of our own bodily temperature rising, because we understand that we can feel hot. How do we analogously feel the rising of the cost of living?

Being conscious of, then, means not only that we know that we are feeling, perceiving, and so forth (although it does entail at least that); it

The Challenge of Psychiatry

also means that we know these things in a special, nonobservational way. We can thus only be conscious of those things of which we have this nonobservational knowledge, this privileged access.

This may seem to return us to the stream of consciousness identification of "conscious of" with the datable mental experiences of our inner phenomenology. It is indeed often the case that when I have nonobservational knowledge it is accompanied by a direction of my attention to those experiences of which I have such knowledge. Such is not inevitably the case, however. One may, for example, have nonobservational knowledge of one's present intention to get a haircut without *having* recitory, haircut craving, or any kind of mental experience. Alternatively, one may have some mental experience, such as feeling quite depressed, and one may have nonobservational knowledge of that feeling, without focusing one's attention on such a feeling. In neither case is the possession of nonobservational knowledge dependent upon one's attention being directed to the relevant mental experiences, nor even on there being such mental experiences.[64]

With these two ordinary senses of being conscious of a mental state, we can easily construct two corresponding senses of mental states being *unconscious*. By "unconscious mental state," we might mean that one did not have one's attention directed to that state. An unconscious pain, for example, would either be an unfelt pain (if this is possible), or a painful feeling to which one paid no attention because one was distracted by some other mental experience. Alternatively, we might mean that the holder of the mental state does not have the capacity to recognize the state that he is in; he cannot describe it even if he attempts to direct his attention to it. An unconscious pain in this sense would be a pain that its holder did not know about, even when his attention is directed toward the question of whether he hurts anywhere.

Freud's Nontheoretical Use of Unconscious

To what extent did Freud's use of unconscious differ from ordinary usage thus far analyzed? Freud in his writings about the unconscious tells us that psychoanalysis progressed through three different usages of the phrase: (1) the purely descriptive sense; (2) the dynamic sense; and (3) the topographical sense.[65] To preview these senses briefly: A "psychic element" was descriptively unconscious for Freud if it could not be described as conscious in the ordinary meaning of the term as Freud analyzed it; dynamically unconscious if it was repressed; and unconscious in a topographical sense if it belonged to "the System Ucs," or, more popularly, the unconscious (used as a noun).

Freud's nontheoretical use of unconscious is to be found in his descriptive sense and in one interpretation of his dynamic sense of the word. It is useful to extract his nontheoretical usage of the word first because doing so isolates those Freudian claims about the unconscious that are not hostage to the more problematic parts of Freud's metapsychology. I shall in the succeeding subsection then discuss the possible, theory-laden interpretations of unconscious brought on by the topographical and dynamic senses of the word.

Freud's descriptive sense of unconscious is simply the negation of the stream of consciousness sense "of conscious of":

> "Being conscious" is in the first place a purely descriptive term, resting on perception of the most immediate and certain character. Experience goes to show that a psychical element (for instance, an idea) is not as a rule conscious for a protracted length of time. On the contrary, a state of consciousness is characteristically very transitory; an idea that is conscious now is no longer so a moment later, although it can become so again under certain conditions that are easily brought about. In the interval the idea was—we do not know what. We can say that it was *latent,* and by this we mean that it was *capable of becoming conscious* at any time. Or, if we say that it was *unconscious,* we shall also be giving a correct description of it. Here "unconscious" coincides with "latent and capable of becoming conscious."[66]

An unconscious mental state, in this descriptive use of unconscious, is simply one that is not now the subject of attention in one's stream of consciousness. One is not feeling it, deliberating about it, or reciting it to oneself, although one is capable of directing one's "inner eye" (of attention) upon it.

This led Freud to distinguish conscious, being that to which one's attention is currently directed, from preconscious, or that which is capable of being recalled but which is temporarily out of the limelight (i.e., not being felt, thought about, etc.). Freud classified as descriptively unconscious that which is preconscious, that is, capable of recall but not now the object of conscious attention.

If this were all that Freud had meant by his "discovery of the unconscious" we should never have heard of him. For it is hardly startling to assert that we are not always, for example, reciting to ourselves our thoughts or intentions. The normal state of affairs would be for us to be unconscious of our mental states much of the time in such a usage. Nor would it be novel to assert that we have many mental states about which *at no time* we deliberate, engage in conscious planning, or have other mental experiences. Freud himself acknowledged this when he wrote that the recognition of such a usage of unconscious "might be considered an uninteresting piece of descriptive or classificatory work,"[67] and that by such work "we should have learnt nothing new."[68] The novel insights, he felt, had to be conveyed by a different meaning of unconscious, that conveyed in the dynamic sense of the term.

The Challenge of Psychiatry

In analyzing the descriptive sense of unconscious Freud was plainly attempting to analyze the ordinary usage of the term. He was seeking to elucidate what we ordinarily mean by unconscious "as a description at once applicable and easy to understand," because familiar, and as having "no theoretical implication,"[69] because as yet unreconstructed in light of his theories. In this he was only partly successful because of his acceptance of the stream of consciousness sense of conscious of as its only ordinary sense.

The other ordinary sense of conscious, and thus of unconscious, Freud only arrived at through his dynamic usage of unconscious. In introducing a dynamic sense of unconscious Freud was formulating two distinct claims. The first is that we are not only unconscious of our mental states in the sense that we are not now directing, or have not directed in the past, our conscious attention to them (Freud's descriptive sense), but that we also are unconscious of some of our mental states in the sense that we are not able to recall them at all, even if we do direct considerable attention to the question of what they were. The second and distinct claim is that there is an explanation for why we at times are unable to bring to mind what our mental states are; we lack such ability because we have repressed such mental states: "The reason why such ideas cannot become conscious is that a certain force opposes them, that otherwise they would become conscious."[70]

Freud consistently wished to express both claims by using a dynamic sense of unconscious, but in fact they are quite distinct. The first is a purely descriptive claim about there being mental experiences or states that are very difficult to recapture through memory. The second is an explanatory claim, purporting to elucidate why the first claim might be true. The first could be true, but the second false. There is no reason to require that both claims be considered together, and so I shall consider the first, the descriptive claim, separately.

The first claim is quite close to the assertion that would be made in ordinary language by describing a mental state as unconscious in the dispositional sense of unconscious, that is, that denies that holders of the state can avow nonobservationally what state they are in. The only difference is in the degree of difficulty Freud thought one had in bringing to mind that which is dynamically unconscious. Both the ordinary, dispositional sense and Freud's dynamic sense are the same in their denial of an ability to say what one's mental state was. Neither merely denies that one had some datable conscious experience to which one's attention was directed.

Freud's *descriptive* distinction between his descriptive and his dynamic senses of unconscious thus closely corresponds to the two senses of unconscious in ordinary speech:

> In order to explain a slip of the tongue, for instance, we find ourselves obliged to assume that the intention to make a particular remark was

> present in the subject. We infer it with certainty from the interference with his remark which has occurred; but the intention did not put itself through and was thus unconscious. If, when we subsequently put it before the speaker, he recognizes it as one familiar to him, then it was only temporarily unconscious to him; but if he repudiates it as something foreign to him, then it was permanently unconscious. From this experience we retrospectively obtain the right also to pronounce as something unconscious what had been described as latent. A consideration of these dynamic relations permits us now to distinguish two kinds of unconscious—one which is easily, under frequently occurring circumstances, transformed into something conscious, and another with which this transformation is difficult and takes place only subject to a considerable expenditure of effort or possibly never at all. In order to escape the ambiguity as to whether we mean the one or the other unconscious, whether we are using the word in the descriptive or in the dynamic sense, we make use of a permissible and simple way out. We call the unconscious which is only latent, and thus easily becomes conscious, the "preconscious" and retain the term "unconscious" for the other."[71]

Freud's only mistake here was to assume that in ordinary language we do not have pretty much the same meaning of unconscious that he thought he was inventing. He thus presented as a conceptual innovation (the dynamic sense of unconscious) what was in fact a refinement of one of the ordinary meanings of the term.

This is hardly to belittle the extent of Freud's empirical discovery that a great deal more of our behavior is explicable by reference to unconscious mental states than we had supposed. All that has been said is that what Freud meant by saying that a mental state was unconscious in his dynamic sense was little more than what one would have meant had one said that a mental state was unconscious in the ordinary meaning of that term. Thus, nothing in Freud's use of unconscious as so far explained is hostage to any dynamic or economic metapsychology.

Does conscious in Freud's usage as the opposite of (dynamic) unconscious have the further implication that it does in ordinary language, namely, the one not only knows one's mental state, but knows it in a nonobservational way? Although Freud is not entirely consistent on this point, there is a strong case to be made that the conscious/unconscious dichotomy in Freud's dynamic sense parallels ordinary usage in this feature as well. One can see this by understanding what it means to "make the (dynamic) unconscious conscious," the early formulated goal of psychoanalytic therapy.

Consider a patient undergoing psychoanalytic therapy who is told by the analyst that he really desires the state of affairs described by q. Although the patient at first rejects such an interpretation, after some further sessions, he states that he too now knows that q was and is the object of one of his desires. In Freud's use, is he now *conscious* of his desire for q? Is this an instance of what Freud meant when he spoke of transforming an unconscious intention into something conscious only with a "considerable expenditure of effort"?

The answer is plainly no. To become conscious that he has a desire for q, the patient does not merely accept that fact intellectually. He does not come to know it by being *convinced* by his analyst. He has to *remember* that q was something he wanted. He has to know it in the same way that he knows his conscious desires, namely, in a nonobservational sense. He cannot merely be convinced by the evidence (e.g., a consistent behavior pattern) or by the authority of his analyst. This would be like knowing what someone else's desires were—from the evidence. And as Freud said, "A consciousness of which its possessor knows nothing is something very different from that of another person."[72] It is different because we know it in a very different way, through the privileged access of remembering what we desired, not through observation.

Only by such recapture through memory will we see the desire as *ours*, as being a part of our person. Memory is one of the critical ingredients in our sense of self-identity.[73] Tying the idea of making the unconscious conscious to memory thus makes our unconscious mental states *ours*, a part of us, in a way impossible if such states come to be known to us only in the ways in which we can come to know someone else's mental states.

Freud often recognized that becoming conscious of one's dynamically unconscious mental states was not simply knowing what they were in the same way as one knows some scientific fact:

> What then have we to do in order to bring what is unconscious in the patient into consciousness? At one time we thought that would be very simple; all we need do would be to identify this unconscious matter and then tell the patient what it was. However, we know already that that was a short-sighted mistake. Our knowledge of what is unconscious in him is not equivalent to his knowledge of it ... we have to look for it in his memory.[74]

Merely telling patients about their unconscious mental states may convey knowledge to them, if they believe it. But:

> There is knowing and knowing; they are not always the same thing. There are various kinds of knowing, which psychologically are not by any means of equal value... When the physician conveys his knowledge to the patient by telling him what he knows, it ... does not have the effect of dispersing the symptoms.... The patient has learned something that he did not know before—the meaning of his symptom—and yet he knows it as little as ever. Thus we discover that there is more than one kind of ignorance.[75]

It would be a mistake to think that this psychoanalytic notion of memory requires that one at some point be conscious of a mental state and then have forgotten it. Although much of what we remember is what we once consciously knew but then forgot, that is not the notion of memory relevant here. The Freudian claim of extended memory is that we can remember many things of which we were never aware. We might, for example, remember our anger at some time in the past without having been aware that we were angry at the time. Lest this claim seem problematic, one might note that all memories of dreams are of this sort.

There is thus a rather complete parallel between the Freudian meaning of unconscious and its ordinary meaning. This point is basic to understanding one thing psychoanalysts can mean by speaking of the unconscious. This nontheoretical idea is simply that persons have many mental states of which they are not aware (in either ordinary sense) but of which they can potentially become aware through their extended memory. This is the "unconscious" of poets, novelists, lawyers, and historians, all of whom (long before Freud) easily spoke of there being mental states that were unconscious in this sense. This nontheoretical notion must be separated from the elaborate, theoretical explanation Freud proposed as to *why* we are not conscious of all of our mental states. That explanation begins with the second claim implicit in Freud's dynamic sense of unconscious and with the claims Freud wished to make by inventing the topographical sense. It is to these that I shall now turn.

Theory-laden Usages of Unconscious

It would be a mistake to think that Freud's dynamic and topographical metapsychology are simply stipulations of two more senses of the word unconscious to be added to the two ordinary senses just explored. Rather, what Freud sought from these metapsychological viewpoints was to *explain* how mental states of various kinds could be unconscious (in the ordinary sense of the word). Such explanations do introduce some theoretical conception(s) of the unconscious that find no parallel with the ordinary conception; nonetheless, such more theoretical conception(s) should be seen as part of the general theory with which Freud sought to explain the existence of unconscious mental states as ordinarily conceived. Such theoretical conception(s) of the unconscious thus stand behind the more ordinary ones in the same way that the theoretical conception of water as H_2O stands behind the ordinary, pretheoretical conception.[76]

The part of Freud's explanatory theory relevant here is centered on three ideas, the ideas of repression, the instincts, and the System Ucs. Repression for Freud was a process that occurred in the history of an individual with regard to certain mental states. A repressed belief, for example, was a belief that was unconscious because it had undergone this process of repression. Such a process occurred not just once with respect to a given idea, Freud thought, but was repeatedly engaged in whenever the situation was otherwise propitious for the belief to become conscious.[77] Such a process is thought to serve a function,[78] namely, the avoidance of the pain a person would otherwise experience if the repressed belief were to reach that person's awareness. Repression is thus part of the Freudian view of persons as pain-avoidance and pleasure-seeking mechanisms.

Unconscious mental states that are repressed need not ever have been the subject of awareness. What Freud called "repression proper" was for those beliefs and the like that were once (usually in childhood) conscious or preconscious; Freud also thought that there was a "primal repression" that kept some mental states from *ever* having been conscious or accessible to consciousness.[79] Both kinds of repression were linked by Freud to his instinct theory. For it was the mental representations of instinctual impulses that were subject to either primal repression or repression proper.

In understanding Freud's instinct theory in the present context it is not so important that one grasp the varying objects Freud at various times proposed as our "ultimate motivations" – whether sexual, aggressive, survival oriented, or the rather grandiloquent "Eros" and "Thanatos" of Freud's last formulations of his instinct theory. Sufficient for understanding Freud's theoretical notion of the unconscious is to understand that it is in large part defined in terms of instincts with *some* limited range of objects as their goals.

The ultimate object of the instincts for Freud (usually called their "aim") was to achieve satisfaction. Such satisfaction was conceptualized by Freud as having some contingent correlation with experienced pleasure; ultimately, however, satisfaction is part of Freud's energy theory that views the human being as an energy-discharging mechanism. Stimulation of various kinds bombards the person. Such stimulation includes the stimuli of the five senses, the kinesthetic sensations of the internal organs, and most important, the stimulations of the instincts themselves. The latter stimulations were conceptualized by Freud as having their *source* in the body and yet as having an *object* in the mind. Freud assumed that instincts were both physiological phenomena of some kind – whether chemical, electrical did not matter – and mental in Brentano's sense of "mental," viz., directed upon an object (or "mental content" or "mental representations").[80]

We encountered this aspect of Freud's theory at the end of Chapter 1, where I gave some reasons for being very suspicious of this attempt to lump physiology with mind via the conceptual cement called *Trieb*, or instinct. Still, to understand Freud's theoretical notions of a dynamic and topographical unconscious, one must at least grasp (even if only to reject ultimately) the rudiments of Freud's instinct theory.

The third crucial idea is the topographical one, the System Ucs itself. The ideas of repression and of instinct allow one to see why Freud thought of the unconscious as a *system*. It was not a system in anatomical terms. Brain anatomy might or might not isolate some portions of the brain that are unconscious in Freud's sense, but nothing in Freud's theory turns on such anatomical discoveries. The reason for this is that Freud's theoretical unconscious is not a hypothesis about physical *structure* of any kind, whether in crude anatomy or in more sophisticated chemical terms. Rather, Freud's notion of system is a *functional* notion (in the sense introduced in Chapter 1 discussing the functionalist view of mind). The mental states that are unconscious could be aggregated into a system, Freud thought, not because of any structural similarity the underlying brain states may or may not turn out to have, but rather because such unconscious mental states serve the same *functions*. That a mental state was unconscious came for Freud to mean not only that such a state was not presently accessible to consciousness but also, and more importantly, that it served the same crucial functions as did other unconscious mental states. As Freud wrote in 1912:

> Unconsciousness seemed to us at first only an enigmatical characteristic of a definite mental act. Now it means more for us. It is a sign that this act partakes of the nature of a certain mental category known to us by other and more important features, and that it belongs to a system of mental activity ... The index-value of the unconscious has far outgrown its importance as a property.[81]

The dynamic and topographical metapsychologies together form Freud's first stab at giving the mind a functional organization. The System Ucs was for Freud a grouping of mental states by the functional role they had in common. That functional role is given by Freud's theory of instincts in continuous conflict with the mental states causing repression. The dynamic balance, in other words, between types of mental states that recurringly conflict is what justified for Freud a systematizing of one pole of that conflict into a System Ucs.

Ultimately, then, Freud gave both a redescription and an explanation of the fact that some mental states are unconscious. The *redescription* was of an aggregate of mental states that not only are unconscious but also serve a common (instinctual) function in mental conflict. The *explanation* why such mental states serving such common function are unconscious was because they are repressed. It is worth reemphasizing that the existence of unconscious mental states is *not* hostage to this particular organization of them, nor to this explanation of them, being true. Freud's dynamic and topographical metapsychologies lay out one attempt among others to organize and explain the apparent fact that there are unconscious mental states.

The Challenge of Psychiatry

Before turning to the challenges the unconscious presents to the legal view of minds and persons, it may be well to review the pretheoretical and the Freudian conceptions of the unconscious and to contrast them with each other and with certain other ideas about the unconscious. We have distinguished two conceptions of the unconscious that are often unnecessarily confused with one another and that have different implications for law and morality.

The first is what I have called the pretheoretical notion of the unconscious. This is the view examined earlier that holds that persons are possessed not only of states that are not the subject of present attention (preconscious), but also of states that are not subject to recall even if attention is directed toward them. Such mental states may exist and they may influence behavior without the subjects being aware of them or of their influence. This pretheoretical conception of the unconscious is completed by the Freudian idea of extended memory, according to which any unconscious mental state is *potentially* accessible to memory if it is a mental state of the person at all. Such recall may be prompted by free association, by reexperiencing the mental state by transference, or by any other memory-jogging technique. Neither such therapeutic techniques, nor the idea of extended memory itself, are dependent upon Freud's dynamic and topographical metapsychologies being true. The idea of extended memory is itself but a natural extension of the psychology of common sense, according to which we each have privileged access to the contents of our own mind.

The pretheoretical notion of the unconscious makes no commitment to there being *some thing* referred to by the noun phrase, the unconscious. The ontological commitment here is only to a universal, not to a particular. The commitment is to there being particular mental states that have the *quality* (property, trait, characteristic) of being unconscious. There need be no commitment to any structurally or functionally defined thing called the unconscious in this ordinary, pretheoretical view. Such I take to be the salvageable point of those ordinary language philosophers who often urged that unconscious should never be used as a noun but only as an adjective or adverb.[82] The unconscious in this ordinary sense is only a conveniently abbreviating expression, and that which it abbreviates are longer-winded expressions that predicate unconsciousness (as a quality) of particular mental states.

The second conception of the unconscious is Freud's theoretical exposition just concluded—what I shall henceforth call the "Freudian unconscious." Here one conceives of the unconscious as an aggregation of mental states that not only share the property of being unconscious but also share a functional role in the conflict-ridden and tension-reducing mechanisms that human beings are posited to be.

In addition to these two conceptions of the unconscious several additional conceptions should be mentioned, if only to serve by way of contrast. One of these is what might be called the "animistic unconscious." One way to view Freud's topographical unconscious is as if there were another person "in" us as well as the self that we experience. One does this the moment one attributes causal agency and practical reason to the unconscious and not to the whole person. This conception of the unconscious I shall discuss shortly when I discuss the alleged disunity of the self, the third main challenge of psychiatry to law.

Another conception of the unconscious stems from the emphasis of Freud's developmental or genetic metapsychological viewpoint on the events (or fantasized events) of early childhood. In the heyday of logical behaviorism it was fashionable to "operationalize" Freudian concepts, including the unconscious, by reducing them to statements about observable stimuli and observable responses.[83] This might be called the behaviorist unconscious. The unconscious, according to such a reductionist scheme, was simply a shorthand for the events of childhood that cause (via unknown physiological mechanisms) adult behavior to be as it is. Since logical behaviorism in general need not be taken seriously, this mechanistic, reductionist conception of the unconscious may also be largely ignored. (I shall return briefly to it in Chapter 7.)

Much more important is what might be called the physiological unconscious. This conception of the unconscious is not explicitly a Freudian notion, although hints of such a conception loom very large behind Freud's theorizing about the unconscious in dynamic, topographical, and economic terms. In such a conception the unconscious refers to those physiological processes and states that must exist in the brain for intelligent functioning to take place but of which the subject is unaware. One example, well developed in the recent psychology of perception, is provided by those normal processes that take place in the preprocessing of information done in the ganglion cells of the eye prior to the sending of a signal up the optic nerve to the brain.[84] Such intelligent functioning involves states of which the person is not aware and of which, *through his memory,* he will never become aware. Such unconscious states are thus distinct from the unconscious *mental* states of a *person* described by the pretheoretical conception of the unconscious.[85] Such states are also separate from the kinds of instinctual, repressed, systematically organized states of the Freudian unconscious. Such perceptual states or processes are not instinctual, not part of "the forces of repression," and, in short, have nothing to do with Freudian dynamics.

More generally, one might well think that all mental states of whatever type must be underlain by physiological goings-on of some kind. (One may hold to such correlations between mental states and brain states no matter where one comes out on the mind/brain identity briefly discussed in Chapter 1; brain/mind *correlations* do not entail any kind of *identity*.) Not only are the visual experiences of persons underlain by complicated physiological processes, but acts of imagination, formation of intention, sensations of pain, use of language, and thinking in general are surely underlain by physiological processes as well. Since all of these processes in the brain are unknown to us, one might well call all of them the unconscious.

I mention such a physiological conception of the unconscious mostly to put it to the side in future discussions. Yet it must be explicitly put aside else it clouds the nature of the challenge the unconscious presents to the legal view of minds and of persons. It is, I suspect, a (largely unconscious) fallback position of Freudians about their theories: Even if the dynamic, topographical, and economic metapsychologies cannot hold their own as *psychological* theories, perhaps physiology will save the day by showing there to be instinctual and repressive forces, and so on, as *physical* processes in the brain.

Much of the temptation that is so common to Freud and his followers, namely, to think that all of conscious mental states are underlain by unconscious mental states, depends upon this physiological reading of "unconscious mental states." There is nothing illegitimate about such physiological speculation. Many others besides Freudians, such as Noam Chomsky and his followers in linguistics, engage in the same kind of speculation about what sorts of physical states and processes there must be if one is adequately to account for intelligent mental functioning.[86] What is important is that such a physiological conception of the unconscious be recognized as such and that it be distinguished from what I have called the pretheoretical and the Freudian conceptions of the unconscious. If one does this it becomes much less plausible that all our conscious mental life is underlain by the unconscious or that the conscious and the unconscious are like a single iceberg, with consciousness being only the small portion above the surface of the water. Such a claim is much less plausible if construed as an assertion that our extended memory can potentially recapture all such underlying structures or processes. It is also less plausible if construed as a claim that *all* of our mental states can be explained by the hidden dynamics of the instincts and their repression, including the most abstract thought processes and the most mundane daily decisions.[87] Only under a physiological conception of the unconscious does Freud's iceberg thesis become very likely.

Also rendered problematic by keeping Freudians to their word of providing a *psychological* theory about the unconscious are Freud's numerous references to an unconscious that extends well beyond the repressed. At the outset of his paper on the unconscious, for example, Freud mentions that "the repressed does not comprise the whole unconscious. The unconscious has the greater compass: the repressed is a part of the unconscious."[88] To the extent that all Freud meant by such a statement is what he later explicitly said—that those mental states in conflict with repressed states may themselves be unconscious[89]—then there is no inadvertent departure from the dynamic metapsychology. Both sides of the hypothesized mental conflict may be unconscious even if only one of them can be assigned to the System Ucs because only it is repressed. Often, however, such exegesis cannot be accomplished on the Freudian corpus, and Freud's omnipresent unconscious is no more than the physiological speculations he purportedly abandoned when he put away his early *Project for a Scientific Psychology* in favor of psychological theorizing.

THE CHALLENGE TO LAW OF AN OMNIPRESENT UNCONSCIOUS

That the legal theory of minds and persons should be severely challenged by the idea of the unconscious may come as no surprise. To any lawyer steeped in doctrines that turn on the intentions of parties when they enter a contract, marry, make a will, or commit a crime, the idea that there are always conflicting sets of intentions, one or more of which may be unknown to its holder, will of course seem more than a little disorienting. What is perhaps surprising is the apparently contradictory implications for law that are thought to stem from the "discovery of the unconscious."

In assessing the seeming impact of the unconscious on responsibility, imagine two sorts of cases. In the first, an actor does not prima facie perform an intentional action. He makes an apparent slip of the tongue, dreams a dream, or performs some seemingly accidental action. If it is known that his slip, dream, or accident was, however, in fact motivated or caused by some desire of which he was not and is not now aware, does this knowledge alter one's assessment of his responsibility for any resulting harm? In the second case, the actor does prima facie perform an intentional action. If it is known that the action is caused by his unconscious mental states, does this affect one's assessment of his moral and legal responsibility for the act?

Interestingly enough, psychoanalysts and others are led both ways as to the effect of the unconscious on responsibility for particular actions. In the first case, it is often said that the individual who is *not* ordinarily held responsible for a particular act is nonetheless shown to be responsible if he acted for motives or reasons, even if they were unconscious ones. On the other hand, in the second case it is often said that the individual who is ordinarily held responsible for some act is nonetheless shown *not* to be responsible if this act is explained by his unconscious mental states.

The paradox is heightened by moving from responsibility for particular *acts* to the responsibility, in the sense of accountability, of *agents*. Again, it is said both that everyone is *more* rational than generally thought, in that even one's dreams and apparent slips are actually rational productions,[90] and that everyone is *less* rational than generally thought, because all of the seemingly rational reasons for conduct are a mere facade or screen behind which operate the primitive, irrational wishes of the primary process. Insofar as rationality is the hallmark of sanity, this means, as is again often said, both that no one is really crazy, and that everyone is really crazy.

A convenient illustration of these two contradictory implications is presented by the well-known case of *State v. Sikora*.[91] Walter Sikora was tried for the murder of someone who had beaten him up in a bar in New Jersey. At his trial a dynamic psychiatrist, a Dr. Galen, proposed to testify that Sikora had to kill his victim because he was under the control of his unconscious. In deciding whether to admit such testimony Chief Justice Weintraub noted the apparently contradictory implications such testimony could have on Sikora's (or anyone's) responsibility. In the first place, "we could say it makes no difference" that it is the unconscious that is in control:

> We could say that in punishing an evil deed accompanied by an evil-meaning mind, the law is concerned only with the existence of a will to do the evil act and it does not matter precisely where within the mind the evil drive resides.[92]

This, Weintraub recognized, could dramatically extend responsibility:

> The possibilities here are rich. It would be quite a thing to identify the unconscious drive and then decide whether it is evil for the purpose of criminal liability.... Shall we indict for murder a motorist who kills another because, although objectively he was negligent at the worst, the psychoanalyst assures us that the conscious man acted automatically to fulfill an unconscious desire for self-destruction?[93]

Alternatively, the implications for responsibility stemming from the unconscious could be quite the opposite. The dynamic psychiatrist "traces a man's every deed to some cause truly beyond the actor's own making, and says that although the man was aware of his action, he was unaware of assembled forces in his unconscious which decided his course. Thus the conscious is a puppet, and the unconscious the puppeteer."[94] As Weintraub further noted, "Under this psychiatric concept [of the dictatorial unconscious] no man could be convicted of anything if the law were to accept the impulse of the unconscious as an excuse for conscious misbehavior."[95]

The same apparently contradictory implications are generated by taking the unconscious into account in the ascription of desert rights. The unconscious might imply an expansion of contract or property rights because we (unconsciously) intend far more than we know. Alternatively, if the unconscious underlies all of our conscious intentions and is really in control, perhaps we never really form the (conscious) intentions we think we do and thus never deserve the property or performances of others that we think we deserve.

The reason for these apparently contradictory implications of the unconscious for the ascription of rights and responsibilities lies in the different conceptions of the unconscious being employed. If one has the pretheoretical conception of the unconscious in mind, then the discovery of the unconscious is the discovery that each of us has more mental states that are truly *ours* – a part of our person recapturable by our extended memory – than we had thought. Such discovery has the potential at least of dramatically extending responsibility and rights, because the conditions under which responsibility and rights are ascribed can seemingly be satisfied on far more occasions than we had thought. Consciously involuntary movements may be actions and consciously unintentional actions may be intentional if unconscious mental states are discovered that are truly part of our selves.

On the other hand, if one has the Freudian unconscious in mind – the dynamic unconscious of repressed instincts – then the apparent implication will be to reduce (or eliminate entirely) desert. In a mechanistic view that we are all puppets blind to the control of the drives that monotonously seek but one thing, the discharge of their psychic energies, the apparent implication will be that no one deserves anything, neither reward nor punishment. For one has truly *done* nothing to merit praise or condemnation; one has only reacted to unconscious forces.

We shall have occasion in later chapters to examine each of these apparent implications for law stemming from the idea of the unconscious. For now it is sufficient to see the inconsistent challenges the two different conceptions of the unconscious present.

The Corporate Self

THE THEORY THAT WE ARE COMMUNITIES OF SELVES

It has long been thought that the findings of psychoanalysis challenge the commonsense idea of the unity of the self. Norman Brown, whose exegesis of Freud once drew quite a following, forthrightly stated this challenge:

> Every person ... is many persons; a multitude made into one person; a corporate body; incorporated, a corporation.... The unity of the person is as real, or as unreal, as the unity of the corporation.[96]

Part of what Brown meant by this can be gleaned from his citation of Joan Riviere. Riviere thought that we build a self out of incorporating others' personalities into our own:

> There is no such thing as a single human being, pure and simple, unmixed with other human beings. Each personality is a world in himself, a company of many ... self ... is a composite structure which

The Challenge of Psychiatry

has been and is being formed and built up . . . out of countless never-ending influences and exchanges between ourselves and others. . . . These other persons are in fact therefore parts of ourselves.[97]

These notions about the etiology of self are also to be found in Freud, particularly in his discussion of how the superego develops by the identification and object relations engaged in between children and their parents. Such etiological notions, however, form only a part of the general conclusion reached by Freud that "our mind . . . is no peacefully self-contained unity." It is, Freud continued, "rather to be compared to a modern state in which a mob, eager for enjoyment and destruction, has to be held down forcibly by a prudent superior class."[98]

The main motive that led Freud to view the mind as a potential battleground between competing mobs was his dominant thesis that persons are conflict-ridden creatures. Such conflict, Freud thought, could be observed in clinical practice by perceiving the *resistance* patients exhibited to getting well, a resistance that flatly opposed their apparently sincere desires to get well. More generally, Freud thought he could detect such conflict between opposed intentions that lay behind slips of the tongue and other parapraxes. Dreams and neurotic symptoms also seemed to exhibit a person as a being whose mental states were in conflict. Such considerations led Freud to generalize even further. Not just in symptom maintenance or symptom formation of neurotics, or in peripheral phenomena such as dreams or parapraxes, was conflict to be found. Psychoanalysis as a general psychology takes all persons to be conflict-ridden.

The two most famous conceptualizations of this view of persons as conflict-ridden creatures are to be found in Freud's topographical and structural metapsychologies. The topographical divisions of the mind—the Systems Csc, Pcs, and Ucs—we have already discussed. As is well known, Freud's structural divisions of the mind into id, ego, and superego grew out of the earlier topographical divisions. The problem that by 1923 (when *The Ego and the Id* was published) had convinced Freud to substitute one division for the other was the failure of the topographical scheme to reflect accurately the conflict he thought he had discovered in the human mind. Specifically, the agency that institutes repression Freud thought to be unconscious. Yet that which such repressing agency opposed (namely, the instincts) was also thought by Freud to be unconscious. Conflict between such systems could accordingly be conceptualized as conflict between a System Csc and a System Ucs only if some of the System Csc was unconscious. Freud understandably rejected the idea of an unconscious consciousness, and so substituted the first person, singular pronoun in German, *Ich,* as the name of the system opposing the instincts. The System Ucs became *das es,* "the it" or "id" that Nietzsche had first coined as the name of ego-alien mental states.

Freud was far from original, either in his view that the human mind is a battleground of conflicting mental states, or in his view that such conflict should be conceptualized as a fracturing of the self. One of Freud's more explicit forerunners was Plato, who held both of these views. In Book 4 of the *Republic* Plato too analogizes the human psyche to a state with conflicting parts and has Socrates expound that

> it is obvious that the same thing will never do or suffer opposites in the same respect in relation to the same thing and at the same time. So that if ever we find these contradictions in the functions of the mind we shall know that it was not the same thing functioning but a plurality.[99]

Since Socrates then proceeds to find such contradictions between desires and that which on occasion restrains us from satisfying our desires, he concludes that there must be at least two parts to the psyche: "that in the soul [psyche] whereby it reckons and reasons the rational, and that with which it loves, hungers, thirsts, and feels the flutter and titillation of other desires, the irrational and appetitive."[100]

There are two distinct steps to the Freud–Plato subdivision of mind. The first harks back to the functionalist view of mind discussed in Chapter 1. For both Freud and Plato arranged their subdivisions of the mind not only as the poles of mental conflict, but also by the different kinds of mental functioning involved. Ego, id, and superego represent Freud's second stab at giving the mind a functional organization. For Freud as for Plato (and for Hume), the basic functional division was between reason and passions: "We might say that the ego stands for reason and good sense while the id stands for the untamed passions."[101] Freud and later Freudians have elaborated on this familiar distinction considerably, however.

The id Freud conceived as "instinctual cathexes seeking discharge — that . . . is all there is in the id."[102] The id was assigned by Freud the sole function of motivating us to do or think anything. It is the ultimate "moving force" behind all we do, guided by but one ultimate aim, the seeking of discharge (or satisfaction — the "pleasure principle"). The ego was assigned a wide variety of functions by Freud, including most of what we would ordinarily think of as intelligent mental functioning. As described by Arlow and Brenner:

> There is no complete list of ego functions. However, any attempt to formulate such a list would have to include the following: (1) consciousness; (2) sense perception; (3) the perception and expression of affect; (4) thought; (5) control of motor action; (6) memory; (7) language; (8) defense mechanisms and defensive activity in general [including most significantly for Freud the instituting of repression]; (9) control, regulation, and binding of instinctual energy; (10) the interpretive and harmonizing function; (11) reality testing; and (12) the

The Challenge of Psychiatry

capacity to inhibit or suspend the operation of any of these functions and to regress to a primitive level of functioning.[103]

The superego for Freud is defined by the functions of self-observation, of conscience, and of maintaining the "ego-ideal."[104]

This kind of functional subdivision of the mind is not only as ancient as Plato but also as modern as the functionalist approach to mind of recent philosophers and workers in the field of artificial intelligence. It is a move that should tempt anyone who sees the conceptual connection between mind and function. The second step in the Freudian subdivision of mind is more problematic: that is, to *personify* each of the mental "structures" that were initially given a functional definition.

One personifies functions, or aggregates of functions in a person, in the same way that one personifies animals, stones, or corporations: One attributes causal agency (autonomy) and practical reason (rationality) to them. Such attributions are rampant throughout Freud's discussion of id, ego, and superego. I refer not so much to the famous likening of the ego to "a man on horseback" in its relation to the id,[105] which has a heavily metaphorical cast to it. Consider rather such attributions of causal agency as Freud's early statement that "control over the body" passes from one's ego, and its will, to an opposing "counter-will" when one performs an erroneous action.[106] Or, "Psychoanalysis . . . can say to the ego:'. . . a part of the activity of your own mind has been withdrawn from your knowledge and from the command of your will.' "[107] Or, "The ego is in the habit of transforming the id's will into action as if it were its own."[108]

Analogously, Freud attributes practical reason—belief/desire sets and intentions—to these subcomponents, as in: "The ego must on the whole carry out the id's intentions."[109] Or, the "superego . . . enjoys a certain degree of autonomy, follows its own intentions."[110] Or, "Resistance can only be a manifestation of the ego, which originally put the repression into force and now wishes to maintain it."[111]

Aside from causal agency and practical reason, other attributes usually reserved for whole persons are also attributed to these subagencies. They have emotions and feelings (in melancholia, "the ego . . . feels itself hated and persecuted by the superego, instead of loved"[112]); they not only operate unconsciously but they also are themselves unconscious;[113] they have a limited character at least ("The ego is peace-loving and would like to incorporate the symptom, to include it in its ensemble."[114]); they have their own self-respect and pride to maintain ("If the ego has successfully resisted a temptation to do something that would be objectionable to the superego, it feels its self-respect raised and its pride increased, as though it had made some precious acquisition."[115]); the id can have rights[116] and the ego, responsibility.[117]

This kind of language goes far beyond the division of mind on functional principles. What such language betokens is personlike agencies within every person. As Freud on occasion admitted, at least with respect to the ego, he had "personified" it and "set it up as a separate organism."[118]

A typical response of modern psychoanalysts is to be somewhat embarrassed by this personification of what were originally functional subdivisions of the mind. Heinz Hartmann, for example, attributes the "accusation against analysis of an anthropomorphization of its concepts" in part to "Freud's liking for occasional striking metaphors."[119] All is well, such analysts assure us, because such metaphor can be eliminated: "In all those cases a more careful formulation can be substituted which will dispel this impression."[120]

Such statements remind one of B. F. Skinner's like claims that *his* extensive use of mentalist vocabulary could be paraphrased away to the austere language of behaviorism, if someone gave him adequate reason to do it.[121] In fact, such eliminations of animistic "metaphor" are not so easy, for either Skinnerian or Freudian psychologists. There are two reasons for this. To begin with, there is Irving Thalberg's point[122] that even a metaphor must point us toward some hidden similarity between two classes of things. The old metaphor, "Man is a wolf," would not pass muster even as a metaphor (to say nothing of passing muster as an original contribution to zoological theory) if there were not some similarity between humans and wolves.[123] As Freud recognized with one of his earlier animistic metaphors, "These crude hypotheses, the two chambers, the doorkeeper on the threshold between them, and consciousness as a spectator at the end of the second room, must indicate an extensive approximation to the actual reality."[124] To make out the personification of ego, id, and superego, even as a metaphor, thus involves pointing out what it is about these structures that makes them very much *like* persons. If such likenesses are that these structures all possess causal agency and practical reason, have a rich emotional life and some character structure, and can meaningfully be said to exercise rights and be held responsible, then by our ideas of personhood this is no metaphor: These structures *are* persons.

The second reason that makes it difficult for psychoanalysts to adopt Hartmann's kind of response is that there is some theoretical necessity for these Freudian animisms' *not* being eliminated. It is costly to Freudians to deanimize Freud's psychic structures. What it costs them is some of the claimed explanatory power of the theory. For if ego, id, and superego do not really have causal powers and practical reason, and do not really enter into the complex "personal" relations Freud ascribes to them, it is very difficult to make out how the structural metapsychology *explains* anything. As a functional organization of the mind such structuralism is unproblematic; but a functional organization is a descriptive, classificatory device, as we saw in Chapter 1.[125] A functional organization does not explain particular

The Challenge of Psychiatry

behavior in the way in which Freud seeks to explain behavior by the animistic interactions between ego, id, and superego. To say, for example, that a corporation failed to seize some opportunity because the board of directors failed to perform its function is explanatory not because the corporation decision-making process can be given a functional organization. It can, but needed to make out this "failure of function" by the board as an explanation for a particular decision by the corporation is that there really be a board of directors composed of flesh and blood people with causal powers and practical reason. "Board of Directors" cannot simply name an aggregation of functions necessary for corporate decision making to take place. Such a functionally defined entity must also have the structure and characteristics of a thing—in this case, a group of people—if it can be cited as a *cause* of some decision by the corporation.

All of this was stated very succinctly years ago by Ernst Nagel. Finding it "tempting to read all this as just metaphorical language, a convenient and dramatically suggestive way of talking," Nagel found nonetheless "such a reading difficult to carry through if one is to make consistent sense of the theory."[126] Such reading is difficult, Nagel said, because "of the causal powers the theory ascribes to its theoretical entities. If these causal ascriptions are themselves construed figuratively, I cannot make ends meet in understanding the theory as a supposedly 'dynamic' account of human personality and conduct."[127]

The short of it is that Freud and his followers not only have personalized what was initially a functionally defined subdivision of the mind, but they also are required to do so if they are to maintain the claimed explanatory power of the structural metapsychology. We shall now turn to the consequences for our pre-Freudian conception of "our selves" that such a disunity of self would entail.

THE CHALLENGE TO LAW OF THE CORPORATE SELF

As stated in the beginning of Chapter 2, we should regard a concept such as "person" as having both criteria for its correct use and legal and moral consequences attached to its use in certain contexts. We should accordingly distinguish two sorts of consequences a radical alteration of that concept would have: the ramifications such alteration would cause in our basic metaphysics about what persons are; and the consequences for the moral and legal doctrines that use the concept. I shall discuss the impact Freud's fracturing of the self would have in each such area.

Metaphysical Consequences of Disunity of Self

"Metaphysical" is not here used in a pejorative sense. All that is meant by the word in this context is to identify those consequences of disunity that would threaten our most general and abstract aspects of ourselves. There appear to be at least three aspects to our nature that seem to demand or make important that we have some concept of the unity of the self. The first stems from the way in which we individuate mental states, on the one hand, and physical states, on the other hand. We individuate mental states such as intentions, hopes, desires, and fears, not only by their contents and the time at which they are held, but also by the person who holds them. Two people who each desire that the very same state of affairs obtain at the very same time still have (numerically) distinct desires. By contrast, we individuate physical states—using the phrase very broadly to encompass dispositional states and functional states as well as straightforwardly physical states—in part by the physical body whose states they are.

If we are "disunified" in what I take to be the basic sense, viz., that there is more than one person per human body, then we may rule out any nondualist solutions to the mind/body problem. Suppose, for example, there were three persons per body. A mental state that we normally would regard as one mental state token, we now must regard as three.[128] Yet the corresponding physical state with which we might hope to identify the mental state in question is only one state (unless perchance there should turn out to be three distinct physical states in the brain for just those mental states we assign to three different people). This would seem to rule out any identification of mental states with physical states and thus preclude adopting any of the three most tempting metaphysical views on the relation of bodies and minds, namely, materialism, behaviorism, and functionalism.[129] Indeed, one would seem to be committed to some form of dualism, with all of the problems so well detailed in the philosophy of mind since Gilbert Ryle.[130] The way not to be saddled with dualist metaphysics is to adhere to the idea of "the unity of the self" in one of its important senses, namely, that there is only one person to be found "in" any given human body.

Analogous problems arise for our basic ideas about human actions if we begin to think of each human being as composed of multiple selves. How one individuates human actions has been a much-debated matter in the contemporary philosophy of action. There are proponents of "fine-grained" modes of individuating, proponents of "coarse-grained" modes, and compromise positions.[131] Taken for granted by both sides of the contemporary debate is that one can individuate *basic* acts, no matter how one comes out on identifying such basic acts with more complex acts. The way in which we individuate basic acts is in part by the person whose acts they are. If two different people perform the very same kind of basic act, those are two distinct acts. By contrast, the bodily movements that in some suitably loose sense "constitute" the basic acts[132] are individuated by the body whose movements they are.

The Challenge of Psychiatry

Again, contradiction seems imminent if we maintain those modes of individuating acts and movements and maintain that there is more than one person per human body. Suppose, for example, some action is a "compromise formation" between the activities of the id and of the ego. There should be two basic acts by these "people," but they have only one body through which they can act. By the bodily movement criterion, this should be one basic act, but by the personal criterion there should be two. The only way for a multiple selves theorist to avoid the contradiction would be to deny that there is any special relation between some particular raising of an arm and the basic act of raising that arm on that occasion. However one comes out on Wittgenstein's famous question of what is left over if we subtract the fact that my arm goes up from the fact that I raise it,[133] it surely is not going to be that the movement and the act bear no intimate relation to one another.[134]

The third of our metaphysical needs stems from the experience we have of ourselves as being the same self both at a time and over time. We usually experience simultaneous perceptions, imaginings, emotions, intentions, inferences, and the like, as being *ours* (and thus of one person); moreover, we remember past experiences as being ours as well. Whether this unity of consciousness can be made into a necessary or a sufficient criterion for identifying persons has been a much-debated matter since Locke.[135] To the extent that there is such an experience of unity—and some of the data of psychoanalytic theory rather directly challenge this—it surely at least inclines us to a view that there is at most one self in our bodies at any given time.

Moral and Legal Consequences of Disunity of Self

Persons as the Holders of Rights: The most basic facts about our nature—our physical embodiment and our possession of consciousness—suggest some doctrine(s) of the unity of the self. In addition to these metaphysical needs for such a doctrine, our moral and legal theories seemingly presuppose the same doctrine. Consider first persons as the holders of moral or legal rights. Each person, for example, has a right to receive justice in the distribution of social goods. Any plausible theory of distributive justice will involve the idea of the equality of persons and their prima facie entitlement to an equal distribution of social goods. Such ideas make sense only if they presuppose some way of individuating persons; the principle of individuation our sense of justice rather clearly employs is one person per body. Otherwise, for example, pregnant women, multiple personality persons, and classical Freudians would all be able to use the car pool lanes reserved for more than one person on the freeways, even though they were, so to speak, "by themselves."

Our assignment of property rights also presupposes some unity of the self. Consider the ownership we each have of our own bodies, a property relation insofar as we can sell our hair or blood, donate our organs, and exclude other persons from contact or intrusion. Suppose one is a Lockean about property rights, so that in the first instance such rights are acquired either by possession or by the mixing of one's labor with the property. If there is more than one self per body, this leads to some very strange results. Suppose, for example, that we were to think of a person with multiple personalities as being different persons at different times. Presumably the first person to "possess" the body gains title to it on the occupation version of Locke's theory. Alternatively, on the labor theory, presumably the first self that improves the body in some way (through a regimen of exercise, perhaps, or the acquisition of a sexual partner) gains the property rights. (Gluttonous selves would, in either version, be excluded from owning the body because of the Lockean proviso against waste.) In any case, however title is acquired, one would want to know what would happen when the owner "left." Should this be treated as an abandonment? Even if it is, perhaps there was fraud on the part of the second possessor (i.e., self-deception), which would vitiate any purported abandonment. Alternatively, suppose the ownership relation continues after the first self leaves. Eventually its title would be lost because of the running of the statute of limitations for the recovery of "personal" property, because typically title is lost to another who takes adverse possession. Of course, one should not be too hasty here, for sometimes the statute of limitations may be tolled if the owner is out of the jurisdiction, which presumably the first possessing self was when another self took charge. Additionally, such a self might again raise a claim of fraud, a good defense to adverse possession, if there is (self-)deception with regard to the intent to remain in possession.

This is admittedly a rather silly story, but like most reductio ad absurdum arguments the point is to thrust the absurdity of the conclusion back on to the premises that generated it. Since neither the Lockean theory of property nor the idea of property rights in a body is *that* silly, that leaves the idea of more than one person per body as the premise that causes all the problems.

Persons as the Subjects of Responsibility: Our moral and legal theories not only assign rights to persons; they also ascribe responsibility. These theories too would be considerably different than they are if we could not assume the unity of the self. One can see this by adverting to the conditions under which responsibility is ascribed, in both morals and law. As examined in Chapter 2, we hold someone prima facie culpable if he per-

The Challenge of Psychiatry

forms an action intentionally causing harm; we hold him actually culpable if, in addition, he lacked any of the justifications or excuses for actions that mitigate or eliminate responsibility.

The notion of multiple selves would make a hash of the conditions under which we ascribe moral fault, for it would lead to contradiction at every turn. Multiple selves, some of whom are knowledgeable and some of whom are ignorant, would result in actions being both intentional (for the knowing self) and unintentional (for the ignorant self) in every case. Indeed, insofar as knowledge is the hallmark of basic actions, every basic act by some subagent would also fail to be a basic act by some other subagent of a multiple-personed body. Such contradictory implications for responsibility would also exist if one had to apply established excuses from responsibility to multiple selves. Consider one excuse, duress, acting under threat by another. Given the dynamic relation Freudian theory posits between the ego and the id, the result would be that one self would be acting under the threat of another self;[136] in such a case, responsibility would be undeterminable, because if there is one self who is threatened and thus excused, there is another self who is the threatener and who would not be excused. So in excuses, as in the prima facie case, there will be no answer to the overall question, Was he (the whole human being) responsible? For in all cases he both was and was not.

Because the ascription of moral fault is a necessary condition to the imposition of liability in criminal law, this quandary about moral responsibility would also be a quandary about legal liability. Unless one could devise punishments that punished only the guilty self in some body, multiple selves within the same body would face the legal system with the choice between a radically extended system of vicarious responsibility, or not punishing anyone ("Better to let ten guilty selves go free than to punish one innocent self?").

Persons as the Subject of Self-Interest: As a last example of the presupposition of the unified self of our moral and legal theories, consider the calculation of self-interest recommended by egoism. Although egoism is not much of a *moral* theory, we all have a special concern for our own self-interest, and so will share any presuppositions of unified selves of this theory. If there are multiple selves sharing the same body, our idea of *self*-interest would be considerably different than it is. We conceive of self-interest in terms of all of our needs at a time. We arrive at our overall self-interest by taking into account all of the needs, desires, and emotions that seem relevant to any particular decision. Yet if my ego, say were a different self than my id, why should the one care about the other? Presumably each—themselves being "egoists"—have that special concern only for their own self-interests.

Regarding some of our mental states as belonging to another would not reflect our experience in taking such interests into account as *ours* in framing our overall self-interest. We weigh such interests and form what, in Chapter 2, we called second-order desires with regard to them, that is, we may discount some desires because we think them less worthy than others. This kind of merging of component wants into an overall want would be impossible if we have separate selves within the body. Rather, "one" (whoever that is) would have to construct either a social welfare function for "interpersonal" utility comparisons, or adopt a scheme of distributive justice between such selves, in order to calculate what we call (overall) self-interest. Not only is the first no more possible for selves within a body than it is for separately embodied selves, and not only is the second inconsistent with egoism, but neither mode of taking into account the differing interests one may have on any particular occasion squares with our experience of forming such components into our own self-interest.

In each of these ways, our moral and legal theories demand that we regard ourselves as unitary. Not surprisingly, this presupposition matches that required by our most basic, metaphysical conception of ourselves. The single self presupposed by our being embodied and having conscious experience is the same single self that can hold rights, be responsible, and maximize its own or others' self-interest. Psychoanalytic theory is as interesting as it is partly because it seems to challenge this very basic presupposition of our metaphysics and morals.

II Rationality and madness

4 Does Madness Exist?

DOUBTLESSLY THE MOST dramatic way to combat the challenge of modern psychiatry's extended view of madness is to adopt a position exactly the opposite of that which one would combat. With a rather nice symmetry one might answer those post-Freudian psychiatrists who urge that we are *all* crazy, by saying that *no one* is crazy. Such an answer not only heightens the disagreement as much as possible, but it also relieves one from the difficult task of drawing any line between the healthy and the ill, the bad and the sick. For in such a view, there is no such line to be drawn.

Such a response is to be found in the work of the "radical psychiatrists," the most prominent and most theoretically ambitious of whom is Thomas Szasz. For over two decades Szasz and his followers have been proclaiming mental illness to be a myth. As might be expected, repetition of this mantra has hardly furthered any serious analysis about the nature of concepts like mental illness or madness, nor about their moral and legal relevance. Indeed, quite the reverse. Answers to essentially ethical and political questions about psychiatric practices or legal doctrines with regard to the mentally ill have been given by trundling out the contemporary shibboleth that mental illness is a myth, rather than in terms of the ethical and political arguments necessary for such answers. There has developed a disturbing tendency to regard complicated legal issues, notably the proper place of mental illness in various legal tests (of insanity in criminal trials, of incompetency to perform various legal acts or to stand trial, the tests for civil commitment), as solved by the new truth that mental illness is but a myth anyway. Equally disturbing is the accompanying belief that problems of social policy and social justice, such as what in fact society should do with dangerous persons who have not committed any criminal acts, can be satisfactorily resolved if legislatures will but recognize mental illness for the sham that it is.

If mental illness were a myth, acceptance of such a truth would provide straightforward answers to such legal, ethical, and political questions. One would not have to muddle along in the grubby details of comparing awful prisons with almost as awful hospitals for the criminally insane. One would not have to grapple with difficult policy issues such as the rationale for punishment generally and its relation to those found not guilty by reason of insanity. For it would be instantly clear that those we call mentally ill should be punished just like anyone else if they commit a criminal act; that they should have all the rights of an accused criminal if society should seek to deprive them of their liberty, no matter how the proceeding or the place of confinement might be named; that legal tests should abolish the phrase; and, easiest of all, that psychiatrists should mind their own business and leave the law to the lawyers.

The problem is that mental illness is not a myth. It is not some palpable falsehood propagated among the populace by power-mad psychiatrists, as Szasz in increasingly strident tones has proclaimed; it is a cruel and bitter reality that has been with the human race since antiquity. This is such an obvious truism that to have stated it thirty years ago would have been an embarrassment. Since the advent of radical psychiatry and its legal entourage, however, such truths need restatement. Even more, they need restatement in a form specifically addressed to the various senses in which mental illness has been thought to be a myth. Since in my reading of the radical psychiatrists there seem to be five distinguishable points they have in mind in thinking of mental illness as a myth, the discussion will proceed by considering them seriatim.

The Mythology of Radical Psychiatry

THE MYTH AS A QUESTION OF ONTOLOGICAL STATUS:
THERE IS NO SUCH THING AS MENTAL ILLNESS
BECAUSE THERE IS NO REFERENT
OF THE PHRASE

Mental illness is a myth because, stated popularly, "There is neither such a thing as 'insanity' nor such a thing as 'mental disease.' These terms do not identify entities having separate existence."[1]

Less popularly: "It is a term without ostensive referrent [sic] and lacking any, it cannot even be said to have outlived its usefulness, because there is no reason to think that it ever had any."[2] Szasz and his psychiatric and legal followers are suspicious of mental illness as an entity or thing; when looking into their ontology they see no such thing. Three points require discussion here.

1. If the argument is that entity thinking *as such* is to be regarded with suspicion, as Szasz at times suggests, then the critique is radical indeed. As Quine has noted, "We talk so inveterately of objects that to say we do so

seems almost to say nothing at all; for how else is there to talk?"[3] "Thing theory" is implicit throughout our ordinary and scientific speech, and it is simply wrong to regard it as some primitive form of speech that is replaced with a more sophisticated mode of talk with the maturity of a science. Thus, Szasz's statement that "entity thinking has always preceded process-thinking"[4] is not an accurate characterization of the development of modern science. In fact, higher-order theoretical statements characteristic of advancing science *increase* the number of entities we admit into our ontology, not decrease it. Forces, fields, and electrons are obvious examples.

2. If the argument is that entity thinking is scientifically legitimate, but only about those entities referred to by terms capable of *ostensive* reference (i.e., things that can be pointed at such as Nixon or St. Elizabeth's Hospital), the radical psychiatrists have a radically impoverished ontology – a nominalist ontology that would not admit the thinghood of abstract entities such as the number 2, squareness, shape, zoological species, or, more to the point perhaps, psychological states. Such a restricted ontology is characteristic neither of science nor of common understanding.

In response to this charge of nominalism, made by me in an earlier article criticizing Szasz, David Levin has urged that "the caution and skepticism of the radical (existential) psychiatrists . . . has nothing to do with a Quinean predilection for desert landscapes."[5] Yet much of the popular appeal of the "There is no such thing as mental illness" slogan stems from just this kind of nominalist understanding of what there is. When Szasz or even his more sophisticated defenders tell us that mental illness does not refer to any "specific, punctuate, somehow localizable entities,"[6] they imply that the phrase must have such a reference on pain of being a myth. This *is* a kind of nominalism about what there is that holds mental illness to a standard that could not be met by the numerous abstract terms of any theoretical science.

Indeed, in such a restrictive, nominalist ontological system physical illnesses would not exist either. For the names of physical illnesses do not refer to concrete entities: "Diseases are not things in the same sense as rocks, or trees, or rivers. Diseases . . . are not material."[7] Although diseases might be *caused* by the presence in the body of some such entity (as a cold may be caused by a virus), and although they might be associated with *symptoms* that are concrete entities (e.g., the fluid present in the sinuses), a physical illness is not (identical with) either its causes or its symptoms. The only thing one can fix as the referent of the names of various physical illnesses are states the ill are in, abstract entities incapable of being pointed at in some ostensive definition.

3. In any case, most of the things people have wanted to say about mental illness can be said without making ontological commitments to any entity, concrete or abstract, referred to by the phrase, and thus any criti-

cism of its use based on its lack of a referent, ostensive or otherwise, is misconceived. In his essay on "Sense and Reference" Frege made famous the distinction between the sense of a term and its reference.[8] The important corollary for our purpose is that words may be used significantly (i.e., they may make good sense) and yet *not refer*. As Quine has elaborated, "Being a name of something is a much more special feature than being meaningful." Even "a singular term need not name to be significant."[9]

This is particularly evident in our use of predicates. We can say "Some dogs are white" or "Some houses are red," without making ontological commitments to (without presupposing there are such things as) whiteness or redness. Similarly, we can say "Some persons are mentally ill" without making ontological commitments to any *thing* referred to by "illness." More colloquially, denial of the existence of anything called mental illness hardly entails a denial of the existence of *persons* who are mentally ill.

In addition to describing people as being mentally ill, we also often wish to explain their behavior as being due to their mental illness. Although such statements as "He did it because of his mental illness" appear to require an entity referred to by mental illness, in fact, such explanations mean nothing more than is conveyed by "He did it because he is mentally ill" — another use of the predicate "is mentally ill" that does not require a reference to be significant.

To the extent that common and psychiatric discourse about mental illness can be paraphrased so as to avoid the hypostasis of an entity named by the phrase, then any criticism that complains that there is no such thing as mental illness is beside the point; for orthodox psychiatry and common understanding can happily agree, but still use the phrase to make significant (albeit nonreferring) statements. We often make use of the names of states, attributes, properties, and traits as if they named some things in our ontology, for economy of speech is often gained by so doing.[10] To be sure, if someone (such as Szasz) makes an issue of the ontological commitments involved in our uses of redness or illness, "the burden is of course on us to paraphrase or retract."[11] But if we can paraphrase the usage into the noncommitting use of "ill," then the phraseology is a harmless but convenient mode of speaking against which the "ontological discovery" of radical psychiatry is irrelevant.

For my own part I think this detour into ontology is a red herring. The lack of any thing one can point to as the referent of mental illness does not do orthodox psychiatry the damage Szasz and others suppose; if mental illness is a myth in this sense, it is in the good company of many other words and phrases useful in science and everyday life that have either no reference or a reference only to abstract entities. That this herring is constantly being dragged across our path is doubtless due to the immense popular appeal of the denial-of-existence idiom in the hands of a skillful polemicist. It makes psychiatry and the study of mental illness *sound* about as useful as "unicornology" and the study of unicorns.

Szasz has accused me generally of putting words in his mouth[12] and has specifically denied that he makes this ontological version of the myth argument:

> I do not assert, as some of my critics claim, that psychiatry is not a science because it deals with non-existent things, such as "mental illness."[13]

This is hard to square with Szasz's repeated assertion of just this argument, as in:

> Psychiatry is said to be a medical specialty concerned with the study and treatment of mental illness. Similarly, astrology was the study of the influence of planetary movements and positions on human behavior and destiny. These are typical instances of defining a science by specifying the subject matter of study. These definitions completely disregard method and are based instead on false substantives ... But suppose, for a moment, that there is no such thing as mental illness and health. Suppose, further, that these words refer to nothing more substantial or real than the astrological conception of planetary influences on human conduct. What then?[14]

In any event, perhaps Szasz and his defenders agree that "it is no part of the radical (existential) position to argue 'occamistically' that ... there is no such thing as mental illness."[15] If so, the ontological status of some *thing* called mental illness is not really at issue here. Other types of arguments must thus be marshaled if mental illness is in some sense to be made out to be a mere myth.

THE MYTH AS AN EMPIRICAL DISCOVERY:
NO ONE IS IN FACT MENTALLY ILL

Often mental illness is said to be a myth, not just in the sense that it does not exist, but also in the sense that no one is in fact mentally ill. The claim, in other words, denies not just that mental illness is a name of some thing, but that mentally ill is ever truly predicable of a person. The claim is that no one is really mentally ill.

This claim that mental illness is a myth is put forward as an empirical discovery: All of those people who have been thought to be mentally ill (i.e., irrational) are in fact just as rational as you and I. Szasz makes this claim when he argues that "insane behavior no less than sane, is goal-directed and motivated," and concludes from this that we should regard "the behavior of the madman as perfectly rational from the point of view of the actor."[16] Braginsky, Braginsky, and Ring purport to have made the same "discovery" regarding schizophrenics:

159

> The residents who remain in "mental hospitals" are behaving in a perfectly rational manner to achieve a personally satisfying way of life—often the most satisfying of which they are capable... in a certain sense an individual *chooses* his career as a mental patient; it is not thrust upon him as a consequence of his somehow becoming "mentally ill." But in just what sense does the individual "choose" his career? In our view, having and maintaining the status of a mental patient is the outcome of *purposive* behavior. Furthermore, given the life circumstances of most of the persons who become and remain residents of mental hospitals, their doing so evinces a realistic appraisal of their available alternatives; it is, in short, a *rational* choice.[17]

The central thrust of this form of the argument is not to claim that mental illness and mentally ill are meaningless—their meaning is assumed to be closely connected with that of irrational—but to dispute as a factual matter that there are persons who fit the agreed-upon definition of mental illness (irrationality). In fact, however, what has been done here is not to present a discovery of new facts, overlooked by orthodox psychiatrists because of their own self-interest or whatever, but rather to stretch our concepts of rationality and purposive behavior to accommodate within their criteria facts well known to orthodox, as well as to radical, psychiatrists. The facts—the behavior of patients—are often undisputed. What is disputed is the precise nature of the criterion to be applied in judging the behavior as rational or not.

As the foregoing quotations from Szasz and Braginsky et al. make clear, the notion of rationality they employ is linked to the actor's having reasons for his actions. As we explored in Chapters 1 and 2, the relationship between an agent's being thought to be rational and his acting for reasons is best brought out by the Aristotelian idea of a practical syllogism. When we explain an action by giving the actor's reason, we refer to a belief/desire set the contents of which fit the form of a valid practical syllogism. To act so as to satisfy *any* valid practical syllogism is to be *minimally* rational as we earlier defined that phrase. There are also, as we explored, several stronger senses of rational that impose requirements of intelligibility on desires, evidential well-foundedness on beliefs, consistency between different beliefs or different desires, transitivity of desires, and the like. We can for now put these stronger senses of rational to the side, because by and large the empirical version of the myth argument is only intended to show that the behavior of the mentally ill is rational in the minimal sense defined earlier; that is, *some* set of beliefs and desires (no matter how bizarre) is furthered by the act in question.

The crunch for even this limited attempt at making out the behavior of the mentally ill as rational comes in making more precise the nature of the beliefs and desires of mental patients in terms of which their actions are to be so adjudged. More specifically, the fudge occurs with the use of *unconscious* beliefs and desires to fill in where we all know that mental patients did not consciously guide their actions to achieve such goals in light of such beliefs. Braginsky et al. are explicit about this: "It is obvious that rational goal-directed behavior does not guarantee that the individual appreciates what he is up to."[18] Szasz's glossing over of this distinction is particularly transparent:

> In describing this contrast between lying and erring, I have deliberately avoided the concept of consciousness. It seems to me that when the adjectives "consciously" and "unconsciously" are used as explanations, they complicate and obscure the problem. The traditional psychoanalytic idea that so-called conscious imitation of illness is "malingering" and hence "not illness," whereas its allegedly unconscious simulation is itself "illness" ("hysteria"), creates more problems than it solves. It would seem more useful to *distinguish between goal-directed and rule-following behavior on the one hand, and indifferent mistakes on the other* . . . In brief, *it is more accurate to regard hysteria as a lie than as a mistake.* People caught in a lie usually maintain that they are merely mistaken. The difference between mistakes and lies, when discovered, is chiefly pragmatic. From a purely cognitive point of view, both are simply falsehoods.[19]

The fudge occurs in the shift from our judgments of rationality being based largely on the agent's conscious beliefs and objectives, to a notion of rationality by virtue of which we adjudge an action as rational if we can *posit* any set of beliefs or objectives with which we can explain the action. The problem is that it is notoriously easy to posit beliefs and desires to explain any finite sequence of the behavior of anything. Simply pick a consequence of the behavior and label it the objective, pick a set of beliefs by virtue of which it would appear likely that such a consequence would indeed ensue as a result of the behavior, and one is then in a position to adjudge the behavior as rational, relative to that objective and that set of beliefs. The shedding of leaves by a tree, the falling of stones, the pumping of blood by the heart, and the most chaotic word salad of a schizophrenic are all "rational" activities, judged by such a standard. The "action" of a tree in shedding its leaves is rational if we suppose that it desires to survive the coming winter, and believes that the only way to do this is to lower its sap level, thereby killing off its leaves. Similarly for stones, hearts, and schizophrenics.

The reason why such explanations are so easy to manufacture lies in the inherent ambiguity of behavior as a criterion for such matters. If we know by some independent means that an agent believes that action A will lead to result R, and he does A, we have good grounds for attributing to him a desire for R; if we know that he desires R and that he does A, we have equally good grounds for supposing that he believes that *A* will lead to *R*. But if we know neither his beliefs nor his desires, but only that he does *A* and that *A* does result in *R*, we have no means of singling out *R* as his motive, for any other consequence of *A* would do as well. "There is nothing in a pure behaviorist theory to prevent us from regarding each piece of behavior as a desire for whatever happens next."[20]

Neither Braginsky's "goal-directed" nor Szasz's "rule-following" criteria are adequate here. As was discussed in Chapter 1, such Wittgensteinian patter fails to distinguish between behavior that happens to have a pattern to it and behavior that has the pattern it does because the actor whose behavior it is *followed* that pattern as he acted. All sequences of behavior have patterns to them; indeed, for any finite sequence there is an infinite number of such patterns (rules) that will fit that sequence. To make rule-following into a criterion with which one can *discover* belief/desire sets, and not merely *posit* their existence, Szasz and company must tell us when an actor truly is following some rule, that is, when he actually has a belief/desire set that includes the rule in its contents.[21] The most plausible candidate as a criterion for such rule-following lies in the actor's first-person knowledge, including his extended memory.[22] But such a criterion gets Szasz back to the consciousness (or the potential for consciousness) criterion that he is so eager to abandon.

Thus Szasz can "avoid the concept of consciousness" only at the price of significance. What he fails to realize is that any behavior can be seen as rational (or as in accordance with rules of a game, or as furthering certain goals—Szasz's substitute criteria for consciousness), if one allows oneself the freedom to *invent* the beliefs and desires in terms of which the behavior is to be so viewed.

On occasion the empirical version of the myth claim is put forward without any extensive reliance on some supposed unconscious beliefs or desires of the mentally ill. R. D. Laing, in particular, explicitly disavows use of unconscious beliefs or desires in reaching his well-known conclusion that "*without exception* the experience and behavior that gets labelled schizophrenic is *a special strategy that a person invents in order to live in an unlivable situation.*"[23] Nonetheless, such studies do not show schizophrenics to be as rational as everyone else, for the conscious beliefs such patients admittedly do have are themselves irrational beliefs; and the actions that are predicated on irrational beliefs, and actors who hold them, are, in common understanding, irrational.

This is quite clear with regard to many of Laing's reported patients. The woman who avoids crowds may be rational in so doing, *given* her belief that "when she was in a crowd she felt the ground would open up under her feet." Similarly, many of the peculiar actions of one who believes that "she had an atom bomb inside her"[24] may be rational, *given* such a belief.

Does Madness Exist?

But the beliefs themselves are irrational, with the result that neither the agent nor the action they explain can be said to be rational. To be sure, Laing's studies of the "social intelligibility" of schizophrenic symptoms do not end with the discovery of such obvious beliefs; Laing often attempts to go further and explain how such beliefs could be formed by an individual in the patient's situation. Yet the explanation Laing typically gives—the patient "adopts" the symptom as the only response to an intolerable situation—involves reference to further beliefs that are also irrational.

A convenient example is the case of "Joan," a catatonic who was not one of Laing's patients but whose case Laing believed to afford "striking confirmation" of his views regarding schizophrenia. Joan's own subsequent avowals were used by Laing in attributing to her catatonic withdrawal a rational basis. She recalled that when she was catatonic, she "tried to be dead and grey and motionless." She thought that her mother "would like that: She could carry me around like a doll." She also felt that she "had to die to keep from dying. I know that sounds crazy but one time a boy hurt my feelings very much and I wanted to jump in front of a subway. Instead I went a little catatonic so I wouldn't feel anything."[25]

Laing finds in such statements the two typical motives for catatonic withdrawal. First, "There is the primary guilt of having no right to life . . . and hence of being entitled at most only to a dead life." Since Joan's parents had wanted a boy, and since "she could not be anything other than what her parents wanted her to be," she sought to be "nothing," that is a passive catatonic.[26] Second, Joan's withdrawal was viewed by Laing as a defensive mechanism to avoid the loss of identity (Joan's metaphorical dying) with which she was threatened by any normal relationship with others: "One no longer fears being crushed, engulfed, overwhelmed by realness and aliveness . . . since one is already dead [by the catatonic withdrawal]. Being dead, one cannot die, and one cannot kill. The anxieties attendant on the schizophrenic's phantastic omnipotence are undercut by living in a condition of phantastic impotence."[27]

None of this would convince us that Joan or others like her were rational in effecting catatonic withdrawal (even if we were convinced that at least in her case the withdrawal was an *action* she performed for reasons at all). Her action (or nonaction) is based on a series of beliefs that are irrational, including her belief in a disembodied self, a belief in her parents' complete determination of her worth, and a belief in her own omnipotence and impotence.

It is sometimes thought that the rationality of beliefs cannot be objectively judged and that calling them irrational is simply a pejorative way of saying they are false. The conclusion in the present context would be that people like Joan are thus as rational as the rest of us, only mistaken about certain facts. The analysis toward the close of Chapter 2 was intended to forestall just such an objection. Prima facie, the most obvious way to differentiate beliefs that are irrational from those that are merely false is by looking, first, at the consistency of the belief with other beliefs of the patient, and second, at the coherence of the belief with all else the patient believes. With regard to consistency, if Joan believes both that she is omnipotent and that she is impotent, one or both of those beliefs is irrational. With regard to coherence, one must look at the influence relevant evidence would have on the holder of the belief. It is characteristic of irrational (incoherent) beliefs that their holders maintain them despite the lack of coherence with other beliefs they have. There is a "fixed" or "frozen" nature about such beliefs, in the sense that they are not corrigible by relevant evidence. Such irrational beliefs are held with a strength (relative to other beliefs the actor has) disproportionate to the evidence known to the actor. Thus, the man "who believes very strongly that his brother is trying to poison him (in spite of appearances) and who believes, rather weakly by comparison, that Boston is north of New York, is likely to be flying in the face of the evidence and the claims that the evidence renders likely."[28] He is likely, in other words, to be irrational in his belief of his imminent poisoning.

The empirical version of the myth argument fails because it is, empirically, false. By our shared concept of what it is to be rational, the mentally ill are not as rational as the rest of the population. Only by muddling the concept of rationality have the radical psychiatrists appeared to call into question this obvious truth. Only by attributing unconscious beliefs and desires to the mentally ill for which there is no evidence, or only by referring to beliefs that are themselves irrational, can motives be found for all of the peculiar behavior symptomatic of mental illness. Neither of these moves satisfies what we usually mean by rational as applied to actions and agents. One may, of course, like Humpty Dumpty, choose to make a word like rationality mean what one pleases, but surely it is unhelpful when one does so to then present the *manufactured* match between the facts and the new criteria for the word as a discovery of new facts, previously overlooked because of the willful blindness of self-interested or power-mad psychiatrists. To do so is to manufacture one's own myths.

THE MYTH AS A CATEGORY MISTAKE: MENTAL ILLNESS IS NOT A PHYSICAL CAUSE

In *The Concept of Mind,* Gilbert Ryle made popular the notion of a category mistake. His motive for using this notion was to avoid having to take a position on the ontological status of mental entities. The dualism Ryle attributed to Descartes, that is, the two-worlds view that there are minds and there are bodies, each in its own species of existence, is difficult to maintain for all of the reasons Ryle recounts throughout the book. Yet neither form of monism—that there are only minds (idealism) or only bodies (physicalism)—seems to do justice to the way we speak of ourselves as persons. We do use mental terms such as belief, desire, or pain in apparently significant discourse, and yet when we attempt to say something about the entities to which such terms ostensibly refer, we are baffled. How do we describe a belief? What properties can we give it? Does it have physical extension? And if it has no such properties, what sort of a thing is it anyway?

Ryle sought to avoid answering these questions about the ontological status of mental entities. One kind of question we do not have to answer is a question that is not meaningful. Ryle sought a way of saying that questions of the form "Are there bodies and minds?" are not meaningful, because a category mistake has been made in conjoining a term in one category (bodies) with a term in another (minds). It is like conjoining hopes, the tide, and the average age of death to say (in the same logical tone of voice) that all three are *rising*. Ryle explicitly avoids the snare of saying that there are two species of existence (which is just dualism); he is operating on the level of language only, claiming that we use the word "exists" in two different senses when we speak of bodies and when we speak of minds.[29] Hence, a difference of linguistic categories for Ryle does not imply a difference in ontological status (nor does it exclude it).

One of the particular category mistakes that Ryle is at pains to correct throughout his book is the assumption that "there are mechanical causes of corporeal movements and mental causes of corporeal movements."[30] For Ryle this statement contains a category mistake because it is a conjunction of words in different categories—specifically, the names of the candidates for mental causes, such as belief, desire, volition, and so on, are in a different category from the kinds of words we use to label mechanical causes. Ryle later brings out this difference: He likens mental words, such as desire or motive, to dispositions, and contrasts them with mechanical causes. His well-known example is the broken window: One way of explaining the shattering of a window is to say a rock hit it; another is to say the glass was brittle, that is, it had a tendency to break when hit by a hard object. The first form of explanation refers to a mechanical cause, the second, to a dispositional property. Ryle construes motive words such as vanity or greed similarly to words such as brittle or soluble: Such words do not cite a cause, but rather a tendency of persons or objects to behave in certain sorts of ways.

By his examples, vocabulary, and explicit citation, Szasz makes it clear the he has read Ryle with approval. Thus he begins Part I of *Law, Liberty, and Psychiatry* by quoting Ryle on the nature of myths: "A myth is, of course, not a fairy story. It is the presentation of facts belonging in one category in the idioms belonging to another. To explode a myth is accordingly not to deny the facts but to re-allocate them."[31] Mental illness is a myth, then, in the same way that other mental terms are myths: It is as improper to place mental illness in the same category with real illnesses (read as physically caused illnesses) as it is to treat belief, desire, and perception as the names of mechanical or paramechanical causes.

Szasz, in fact, makes a number of distinct uses of the doctrine of categorical differences in his attack on mental illness as a myth.

1. His primary use is to focus on mental in mental illness and to argue that mental illness is a myth because mind is a myth (and hence a sick mind is a myth).
2. He also focuses on illness, to argue that the term necessarily refers to physiochemical events going on in the body; thus, to say that a *mind* could be ill is absurd because only physical bodies can be ill (in the ordinary meaning of the word).
3. Szasz also utilizes the doctrine of category difference to inveigh against any use of the names of particular mental illnesses, such as schizophrenia or hysteria, the argument here being that the symptomatologies of particular illnesses illicitly conjoin words referring to behavioral tendencies with words referring to physiological happenings in the brain, as well as with words whose only reference is to mental experience—a clear example, for Szasz, of a category mistake.
4. Finally, because of the categorical differences between mind words and brain words, Szasz appears to believe that it is logically impossible to establish correlations between the mental and behavioral-based syndromes we call mental illnesses and the brain events that may cause them; hence, the scientific aspirations of psychiatry and the medical treatment of mental illness are forever condemned to frustration because the aspirations themselves are logically absurd.

It should be noted that the first two of these arguments deal with mental illness in general, the second two with the names of particular illnesses. For clarity, it helps to keep these two discussions separated, even though they are obviously related. Thus, I shall proceed to discuss Szasz's use of the doctrine of categorical differences in the foregoing four-part order. The ultimate conclusion of all of them, it is worth emphasizing, is that mental illness, and mental illnesses, are myths.

1. What is a sick mind? Surely a large part of the appeal of the myth argument stems from the difficulty one has in answering this question.

Does Madness Exist?

One may indeed be tempted by the radical psychiatrists' reply that only bodies can be sick and that minds are not the sorts of things that can be either healthy or ill. Yet a good deal of the attraction of this argument should be eliminated once it is realized that the difficulty we have in saying anything very intelligible about what a sick mind is stems directly from the difficulty we have in saying anything very intelligible about what a mind is. For unless we are prepared to jettison our talk about minds in toto—as Szasz plainly is not—merely pointing out that mental illness has no clearer reference than does mind itself is hardly a sufficient basis for labeling it a myth.

Fixing the reference of mind, and mental words generally, is notoriously difficult. Yet, in fact, we can leave the question of reference open and still see that in no pejorative sense is a sick mind a myth. One may adopt any nondualistic position on the ontological status of mental entities (the popular ones presently being logical behaviorism, which asserts that minds are hypothetical constructs from behavior; materialism, which asserts that minds are [identical with] an as yet unknown set of physiological phenomena; functionalism, which contends that minds are functional states of physical systems; or Ryle's own position that one may avoid the question because it cannot be meaningfully framed). Perhaps mind and other mental terms are not even referential in character, as has also been suggested,[32] so that we need not worry about what sorts of things minds are. Whichever of these positions one adopts, one is immune to the kind of criticisms Ryle directed against Cartesian dualism (and which Szasz and others would redirect against the supposedly dualistic assumptions inherent in the term mental illness); for in none of them does one presuppose the existence of some funny, nonmaterial mind substance. In none of them need one who speaks of mental illness be committed to "paramechanical myths" about ghostly mind things being "injured" in some nonspatial way. Mental illness can make perfectly good sense—as much so as mind and mind words generally—no matter which of these general positions one takes as to the reference of mental terms, even if the position adopted is that none of them refer to anything.

The question "What is a sick mind?" can be left aside in favor of a more useful question: Does mental illness have as significant a descriptive/explanatory use as other mental expressions? If it does not, then "myth" is as good a pejorative label as any; but if the phrase does have a significant use, then no amount of Rylean exorcism as to the phrase's supposedly ghostly referents can suffice to eliminate it from our vocabulary.

Our mentalistic vocabulary may conveniently be divided between experiential terms and those terms we use to describe and explain human actions. Thus, when we predicate "is in pain," "is feeling tired," or "is seeing an orange afterimage" of another, we are ascribing mental experiences to him; when we predicate "is murdering," "is hiding," "is trying to hide," or "wants a yacht" of another, we describe his doings as actions and explain such actions by his (mental) intentions, desires, beliefs, motives, and so on. Since the concept of mind is intimately connected with our concept of what it is to be a person, predicating mental experiences, actions, and intentions of another being is necessary not only for saying that he has a mind, but also for thinking of that being as a person.

Mental illness is used to deny that part of our mentalistic vocabulary, namely, the action/intention predicates, is as regularly or as properly applicable to the mentally ill as it is to more normal persons. This is merely a corollary of saying that the mentally ill are not as rational as the rest of us, in the senses of rational discussed in Chapters 1 and 2. For those senses of rationality are all linked to our usage of the action/intention predicates. If an individual is irrational in the sense that his desires or beliefs are unintelligible, inconsistent, intransitively ordered, or incoherent, then the action/intention mode of explanation begins to break down. If the individual is so far gone that for some of his actions we are unable to make out any set of beliefs or desires, no matter how bizarre or inconsistent, then this mode of explanation breaks down entirely. Although no one would deny that the mentally ill have mental experiences (indeed, they may have something of a surplus), the diminished rationality of the mentally ill does entail a diminished applicability of the other part of our mentalistic vocabulary, the action/intention predicates.

If enough of the observed behavior of the same individual resists application of the action/intention predicates, we will come to regard that individual as different from most of our fellows, different because we lack *the* form of description/explanation of his behavior by virtue of which we understand ourselves and others in daily life. To identify another being as a person fully like us, we need to be able rather regularly to see his actions as promoting desires we find intelligible in light of beliefs we find rational.

A sick mind is thus properly predicated of an individual when we are unable to presuppose his rationality to the same extent we do for others. A sick mind is an incapacity to act rationally, which, in the senses of rational used here, means an incapacity to act so as to further rational desires in light of rational beliefs.

In so using mental illness one is thus committed to no funny, nonmaterial substances that are in some nonspatial way injured or impaired. Mind and other mind terms may not refer to such paramechanistic myths, but then mental illness does not either. To say that someone's mind is ill is only to say that his capacity for rational action is diminished, that the subject himself is irrational. Since mind in Ryle's own analysis is the name of all such capacities for intelligent performances, a lack of some of them may as properly invoke mind words as may the possession of them. To the extent that one is willing to say of another, "He has a mind" (or "He is a person"), then to the same extent one should be willing to say, "His mind is defective" (or "He is not fully a person"), if he in fact lacks the relevant capacities.

2. Of course, if illness meant "deviation from an anatomical or physiological norm,"[33] as Szasz believes, then *mental* illness would still make no sense—for how can a mind (or capacities for intelligent performances) deviate from physical norms? Minds cannot be normal or abnormal vis-à-vis such physiological norms, and, Szasz argues, beliefs to the contrary are simply category mistakes.

Does illness properly predicated of a person mean that that person's bodily structure is abnormal in comparison with other people's bodily structures? The first thing one wants to say is that illness was a word in the English language long before anyone knew very much about anatomy or physiology, and thus, the meaning of the word cannot be a matter of statistical deviation from a physiological or anatomical norm (else the word would have had no use prior to knowledge of such norms and such deviations). Still, one might think that our ancestors had a different concept of illness from ours. So, to move on to contemporary thought experiments, imagine an individual possessed of a cubical stomach. This stomach, although abnormal in its physical structure, functions perfectly efficiently in digesting foods; it thus allows its owner as long a life as people with normal stomachs. Suppose further it causes him no discomfort and that it allows him to eat and drink the variety and quantity of foods available in his society. Despite the presence of an abnormal physical condition, no one would call this individual ill.

What such a thought experiment shows is that physical abnormality is not a sufficient condition of being properly adjudged ill. Is such abnormality even a necessary condition of illness? Imagine an individual who possesses a small gland common to all people. As with everyone else, this gland causes him pain, increases his chance of early death, and prevents him from eating a large number of foods. Despite the fact that this physiological condition (until corrected by surgery) is universal, I should think we would want to label the state caused by it an illness, similar to the universal illnesses from which we all might suffer after a nuclear war.

What these examples show is that being ill, even physically ill, is not the same as being in a certain physical state, even if that state deviates widely from what is normal for human beings. It is not a state in which one's bodily structure deviates from a statistical norm, as Szasz argues throughout his work.[34] Deviance from a physiological norm is in itself neither a necessary nor a sufficient condition of being ill. It is at best an indication that someone *might* be ill because some physical abnormalities are correlated with some diseases (and thus with being ill).

Saying what illness does not mean is considerably easier than saying what it does mean. Yet as we shall explore in the next chapter, being ill seems to involve something like being in a state of pain or discomfort, which, if not removed, may lead to premature death, and which for its duration incapacitates the patient from certain activities thought normal in or society.[35] One might assume that such states are physically caused, but such assumptions are irrelevant to what we mean by illness. There are presumably physical causes for our being in all kinds of states, such as being a thousand miles from Paris or for being alert or angry. *Whether* there are physical causes for such states, and if so, *whether* they are manifested by abnormal physical structures, is irrelevant to whether or not one is ill, alert, angry, or a thousand miles from Paris. Merely discovering a physical deviation in no way tells us that the person whose body it is that deviates is ill. Rather, properly to predicate illness of another we need to know such things as whether he is in pain, is incapacitated, or is dying.

The reason why this has been so well camouflaged by the radical psychiatrists is that the names of *particular* illnesses, such as polio or pneumococcal pneumonia, do involve knowledge of physical causes (as discussed at the end of this section). Whether one has polio or pneumococcal pneumonia is determined in part by knowledge of the bacterium or virus involved. Yet whether one is ill (in general) is *not* determined by such causes; whether one is ill in general is determined by wholly different criteria, seemingly connected with pain, incapacitation, or hastened death.

Once one appreciates this, then the propriety of terming hysterics (mentally) ill is also evident. The activities for which one is incapacitated by a paralyzed arm do not differ a whit whether the paralysis is anatomical or hysterical; in neither case can one play baseball, tend father effectively, etc. The admittedly sincere reports of pain of a hysteric throat irritation are as good evidence that the hysteric feels pain as are such reports of one whose C fibers are really jingling with physiological pain signals due to a physically caused throat irritation. More generally, those whose capacity to act rationally is diminished because their memory, perception, reasoning abilities, or other mental faculties are impaired are incapacitated from a normal life in our society no less than is, for example, the chronic alcoholic whose short-term memory banks have been physically damaged by his long-term drinking habits (Korsakoff's syndrome).

Being in a state properly called ill, then, does not depend on one's knowing, or even in the first instance on there being, any particular physiological condition. It depends on one's being in a state characterized roughly by pain, incapacitation, and the prospect of a hastened death. There is nothing mythical about such a state, whether it be due to a broken leg or a broken home.

3. If mental illness is not a myth, that is not yet to say that psychiatry is

the scientific way to go about studying it. The claim of orthodox psychiatry to scientific expertise, in other words, rests on there being not only a nonmythical subject of study (mental illness), but also scientific knowledge about it. Some of such knowledge is to be found in the diagnostic categories of orthodox psychiatry.

It is for this reason that it has been important for radical psychiatrists to attack the validity of the traditional diagnostic categories. Szasz's version of the attack is based on Ryle's category distinctions. Szasz's primary use of the doctrine of category distinctions here is as a reminder that schizophrenia, hysteria, and so on do not presently refer to known events in physiology that cause behavior. But this is undisputed and provides no grounds for saying that schizophrenia or hysteria are mere myths, or for denying that such words have a significant use. Understanding that schizophrenia is on a par with some of our other mental-conduct terms, in that we do not know whether it refers to any set of mechanical or paramechanical causes, is not to eliminate it from our vocabulary but to "reallocate it," in the language of Ryle. The syndrome we call schizophrenia may currently explain behavior only in a way analogous to explanations in terms of character traits, that is, in terms of dispositions themselves implied from the pattern of a person's prior behavior, and not by reference to any set of physiological conditions. Yet as Ryle points out, we engage in the same construct building when we explain the breaking of glass, or the dissolution of salt, by citing the dispositional properties of brittleness or solubility. Significant explanatory (albeit nonmechanistic) truths can be framed with all such terms, and no one goes around writing books on "the myth of brittleness" or "the myth of greediness."

Szasz, however, presses the argument to claim that schizophrenia and other terms are logically absurd in ways that brittleness is not. There seem to be two versions of the category-mistake argument here. The first is the juxtaposition of behavioral symptoms and brain symptoms in the same classificatory scheme:

> Consider, for example, general paresis. This diagnosis refers to a physiochemical phenomenon. The term does not describe any particular behavioral event. How then can we hope to bring it into a meaningful relation with other psychiatric diagnoses that refer only to behavioral events, such as hysteria, reactive depression, or situational maladjustment? It is as if, in the periodic table of elements, we would find coal, steel, and petroleum interspersed among items such as helium, carbon, and sulfur. This is the main reason the taxonomic system known as psychiatric nosology does not work.[36]

Second, at other points in his works Szasz puts forward the rather curious argument that psychiatrists cannot classify human behavior because human beings react to the classificatory labels placed upon them whereas stones, plants, and stars do not. This error is not "due to any lack of humane feeling in psychiatrists, but rather to the fallacy of thinking in terms of natural science." Such an approach ignores "the differences between persons and things and the effects of language on each." In the orthodox account of mental disease, Szasz asks: "What is the status of human action? The answer is: none. There is no such thing as action to attain a goal—only behavior determined by causes. Herein lies the fundamental error of the medical and mechanomorphic approach to human behavior and to psychiatric classification."[37]

The first of these two additional attacks on the classificatory scheme is mistaken for the reasons discussed in the following subsection: There is no logical error in supposing that mental incapacities can be *correlated* with brain events to form composite symptomatologies, even if minds are not *identical* with brains. Discussion of this will be deferred briefly. The second of Szasz's arguments here obviously has nothing to do with "the logic of classification," as Szasz sometimes terms his Rylean weaponry. The blunt fact of the matter is that in everyday life and in social science we do classify human behavior all the time, and the fact that those labeled patriotic, ambitious, greedy, or schizophrenic may not care for the label has nothing whatsoever to do with their propriety for descriptive or explanatory purposes. One might have *ethical* qualms about *telling* the subjects they are being so classified, particularly if one has the authority of a psychiatrist in a mental hospital to make the label stick; such ethical qualms, or their associated therapeutic concerns, are totally beside the point if one is judging psychiatric classifications of behavior by their logical or scientific methodology. The error, if there be any, is more akin to that of a nuclear physicist working on the atomic bomb—a mistaken sense of personal value, perhaps, but hardly a mistake in the scientific methodology of nuclear physics.

There are questions that might be raised about the diagnostic categories of psychiatry, but they are not questions of category difference. The aggregation of symptoms into particular syndromes associated with hysteria, schizophrenia, and so forth forms inductive claims whose nature is clear— as clear as the nature of the claim that people who tend to look in the mirror often also tend to feel pleased when flattered and avoid conversations in which others are praised (Ryle's partial unpacking of the character trait of vanity). There is nothing logically suspect about the inductive process by which we initially classify familiar as well as bizarre behavior into character traits and mental diseases. Nor is there anything illegitimate in our seeking to find the hidden natures of either mental diseases or character traits in physiology.

4. The heaviest burden placed by Szasz on the category-mistake version of the myth argument comes in another of his uses of it, viz., his attempt

Does Madness Exist?

to construct a logical chasm out of Ryle's categorical distinctions. For Szasz not only asserts that schizophrenia and other syndromes are not currently to be explained by reference to mechanical causes, but also appears to insist that such explanations cannot be given, no matter what medical discoveries might be made. Unlike physical illnesses, those syndromes we call mental illnesses cannot be caused by some set of physiological events. In this logical claim he is surely in error.

What Szasz has in mind here is the Wittgensteinian distinction Richard Peters drew between actions and movements, and between reasons and causes.[38] Physical bodies, including the physical bodies of human beings, move through space in a manner describable by physical descriptions in terms of velocities, accelerations, spatial coordinates, directions, and so on. According to Peters, such movements of the human body constitute *actions*, however, only if they are seen in the light of human conventions: The physical movements of the arm and fingers in moving wooden figures on a checkered board only constitute the action of "castling the king" in light of an intelligent agent following the rules of chess. Further, in the Peters view, only physical movements can be explained by the mechanical causes provided by the laws of physics, whereas for actions only reasons (purposive rule following) are appropriate. One neither explains the orbiting of the planets by reference to their motives nor explains why another human being castled his king by reference to his synaptic firing patterns.

While I do not think Peters's or (Szasz's) rule-following analysis is adequate as a general account of human action, but rather represents an analysis of one species of *complex* actions, this does not matter for present purposes. For Szasz and Peters were struggling to express a thesis that might better be defended on other grounds. The thesis is the irreducibility thesis we encountered in Chapter 1, according to which no Intentional discourse (such as is involved in reason-giving explanations) can be reduced to the non-Intentional discourse of natural science. In numerous ways philosophers have sought to capture the striking fact that the words we apply to describe and explain the doings of *persons* differ significantly from the words we use to describe and explain natural phenomena. The analytic philosophy of the last twenty-five years has variously polarized these differences as being between actions and movements, reasons and causes, teleology and mechanism, Intentional idioms and the non-Intentional, intensional talk and extensional, the language used to describe meaningful behavior and that used to describe the inanimate, those claims known with certainty and those claims supported only by fallible, inductive inferences as in science.

In Chapter 1 we left open whether any of these differences justified the permanent nontranslatability of mental words to brain words that the irreducibility thesis entails. We granted only "provisional independence" to reason-giving accounts from underlying physiological accounts. Such a tentative separation of mind from brain cannot, of course, justify the belief that it is some kind of logical mistake to think that mental illness may be physically caused, as Szasz believes. And even if one grants that there is permanently, and not merely provisionally, some fundamental cleavage in one's speech and its irreducibility, that does not mean (contra Peters and Szasz) that the various mental illnesses may not be explained by reference to physiological events or any other mechanical causes. What the irreducibility thesis entails is that one cannot *identify* mental entities such as beliefs, desires, or pains with physical events, either behavioristic or physiological.[39] It does not entail that one may not *correlate* the mental experience of pain with certain physiological events (e.g., the stimulation of c fibers in the brain). Nor does it entail that schizophrenia may not be correlated with some sorts of events in the brain.

None of this is to say that such correlations between the aggregations of symptoms we label as mental illnesses of various kinds and physiology do exist, for one cannot tell in advance what slices of behavior can be correlated with what slices of physiology (this is true no matter how strictly one subscribes to determinism). It is a question for empirical discovery, and logical arguments either way are not decisive. The correlations between the disposition to bleed profusely and certain chemical states of the blood (hemophilia), violent character and XYY genetic makeup, and certain addictions (dispositions to act in certain ways) and the events in physiology that cause them are still suggestive examples. Whether similar correlations can be found between, for example, schizophrenia and certain happenings in physiology[40] is a matter for painstaking research, not for the armchair guesswork more frequently found in philosophy than in medicine.

It might be argued that it is illegitimate for psychiatrists to anticipate such discoveries before they are made, by using implicitly causal disease words such as schizophrenia or kleptomania. Szasz argues, for example, that it is "faulty reasoning to make the abstraction 'mental illness' into a cause of, even though this abstraction was originally created to serve only as a shorthand expression for, certain types of human behavior."[41]

Yet this is done all the time in "real" medicine as well as in psychiatry. Clusters of symptoms are thought to be due to an underlying condition, named and treated as illnesses, well before one could identify the cause of such symptoms. Polio was a disease before one discovered its virus origin. Moreover, we say that such diseases are (causally) responsible for the cluster of symptoms; even without knowledge of the cause, and knowing only the behavioral symptoms, we still do not mean that polio is just the symptoms by which we diagnose it. If we had meant this prior to knowing the causes of polio, no doctor could "ever [have] said (and many did) 'I believe this may not be a case of polio,' knowing that all of the text-book

Does Madness Exist?

symptoms were present."[42] By polio we meant *whatever* was responsible for the symptoms doctors observed, assuming that, in time, scientific research would tell us what the "whatever" might be.

Unless one can show some good reason to suppose that the symptoms of the various mental illnesses may not be caused by some kind of events in physiology (which I have attempted to show cannot be done, at least on logical grounds), then schizophrenia and other mental illnesses are no more myths because of the lack of any presently known physical causes than was polio a myth in the absence of similar knowledge.

THE MYTH AS A DEDUCTION FROM EPISTEMOLOGICAL RELATIVITY:
WE ARE EQUALLY MAD FROM THE EPISTEMOLOGICAL POINT OF VIEW OF THOSE WE LABEL MAD

"The quality of myth," Quine tells us, "is relative . . . to the epistemological point of view."[43] Mental illness is a myth in the interpretation discussed here, because our current epistemology, in which we have concepts like mental illness, is itself a myth — judged, of course, from another epistemological point of view, not from our own. If one subscribes to the view that there is no judging between such basic points of view, then the argument of R. D. Laing and others — that from the point of view of those we label insane we are insane — has some sting. Attribute to those we label as mentally ill an epistemology; grant that, although it differs from ours, the relative merits cannot be judged. Our labeling of others as mentally ill thus is a myth because it presupposes what it cannot have, namely, a standard of judgment applicable to those judged as well as to those judging.

Aside from Laing and his glorifying of the "schizophrenic voyage," one may perhaps find this version of the myth argument in the existential analysts. Manfred Bleuler, for example, characterizes existential analysis as treating

> the patient's utterance quite seriously and with no more prejudice or bias than in ordinary conversation with ordinary people. . . . Existential analysis refuses absolutely to examine pathological expressions with a view to seeing whether they are bizarre, absurd, illogical or otherwise defective; rather it attempts to understand the particular world of experience to which these experiences point . . . The existential analyst refrains from evaluations of any kind.[44]

It is tempting to treat this as no more than "the most promising therapeutic approach," as does David Levin.[45] The success of such therapeutic approaches is, of course, irrelevant to our epistemological concerns here. One may well be called upon to be very empathetic to the patient's point of view in therapy; one may also need such empathy to understand "the patient's world" for any purpose, therapeutic or explanatory. To make out the version of the myth argument here considered requires more, namely, that one *cannot* (not *will* not) judge the patient's point of view as "bizarre, absurd, illogical or otherwise defective."

The problem with this version of the myth argument is the premise with which it begins, namely, epistemological relativity itself. More specifically, the error of the relativists is their assumption that to have the capacity to judge another's entire system of beliefs one must have the ability to stand outside one's own beliefs. The general idea is that objective knowledge about anything requires that one have the ability to stand outside all human convention, to gape at reality unmediated by the distortions of such conventions. Since no person can do this—it is doubtful that any god could, since the idea is probably self-contradictory—the relativist concludes that there can be no objective knowledge.

Yet our capacities to judge another point of view are not hostage to our attaining this unattainable convention-free stance. We admittedly view the world, scientifically and morally, by the conventions involved in our society's shared set of beliefs, and we make our judgments accordingly. Yet this is no embarrassing concession for realists to make, for they are only committed to saying that we can alter those conventions to better fit the real nature of the world as we progressively experience it. The "conventions" of our shared beliefs are in effect part of our collective *theory* about how the world really is.[46] When we come across a radically different system of beliefs, following different conventions, we do not have to grant it some kind of epistemological parity. It may be an equally plausible theory, in which case we should consider it a supplement or a replacement of our own; or, as in the case of the insane, it may be a wildly implausible theory. In either case, such beliefs form a *theory* that competes with our own; to the extent a rival system of beliefs fares badly in such competition, we are perfectly entitled to judge it to be false. If it is not only false, but obviously false in the face of overwhelming evidence, it is also a "crazy" system of beliefs to adhere to, and those who adhere to it nonetheless are themselves quite properly judged to be crazy.

The relativists are hard put to disagree with the foregoing. For what could their disagreement come to? They cannot get free of their conventions in order to tell us how things really stand with competing epistemologies. Their statement that all beliefs are relative to the system of beliefs of which they are a part is, *by their criterion,* a relative statement. By the realists' criterion, on the other hand, it is not a relative statement—it is a false one.

In addition to these general philosophical difficulties, any mythicist who urges this version of the myth argument has the challenging task of showing that the beliefs of the severely disordered are sufficiently *systematic* that one could call them an epistemological point of view. For the fragmented beliefs of such human beings can only with the broadest tolerance for contradiction be cohered into much of a system at all. There is something almost cruel in Laing's glorifying of the experience of schizophrenia into a voyage of self-discovery by someone too virtuous to adhere to the epistemology of a sick society. Such awe for the insane, typical in primitive peoples, belongs with other primitive beliefs: as myths that should no longer command our respect.

THE MYTH AS AN EVALUATION MASQUERADING AS AN EXPLANATION: THE ABUSE OF THE NORMATIVE FORCE OF MENTAL ILLNESS BY ORTHODOX PSYCHIATRY

Sensitivity to the normative connotations of the concepts of mental health and mental illness is, I suspect, rather widespread. When one of the psychiatrists at the annual meeting of the American Psychiatric Association some years ago loudly diagnosed a radical feminist who was disrupting the meeting as a "stupid, paranoid bitch," something other than a value-neutral explanation of her behavior was intended. The same suspicions are engendered when psychiatrists label homosexuals as mentally ill, or when mental health is used as a synonym for whatever way of life is adjudged good. The radical psychiatrists build on these kinds of examples to argue that mental illness and the predicate mentally ill are used *only* to make evaluations of others' behavior, and that these terms are particularly effective as evaluations because they are paraded as value-neutral, scientific explanations: "While allegedly describing conduct, psychiatrists often prescribe it."[47]

> The masquerading of promotive assertions in the guise of indicative sentences is of great practical significance in psychiatry. Statements concerning "psychosis" or "insanity"... almost always revolve around unclarified equations of these two linguistic forms. For example, the statement "John Doe is psychotic" is ostensibly indicative and informative. Usually, however, it is promotive rather than informative.[48]

It may seem curious to claim that mental illness is used like "bad" or "wrong" — that is, used to pass moral evaluations — when by our shared notions for moral responsibility we use the same phrase to *excuse* those who are mentally ill. To attribute a harmful action to the actor's mental illness, then, cannot always be exactly the same as attributing it, say, to his "murderous personality." What Szasz *sometimes* has in mind in saying that mental illness is used prescriptively or promotively is not that moral judgments are made with such use; rather, psychiatric usage of the phrase is often promotive in the quite different sense that the capability of being morally responsible is denied. Mental illness for Szasz is evaluative often only in the sense that the term denies the personhood of those to whom it is applied: "What better way is there . . . for degrading the culprit than to declare him incapable of knowing what he is doing . . . This is the general formula for the dehumanization and degradation of all those persons whose conduct psychiatrists now deem to be 'caused' by mental illness."[49]

Although needlessly stated in inflammatory terms (as if orthodox psychiatry were universally motivated by a desire to degrade the mentally ill), Szasz here suggests a very important feature of mental illness. Insanity and mental illness mean, and historically have meant, irrationality; to be insane, or to be mentally ill, is to fail to act rationally often enough to have the same assumption of rationality made about one as is made of most of humanity. And without that assumption being made, one cannot be fully regarded as a person, for our concept of what it is to be a person is centered on the notions of rationality introduced earlier. Unless we can perceive another being as acting for rational ends in light of rational beliefs, we cannot understand that being in the same fundamental way that we understand each other's actions in daily life. Such beings lack an essential attribute of being a person. It is thus easy to appreciate that the insane historically have been likened to young children, the intoxicated, and wild beasts, as we noted in Chapter 2. For lacking rationality, the mentally ill are, as Bleuler said of his schizophrenic patients, stranger to us than the birds in our gardens.

Such statements are, of course, offensive to the ears of those concerned about the moral claims and legal rights of mental patients. Yet unless radical psychiatry and its lawyerly following can show, as I have argued earlier in this chapter it has not, that those we label mentally ill are just as rational as everyone else, part of our fundamental explanatory scheme and part of our fundamental notion of personhood are not applicable to the mentally ill. This includes notions about their lack of responsibility and inability to choose and act upon their own conception of their good. If one believes (contra Szasz et al.) that there are in fact people who do not act rationally often enough for us to make the same assumption of rationality for them as we do for most of our fellows, then this evaluative force customarily attached to the use of mental illness in certain contexts is accurate enough in its reflection of how the mentally ill fit into our fundamental conceptual scheme.

Szasz at other times seems to have in mind a second kind of normative force that we do on occasion attach to mentally ill, in everyday expressions such as "That was an insane thing to do" or "That's crazy!" In such usages we may express disapproval of the agent's ends and actions, recommending that one ought not to do such things or seek such ends. Thus

Szasz is also right to note that *at times* mentally ill or insane can be used as terms of general disapproval: "The difference between saying 'He is wrong' and 'He is mentally ill' is not factual but psychological."[50] Other examples with which we began this section were the spot "diagnosis" of the radical feminist and the use of "mental health" by some psychoanalysts, such as Erich Fromm, as if it were synonymous with "good."

To the extent that orthodox psychiatry uses these words in this way it is plainly abusing them. The phrase mental illness and its companions are so abused not by being applied to those who are in fact irrational, but by being applied to persons who are rational but of whose values prevailing psychiatric opinion does not approve. An action that is fully rational in each of the senses examined earlier cannot, without ignoring the meaning of the words, be said to be insane or due to mental illness, no matter how deviant the end pursued may be. The fact that homosexuals have a preference for a sexual relationship not shared by most of the populace is hardly grounds (as the APA, with strong dissent, implicitly recognized in its deletion of homosexuality as an illness) for labeling that preference irrational (ill). Homosexuals may (sometimes, often, or always) be mentally ill, if their capacity for rational action is significantly diminished below our expectations. Such irrationality is hardly shown, however, by their unpopular sexual desires alone if those ends are pursued on the basis of rational and consistent beliefs, without conflict with other strong desires, and by relatively efficient means.

The mistake of radical psychiatry is to assume that mental illness is a myth just because the phrase can be so abused. The mistake is to assume that because words such as murder, greediness, mental illness, or even good can be used to express attitudes, kindle emotions, pass evaluations and the like, they cannot also be used at the same time as a legitimate form of explanation or description, or at different times only as a description or explanation.[51] Those moral philosophers who purported to discover another logical gulf, this time between evaluative and descriptive statements, ignored the relatively obvious fact that words used in evaluations can also be used to express descriptions. Merely because a woman may call the doctor who, through surgical error, kills her husband a murderer, despite the fact that one of the main criteria for that term's proper use is not met (viz., *intentional* killing), is not sufficient to show that murderer cannot have legitimate descriptive and explanatory uses.

Szasz's essential confusion here is between the *force* of a term and its *meaning*. Szasz appears to believe that if a term has an evaluative force it cannot also have some descriptive meaning. Although Szasz here has some respectable company in the emotivist moral philosophy of the 1940s and 1950s, no one, I think, takes such analyses very seriously any more. Since J. L Austin's important work on speech acts,[52] few would believe that because a word has a conventional force—say, of condemnation—it cannot also have descriptive content. Murderer is just such a term.

Mental illness is perhaps a dangerous term because its normative force makes possible the kind of abuse mentioned earlier; but the same also can be said of many of the terms with which we describe and explain human action, such as greedy, stupid, murder, or manipulative.

In the earlier paper from which this chapter was derived,[53] I thought that Szasz himself should not be accused of making this mistake. Having read my earlier paper, Szasz now wishes to make it clear that he claims this mistake as his own. For he has recently urged at length that one of the principal difficulties with the concept of mental illness "is that although 'mental illness' is a prescriptive term, it is usually used as if it were a descriptive one."[54] From this, he concludes that "psychiatry is not a science because its practitioners are basically hostile to the ethic of truth-telling," truth telling for Szasz being linked to *descriptive* use of language only.[55]

What Szasz has failed to recognize is that no amount of haranguing about the various normative forces conventionally attached to mental illness can convince anyone that the phrase has no descriptive meaning. Needed is some independent argument to establish that there is no descriptive meaning for such phrases. Such arguments as are to be found in the literature of radical psychiatry—the four previous versions of the myth argument—are insufficient for this purpose. With their collapse must also fall this fifth and final version of "the myth of mental illness."

Conclusion

The disease that radical psychiatry has contracted (and that appears to be contagious, at least for those lawyers who always knew that psychiatry was pseudoscience anyway) is the temptation to regard complex legal, social, ethical, and conceptual problems as solved once it administers a sufficient amount of antimyth antidote. In Szasz's case in particular, it is an attempt to use the therapeutic tools of modern philosophy to dissolve the problems, not to solve them.

If indeed one believes that there is no such thing as mental illness, that those we call mentally ill are fully as rational as anyone else, only with different aims, that the only reason anyone ever thought differently was because of unsophisticated category mistakes or because of his adherence to the epistemology of a sick society, and that the phrase accordingly is only a mask used to disguise moral judgments in pseudoscientific respectability—if, in other words, one accepts the myth thesis—one will necessarily also believe that one wields an Alexandrian sword with which to cut through the knotty legal problems surrounding the treatment of the mentally ill. For once one subscribes to these versions of the myth argument a number of radical consequences for the present treatment of the mentally ill are self-evident truths to all but the uninitiated: Either the insanity defense should be abolished and those we call mentally ill punished like anyone else, or at the very least the phrase should play no part as a separate defense; the incompetency plea should either be abolished or highly limited; those we call mentally ill should be sued for breach of contract like anyone else, not excused from their contractual obligations because of supposed incapacity to contract; no one should be civilly committed for mental illness, for the mentally ill know their own good and have the capacity to act in accordance with such a conception no less than anyone else, the state thus having no parental role to play here; anyone inside or outside a mental hospital should have the full civil rights of any citizen because he is just like any citizen. In short, one who subscribes to the myth arguments will believe that "we abolish the problem of mental illness by abolishing the concept of mental illness."[56]

This is, of course, preposterous. The mentally ill and their attendant problems will not go away this easily. Neither will the conceptual problem that is the topic of Part II of this book: How does one draw the line between ethics and psychiatry, the bad and the sick? Mythicists such as Szasz would dissolve this problem with the stunning simplicity of denying that there is any such line to be drawn, for none of us is mentally sick.

If only mental illness could in any significant sense be said to be a myth. But it cannot. It has been the central thrust of this chapter that a critical reading of Szasz in terms of the philosophers on which he relies renders the myth of mental illness as itself a myth, useful perhaps as a battle cry, but hardly the starting point for any serious consideration of how mental illness is to be conceptualized. I shall accordingly put Szasz and the mythicists aside as we search for the elusive line between the sick and the bad. Such mythicists, because of their polemics and their lack of rigor, cannot help us even though their problem is our problem in this Part II: How to keep post-Freudian psychiatry, with its bloated ideas of mental illness, from eroding the presuppositions necessary to attribute rights and responsibilities to persons.

5 Psychiatry and the Concept of Mental Illness

IN GENERAL, there are two ways of proceeding when one defines a phrase such as mental illness. The first is an analysis of what the phrase means as it is used in a body of discourse. One proceeds by analyzing the various ways in which a phrase is employed, either in the general population or within some subgroup, and one attempts to isolate the criteria *implicit* in such ordinary usage as the meaning of the term. Such discovered criteria are usually called "lexical" definitions.[1]

The second mode of definition proceeds by disregarding the ways in which a phrase is actually used in a body of discourse and focuses on how it ought to be used. One defines a phrase, in other words, by making a proposal as to what it ought to mean to people. Let us call these "stipulative" definitions, because in making them one stipulates (as opposed to discovers) the criteria that are henceforth to govern the use of a term.

In this chapter we shall be concerned with both kinds of definitions of mental illness. I shall begin with an attempt to tease out a lexical definition of the phrase from its usage in ordinary speech. I shall then ask what reasons psychiatrists might have for proposing a different meaning of the phrase. I shall close the chapter by urging that broad psychiatric definitions—such as those we encountered in Chapter 3, but including some that are less broad—have little warrant even for psychiatric purposes (let alone legal purposes, the subject of Chapter 6).

The Ordinary Meaning of Mental Illness

A natural way of proceeding into an analysis of the ordinary meaning of mental illness would seem to be to analyze the meaning of each of its conjuncts, mind and illness, and then to see what the two might mean when conjoined.

THE MEANING OF MIND

One's idea of what constitutes a sick mind can be no better than one's idea of what a mind itself might be. Sir James Stephen, a noted nineteenth-century criminal lawyer, preceived this: "What is the meaning of the word mind? What is a sane and what is an insane mind? ... Difficult and remote from law as some of these inquiries may be, it is impossible to deal with the subject at all without entering to some extent upon each of them."[2]

In answering the question "What is a mind?" in its most obvious sense, one runs immediately into a centuries-old philosophical thicket; that is, the ontological status of mind (and of all of the "furniture" of the mind, such as intentions, pains, and perceptions). The modern positions in this debate seem to be four in number:

1. The *dualist* tradition of Descartes asserts that apart from the physical world there exists the mental world, not existing in space but only in time, accessible only by the reflexive of consciousness. Mental phenomena, accordingly, are irreducible to physical phenomena, and an independent science of the mind, with an elaborate deductive structure mirroring the theoretical structure of physical science, is thus a legitimate enterprise.
2. The *physicalist* tradition in its modern form asserts that mind and brain are identical. There is just one species of existence, that of the physical world, in this view, and the ultimate reference of mental words would be found to be either physical things or states of physical things.
3. The *(logical) behaviorist* tradition interprets all reference to mind as constructs out of behavior. In such a view, mind is in one sense no thing at all, in the same sense that force is no thing at all for "instrumentalists" discussing theoretical entities in the philosophy of science. Mind and its furniture, such as intentions, sensations, and beliefs, are only explanatory constructs, a collection of dispositions to behave in certain ways that explain behavior in the way the dispositional properties explain instances of the disposition in question for natural objects.
4. The most recent variant, *functionalism,* asserts that minds are logical or functional states of physical systems. The analogy often drawn by proponents of this view is to a Turing machine, a machine whose states are defined by a machine table such that physical structure is left unspecified; that is, the machine may be said to be in a certain state by meeting criteria that have nothing to do with the machine's physical configuration. Mental states, analogously, are functional states of a person, the criteria of which are intimately connected to his linguistic abilities, but whose physical realization is unspecified and perhaps unspecifiable in any one-to-one correspondence with his functional states.

Each of these views is not, as its counterpart in psychology might be, a "theoretical perspective" or research strategy. Rather, each purports to tell us what we all ordinarily think, as presupposed in our ordinary speech, a mind is. They are, in other words, analyses of our shared conceptual system; not theoretical postulates in some new conceptual system. Thus, if correct, each of them would be the first step in an analysis of our ordinary concept of mental illness.

In light of the well-charted difficulties with each of these positions, some way of avoiding a general defense of one of them would seem desirable.[3] One avenue of avoidance is that of "semantic ascent": If we do not wish to talk about the thing itself, we may still talk about our talk about the thing. Indeed, much of the philosophy of mind prior to the emphasis of the last fifteen years or so on the mind/body relationship is engaged in this kind of conceptual analysis: showing not what a sick mind is in terms of its relationship to physical bodies, but by analyzing mental illness in terms of its relationships to other mental terms. We may leave the question of the reference of all mental terms open and still say something about the internal relationships that hold between them.

In examining our mentalistic vocabulary, it is doubtlessly not necessary to fix the precise boundary we use to mark off such vocabulary from the rest of our language. This is a matter of some dispute in philosophy, and for our purposes a precise demarcation is not in any event necessary. Paradigmatically mental are words such as belief, knowing, motive, intention, imagining, perceiving, angry, depressed, and the like.

One set of characteristics of mentalistic expressions that some philosophers believe to be "the mark of the mental" has to do with certain peculiarities of our first-person usage of many mental terms. These we shall examine in some detail in Chapter 7. Preliminarily, however, we may distinguish three claims usually being made here. First of all, most of our vocabulary of mind is asymmetrical with respect to the modes of its verification in its first- and third-person usages. Contrary to the claims of behaviorists, I do not always or even typically come to know my moods, emotions, motives, pains, imaginings, or whatever, in the same way that other people do; I do not, for example, observe myself saying "Ouch," or observe my hand being removed from the hot stove, in order to conclude that I am in pain. I know that I am in pain in an immediate way without resort to such observations, and my statement that I am in pain is thus verified in a way quite different from a similar statement made by someone else about me in the third person, namely, "He is in pain." Our mentalistic vocabulary, in other words, reflects a seeming *privileged access* that we each have to our own mental states, privileged in the sense that first-person claims to knowledge about mental states are not subject to the usual demands for evidence from observation.

The Concept of Mental Illness

Second, our language of mind is such that the words we use to describe many mental states make them seem *self-intimating;* it may seem plausible to claim, for example, that if I am in pain, I must know it. It sounds a bit odd to ask oneself whether one is in pain. Third, our mentalistic vocabulary seems to imply that we are *incorrigible* in our statements about being in mental states. The claim here is one of infallibility about the contents of one's own mind: If I think I am in pain, I am; if I think I intend to do some action A, I necessarily intend to do A. Such supposed infallibility in our knowledge of our own mental states is reflected in the oddness of questioning first-person, present-tense descriptions of them on grounds other than sincerity.

These three related epistemic claims about the vocabulary of mind—privileged access, self-intimation, and incorrigibility—are not all, as we shall see, true. With regard to self-intimation and incorrigibility in particular, there are at most supporting hints of such claims in ordinary usage. With regard to mental illness, however, there are not even such hints. Mentally ill persons do not have some privileged access in determining whether they are mentally ill. If a person is going to describe himself as being mentally ill, he will have to make the same sorts of observations a third-person observer would have to make and does not have some noninferential, nonobservational way of knowing that he is mentally ill. The inference involved is shown directly by such common expressions as, "I must be insane" (compare: "I must be in pain"). Similarly, there is no hint that the state of being mentally ill is self-intimating. A person who is mentally ill need not necessarily know that he is mentally ill; often, mentally ill persons go to great lengths to resist that conclusion. Finally, there is no hint that one is incorrigible with respect to thinking that one is mentally ill. One can believe oneself to be mentally ill, and not be mentally ill at all. A psychiatrist need not accept at face value a patient's sincere description of himself as mentally ill.

In this respect, mental illness is like another class of mental words, namely, those words with which we describe the character traits of normal people, words such as greediness, vanity, or stupidity. For there is also no hint of privileged access, self-intimation, or incorrigibility in our first-person use of character-trait words either. We must observe our own actions and their motives to see if we are, for example, vain or greedy; we can easily be wrong if we think we are vain, and ignorant of the fact that we are greedy.

This parallel suggests that mental illness, like the words we use to describe character traits, is fundamentally connected to behavior and not to mental experience. For words of character are behavioral in their criteria, and this is reflected directly in the fact that first-person usage of such character words is not even arguably incorrigible, nor is there privileged access, nor are such states self-intimating.[4] Mental illness, sharing those same features, would seem to indicate a similar lack of connection to mental experience, but rather a connection to behavioral criteria in an application of the term. This is not to deny that being mentally ill may not involve characteristic mental experiences; it denies only that those experiences are themselves the criteria of the word. There may well be mental experiences characteristic of being greedy or vain as well; yet it is greedy and vain behavior, not those experiences, that entitle both the actor and the observer to so describe the actor's character.

To say that mental illness is, in the first instance, connected to behavior is not yet to say what it is about the behavior of persons we label mentally ill that enables us to so label them. We must defer this inquiry until we have first ascertained something of the ordinary meaning of the word "ill," to which I now turn. Preliminarily, however, this third-person aspect of "mental illness" may reflect the deep-seated "we/they" attitude inherent in the popular understanding of the mentally ill; perhaps because "mentally ill" is a label we have invented principally to apply to other people who are different from us and not to apply to ourselves.[5]

THE ORDINARY MEANING OF BEING SICK, ILL, OR DISEASED

Illness and the Body

A misconception about our shared concept of illness that is easy to fall into is that to be ill one's bodily structure must deviate from a physiological or anatomical norm. This is the Szaszian claim examined in the last chapter. The two distinguishable claims made here are: (1) that illness is necessarily *caused* by something physical—if not some invading thing, like a spirochete in general paresis or a virus, then some physiological deviation of the subject's body, such as chemical imbalance in the neurotransmitters of the brain; and (2) that illness is necessarily *manifested* by deviant physiological structures, such as high blood pressure or inflamed joints. There must be, in other words, physical symptoms and/or physical causes.

Neither of these claims squares with the ordinary way in which we use "ill." It is easy to see that such deviant physiological structures cannot be a sufficient criterion of being ill, else people with large heads, long noses, or abnormally structured bodily parts of any sort would all be ill. Yet many deviant structures are simply irrelevant to health or illness, and indeed some of them may make a person healthier.[6] More pertinently, such deviant physiological structures are not even a necessary criterion for being ill. Historically this had to be true; people were said to be ill long before anyone knew about the deviations of bodily structure that may accompany illness. Even today, when ordinary usage has had time to accommodate itself to the influence of medicine, we would describe someone as ill even if his bodily structure were completely nondeviant from that of the rest of the population. The survivors of a nuclear war may all have physical structures (statistically normal for them) that incapacitate them from many activities, hasten their death, and cause a great deal of discomfort. The fact that such persons' bodies are statistically normal would not prevent us from saying that these individuals are ill.

None of this is as true of the word "disease" as it is of "ill" and "sick." For many doctors, "the term 'disease' is traditionally identified with pathology of tissue."[7] This medical assumption is reflected in ordinary usage in two ways: First, we more often speak of a person's *having* a disease, something he possesses, than of his *being* diseased; second, the normal subject of the "diseased" predicate is not persons but their bodies or some part of their bodies. I shall pursue each nuance of ordinary usage separately.

We quite readily say of someone that he has a disease; we do not as readily say he has a sickness or he has an illness. We are more likely in the latter case to say he is sick or he is ill. This reflects the fact that the concept of disease is linked to the classificatory systems of medicine more than are the concepts of being sick or ill. To say of someone that he has a disease implies that he has some one disease among others. Saying that someone is ill or is sick in general does not presuppose he has some one sickness or some one illness among a host of classified illnesses and sicknesses.

The importance of this link of the concept of disease to systems of classification in the present context is this: Classificatory systems are often built on implicit causal hypotheses, and the notion of disease reflects this origin. It sometimes is thought that diseases are classified by the recurrence of a pattern of symptoms alone: "The term ['disease'] refers to a pattern of factors which somehow hang together and recur, more or less the same, in successive individuals. Thus, pain in the right lower quadrant of the abdomen, with nausea, vomiting, fever, and a high white count, spell out the features of acute appendicitis."[8]

Yet this kind of aggregation of symptoms into a recurring pattern is only the first step in classifying diseases. Such correlations are made with the hope of finding a "hidden nature" to such diseases, a hidden nature not to be found in the cluster of symptoms themselves.[9] Once we discover such hidden natures (e.g., a ruptured appendix), their presence or absence determines whether a given individual has that disease; an individual who manifests identical symptoms without having a ruptured appendix does not have appendicitis. Moreover, our intention when we use words such as polio or multiple sclerosis is to refer to such hidden nature, even if we do not know it. The point, in other words, is not that we change the meaning of disease words when we discover physical causes, but rather that we intend by using such words to refer to some such set of causes, leaving to science to discover their actual nature.

We use the word "disease," then, in light of a set of background beliefs about there being discrete diseases, separate from one another, not only by their differing cluster of symptoms but also ultimately by their physical causes. There is thus at least a suggestion in ordinary usage that having a disease means that something is wrong with one's body.

The second nuance of ordinary usage of disease is that we freely predicate "is diseased" of bodies and parts of bodies. We do this more frequently, indeed, than we speak of persons' being diseased. We may say that his brain is diseased, or that he has brain disease, or that his body is "rife with disease." With "ill" or "sick," this is not the case: We do not usually say of someone that his body is sick or that his liver is ill—as if *he* were not. The general predicates "is ill" or "is sick" have persons as their normal subjects. Disease in ordinary understanding is thus prima facie an attribute of bodies directly; one would thus expect the symptoms and causes of the disease to be of a physical sort.[10]

For each of these reasons, disease does suggest physical symptoms and physical causes.[11] Does this implication of physical causation infect our use of the general predicates "is ill" or "is sick"? It might seem that one cannot be ill without having a disease, that is, without having something wrong with one's body. Yet, in fact, the assumption of physical causation is not contagious. In the law of torts the late William Prosser once said that there is no requirement whatsoever that a tort have a name, meaning that any personal injury caused by the culpability of another ought to be a compensable tort irrespective of whether or not it happened to fit the existing classification of causes of action that tort law has set up. A similar slogan regarding diseases would be appropriate: One can be ill without having any recognized disease. One is ill by virtue of being in the state characterized in the next subsection, a state principally characterized by incapacitation, and in some cases connected to pain and death as well. Only if one were to equate the general state of being ill with the more specific one of having some medically recognized disease would the implication of physical causality be proper.[12]

Being ill, then, is independent of having some specific disease of the body, or of physical causation and symptomatology in general. In light of this, the common opposition of mental and physical illness can be misleading insofar as it suggests that real illnesses are physical illnesses, and that mental or functional illnesses are illnesses only by a rather weak analogy. Rather, people are just plain ill; if we wish to subclassify by causes or symptoms, all well and good. Only, one should not mistake the principle by which we make such subclassifications for the general criteria for being ill to begin with.

The Concept of Mental Illness

Imagine a state, call it state A, defined by one criterion: being in the water 200 miles from the center of some island. Suppose further that this is thought to be an undesirable state to be in so that a profession is begun whose principal responsibility is to prevent people from getting into such a state. We find a number of persons who are in state A, that is, they are out in the water somewhere on the circumference of a circle whose center is the island, and whose radius is 200 miles. We would doubtlessly be curious about how they all got there; indeed, to the professional group dedicated to preventing it, this knowledge of causation is crucial. We discover that some got there by shipwreck; for the rest, we can discover no means of transportation (perhaps we do not know about airplanes or submarines). We may classify all such persons as being in "shipwreck state A" and "other state A." Both such groups of persons, however, are plainly in state A. How they got there is a very interesting question around which we may build a classificatory system, but it is also quite distinct from whether or not they are there, the sole defining characteristic of being in state A.

On Being Ill

If "being ill" predicated of a person does not mean that the person's body deviated from some physiological norms, what does it mean? Under what conditions do we say of someone that he is ill or sick?

The central idea behind illness is that of impairment: To be ill is to be impaired from functioning in some of the wide varieties of ways we think to be normal. Often such impairment may be accompanied by pain or other forms of distress; sometimes such impairment may be accompanied by an increased likelihood of death (which I suppose could be viewed as the limiting case of impairment of functioning). Each of these has been suggested as a supplementary criterion for being considered ill. But the central criterion of being ill seems to be that the person so described is incapacitated in some ways yet to be specified.

Functional impairment can occur at either of two levels: at the level of specific diseases of bodily parts, or at the level of the total functioning of the person in his society. Ultimately, the first depends on the second; that is, we judge someone to have a bad heart only by virtue of the heart's not being able to perform its function properly, and we can judge whether or not the heart is properly performing its function only by knowing whether or not the person is or is not functioning properly.

To see this, imagine someone who has a heart with a valve such that the tissues in various parts of his body receive an inadequate supply of blood so that he is seriously incapacitated; we will say of such a person that his heart is not performing its function properly. For the function of the heart is to circulate the blood, which, by hypothesis, it is not doing.

How we ascertain what the function of the heart is, and once having ascertained that, how we further ascertain whether it is adequately performing that function, illustrates the dependence of the notion of a properly functioning heart on the notion of a properly functioning (i.e., healthy) person. As set forth in Chapter 1, the information content of function statements is that the process to which a function is assigned (the heart's beating) has as one of its effects the activity identified as the function (the circulation of blood). Yet the assignment of functions to parts of a system cannot be made simply on the basis of this sort of causal information. Simply because the circulation of the blood is one consequence of the heart's activities does not entitle us to label that consequence as the heart's function. For the heart's beating has a number of consequences in addition to the circulation of blood — for one thing, it makes some noise. Absent some other criterion of function assignment, we are equally free to say that the function of the heart is to make noise in the chest cavity.

The criterion by virtue of which we select one consequence of the heart's activity as its function is that we already have some further end state in mind toward which that consequence itself contributes. Because the circulation of blood itself causally contributes to the maintenance of the end state of the person's properly functioning, it, rather than the noise, is assigned as the function of the heart. Similarly with the determination of whether the heart is *properly* performing its function: The amount of blood that is the heart's function to circulate is whatever amount is necessary for a human being to function properly.

To ascertain whether someone is ill, then, ultimately involves us in ascertaining whether he is incapacitated from functioning properly; even if his specific complaint involves some bodily defect, we will judge that defect to be a disease, and the person to be ill, only if *he* is not in good working order.

How do we judge whether someone is in good working order? More specifically, what sorts of things must one be capable of doing in order to be not ill (i.e., healthy)? Many people are incapable of distinguishing good wines from mediocre ones; others seem to be incapable of experiencing orgasm in heterosexual relationships; others are incapable, because poor, of going to expensive artistic performances, and some are incapable of appreciating them if they were to go; still others are left-handed or stutter. Yet surely none of these incapacities makes one ill.

Our ordinary conception of health, or of proper functioning, avoids the pitfalls of equating health with happiness or with human flourishing in general, and of thus equating illness with any form of incapacity for happiness and flourishing, such as those involved in poverty, ignorance, and cultural deprivation. When we say of someone that he is ill, we mean he is incapacitated from pursuing those basic activities that are necessary to any

The Concept of Mental Illness

person's conception of the good life. (These activities I later discuss as the "thin theory" of the good.) In terms of our heart patient, he is ill if he cannot move about the world as well as most people without keeling over — in short, if he cannot do some wide variety of things we all do in our daily lives in order to get by. If he can do these basic things, he is healthy, in the negative sense of the word, that is, he is not ill.

There is, of course, a wide variation in the judgments people make about the good life. There is much more agreement on the capacities necessary for the wide variety of conceptions of the good life that people hold. We have good agreement that the ability to control one's body in the world, for example, is necessary; probably equally good agreement about the ability to think and reason coherently. We can imagine other societies in which even these basic capacities were not valued because the goods they made possible were not valued. In a society in which physical movements requiring any exertion were thought undesirable, for example, health would not require the same sort of capacities as it does in our world. Our hypothetical heart patient would not be ill, nor his heart functioning improperly, just because he could not run up stairs, play football, and so forth (although it is hard to imagine that he would not be incapacitated from some sort of activities thought to be desirable). All judgments of illness and improper functioning of body parts are thus normative in the sense that they are dependent on value judgments about what sort of basic capacities are desirable for any being who is a person.

Yet this value-laden feature of the ordinary conception of illness hardly collapses all judgments of goodness into judgments of health, nor all judgments of badness into judgments of illness. The normative judgment involved in attributing illness concerns the desirability of certain basic capacities being essential to the good life, however conceived, of any human being in our society; such normative judgment is not the all-out judgment of what is good for persons. It is only by leaving the ordinary conception of health, by expanding it to include all capacities one might think desirable in order to lead a fulfilled or happy life with a corresponding expansion of illness as anything less than such a life, that some psychiatrists and followers of naturalistic ethics make the normative aspects of health and illness troublesome.

There is, of course, some vagueness inherent in distinguishing one kind of normative judgment from another in order to maintain the line between ethics and medicine. Recognizing this, a number of writers have sought to show that judgments about illness (or at least disease) are not based on any normative judgments at all. If this were right, then the line between ethics and medicine would be even clearer than it is, for medical judgments would not be (or presuppose) value judgments of any sort. One example of this view is Louis Swartz, who urged that the line between ethics and medicine has been drawn between *total* functioning (a value judgment) and the functioning of parts or subdivisions of the human organism (supposedly a factual judgment):

> Traditionally, disease has meant the disturbance of some subdivision of total human functioning, such as respiration, rather than total functioning, or conduct. Whatever the historical basis of this view point, it ought to be retained. It is a useful means by which to differentiate problems of malfunctioning from the moral issue of what is good or evil.[13]

There is no doubt that we can distinguish questions about the function of persons from questions about the function of their bodily parts. Yet, as we have seen, *ultimately* to assign a function even to a body part *is* to make some (value) judgment about basic capacities a properly functioning person must possess. Only if Swartz and others like him[14] can develop some nonnormative basis for judging the proper end state for persons that allows function assignments to be given can this line between ethics and medicine be drawn.

I argued in Chapter 1 that there is an alternative way of defining end states that makes function assignments significant. Where there are homeostatic mechanisms at work such that the system in question tends to maintain itself in certain states, despite disturbances, then such states can be used as the relevant end states for the assignment of functions. Whether a given system tends to maintain certain states is a factual question and need involve no value judgment.

Just such a point has been made recently by Christopher Boorse in his argument that the ordinary meaning of disease is value-free:

> It seems clear that biological function statements are descriptive rather than normative claims. Physiologists obtain their functional doctrines without at any stage having to answer such questions as, what is the function of a man? Or to explicate "a good man" on the analogy of "a good knife." Functions are not attributed to the whole organism at all, but only to its parts, and the functions of a part are its causal contributions to empirically given goals. *What goals an organism in fact pursues . . . can be decided without considering the value of pursuing them.*[15]

From this Boorse concludes that disease, being impaired functioning of bodily parts, is a value-free concept.

The problem for this value-free account of disease or illness is not that it has hidden values in it. Rather, the problem is that it is not an accurate account of disease or illness. Consider first disease, even when that term is limited to diseased body parts. The homeostatic mechanisms that do exist in the body are evolutionarily generated features that tend to produce one effect, survival (either of the individual or the race).[16] Although there is no dearth of attempts to analyze disease in terms of survival,[17] such analyses fail to account for our broader use of this term. One might urge, as has Joseph Margolis recently, that death is never a sufficient criterion of disease:

> There are diseases that are lethal but *there are no diseases that are classified as such merely because they result in death*. On the contrary, the most interesting general feature about disease is that it is a disorder or the cause of disorder of a certain sort *within the functional range of ongoing life*.[18]

As an analysis of our ordinary usage this seems wrong. Consider what we would say of a man who drops dead suddenly without a day's incapacitation or a single painful sensation. If he died from a slowly growing cancer in the lung, but had no pain or incapacitation, was he diseased before he died? We would clearly say he was diseased, or that he had a lung disease, or that his body was rife with disease. Suppose further that the condition this man had is *never* accompanied by any form of incapacitation or pain. I think it plain we would still call such state a disease.

Hence, the survival value of some end state is perhaps a sufficient basis on which to seize upon such an end state as the basis for assigning functions (and thus, for judging *dysfunction*). But it surely is not a necessary one. Diseases need not *ever* be lethal to be diseases. They need only be incapacitating from a wide range of desirable activities. The survival-based homeostatic balances can thus only be a partial criterion for deciding the end states necessary for assigning functions to body parts. For most (if not all) diseases some normative judgment about what minimal capacities a person should possess must be made.

This is, of course, more obviously true when one speaks of *mental* diseases. It remains to be shown that there are any naturally occurring homeostatic balances maintained in the mind.[19] Yet without such balances, there can be no value-free definition of disease. Even more clearly here than for diseases of bodily organs, one must make some limited normative judgment about what basic mental capacities are needed in a person.

This need for some normative judgment is even more obvious for illness than for disease. For illness does not have the tie to pathology of tissue that disease has. There is thus even less temptation to assume that there are some natural functions that can be discovered, impairment of which constitutes illness.

The upshot is that judgments of illness and disease presuppose certain value judgments. If I am wrong in this regard, so that judgments about health, disease, and illness are value free, then so much the better for the ultimate thesis of this chapter, namely, that there is a significant line to be drawn between health and goodness, illness and badness. In such a case the line to be drawn would be between facts (about function assignments) and values. Alternatively, on the assumption that judgments of illness are value laden, this does not mean that they are the same as our general value judgments about bad persons and actions. Presupposed by our ordinary notions of illness and disease is the limited value judgment that certain basic capacities are desirable for a person, no matter what his conception of the good life. It is impairment of these capacities that constitutes illness and disease. It is not failure to realize some conception of the good life itself that is illness or disease. Only in the latter case would there be no line between ethics and medicine to be found in the ordinary conceptions of health and illness.

There are a number of supplementary stipulations that one must make in order to narrow the extension of "impaired basic capacities" to be equivalent to that of "ill." To begin with, we do not ordinarily think that permanent disabilities are illnesses. Persons who are born blind or deaf are not ill. We distinguish congenital conditions, no matter how seriously disabling, from illnesses. Second, we also seem to distinguish injuries from illness. The victim of an automobile wreck, no matter how incapacitated, is not in ordinary understanding ill, although he obviously is not healthy either. These distinctions are reflected in the criminal law's distinction between disease and defect:

> We use "disease" in the sense of a condition which is considered capable of either improving or deteriorating. We use "defect" in the sense of a condition which is not considered capable of either improving or deteriorating and which may be either congenital, or the result of injury, or the residual effect of a physical or mental disease.[20]

There are doubtlessly other limitations as well that must be pursued in a thorough ordinary-language analysis of the meaning of ill. One would need to exclude some conditions capable of improving that do involve basic incapacities, such as pregnancy and perhaps extreme obesity. More important in the present context is the further alleged nuance of the ordinary meaning of illness that I mentioned in Chapter 3. This was the suggestion of lawyers, philosophers, and psychiatrists that to be ill is to be nonresponsible for the symptoms of one's illness. Becoming ill, it is often thought, is necessarily something that happens to one, not something one brings on oneself.

There are in fact two limiting conditions on the meaning of illness implied in such a claim: (1) that if a person by his voluntary act brings on the condition, he is not ill; and (2) if one can remove the condition by voluntary act, he is not ill. Neither of these conditions is part of the ordinary meaning of illness. If they were, people who have lung cancer due to smog would be ill, but those who have the identical condition exclusively because of smoking would not. Similarly, people who have curable diseases would not be thought to be ill if they continued in their state for

The Concept of Mental Illness

voluntary failure to take the known cure; indeed, this would seem to have the curious result that Christian Scientists are never ill except when afflicted with incurable diseases.

Although the central idea of illness is the impairment of function, the abilities that are impaired when one is said to be ill do not necessarily include the ability to get rid of the condition one has. That ability is possibly relevant to the medical profession's determining whether drug addicts and alcoholics are worthy of medical attention; it is possibly relevant as well to the law's concern about the fairness of punishing someone for having a condition he cannot help. The only point here is that the possession of that ability is not denied simply because one is properly said to be ill.

ON CONJOINING MIND AND ILL: THE ORDINARY MEANING OF MENTAL ILLNESS

What do we add to the meaning of ill when we describe someone as being *mentally* ill? The first question to be resolved is whether "mental" describes the symptoms of an illness, or its causes. It is often assumed by those hostile to the idea of mental illness that the classification is by causes. Thus, the arguments of Szasz are proffered against those psychiatrists who believe physical causation to underlie mental illness: If there are such physical causes, according to Szasz, then we have brain disease, not mental illness.[21]

It is odd to think that something of such long standing as our concept of mental illness could be the hostage of physiological research in this way; that is, that such research could show us, not more about mental illness, but that it really does not exist. If the hope of nineteenth-century psychiatry were realized so that every person we call mentally ill possessed within his body some identifiable physical condition, surely we would say that we have discovered mental illness to have physical causes, not that it did not exist.

This suggests, although it does not prove, that the classification of illnesses as mental is related in some way to the symptoms exhibited by the person, not to the species of causation involved. What sort of symptoms lead us to classify an ill person as being *mentally* ill? It is that set of symptoms showing some impairment of those abilities we think of as mental abilities. Our mentalistic vocabulary is rich in words labeling, by some functional division, various mental powers. We have capacities of perception, of memory, of imagination, of learning, the basic capacities of reasoning and thinking, the capacities to feel emotion, and the capacities of will to have one's emotions and desires issue in one's actions. It is the impairment of these mental functions that we first and foremost have in mind when we speak of someone as being mentally ill. Thus, the ancient synonym of mental illness: the "loss of reason."

Recalling the behavioral bias of our criteria in applying mental illness, it would seem that the kinds of symptoms we should look to first that would exhibit in a relevant way the sorts of mental incapacities we have in mind when we call someone mentally ill, are the behavioral symptoms. Although psychologists or others might test mental capacities in ways quite different from simply observing daily behavior, and while it is doubtlessly a legitimate enterprise to attempt a phenomenological description of what it is like to experience going crazy, the principal criteria by which we ordinarily apply our notions of mental illness should be in some way linked to the behavior of the person whom we can call mentally ill.

Perhaps the analogy to character traits will again prove fruitful. When we say of another that he is greedy or vain, we have necessarily generalized about large aggregations of his observed behavior. We are claiming to have observed a consistency in his actions, namely, that he characteristically performs greedy or vain ones. Further, we are claiming in our description of him as greedy or vain that he is disposed to do similar sorts of things in the future. We thus both find an intelligible pattern to his past actions, and make a hypothetical assertion about what he will do if he gets the chance in the future.

Mentally ill is constructed somewhat similarly. We apply the label to a class of persons whose actions follow a certain pattern. Unlike words of character, however, we predicate "mentally ill" of a person whenever we find his pattern of past behavior unintelligible in some fundamental way; or, perhaps because of the unintelligibility of his acts, the only pattern we discern is that there is no pattern at all, and thus we think such an individual to be unpredictable as well.

When is there this fundamental failure of understanding of a fellow human being? The answer lies in those attributes that allow us to see another member of the human species as a person, that is, the attributes of autonomy and rationality. If we came across a being to whom we were not even willing to attribute causal agency (and thus would not consider him the author of his own actions), we would see him as fundamentally different from us. I doubt that even for the craziest of human beings there is such a radical suspension of personhood. Rather, it is the lack of rationality that prevents us from understanding mentally ill human beings to the same extent that we understand more normal persons.

The unintelligibility of the actions of the mentally ill stems from the fact that *the* rationalizing form of explanation, in terms of reasons for action, is not as regularly available to explain their actions as it is to explain the actions of the rest of us. More specifically, this form of explanation may break down in one of two ways.

The Concept of Mental Illness

In extreme cases, we may be unable to make out any set of beliefs and desires by virtue of which we may view an action as rational. For example, the bodily motions of epileptics during a grand mal seizure or perhaps the word salads of schizophrenics would seem to be nonrational activities in this sense. In such cases we are unable to see the action as even the *minimally* rational thing to do in light of any set of beliefs and desires we can reasonably ascribe to the agent. Second, to say that a person's action is irrational may be to deny the rationality of the beliefs or of the desires on which the action is based. The individual who avoids all contact with people because he believes he is made of glass and will shatter if touched behaves in a minimally rational manner in light of his desire not to shatter and his belief that he is made of glass and will shatter if touched. But the belief itself is irrational, and actions predicated on irrational beliefs are themselves, in ordinary understanding, irrational actions. Likewise, we may find the agent's desires defective, either because they are not intelligible to us as ends of action or because they are inconsistent with one another. The mentally ill often have conflicting desires: By acting to fulfill one desire, they often frustrate another. While this circumstance is true for most of us some of the time, more of the mentally ill's desires are unconscious and, being unconscious, cannot be resolved into a transitively ordered or consistent set of wants. Acting on such unresolved conflicts of desire cannot be fully rational, because such actions necessarily frustrate some things one wants a great deal, although perhaps unconsciously.[22]

When explanations of the actions of another human being break down in these ways, we say that he is irrational. We mean by irrational just that some significant portion of his actions pursue irrational ends, are predicated on beliefs themselves irrational, or are not based on desire/belief sets at all.

This kind of pattern of irrational action is the primary symptom of the mental incapacities we label mental illness.[23] For the mental abilities of perception, memory, imagination, and particularly reasoning are necessary in the acquisition of rational beliefs and in maintaining consistency between belief sets and desire sets. Rationality is one of the fundamental properties by which we understand ourselves as persons, that is, as creatures capable of adjusting our actions as reasonably efficient means to rational ends. Being mentally ill means being incapacitated from acting rationally in this fundamental sense.

There are obviously degrees of irrationality. How irrational must one be to be mentally ill in the popular understanding? Psychiatry in this century has doubtless influenced the popular understanding of the concept of mental illness. We are all to some degree irrational in our conduct; we are thus tempted to say that we are all a little bit crazy.

Yet side by side with this sophisticated, educated view there exists our ancient paradigm of mental illness: It is not manifested by the occasional irrationality we all exhibit. It is reserved for those gross deviations from intelligibility we still capture with the more severe statements, "He is crazy," or "He is insane," or "He is mad." Those idioms capture the essential notion of the ancient conception of mental illness as madness: that mentally ill people are different from us in ways we find hard to understand.

The National Opinion Research Center at the University of Chicago, in surveying the public's ideas about mental illness, found that "there is an old, socially-sanctioned, well-established set of views which supports the identification of mental illness only with the violent, extreme psychoses and, within this context of ideas, mental illness emerges as the ultimate catastrophe that can happen to a human being."[24]

The Purposes Behind Psychiatric Redefinition of Mental Illness

The seeking of a lexical definition such as the foregoing can be justified by the goal of clarity. For in seeking such a lexical definition one seeks to make explicit and clear what was only implicit and perhaps unclear in one's ordinary usage of a term or phrase such as mental illness. Justifying a (stipulative) redefinition of a well-known phrase is a different matter, however. When psychiatrists arrogate to themselves Humpty Dumpty's freedom to "make a word mean what we please," they also accept the burden of detailing the ends they seek to achieve by redefining a phrase one way rather than another. With the freedom to define as one pleases comes the responsibility to defend what it is one pleases to say.

To begin with, two questions need to be distinguished here. The first is: What purposes are served by classifying mental disorders into the various categories of schizophrenia and so forth? The second is: What purposes are served by going further and attempting to define mental illness in general (as opposed to defining schizophrenia, antisocial personality, etc.)? It is easy to conflate these two distinct concerns, but they are in fact quite different in the justifications that might plausibly be offered for each.

There are doubtless a number of legitimate reasons why doctors generally, and psychiatrists in particular, seek to classify disorders. The scientific and therapeutic concerns of medicine have for centuries dictated that symptoms that recur together, develop in an established course, and so on be provisionally linked as separate disorders. Such inductive procedures would seem to be a necessary first step in seeking the sorts of causal accounts themselves necessary to discover and justify effective therapies.

Those sorts of reasons, however, do not justify going beyond the task of classification and attempting the different task undertaken when psychiatrists purport to tell us what the general phrase mental illness should mean. There must be purposes other than those behind classificatory schemes that justify this more general definitional effort.

There are seemingly four possible purposes to be served by psychiatrists' attempts to stipulate some general definition of mental illness. The first I shall call a jurisdictional purpose: A definition of mental illness should mark clearly the sphere of proper concern – the jurisdiction – of psychiatry. To serve this purpose, a definition of mental illness should include all and only those conditions that are properly the subject matter of treatment by psychiatrists.

The second possible purpose for defining mental illness is a kind of social strategy. Once one perceives that illness is widely regarded as a condition for which one is not responsible, one might guide one's definition of mental illness to cover just those conditions to which one thinks the sick role is the appropriate social response.

The third possible purpose is one I shall call the "hard cases" purpose of giving a definition. It was a hard case such as homosexuality that most recently generated the discussion about what is a mental illness. Such hard cases can be resolved, or even intelligently debated, only if one has clearly in mind what it is one is claiming when one asserts that homosexuality, for example, is or is not a mental illness. Hence, the hard cases purpose: A definition of mental illness should allow us to resolve cases (or at least know what we are arguing about if we cannot resolve them) when we are unsure of whether to classify a condition as a mental illness.

The fourth purpose behind such general definitional efforts is what I shall call the legitimization purpose served by such definitions. The purpose of defining mental illness on this rationale is to legitimate psychiatry as a genuine branch of medicine. A definition of mental illness serves this purpose only if it shows mental illness to be a species of the genus, medical illness.

Before one critiques various definitions in light of these purposes, one first must ask whether these are legitimate purposes for defining mental illness. Would any definition that satisfied them be useful? Can any definition in fact accomplish all of them? Let me reexamine them one by one.

JURISDICTIONAL PURPOSE

To stipulate a definition of mental illness so as to serve the jurisdictional purpose is to focus on one typical consequence of someone being authoritatively labeled mentally ill: He is the appropriate subject of treatment by a psychiatrist. In such a case, one defines mental illness so that it can be used as a kind of trigger for psychiatric treatment: To be mentally ill (as redefined for this purpose) is to require the services of a psychiatrist, and vice versa.[25]

To define mental illness solely with this "trigger of treatment" rationale in mind would require that one include in mental illness all and only the conditions that psychiatrists properly treat. Treatable by a psychiatrist, in such a case, becomes both a necessary and a sufficient condition of being mentally ill. Some psychiatrists who have seen this requirement have thought that they could take "treatable by a psychiatrist" as the sought-after definition of mental illness itself. E. Jellinek, for example, once concluded that alcoholism was an illness because the medical profession treated it as one;[26] similarly, F. Kaupl Taylor once equated being diseased with "patienthood," and the latter with expression of therapeutic concern by doctors.[27]

Even if one's exclusive concern in defining mental illness is jurisdictional, one cannot use the desired consequence of the definition as the definition itself. It is perfectly trivial to assert that to be mentally ill is to be the subject of treatment by psychiatrists—if one's only definition of mentally ill is "treatable by a psychiatrist." To avoid such triviality one needs to spell out in the definition what kinds of conditions are the appropriate subjects of treatment by psychiatrists. To do otherwise is to be like the aforementioned mortician who, much concerned to define the domain of his professional concern by giving a definition of "dead," ends up defining it as: "a state that is the appropriate subject of the professional concern of a mortician."

One must thus bring into the definition some content, and not give a "definition" that only points out the desired consequence one hopes to achieve from the completed definition. But where is such content to come from? There are two different sources, relating to two different kinds of jurisdictional definitions, one descriptive and the other normative. The descriptive branch would simply look at the conditions psychiatrists do treat and ask, What do these have in common? It is true that one could accomplish this descriptive task simply by pointing to the classified disorders of psychiatry, such as those listed in the third edition of the American Psychiatric Association's *Diagnostic and Statistical Manual* (DSM-III) and saying, "Psychiatrists treat whatever conditions are listed therein as mental disorders." Indeed, as a former president of the American Psychiatric Association once pointed out,[28] that is in fact how many psychiatrists do define the domain of their concern. Although one could do this, surely it is a legitimate enterprise to attempt to discover what all such conditions have in common that makes psychiatrists think of them as mental disorders. It may be that there is no unity to the various conditions psychiatrists have classified as mental disorders; perhaps psychiatrists treat so many different conditions that nothing of interest can be said about them in general. That would not show psychiatry to be without a jurisdiction; it would have as many jurisdictions as there were different mental disorders. But it surely would be troubling to think that one's profession deals with a large number of different things that have nothing in common with each other, other than the juxtaposition of their names in a manual issued by the professional association.

The normative branch would seek to give content to mental illness by looking to the conditions psychiatrists *ought to treat* (which may or may not be the same as the ones they *do* treat). Here one takes a position about who psychiatry can help and defines the mentally ill so that they and only they are in that class. One's theory about what makes some conditions treatable by a psychiatrist will, in such a case, give content to one's definition of mental illness.

Seeking to accomplish either the descriptive or the prescriptive task of making out psychiatry's jurisdiction can potentially generate very broad definitions of mental illness. On the descriptive branch, if it turns out that a lot of people with minor problems seek treatment from psychiatrists, mental illness will include such minor problems. One may well approach the breadth of something like Fromm's definition, with mental health being an ideal state of human happiness and flourishing that few if any attain and mental illness being the state of most of us as we muddle through this life. On the normative branch, if one thinks oneself possessed of a general theory of human behavior, such as Freud's metapsychology purports to be, one may well think that most people could be helped by seeing a psychiatrist. Accordingly, most people should be included within the extension of mentally ill because they are the appropriate subjects of psychiatric treatment.

For my own part I think that there is little to be gained even if psychiatrists were to succeed in either of these definitional tasks. Once one successfully completes them, one may then have a convenient label for the conditions psychiatrists either do or should treat, a label underlain by some theory about what all such conditions have in common. Yet in ordinary medicine there is no felt need to connect treatment and illness: Doctors treat matters that are not illnesses (e.g., delivery of babies, cosmetic surgery, circumcision, and matters of family planning), and there are some illnesses (the terminal ones) that doctors cannot treat.

It is unclear why psychiatrists should seek a tighter connection of illness to their treatment than other medical doctors. One suspects that it is because such a definition of mental illness can serve the legitimization function discussed shortly. Yet this is plainly not so if one defines mental illness just so it fits conditions psychiatrists do or should treat. One cannot then turn around and justify medical treatment because of some mental illness, so defined.

Such circular "justification" for medical treatment (in terms of patients being "ill") is in any event unnecessary. Medical treatment of various conditions can be justified in consensual relations by the fact that it works to the patients' satisfaction in alleviating what bothers them. Psychiatrists, like other doctors, do not need an illness to trigger their professional concern—any more than lawyers need a "legal problem" to trigger their professional concern. The justification for professional services generally is that one can help clients to a position that they, with full information, think to be better.

The jurisdictional consideration accordingly gives little reason to stipulate a broader sense of mental illness than is found in our ordinary conception. If this were the only consideration, psychiatrists could well eschew special definitions of a familiar phrase, since such special definitions always generate some confusion in various audiences (including, often enough, those who do the defining).

THE STRATEGIC PURPOSE

Psychiatrists who would define mental illness so as to serve what I have called a strategic purpose make the following sort of calculation. Since illness generally carries with it a set of exemptions from social responsibilities that Talcott Parsons called "the sick role,"[29] one could guide one's definition of mental illness to include all and only those conditions for which one thinks the sick role exemptions to be appropriate. One looks, for example, at narcotics addiction and judges that for various reasons narcotics addicts should not be held responsible for causing their condition, for not ending it, or for their acts of using narcotics while in it. One accordingly classifies narcotics addiction as an illness just so addicts are given the exemptions the sick role is thought to afford from these responsibilities. As Robert Veatch has noted, "The attempt to place narcotic addiction, violence associated with rage, and larceny and assault by children into the medical model is in large part a move to remove blame."[30]

Fastening on to the social consequences often attached to being ill, and defining mental illness so as to achieve those consequences, is no proper part of psychiatry. It is a political strategy, pure and simple. There may be solid reasons for exempting addicts and others from responsibility. But one must argue for those exemptions on morally relevant grounds, say, the compulsive nature of addiction. It adds not a whit of persuasive power to any such argument to classify the condition as an illness, when by illness one means "exempt condition." Such a strategic purpose thus should not justify any definition of mental illness by psychiatrists.

THE HARD CASES PURPOSE

A relatively straightforward purpose served by psychiatrists attempting to give a general definition of mental illness is to aid in the debate about whether particular conditions are or are not to be classified as mental illnesses. As was illustrated by the vigorous disagreements of a decade ago

The Concept of Mental Illness

about whether homosexuality is a mental illness, one does need to know what one is arguing about (what the characteristics of a mental illness are) before one can even intelligently disagree about whether some particular condition is or is not a mental illness. In law, cases that are difficult to decide are often termed hard cases, and thus I call this justification the hard cases purpose in seeking to stipulate some general definition of mental illness. It might be thought that one can argue by analogy in such cases; for example, "homosexuality is like sterility because both render one unable to reproduce." And, indeed, one can meaningfully debate borderline cases in such ways; only, when one does so, one does unsystematically what a general definition would allow one to do systematically, namely, articulate the criteria by which such analogies hold.

It is sometimes objected that seeking a general definition in order to classify hard cases is a viciously circular enterprise because the definition itself is derived from labeling particular conditions as mental illnesses; and without the general definition, it is asked, how could one know that these particular conditions were mental illnesses?[31] Yet there is in fact nothing suspect in seeking a definition in this way. We are often much more confident of our judgments about the application of words to particular things than we are of some general definition of those words. We may know the meaning of the word "obscene," for example, without knowing any definition of the word; we know its meaning nonetheless in the sense that we can correctly identify obscene motion pictures. There is nothing illegitimate in seeking to abstract from the particular cases we are sure about what they have in common that justifies our calling anything obscene. In such a way we may construct a definition, which we can then use to debate hard cases.

One may have noticed that when seeking a definition for the hard cases purpose, one is no longer stipulating a new meaning of mental illness so as to achieve some desired consequence. For there is a body of judgments to which any hard cases definition must conform; namely, it must fit the particular judgments that some conditions are clearly mental illnesses. Thus, here one is seeking a *lexical* definition of mental illness. Moreover, it does not seem likely that the clear cases or paradigm examples of mental illness differ much between psychiatric and popular opinion. The extreme psychoses are the clear cases of mental illness for everyone. Accordingly, the body of usage to which any psychiatric definition of this sort must conform should differ little from ordinary usage.

THE LEGITIMIZATION PURPOSE

As we examined in Chapter 4, the very idea that there are illnesses of the mind has been under severe attack from numerous directions in the last two decades. Can a definition of mental illness serve as an argument against this attack?

It may sound odd to think of a definition as constituting an argument at all. If psychiatrists were merely *stipulating* a meaning of mental illness to serve the first two purposes, then such a definition by itself would not be an argument. Yet the psychiatric literature is rich in attempts to *analyze,* not stipulate, the meaning of mental illness. The strategy is a familiar one in the literature: One first analyzes what illness means in medicine generally, and then stipulates that the only conditions properly thought of as *mental* illnesses are those that are illnesses by some general medical criterion, only of a mental sort.[32] If successful, one does show that mental illness as defined is a species of the genus, illness. One has thereby legitimated the idea that there are illnesses of the mind, because by definition the only conditions properly so called are all illnesses to start with.

It is worth stressing that this purpose requires an accurate analysis of the general criteria that we all implicitly use to decide what is and what is not an illness generally. One necessarily gives up Humpty Dumpty's freedom to make a word mean what one pleases, for that part of the definition defining illness is not free from factual inquiry. A successful definition of illness will classify as such all and only those conditions that are illnesses. It is thus a legitimate form of objection to this part of the definition to argue by counterexample: If the criteria suggested include conditions most of us do not regard as illnesses, or if the criteria suggested exclude conditions most of us do regard as illnesses, the criteria are wrong—"wrong" in the sense that the definition cannot then serve this legitimizing purpose.

The Expansive Psychiatric Definitions of Mental Illness

We are now in a position to judge the extended view of madness of modern psychiatry. What justification is there to transform the ordinary notion of mental illness as madness into the broad psychiatric conceptions we examined in Chapter 3?

Insofar as the likes of Fromm and Menninger define mental illness merely as the name of all conditions modern psychiatrists either do or can treat, one can have little quarrel with the expansive notions of illness they propose. As pointed out earlier, people who are unhappy for a wide variety of reasons seek psychiatric treatment, and, arguably at least, psychiatrists can and should give such treatment. I argued earlier that mental illness is a confusing label for these conditions and that psychiatrists need it about as much as lawyers need some concept of legal disease to trigger their respective professional concerns. We may bypass this last objection, however, for we may grant the propriety of expansive psychiatric definitions for jurisdictional purposes and still resist any use of such definitions in law, morals, or everyday life.

If psychiatrists wish to mark out the domain of their professional concern by a definition of mental illness, such jurisdictional claim can hardly amount to a claim of *exclusive* jurisdiction of the conditions included. Psychologists, social workers, ministers, priests, rabbis, and lay persons, for example, may also have skills relevant to the treatment of such conditions. More pertinently, lawyers may also "treat" these same conditions, even if the legal "treatment" is in terms of punishment or civil damage judgments. Thus, if psychiatrists include alcoholism, drug addiction, or homosexual behavior in the extension of mental illness because they think they do or should treat such conditions, such labeling is not relevant to the questions of whether such conditions are morally culpable and legally punishable. Nor can the inclusion, for example, of antisocial personality as a mental illness determine whether such condition should constitute an excuse from punishment. Each discipline or profession may have its own purposes for distinguishing some conditions from others. There is little reason to think that "treatable by a psychiatrist" is a factor very relevant to determining moral culpability, deterrability, or any of the other purposes served by criminal law and the law of torts.

Even less relevant are those psychiatric definitions of mental illness that are motivated by strategic purposes. When mental illness is used as a kind of conceptual pawn in political advocacy, it is only a distraction. If someone such as Menninger believes that criminals are what they are through no fault of their own, that they are controlled by unconscious forces, an unhappy childhood, compelling drives and the like, responsibility issues should be argued in those terms. Stretching our ordinary notions of illness so as to play on the usual exemptions granted those who are sick, is simply a distraction, a debater's device to be shunned in serious thought about these issues.

The heart of our concerns in this chapter is reached when we consider broad psychiatric definitions, not as *stipulations* for jurisdictional or strategic purposes, but as *analyses* of what mental illness means. As such, broad definitions such as Fromm's or Menninger's become descriptive claims that we can test against our own understanding of the meaning of mental illness. Does illness generally, or the clear examples of *mental* illness in both psychiatry and ordinary thought, contain within them the features that could justify categorizing criminal behavior, for example, as an illness too?

It is worth reviewing from the earlier half of this chapter what such features are. There are two. First, the clear cases of *mental* illness are characterized by extreme irrationality in the behavior of those we call mentally ill. Second, the irrational behavior evidences *illness* because it is underlain by functional impairment. To the extent that mind as well as body can be given a functional organization, illness is the correct name for the impairments in mental functioning thought to underlie irrational behavior.

To what extent do failures to realize Fromm's "productive orientation" (i.e., failures to realize the human potential for happiness Fromm and company envision as objectively desirable for all persons) fit the two features licensing application of mental illness? Taking them one by one, consider first the rationality of the behavior of such "less than ideal" people. One has to stretch our notions of irrationality considerably if one is to accommodate such failures at achieving happiness as mental illness. One way to do this is by playing on the *vagueness* of rational. Rational is a degree-vague word, like many other words, such as red. Things can be more or less red; human beings can be more or less rational. The obvious way to extend our notions of mental illness is to allow that even the minor irrationality we all can exhibit on occasion can count as mental illness.

A less obvious way to extend mental illness is to play on the *ambiguity* of rational. Instead of judging the rationality of a person (in part) by the intelligibility, consistency, and transitivity of his values and desires, one judges the person by the correctness of those values and desires. For someone such as Fromm or Aristotle, who believe that there is an objectively right way for persons to be, discoverable through reason, failures to act on desires that are correct might (as we observed at the end of Chapter 2) be termed irrational and thus, mentally ill.

Neither of these stretches of irrationality is a legitimate move for a psychiatrist seeking to define mental illness for the hard cases or the legitimization purposes. The play on the vagueness of irrational can only seem tempting because of the lack of any crisp line between the seriously irrational (the mentally ill) and the less seriously irrational (normal persons). Yet no word that is degree vague has any crisp lines. Red, for example, is vague and has no such lines separating it from orange and purple. The lack of any clear lines, however, does not mean one cannot say, "Most items are not red," any more than the lack of any line should prevent one from saying, "Most people are not irrational" (mentally ill). And if one is attempting to legitimate one's application of red to some object, such task is not aided in the least by extending red to include the entire spectrum of visible light on the theory that no significant line can be drawn between red and the other colors. That there is no one place that can be shown to be better than another as the boundary of what is red hardly entitles one to have no boundary at all. Yet this seems to be the reasoning of those who would extend irrational to cover all persons just because there is no one place that can be shown to be *the* place to draw the line between the seriously irrational (the mentally ill) and the normal.

The play on the ambiguity of rational is even more suspect. As we men-

The Concept of Mental Illness

tioned at the end of Chapter 2, there *is* a sense of irrational such that desires or values can be said to be not only unintelligible, inconsistent, and intransitive, but also incorrect. Indeed, an objectivist in ethics is probably committed to there being false (and thus irrational) moral beliefs, desires, and values just as there are false (and in the same sense irrational) factual beliefs. Nonetheless, it is important to see that our ordinary notion of mental illness does not include the latter kind of irrationality. Nor is the difference between judging a desire to be unintelligible, and judging a desire to be false or incorrect, some minor difference of a conventional and arbitrary sort. We judge a desire to be unintelligible when we reach the limits of our empathetic understanding, that is, where we cannot understand how any *person* could want what he claims he wants. Intelligibility of desires is, in other words, one of our important boundaries of personhood.

Such limits are educable; familiarity with different persons, and different cultures, can make one less parochial in the limits of this kind of empathy. Yet some states of affairs remain outside the bounds of things a person could intelligibly want and still remain a person. The presence of such desires (along with inconsistency, irrational factual beliefs, lack of minimal rationality, and lack of a transitively ordered set of preferences) is an indicator of the kind of irrationality we call mental illness.

Nonparochial judgments of unintelligibility will not be at all the same kind of judgments as those that characterize values as wrong, false, or irrational (in the ethical objectivist's sense of irrational). For to say that a value is wrong, false, or irrational is not at all to say that one cannot understand how a person would hold it. The killer for hire has the wrong set of values. An ethical objectivist will also believe that the killer for hire has values that, if he were rational, he would change—he has "irrational values." The killer for hire has intelligible desires or values nonetheless. We can understand the heightened importance he attaches to money, and the lack of importance he attaches to human life, even while we think such values to be wrong, irrational, and evil. Such values are not outside the pale of what a person could want. Put another way: There is such a thing as evil in the world. Believing this, it becomes important not to confuse unintelligibility (madness) with incorrectness (badness) in the major premises of the practical reasoning of human beings.

In terms of our main indicator of mental illness, irrational behavior, there is thus a significant line to be drawn between serious irrationality, on the one hand, and either occasional irrationality or the irrationality of incorrect desires alone, on the other. One cannot gloss over this difference by playing on either the vagueness or the ambiguity of rational. This same line reappears when we turn (as we now do) to the second feature of mental illness, that of impaired functioning.

The clear cases of mental illness are clearly *illnesses* not only because there is severely irrational behavior, but also because that behavior is underlain by impairment in various functions of the mind. There is no such impairment of function when someone arrives at the wrong value judgments. This is true even if one is an objectivist about values so that there are such things as irrational or wrong values to hold.

The reply that psychiatrists in the Aristotle/Fromm camp might make here is to assert that there *is* some impaired mental functioning when persons (such as the killer for hire) make gross mistakes in their value judgments. One would accordingly urge that such persons are properly categorized as mentally ill because they share this essential feature of the clear cases of both illness and of mental illness. Such a reply challenges any attempt to specify functional impairment in a way that does not include the defects in moral reasoning one might plausibly think to underlie mistaken (irrational) values.

To assess this reply, let us reexamine the idea of functional impairment itself. One can meaningfully talk of functional impairments of systems to which one has already given a functional organization. The assignment of functions to mental states or body parts constitutes giving mind or body a functional organization. As we saw in Chapter 1, such assignment of functions makes sense only relative to some end state of the system itself. Hence, our idea of functional impairment is itself dependent on some end state being defined for persons.

How much one packs into mental health, the end state around which one gives the mind a functional organization, determines what will count as functional impairment. Fromm, Aristotle, "third force" psychology, and the positive mental health movement pack a great deal into their definition of this all-important end state, as we have seen. For in their idea of mental health is their vision of the good life for persons, the complete taxonomy of the virtues. If one gives the mind a functional organization based on such an end state, one will naturally include in one's idea of a properly functioning mind those mental states (moral beliefs and emotional states) necessary to reach correct moral conclusions.

The debate here thus focuses ultimately on the propriety of including such value judgments in the end state of health. As we have seen, value judgments are ineliminably mixed up in *all* definitions of end states to be used in giving functional organizations—as true of bodies as of minds. Yet the value judgments behind the ordinary notion of (mental and physical) health are of an extremely limited kind. They form a kind of "thin theory" of the good, as John Rawls uses the phrase—a kind of theory about what all persons would value, no matter what else they might value.[33]

Rawls uses this notion for his own heuristic purposes in constructing a theory of justice. As a thought experiment to aid us in articulating our moral intuitions about justice, Rawls imagines a person in what he calls

The Concept of Mental Illness

the "original position." The person has to decide between competing conceptions of social justice while behind a "veil of ignorance," that is, while he does not know his own conception of the good. He only knows he has some conception of the good, a theory of the virtues, but he does not know what it is. Despite such ignorance, Rawls tells us, we would all nonetheless reason from a set of "primary goods." These are very broadly characterized by Rawls as consisting of rights and liberties, opportunities and powers, and income and wealth. Primary goods, Rawls tells us,

> are things which it is supposed a rational man wants whatever else he wants. Regardless of what an individual's rational plans are in detail, it is assumed that there are various things which he would prefer more of rather than less. With more of these goods men can generally be assured of greater success in carrying out their intentions and in advancing their ends, whatever these ends may be.[34]

Rawl's thin theory of the good is the limited moral theory that justifies certain things being primary goods in this sense, that is, goods valued by all persons no matter what their conception of the good might be, because such goods are necessary to *any* conception of the good.

Liberty, for example, is something one might well believe all persons with *some* conception of the good life would value, because a right to liberty is necessary for one to carry out *any* life plan that one might think to be good.

Our ordinary notions of health (and thus of function assignment, functional organization of mind and body, and functional impairment) are built on such a thin theory of the good. A body that is relatively free from pain, that allows one to move about, and the like, is part of such a thin theory because all persons would value such a body as necessary to whatever else they want. Likewise, a mind that is relatively free from elementary logical errors, that by and large forms factual beliefs in proportion to the evidence available, that has capacities of imagination, and so on is also part of such a thin theory of the good. Such a mind is to be valued by all persons, no matter what else they might think virtuous.

The functional impairment on which our ordinary notions of mental illness are built is value laden only in the sense that it depends on this thin theory of the good. Anyone who wishes to extend this idea of functional impairment to include a *full* theory of the good for people must show that there really is no line between a "thin" and a "full" theory of the good; put another way, there are no things that are good "no matter what else one thinks to be good." Masochists value pain, and slaves might love being enslaved. Bodily health and liberty, one might think accordingly, are not part of any thin theory.

If this were true, Fromm and others would have good grounds for extending our ordinary notions of functional impairment by extending the notions of health on which it is based. The argument would be that the distinction between medicine and ethics is an arbitrary one because only a *non*separable part of our values is included in the definitions of health and impairment.

Yet the distinction between a thin and a full theory of the good is neither undrawable nor arbitrary. The distinction is in fact the same that we discussed before, between values that are unintelligible for a person to hold and values that are incorrect (irrational). A thin theory of the good tells us what things are necessary for the attainment of any (more particular) values a *person* might *intelligibly* hold. It is true that one can imagine beings who might value anything. Their entire lives, for example, might be oriented toward placing their left elbows in mud for as long as possible. If such states of affairs are included as possible motives, then, of course, there can be no thin theory of the good. It is only because we have limits on the states of affairs that *persons* can desire—limits of intelligibility—that a thin theory of the good is possible. Simply because persons do not intelligibly want just about anything, it is possible to develop a limited set of goods that are necessary for all things persons do want.

A full theory of the good makes choices between the numerous conceptions of the good life that are intelligible conceptions. The value judgments such a theory makes are accordingly different from the highly limited value judgments of a thin theory. It is thus no minor shift in our idea of functional impairment to seek to include within the end state that ultimately defines it a full theory of the good and virtuous person. Our ordinary notions of mental health and mental illness do not suggest such a move as a natural extension of the ordinary meanings of those phrases. If psychiatrists are going to plump for such expanded notions, they cannot do so in the guise of an *analysis* of the "essence" of illness or of mental illness, an essence of which only *they* have seen the full implications. They must seek reasons justifying a major *redefinition* of our notions of health and illness. Such reasons, as we have seen, are not themselves very persuasive. Ethics, in short, does not collapse into medicine by any kind of conceptual inertia or manipulation.

To reject the attempted medicalization of morals of the psychiatric turn is not, of course, to deny that health and mental health are good. What is denied is that health is the only thing that is good, that it can be conceived so broadly that it *constitutes* the good. One draws the line between ethics and medicine only by denying this latter claim, not the former evaluation of the goodness of health.

A More Moderate Psychiatric Definition of Mental Illness

The psychiatric turn sometimes takes less dramatic form than that examined in Chapter 3. One such very recent example is provided by Robert

The Concept of Mental Illness

Spitzer, the psychiatrist principally responsible for the third edition of the American Psychiatric Association's *Diagnostic and Statistical Manual*. Spitzer was chairman of the APA Task Force on Nomenclature and Statistics that drafted this official psychiatric taxonomy of mental illnesses. While chairman he proposed a general definition of mental disorder to accompany DSM-III,[35] and in closing the chapter I shall consider the problems presented by even this much more moderate and carefully constructed definition.

Spitzer has been explicit about the reasons for psychiatrists to seek a general definition of mental illness and in one way or another mentions each of the four reasons discussed earlier. The definition proposed follows the classical, Aristotelian pattern of definition,[36] which comes in two steps: One first specifies the genus, or the larger class of things, to which the item to be defined belongs (here, medical disorders); one then states the principle that differentiates the item to be defined within that larger class (for Spitzer, psychological symptoms or comprehension only in psychological terms). If successful, one shows all *mental* disorders to be a species of the genus, *medical* disorders.

Spitzer's own summary of both parts of his complex definition is as follows:

> A medical disorder is a relatively distinct condition resulting from an organismic dysfunction which in its fully developed or extreme form is directly and intrinsically associated with distress, disability or certain other types of disadvantage. The disadvantage may be of a physical, perceptual, sexual or interpersonal nature. Implicitly there is a call to action on the part of the person who has the condition, the medical or its allied professions, and society.
>
> A mental disorder is a medical disorder whose manifestations are primarily signs or symptoms of a psychological (behavioral) nature, or if physical, can be understood only using psychological concepts.[37]

The heart of this definition lies in the first part, defining medical disorder. The principle of differentiation, dividing *mental* disorders from *medical* disorders, is much less problematic once one shelves Szaszian concerns about conjoining mental with disorder or illness.

It is worth noting in passing that there is an issue lurking here: Should one classify as mental disorders those with mental *causes,* or those with mental *symptoms?* It is a common assumption that the difference between physical and mental illness lies in the species of causality involved. For the reasons given earlier, I think Spitzer is correct in classifying by symptoms and not by causes.

Turning to the main part of Spitzer's definition (that which defines the class of medical disorders), this definition comes in three parts: (a) organismic dysfunction that causes (b) negative consequences, which in turn give rise to (c) a call to action on the part of patients, doctors, and society. This nominally three-tiered structure obscures, I think, the true nature of the definition and is in any event unnecessarily complicated.

Taking the third part first, what Spitzer has in mind here as calls to action by various groups are the kinds of things we have discussed earlier. The call to action to patients is to seek treatment by doctors, the call to action to doctors is to treat, and the call to action to society is to grant the exemptions of the sick role. There are two questions one should distinguish in order to see that none of these calls to action is properly part of the definition of medical disorder. First, is it true that if and only if there are the calls to action Spitzer describes, there is a medical disorder? Second, even if it is true, is the fact that there is such equivalence any reason to suppose that part of the meaning of medical disorder is that calls to action exist?

The first question we have already discussed. To repeat what was concluded there: It is not true that if doctors treat a condition, that condition must be classified as a medical disorder. Nor is it true that if a condition is classified as a medical disorder, then such condition exempts one from responsibility, entitles one to third-party payment, and so on. In some of the cases doctors treat there may be such a call to action on the part of society to react to the patient in certain ways, but whether there is will be determined by purposes other than those justifying medical classification.

Second, even if it were true that society exempted persons from certain responsibilities if and only if they had a medical disorder as defined by doctors, surely such exemption is not part of anyone's meaning of medical disorder. To say otherwise is to confuse mere equivalence (p is true if and only if q is true) with "meaning the same as." Consider the *Oxford English Dictionary's* former definition of gold as "the world's most precious metal." Suppose that these expressions are equivalent, that is, whenever "gold" is used, "the world's most precious metal" could be substituted without change of the truth value of the expressions in which they occur. Such equivalence does not show gold to mean the world's most precious metal. To say that the word does mean this reduces the statement that gold is the world's most precious metal to an analytical truth, when, in fact, a rise in the price of silver could make it false. Gold does not mean the world's most precious metal, even if it is a contingent truth about gold that it is currently the world's most precious metal.

As a second example, consider the following definition of death (a condition doctors, lawyers, and philosophers are currently much concerned to define): " 'Death' means to be buried by a mortician." Suppose it were true in our society that all and only dead people are buried by morticians (i.e., "dead" and "buried by morticians" are extensionally equivalent expressions). Even so, the definition misses entirely the meaning of death; otherwise, the idea of being *buried alive* could not constitute the plot of a chilling horror story but only a conceptual impossibility imagined by someone who did not know the meaning of death.

In short, the calls to action are not part of the meaning of medical disorder. They may be consequences of having a medical disorder (although I have argued that one of them, the call to society, is not even that); they may be one of the purposes of giving the definition, as I have argued the triggering of treatment rationale could be; but they are not themselves part of the meaning of medical disorder as doctors or anyone else employ the phrase.

The first of these three tiers, organismic dysfunction, is included by Spitzer as a reminder that the essence of illness is functional impairment. The trick, as Spitzer recognizes, is to specify the end state around which one can judge whether there has been functional impairment or not. Spitzer eschews any of the broad conceptions of such an end state, because he believes there is no consensus "on what represents optimal psychological functioning."[38] He accordingly seeks to define such an end state by saying what it excludes: It excludes distress, disability, or disadvantage, the three negative consequences of organismic dysfunction that form the second of his three tiers. Thus, the content of this definition ultimately comes from these three criteria for being ill.

Distress is defined to include not only physical pain, but also psychological states such as anxiety and anger. Disability is defined as impairment in a "wide range of activities."[39] The third D, disadvantage, is Spitzer's catch-all category. It is, he recognizes,

> heavily dependent on social definitions of the degree of the disadvantage, the undesirableness of the behavior, and other considerations as to the consequences of considering the condition as a medical disorder. For these reasons, all the conditions considered medical disorders on the basis of this criterion *alone* are the ones that are most apt to be a source of intense controversy, particularly those regarded as mental disorders.[40]

The reason for the controversy about this third criterion, disadvantage, is easy to discover. For disadvantage, as used by Spitzer, is far removed from its usage in the literature as a traditional criterion of illness or disease, where it refers to the ability to function effectively, to survive, or to reproduce.[41] The most critical difference from this traditional usage is Spitzer's willingness to allow the adverse reaction of society to count as placing the individual at a disadvantage. Sexual sadism, kleptomania, and pathological gambling are said to disadvantage the individual because such activities lead to painful consequences; namely, the police pick you up. If one were to keep extending such examples, one would include all seriously immoral or illegal activity as leading to painful consequences in all cultures and thus to disadvantage, and thus all dispositions to such activity as medical disorders.

Spitzer recognizes as much when he acknowledges that "a large proportion of individuals involved in criminal behavior meet the criteria for antisocial personality disorder"[42] (itself included as a medical disorder). Homosexuality, although "frequently lead[ing] to painful consequences in environments which demand heterosexual functioning or punish homosexual behavior," is not included only because there are social "environments which support or are indifferent to such behavior [so that] there is no necessary association with a painful outcome."[43]

Surely psychiatrists do not want to say this. One does not want to give up the line between medical judgment and moral evaluation this easily. It strikes me that we might well wish to consider some forms of theft, sexual brutality, or gambling as forms of medical disorder, but not because well-ordered societies necessarily attach painful consequences to these activities. After all, all well-ordered societies attach such painful consequences to many forms of these activities that no one would want to consider as disorders, for example, organized car theft. Surely it is something else about kleptomania, sexual sadism, or pathological gambling that inclines us to regard them as disorders, something other than the fact that no society can tolerate such activities.

The "something else" that suggests itself is to be found in the compulsive and irrational nature of the activities. It would seem that kleptomaniacs might be regarded as having a mental disorder because they do not know why they steal what they do, and they find it difficult, if not impossible, to stop. The difference between a kleptomaniac and a habitual thief would seem to lie, as Max Friedemann once suggested, in these two dimensions, lack of rational motive and compulsion.[44] If so, kleptomania could seemingly be regarded as a disorder under the first two criteria, distress and disability, for those who are irrational and compelled are necessarily those who are impaired from acting in ways in which both they and society would wish them to act. That would seem to qualify as a disablement (the second criterion), usually leading to distress (the first).

One would doubtlessly wish to do further analysis in order to make out the last thesis. To accommodate these cases of compulsion, one might want to modify the range of activities required to be impaired before one is said to have a disorder. One would also want to be clear on the distinction between compulsion and mere causation, so that one is not led to the error of thinking that because one is merely caused to act in certain ways one is therefore impaired in the relevant sense from acting otherwise. Still, this approach seems more promising than does the open invitation Spitzer's notion of disadvantage gives to all who wish to argue that psychiatry is covert moral philosophy, thinly disguised as science.

The Concept of Mental Illness

Another subcategory of disadvantage for Spitzer is "marked impairment in the ability to form relatively lasting and nonconflictual interpersonal relationships" and "impairment of the ability to experience sexual pleasure in an interpersonal context." These are expressly included by Spitzer as disadvantages, not disabilities, because of their normative nature. Yet as we have seen, in a nonharmful sense all medical classification is normative because of its dependence on some desirable end state around which a functional organization can be given to a person; that includes what we call disability no less than the things Spitzer calls disadvantage. Thus, these items, if they are to be disorders at all, should be handled as disabling conditions under the disability criterion. If they cannot be fitted there, perhaps one should simply recognize that psychiatrists, like all doctors, treat conditions that are not disorders.

This problematic third criterion, disadvantage, which stretches mental illness to include much that is criminal or immoral, should be eliminated. Preferable is the definition of mental disorder (also drafted by Spitzer) that finally won its way through the American Psychiatric Association's committee for inclusion in DSM-III:

> In DSM-III each of the mental disorders is conceptualized as a clinically significant behavorial or psychological syndrome or pattern that occurs in an individual and that is typically associated with either a painful symptom (distress) or impairment in one or more important areas of functioning (disability). In addition, there is an inference that there is a behavioral, psychological or biological dysfunction, and that the disturbance is not only in the relationship between the individual and society. (Where the disturbance is *limited* to a conflict between an individual and society, this may represent social deviance, which may or may not be commendable, but it is not by itself a mental disorder.)[45]

This semiofficial definition of mental illness for the psychiatric profession has the virtue of eliminating the concept that makes it difficult to maintain any line between the sick and the bad, namely disadvantage. Retained from Spitzer's earlier definition are the crucial notions of functional impairment (dysfunction) and disability.

Such a definition, like Spitzer's preceding definition, does not by itself say much. It is mostly an expression of an intention to keep the term mental illness from engulfing all socially undesirable behavior. It also focuses our attention on the right concepts to be used in charting the limits of mental illness, disability, and dysfunction. To give any real content to such definition one must undertake the twofold task outlined in the last section: (1) to articulate the degree of irrationality (and its difference from the irrationality of wrong desires and of false beliefs) that makes an actor mad; and (2) to specify the thin theory of the good by which a person's mental abilities can be given a functional organization.[46]

Spitzer in his earlier efforts has obliquely hinted at each of these tasks. With regard to the first, he recognized that "when individuals undergo deprivation and distress in order to obtain some *understandable* positive goal, we assume that the organism is working and do not infer a dysfunction."[47] This is to use, and to use appropriately, intelligibility as the standard to be applied to desires before they can give rise to an inference of mental illness. With regard to the second, Spitzer defines disability as an indication of illness only if it incapacitates from a "wide range of activities." "Wide range" is Spitzer's substitute for what I have called the thin theory of the good, which psychiatrists must develop to have any meaningful definition of mental illness. "The reason," Spitzer tells us, "that a wide range of activities needs to be affected [before we should consider an impairment to be an illness] is to avoid *a priori* decisions as to what areas of human activity are 'basic' or 'essential.' "[48] One of the important theses of this chapter is that one needs precisely a theory of what capacities are basic or essential, in the sense that such capacities would be valued by all persons no matter what else they might intelligibly value. Such normative judgments do *not* collapse psychiatry into covert moral philosophy. They do not because the thin theory of the good behind such judgments is not at all the same as a full-blown theory of the good for persons.

6 The Legal Concept of Insanity

THE CONCEPT OF mental illness figures in both of the legal contexts we distinguished in Chapter 2. Not only is mental illness relevant to responsibility in the law of crimes and torts, but mentally ill human beings also may not be regarded as sufficiently responsible to manage their own property, to make their own contracts, wills, or marriages, to be granted custody of their children in a divorce, or even to make fundamental decisions such as those concerning their liberty or whether they wish to be medically treated in one way as opposed to another. In each of these cases, the law does not regard the mentally ill as having the full rights accorded to legal persons.

These two legal contexts do not exhaust the ways in which the concept of mental illness may come before the courts. When the state civilly commits mentally ill human beings on grounds of dangerousness to others (as opposed to the paternalistic grounds of dangerousness to self or the need for treatment, the other two traditional grounds of commitment), mental illness is relevant in a way different from these two contexts. Because of this difference, however, it has been persuasively argued that civil commitment on grounds of dangerousness to others ought not to use the concept of mental illness at all, and that any individual, mentally ill or not, about whom a reliable prediction of dangerousness can be made, should be detained. The concept of mental illness enters the law at other miscellaneous points as well, including: (1) workmen's compensation law where the issue is whether mental illnesses qualify as compensable injuries; (2) insurance clauses regarding illness must be construed as to their inclusion of mental illness; and (3) malpractice suits in tort law against doctors for failure to diagnose certain mental conditions as illnesses. The main point is preserved, however; legal definitions of mental illness have by and large arisen from one of the two contexts described in Chapter 2, contexts in which the responsibility or the rights of an agent are in question. The concept of mental illness that the law has developed must be seen in this light.

Rationality and Madness

I will not survey each of these branches of the law for differences in the kinds of conceptions of mental illness that courts and legal scholars may have utilized. Instead, I shall focus on one such area of law, that which is the central focus of the context of responsibility assessments: the defense of insanity in the criminal law. Legal insanity in some form has been an excuse from criminal responsibility for centuries. Its proper definition has been extensively debated, by psychiatrists as well as by lawyers; it has by far the richest history of any legal attempt to deal with the concept of mental illness. It is thus an appropriate context in which to assess the relations between the psychiatric and the legal conceptions of mental illness.

The Insanity Tests and Their Underlying Moral Bases

A BRIEF SKETCH OF THE INSANITY TESTS

Insanity, as we noted in Chapter 2, was an excuse in most ancient systems of law. The two analogies that dominated the earliest ideas about insanity were the analogies of the insane to both children and to animals. In the nineteenth and twentieth centuries, however, four tests have dominated Anglo-American law on insanity. I shall briefly summarize these tests and then analyze what I take to be their underlying moral bases.

The M'Naghten Test

In 1843, Daniel M'Naghten shot and killed Edward Drummond, private secretary to the prime minister, Robert Peel. M'Naghten was under the delusion that he was being persecuted by a host of individuals throughout England and Scotland, including, he thought, the prime minister. At his trial he successfully raised the defense of insanity. Given the political unrest at the time, the suspicion that M'Naghten was merely feigning his illness, and the fact that she herself had recently been the target of an assassination attempt for which the assailant was excused by reason of insanity, the queen was outraged at the result of excusing M'Naghten from criminal responsibility. The House of Lords accordingly asked the judges to appear before them as a group and explain the proper tests of criminal insanity. The *M'Naghten* rules originated in the judges' answers to questions put to them by the House of Lords. The much-quoted and operative language of the judges' answers was that:

> to establish a defense on the grounds of insanity, it must be conclusively proved that, at the time of the committing of the act, the party accused was laboring under such a defect of reason, from the disease

The Legal Concept of Insanity

of the mind, as not to know the nature and quality of the act he was doing; or if he did know it, that he did not know what he was doing was wrong.[1]

The *M'Naghten* test quickly became the leading test for insanity in England and America. It is still the exclusive test for insanity in many American states and part of the test of insanity in many others.[2] The essential elements of the test, about which so much has been written, are three: first, that one suffer from a defect of reason; second, that such defect stem from a disease of the mind; and third, that one lack knowledge of some kind, either the knowledge of what one is doing or the moral knowledge that what one is doing is wrong.

The Irresistible Impulse Test

One of the persistent criticisms of the *M'Naghten* test in the nineteenth century, and continuing to this day, is that it does not excuse from criminal responsibility a large enough class of persons. More specifically, the *M'Naghten* test was thought not to excuse those mentally ill persons who knew what they were doing and that it was wrong, but who nonetheless, because of their mental illness, did not have the ability to control their behavior. The distinction often made was between cognitive incapacity and volitional incapacity. The irresistible impulse test was formulated as a response to this criticism of *M'Naghten*. Although no one case gives a classic definition of legal insanity as irresistible impulse, one of the leading cases defined the defense as follows:

> Did he know right from wrong, as applied to the particular act in question... if he did have such knowledge, he may nevertheless not be legally responsible, if the two following conditions concur: (1) if, by reason of the duress of such mental disease, he had so far lost the power to choose between the right and wrong, and to avoid doing the act in question, as that his free agency was at the time destroyed; (2) and if, at the same time, the alleged crime was so connected with such mental disease, in the relation of cause and effect, as to have been the product of it solely.[3]

As Abraham Goldstein has pointed out,[4] the common label for this test — "irresistible impulse" — is misleading. The essential notion of the test is that, because of mental illness, one has lost the power to control himself. The test might more properly be called a "loss of control" test.

The American Law Institute's Definition of Legal Insanity

In the 1950s the scholars and judges comprising the American Law Institute proposed a Model Penal Code for adoption by state and federal jurisdictions. Section 4.01 of the code included a new definition of legal insanity: "A person is not responsible for criminal conduct if at the time of such conduct as the result of mental disease or defect he lacks substantial capacity either to appreciate the criminality of his conduct or to conform his conduct to the requirements of law."[5] This test, or some variant of it, has been adopted within the last twenty years by all of the federal courts of appeals and by a substantial number of states.

The New Hampshire and Durham Experiments

As I shall describe in much more detail shortly, the District of Columbia (between 1954 and 1972) and New Hampshire adopted as their criterion of legal insanity the following: "An accused is not criminally responsible if his unlawful act is a product of mental disease or of mental defect."[6] This test is traditionally analyzed as having two elements: first, that the accused be suffering from a mental disease or mental defect (mental disease being used in the test as a synonym of mental illness[7]); and second, that his criminal act be the product of that diseased or defective condition.

THE MORAL AND PSYCHIATRIC PARADIGMS UNDERLYING THE INSANITY TESTS

Writers in the area of legal insanity have sometimes conflated two quite distinct concepts: legal insanity and mental illness.[8] Although I shall argue ultimately that the two ought to be equated and legal insanity defined as mental illness (at least as the mental illness of the popular moral paradigm I analyzed in Chapter 5), it is nonetheless essential at this stage to keep the two distinct.

Some order can be brought into these tests by observing the relationship between mental illness and legal insanity. To be legally insane is to be excused from criminal responsibility. Each of these definitions of legal insanity thus is a test determining when an accused is or is not responsible in the criminal law. Each of the tests, it will be observed, has mental illness or some related concept as one of its elements. With the exception of *Durham* and the New Hampshire rule, however, the definitions of legal insanity typically do not equate insanity and mental illness, but use mental illness as only one element, one criterion, to determine when someone is legally insane. To be legally insane under *M'Naghten*, irresistible impulse, or the American Law Institute test requires, in addition, that certain other criteria be met. The imposition of these additional criteria should be seen as attempts by lawyers to relate psychiatric views about mental illness prevailing at the time the tests were adopted to well-established moral and legal paradigms of excuses from responsibility. To see this we must return to the taxonomy of excuses in Chapter 2.

The Legal Concept of Insanity

In criminal law, as in morals, two general sorts of conditions excuse: ignorance that is not itself culpable, and compulsion. Such excuses are distinct from other modes of defeating the ascription of legal or moral responsibility known as justification, such as self-defense. These two moral excuses are as old as Aristotle and are embodied in contemporary criminal law.[9] If one makes a mistake of fact about a material element of a crime (e.g., one believes some substance to be harmless food coloring when, in fact, it is poison), one is not held liable to punishment; similarly, those who act under duress (threats by others), or those who act in response to their victims' provoking acts, are also fully or partially excused from punishment.

It is these two traditionally excusing conditions that have been adapted by lawyers and judges as they have added criteria to legal insanity beyond the requirement that an accused must be mentally ill. There are thus basically two kinds of traditional insanity tests: those based on the ignorance of the mentally ill accused person; and those based on some notion of his being compelled to act as he did.[10]

The *M'Naghten* formulation quite obviously is of the first type, which turns on the ignorance of the accused about what he is doing or its moral status. The *M'Naghten* opinion was written, and its rules adopted by other courts, at a time when delusions were thought to be the prominent symptoms of mental illness. Indeed, many judges and lawyers thought that the presence of delusions was the only criterion for being mentally ill. As Sir John Nicholl stated in *Dew v. Clark:*

> The true criterion, the true test of the absence or presence of insanity, I take to be the absence or presence of what, used in a certain sense of it, is comprisable in a single term, namely, "delusion". . . . I look upon delusion in this sense of it, and insanity, to be almost, if not altogether, convertible terms.[11]

It is thus not surprising that a test should have evolved that combined this conception of mental illness—as delusion—with the long-existing moral paradigm that ignorance was an excuse. Although the old language about moral knowledge was retained, the rationale for the language was forgotten; as transformed by the *M'Naghten* rules, the knowledge required was not the general knowledge that was the measure of when a child or an insane person has the mental capacity to be treated as a responsible agent, but was rather the knowledge relevant to determining whether one could avail oneself of the excuse of ignorance of fact or law, an excuse available to sane as well as insane persons.[12]

The irresistible impulse test also represents this fitting of psychiatric insight into an already existing paradigm of moral excuse. It was principally Isaac Ray's criticism of the *M'Naghten* test in the nineteenth century, to the effect that delusion was not the only symptom of mental illness, that persuaded courts to frame an alternative definition of legal insanity around the other existing paradigm of moral excuse, compulsion.[13] Whether a person had lost his ability to control himself, a "volitional incapacity" as opposed to a "cognitive impairment," was the essential question under the irresistible impulse test. Such a test received further impetus with the prevalence of psychoanalytic theories in the 1920s, whose talk of instinctual drives, energies, and forces all at least seemed to add to the idea that mentally ill persons are in some fundamental sense compelled to act as they do and are thus not responsible.

The American Law Institute's test is simply a rewording of each of these aspects of the nineteenth-century tests of legal insanity and their joinder into a single test. Instead of focusing on "knowledge," as in *M'Naghten*, the ALI test talks of "appreciating" the criminality of conduct; in place of irresistible impulses and inabilities to control, the ALI talks of a lack of substantial capacity to conform conduct to requirements of law. The moral paradigms invoked are wholly the same.

Each of these three tests shares a common and fundamental defect: They assume that legal insanity is an *excuse* for the particular acts done, not a general *status* attached to a class of human beings who are not accountable agents. Worse, they assume that insanity is not even a special excuse but is collapsible into the traditional excuses of ignorance or compulsion. There is, in such a view, nothing special about being crazy; one's responsibility is affected only if one can avail oneself of one of the two traditional excuses.

A similar misunderstanding pervades yet another test for insanity often proposed but not yet widely adopted. This view, often called the "elements" approach, also urges that mental illness is not an excuse. Rather, this view urges, it is only relevant to responsibility when it negates the *mens rea* element required for most crimes. Since the *mens rea* requirement for most crimes is intentionality (in Bentham's sense of purpose *or* knowledge), this view usually asserts that mental illness reduces responsibility only when it can be shown to have prevented an accused from forming the intention required for criminal liability. This view, although long accepted by some legal theorists and psychiatrists,[14] and although increasingly proposed as the best test for insanity, currently has its doctrinal home in the related diminished capacity defense.[15]

The problem with each of these views is that they fail to capture our moral intuitions about what it is about crazy people that precludes responsibility. Consider Daniel M'Naghten himself, who manifested some of the classic symptoms of paranoia and who would be considered in popular understanding as quite crazy. First of all, M'Naghten had the *intent* required for murder in England: He shot the gun with the purpose of killing another human being. True, he thought he was killing Prime Minister Peel

The Legal Concept of Insanity

when in fact he was killing Peel's secretary, Drummond. But such mistakes about the identity of the intended victim never excuse in law, as the doctrine of "transferred intent" has long established. In every ordinary and legal sense of the word, M'Naghten *intended* the death of another. Similarly, he knew the "nature and quality of his act"; he knew its wrongfulness; he "appreciated its criminality." He made no *mistakes* about what he was doing – he knew he was shooting, and he knew that he was killing – nor was he ignorant of the legal and moral prohibitions against killing. Finally, there is no very persuasive case for saying that M'Naghten was *compelled* to do what he did. True, under the facts as he believed them to be, he had a hard choice to make. He believed that he was being persecuted by Peel and others and that if he did not strike first, he himself would be hurt or worse. Yet for a sane person such beliefs, even if true, would not give rise to any valid duress defense (there being no threats of immediate harm), nor can such preemptive strikes be justified as self-defense.

The short of it is that M'Naghten should flunk not only the test that bears his name, but all of the standard insanity tests with the exception of *Durham*. Yet I think our intuition is that someone like M'Naghten, who was very crazy, should not be responsible. It is true that we do get angry with even very crazy people when they do illegal acts. But we should not regard such anger as any more than our temporary emotional reaction to having been harmed, either actually or vicariously. After all, we also get angry with our children or our pets when they do things we dislike. Indeed, we even get angry at the chair on which we stub our toe. In all such cases, however, we should not mistake such anger for moral insight into such a being's responsibility. On reflection we should see that the insane, like the very young, are not sufficiently rational to be fairly blamed or punished. If this is so, then lawyers should give up their attempts to define legal insanity in a way that collapses it into some traditional excuse. Crazy people are not responsible because they are crazy, not because they always lack intentions, are ignorant, or are compelled.

The upshot of this is to incline one toward the New Hampshire and *Durham* formula of legal insanity, for this definition equates legal insanity with mental illness. Rather than incorporating long-existing paradigms of moral excuse from other areas of criminal law into a definition of insanity, the New Hampshire and *Durham* definitions regarded mental illness as itself an excusing condition, even if not accompanied by ignorance or compulsion.

Justice Doe, the originator of the New Hampshire test in the nineteenth century, thought that he was returning to the ancient ideas about legal insanity, namely, that mental illness itself excuses. In this respect he was correct; the status of being mentally ill, just like the status of being a child, itself excuses one from responsibility. Unfortunately, however, Justice Doe of New Hampshire and Judge Bazelon of the District of Columbia Court of Appeals were both also heavily influenced by the psychiatric theories of mental illness with which they were contemporary. Their interpretations of their respective definitions of legal insanity were thus more influenced by the prevailing psychiatric theory than by the ancient paradigm to which, on occasion, Justice Doe thought he was returning.

The influence of psychiatry and contemporary opinions about mental illness on the judges who wrote the New Hampshire and *Durham* tests is complicated and will be treated separately below. The history of the origins and administration of the insanity test in those jurisdictions illuminates the influence psychiatric definitions have had on the legal definition of mental illness.

Two Experiments in Merging Legal and Psychiatric Definitions of Mental Illness

THE NEW HAMPSHIRE EXPERIMENT

In 1838, a little-known physician in Maine, Issac Ray, published *A Treatise on the Medical Jurisprudence of Insanity*.[16] The book quickly became the authority in its field and remained the seminal work in forensic psychiatry in the nineteenth century. The book was relied on heavily, for example, by the trial judge in M'Naghten's case (although ignored in the formulation of the *M'Naghten* rules in the House of Lords).[17] Ray's work was also highly influential on those early courts in America that adopted the irresistible impulse test.[18] More pertinent to our immediate concern, however, is Ray's direct and well-documented influence on the development of the definition of legal insanity in New Hampshire.

Ray, like most nineteenth-century psychiatrists, was convinced that mental illness was in essence a brain disease, and that lesions in the brain would eventually be discovered as the cause of mental disorders:

> It is undoubted truth that the manifestations of the intellect and those of the sentiments, propensities, and passions, or generally of the intellectual and affective powers are connected with and dependent upon the brain. It follows, then, as a corollary, that abnormal conditions of these powers are equally connected with abnormal conditions of the brain; but this is not merely a matter of inference. The dissections of many eminent observers ... have placed it beyond a doubt; and no pathological fact is better established—though its correctness was for a long while doubted—than that deviations from the healthy structure are generally presented in the brains of insane subjects.[19]

The Legal Concept of Insanity

This view of mental illness was eventually accepted by Justice Doe of the New Hampshire Supreme Court.

Early in his career Justice Doe sought out the views of Ray on insanity, via the good offices of a Dr. Tyler of Harvard Medical School. The three entered into a lengthy correspondence on the proper definition of legal insanity. Early in the correspondence, Doe asked Tyler:

> Is it now the settled opinion of the scientific world that insanity is only a physical disease, or the result of physical disease?[20]

If the answer were yes, Doe went on,

> Why should the court ever say to a jury more than this in cases of alleged mental aberration or active insanity: "If the disposition of property was the offspring or was caused or affected by mental disease, then it is not the will of the testator—the result of disease cannot have any effect in law."[21]

Both Doe and Ray believed mental illness to be a physical disease. From this premise, it was self-evident to Justice Doe that the following definition of legal insanity should be adopted (as it eventually was in New Hampshire):

> If the homicide was offspring or product of mental disease in the defendant he was not guilty by reason of insanity.[22]

The reasoning to this conclusion was based on a confusion continuing to this day: that if physical causes of behavior are discovered, the actor is *ipso facto* not responsible for that behavior. Doe thought that if the abnormal physical condition of a defendant's brain caused him to commit the criminal act, then necessarily his will, his power to choose, was extinguished; that is, it was not his act:

> For if the alleged act of a defendant was the act of his mental disease it was not in law his act, and he is no more responsible for it than he would be if it had been the act of his involuntary intoxication or of another person using the defendant's hand against his utmost resistance . . . [W]hen a disease is the propelling, uncontrollable power, the man is as innocent as the weapon—the mental and moral elements are as guiltless as the material. If his mental, moral and bodily strength is subjugated and pressed to an involuntary service, it is immaterial whether it is done by disease or by another man or a brute or any physical force of art or nature set in operation without any fault on his part.[23]

The confusion inherent in this chain of reasoning stems from the nature of the language we use to ascribe responsibility, in morals as well as law. As we discussed in Chapter 2, the words with which we describe human actions imply the causal agency of the actor; to be an action at all (as opposed to a mere bodily movement), we must be able to assert that the agent (or the self, the mind, the will, or what have you) was causally responsible for the bodily movements. If we are told that something else caused the bodily movement, then it seems that the person was not causally responsible; for if some other set of conditions, such as an abnormal condition of the brain, was sufficient, that seems to imply that nothing else, such as the will of the actor, was even necessary.

The problem with such a view lies in the failure to see the possibility of there being differing sets of equally sufficient conditions existing to cause the same event. To say that a bodily movement is the product of an abnormal condition of the brain does not preclude one from describing that movement as an action performed by an agent for reasons. We have two vocabularies: that of movement and mechanical causation, and that of actions and reasons. Merely because scientists may discover lesions in the brain is not to preclude the application of the language of action and reasons. When there are mechanically caused movements there may nonetheless be intelligent actions.[24]

It is the language of actions and reasons with which the law deals. In ascribing responsibility, the law adopts with little change the conditions we all use to ascribe moral responsibility in everyday life, conditions framed in the language of action and intentionality. Once one perceives the "provisional independence" (discussed in Chapter 1) of this language from the language of natural science, then assumptions such as those of Doe and Ray become irrelevant to the proper definition of legal insanity. Mental illness may be a physical disease—that debate is certainly still alive—but for legal and moral purposes, the outcome is irrelevant. If mental illness excuses, it is not because it is the name of an as yet unknown physical cause.

Despite their now-questioned assumptions that mental illness is brain disease, and despite their further erroneous assumption that it is only because of such causal role that mental illness excuses, Doe and Ray were on the right track. For what they perceived to be inadequate about the *M'Naghten* test was its failure to recognize the responsibility-precluding nature of mental illness itself. Although for the wrong reason (physical causation), Doe and Ray believed that legal insanity should be equated with mental illness because mental illness by itself precludes responsibility. In that latter belief they were correct.

Their assumption that mental illness was a brain disease, however, led them into a further error for which they have been amply criticized by a century of legal scholars. Because of the assumed physical nature of mental illness, they thought that mental illness was a concept only scientists could meaningfully employ, and that accordingly, those scientists on the frontiers of investigating it—namely, psychiatrists—were the ones to inform the court on whether or not a particular defendant did or did not have those abnormal brain conditions amounting to mental illness. Again and again in their correspondence and elsewhere, they reiterated the notion that the presence of mental disease was a fact to be testified to by medical experts. As Doe put it in an early dissent:

> Insanity... is the result of a certain pathological condition of the brain... and the tests and symptoms of this disease are no more matters of law than the tests or symptoms of any other disease in animal or vegetable life.[25]

In their correspondence, they argued:

> The law does not define disease—disease is so simple an expression that the law need go no further. What is a diseased condition of mind is to be settled by science and not by law—disease is wholly within the realm of natural law or the law of nature.[26]

Such views finally found authoritative expression in the New Hampshire Supreme Court's opinion in *State v. Pike*:

> The legal profession, in profound ignorance of mental disease, have assailed the superintendents of asylums, who knew all that was known on the subject, and to whom the world owes an incalculable debt, as visionary theorists and sentimental philosophers attempting to overturn settled principles of law; whereas in fact the legal profession were invading the province of medicine, and attempting to install old exploded medical theories in the place of facts established in the progress of scientific knowledge.[27]

The result of this view was clear: Psychiatrists would have the authoritative voice about who was legally insane and thus to be excused from criminal responsibility.[28]

The problem with such a result has been restated many times. The criteria of legal responsibility are for the law to settle. Even if mental illness is equated with legal insanity, its definition necessarily is a legal matter. It would be a pure coincidence if the concept of mental illness adopted by psychiatrists for the various purposes discussed in Chapter 5 were the same as the concept suitable to isolate the class of offenders who ought, consistently with the purposes of punishment, to be excused. Indeed, the point is quite general: The law must define legal concepts for itself in light of legal purposes. The law cannot simply adopt a concept developed by psychiatrists for therapeutic purposes, or for that matter any concept developed by any social scientists for explanatory purposes. The purposes of the law in question must govern the definition of any term appearing in that law; no other discipline's conceptualization can safely be adopted and plugged into a legal formula.

The psychiatrists at the state hospital in New Hampshire had the good sense to perceive that they could not have been asked under the New Hampshire test to incorporate their therapeutic notion of mental illness into the formula defining legal insanity. In fact, the concept of mental illness they used in their testimony about criminal defendants was not the same as the concept they used in classifying their patients for treatment purposes. They had to take upon themselves the task Judge Doe and his successors on the New Hampshire bench should have undertaken; namely, to give a separate, legal definition of mental illness as a legally excusing condition.[29]

THE *DURHAM* EXPERIMENT

This fundamental lesson had to be relearned when the Court of Appeals for the District of Columbia decided *Durham v. United States* in 1954. The *Durham* rule regarding insanity, thought by the court to be "not unlike that followed by the New Hampshire court," was also that "an accused is not criminally responsible if his unlawful act was the product of mental disease or mental defect."[30] Unwittingly, the court followed in the steps of the New Hampshire court, both by relying initially on a medical conception of mental illness and by accepting the seeming consequence of the conception, namely, that causation was the real issue involved in the insanity defense. Each aspect of the court's reliance on the psychiatric paradigm of mental illness will be pursued separately.

Defining Mental Disease

Durham was decided explicitly to facilitate psychiatrists in placing their knowledge before the court, which they felt they could not do under the *M'Naghten* test. The influential Group for the Advancement of Psychiatry had earlier written a preliminary version of its report on criminal insanity, cited and relied upon in the *Durham* opinion. This report complained about "a barrier of communication which leaves the psychiatrist talking about 'mental illness' and the lawyer talking about 'right and wrong.' "[31] The test proposed by the committee, and in essence adopted in *Durham*, allowed psychiatrists to testify directly to the presence or absence of mental disease because the test was framed in terms of mental disease itself.

The problem, however, was the same as that which arose in New Hampshire almost a century earlier: Not every medically recognized mental disease could have been intended. Something more restrictive must have been intended by the phrase "mental disease or defect" in the *Durham* rule.

This problem became particularly glaring with regard to sociopaths, a diagnosis that had been applied to Monte Durham himself. Shortly after the *Durham* decision, the staff at St. Elizabeth's Hospital, which was composed of those psychiatrists most often called to testify in District of Columbia criminal cases, made a policy decision that sociopathic or psychopathic personality disturbances would not be regarded as mental illnesses within the meaning of the *Durham* rule. Psychiatrists from St. Elizabeth's Hospital thereafter so testified in District of Columbia cases. Three years later, however, at a weekend meeting, the staff changed the policy, and decided that henceforth, psychopathic or sociopathic personality disturbances would be considered mental diseases for legal purposes. The Court of Appeals for the District of Columbia deferred to this psychiatric judgment, granting a new trial in one case involving a sociopathic individual because, having been tried before the change in classification by the psychiatrists, he was deprived of "new medical evidence ... on an issue vital to his defense"[32] (namely, whether he was mentally ill). As Warren Burger, then a circuit judge who participated in that decision, later noted, "We tacitly conceded to St. Elizabeth's Hospital the power to alter drastically the scope of a rule of law by a weekend change of nomenclature."[33] This illegitimate transfer to psychiatrists of the power to decide the meaning of a legal rule on criminal responsibility resulted directly from the assumption of the District of Columbia judges that mental illness, as used in the rule, was the same concept as that used in medicine. This assumption, implicit in *Durham* itself, had been made explicit shortly after *Durham* was decided when the court of appeals held that

> mental "disease" means mental illness. Mental illnesses are of many sorts and have many characteristics. They, like physical illnesses, are the subject matter of medical science.... Many psychiatrists had come to understand there was a "legal insanity" different from any clinical mental illness. That of course was not true in a juridical sense. The law has no separate concept of a legally acceptable ailment which per se excuses the sufferer from criminal liability. The problems of the law in these cases are whether a person who has committed a specific criminal act ... was suffering from a mental disease, that is, from a medically recognized illness of the mind.[34]

Perceiving that surely not every "medically recognized illness of the mind" excuses from criminal responsibility, psychiatrists in the District of Columbia, as those in New Hampshire before them, took it upon themselves to work out a legal concept of mental disease, first excluding, then including, sociopathic or psychopathic personality disturbances.

Eight years after *Durham* was decided the court of appeals came to recognize that "what psychiatrists may consider a mental disease or defect for clinical purposes, where their concern is for treatment, may or may not be the same as mental disease or defect for the jury's purpose in determining criminal responsibility."[35] The court therefore attempted a legal definition of mental disease for the first time: "A mental disease or defect includes any abnormal condition of the mind which substantially affects mental or emotional processes and substantially impairs behavior control."[36]

The court of appeals thus finally undertook a task it should have undertaken originally: to give legal meaning to mental disease or defect as the phrase occured in the legal rule of responsibility. Unfortunately, however, the definition adopted is simply a regression to the more traditional types of definition of legal insanity. Mental disease is not itself actually defined, except insofar as a vague synonym is supplied: "abnormal condition of the mind." The informative part of the definition, which qualifies abnormal condition of the mind, is simply a reversion to those ancient moral paradigms already incorporated in the *M'Naghten* test, the irresistible impulse test, and the American Law Institute's test. Instead of "lack of knowledge" of the nature or quality of the act or its wrongfulness (*M'Naghten*) or the "substantial capacity to appreciate the criminality of conduct" (ALI), we have "substantially affects mental or emotional processes"; instead of language about acting under an irresistible impulse or lacking "substantial capacity to conform his conduct to the requirements of law" (ALI), we have "substantially impairs behavior controls." Instead of really giving a legal definition of mental illness, the court of appeals in *McDonald* abandoned the attempt by following the traditional formula for legal insanity: Mental illness, or some vague synonym for it, is only one element; added to it is some other traditionally excusing condition.[37] In doing so, the court of appeals abandoned the essentially correct insight behind the *Durham* case: that there is something about mental illness itself that precludes responsibility, irrespective of there being any ignorance about the nature of the particular crime or its prohibited nature, and irrespective of there being any excuse of compulsion.

The "Albatross" of Durham: That Mental Illness Be the Cause of the Crime

In 1972 the Court of Appeals for the District of Columbia abandoned the *Durham* rule entirely and adopted the American Law Institute's definition of legal insanity.[38] One of the principal reasons for doing so was the problem that court had been having with the "product" portion of the *Durham* rule: Psychiatric witnesses came to substitute their own judgments of the responsibility of the accused for that of the jury, and to phrase their conclusions on that ultimate issue in terms of whether or not the criminal act was the *product* of disease.

Contrary to some commentary on *Durham*,[39] this problem did not stem from the inherent lack of meaning that one can assign to the idea of mental illness causing crime. The concept of causation adopted by the court was unproblematic and consistent with the analysis of the causal relationship in

The Legal Concept of Insanity

many areas of law and much of contemporary philosophy.[40] The concept of mental illness as naming the sort of thing that could properly be said to be a cause of behavior was more problematic; for Judge Bazelon, the author of *Durham*, clearly did not believe that mental illness was necessarily some brain condition that caused behavior in some mechanical way.[41] Presumably he and other members of the court meant to invoke psychological (as opposed to physical) theories of causation in thinking of the mental conditions of the mentally ill as a cause of their behavior. The court certainly invited expert testimony in terms of such psychological theories: "Description and explanation of the origin, development, and manifestations of the alleged disease are the chief functions of the expert witness. . . . The law wants from the medical experts . . . expert medical opinion as to the relationship, if any, between the disease and the act of which the prisoner is accused."[42]

The court got more than it wanted of such expert medical opinion. By 1967 it became clear to the court that psychiatric conclusions about "product" were often disguised moral judgments about the culpability of the accused, so the court flatly prohibited psychiatric testimony in terms of product, or cause and effect.[43] It never became clear to the court why psychiatrists were substituting their moral judgments for those of the jury, other than some speculations about defense counsel's strategies. For, if causation were a straightforward scientific question, why were the relevant scientists unable to testify to it without infecting their scientific judgments with their moral judgments?

The initial answer lay in the fact that causation was not an issue on which psychiatrists could be at all helpful, given the deterministic assumptions of modern psychiatry. For if psychiatrists, particularly those of a dynamic persuasion, took the causation test literally, then in every case in which a mentally ill person committed a crime they would have to find the crime to be caused by the disease. One accustomed to thinking in terms of the unified personality, of basic instinctual drives underlying all conscious motivations, of the pervasiveness of unconscious influence, and of the displaceability of psychic energy among seemingly unconnected objects could reach no other conclusion. Accordingly, any distinction psychiatric witnesses might make between mentally ill defendants would have to be made covertly on noncausal grounds.

What psychiatry essentially lacked—and still lacks—was any reconciliation of its own deterministic assumptions with the concept of responsibility. If mentally ill persons are excused because of their lack of "free will" (in a contracausal sense), then psychiatry could be of no help, for its theoretical commitment is that none of us enjoys the freedom the mentally ill are supposed to lack. Judge Bazelon himself ultimately came to wonder "how medical experts can be expected to provide information about the impairment of free will, when free will would seem to be a philosophical and not a medical concept."[44]

The ultimate reason for the psychiatric unhelpfulness was that causal connection, in the sense used by the court, was not the issue anyway. Mental illness is not an excuse from responsibility because it causes criminal actions. This is true no matter if mental illness is construed as the name of some subset of physical causes themselves part of a general mechanistic account of human behavior — the nineteenth-century view — or if mental illness is thought to name some subset of psychological causes themselves part of a general, paramechanistic account of human behavior — a twentieth-century, Freudian view. In either case, the theories involved would excuse us all if such causation excuses the mentally ill. Psychiatric theories about causation, this time in their much less precise twentieth-century form of "psychic determinism," could accordingly only be a distraction from the actual criteria by virtue of which we separate the nonresponsible from the responsible in law and morals.

Had the court paid more attention to the meaning of mental illness and ignored any psychiatric theories of causation, it might have been able to have developed a meaningful idea of the relationship between the illness and the act. As is argued in Chapter 5, mental illness in ordinary understanding means an incapacity for rational action. One may do a certain act in a certain way because of such incapacity, but the "because" need not be construed on the model of mechanical or paramechanical causation.

A bridge may collapse because its materials lack the tensile strength to hold it up; a person may fail a test because he is stupid. In neither case have we cited an event, contiguous in space and time to another event, such that the first can be said to cause the second. The bridge's falling and the person's failing the test are events symptomatic of the general dispositional properties cited to explain them. Similarly, the relationship between illness and act the court might have sought was that the criminal act was symptomatic of the general incapacity for rational action of the mentally ill defendant. Because of its failure to work out an adequate legal definition of mental illness, however, the court could not reach this result but was bound to the psychiatric paradigm of mental illness it had adopted, that of a mechanical cause of behavior.

The Purposes Behind a Legal Definition of Mental Illness

The lesson of New Hampshire and *Durham* is plain: The law must give a legal definition of mental illness in light of the purposes behind the rule of which the phrase is a part. Only in the event that those legal purposes coincided with the purposes underlying psychiatric definitions of the phrase could the wholesale adoption of the psychiatric definitions into law be appropriate. It is not impossible that there be such an overlap of legal and psychiatric purposes. If one's theory of punishment were purely rehabilitative, so that punishment was justified if and only if it was the best way of making an offender a better person, then there could be some overlap. For one of the purposes guiding psychiatric definition (to define conditions treatable by psychiatrists) could then also guide the definition of a class of offenders (the insane) who are not best rehabilitated by punishment. If punishment rarely cures, then anyone who can best be cured of his criminal tendencies by psychiatric treatment should, in a purely rehabilitative theory of punishment, be excused from punishment in order to obtain the more efficacious psychiatric treatment.

To see whether there really is any such overlap between the legal purposes in defining mental illness and the psychiatric purposes in defining the phrase, we must take a brief excursion into punishment theory. One can understand how mental illness should be defined in the criminal case law only if one first understands the purposes for punishing and for excusing from punishment.

A TAXONOMY OF PURPOSES OF PUNISHMENT

The Prima Facie Justifications of Punishment

There is by now a familiar list of prima facie reasons given to justify the institution of punishment. Such a list standardly includes incapacitation, special deterrence, general deterrence, denunciation, rehabilitation, and retribution. A word about each of these reasons is in order. Incapacitation is the simplest of theories, because, as the name suggests, the good punishment achieves is that it incapacitates offenders by locking them up and preventing them from committing further crimes. Special deterrence has a similar aim: Punishing offenders deters them from committing further crimes upon their release. Likewise, general deterrence aims at the prevention of crime by punishing offenders, except that those who are deterred are others in the general population rather than the offenders themselves. All three of these traditional theories of punishment share a common goal thought to justify punishment, namely, the reduction of crime.

The ideas captured in the theory labeled "denunciation," sometimes called the expressive theory of punishment, are somewhat more complicated. One strand of this theory urges that punishment must express society's condemnation because doing so educates citizens in the wrongfulness of the conduct that the criminal law attempts to discourage. So stated, the denunciation theory is no more than a somewhat broader form of the general deterrence theory: Both aim at the prevention of crime, one by scaring people out of it and the other by more subtle educational techniques. Another strand of the denunciation theory asserts that denouncing crime via symbolic blaming coupled with harsh treatment serves an end distinct from the prevention of future criminal conduct. Theorists of this stripe urge that crime must be denounced by punishment, because doing so maintains a sense of social cohesion. If punishments are inflicted, then citizens do not have the sense that the social contract has been broken with impunity by others. The good achieved on this branch of the theory is not the prevention of future crimes; rather, it is thought that a sense of community is itself a good thing that punishment helps to achieve.

Rehabilitation is perhaps the most complex of the theories of punishment, because it involves two quite different ideals of rehabilitation that are usually confused. These two rehabilitative ideals can best be separated by thinking about two different ways of rendering offenders nondangerous. First, imagine that what is done is to place offenders in extraordinarily awful places of detention, with harsh treatment by inmates and guards. Here, nondangerousness is achieved because such offenders either become "penitent," or they are no longer willing to commit crimes because they are unwilling to risk again such awful treatment. For comparison, imagine that the same level of nondangerousness can be achieved if prisoners are placed in much nicer facilities, with kinder personnel (all of them soft-spoken, in white coats, and manifesting sincere concern), a place in which extensive therapy programs are undertaken. Imagine further that the second such program, although much more expensive than the first, not only makes offenders nondangerous, but also makes them flourishing, happy, and self-actualizing members of our society.

The first sort of rehabilitative ideal is one that is achieved when we make criminals safe to return to the streets. This sort of rehabilitative theory justifies punishment, not by appeal to how much better off criminals will be at the end of the process, but rather by how much better off all of us will be if "treatment" is completed because the streets will be that much safer. Such a theory seeks to rehabilitate criminals only as a cost-effective means of shortening the expensive incarceration that would otherwise be necessary to protect us all against crime. The second sort of rehabilitative ideal, by way of contrast, is a paternalistic theory. It seeks to rehabilitate offenders not just so they can be returned safely to the streets, but so they can lead flourishing and successful lives. Such a theory justifies punishment, not in the name of all of us, but rather in the offenders' own name; since it does so in their name, but contrary to their own expressed wishes (few offenders want to be punished), this kind of rehabilitative theory is paternalistic in character.

This paternalistic type of rehabilitative theory has no proper part to play in any theory of punishment, even in the minimal sense of constituting a prima facie justification of punishment. There are three reasons why this is so. First, such a paternalistic reform theory allocates scarce societal resources away from other, more deserving groups that want them (such as retarded and autistic children or the poor), to a group that hardly can be said to deserve such favored status and, moreover, does not want such "benefits." As a simple matter of distributive justice it is difficult to argue that criminals should be favored in the allocation of scarce social resources in these ways. Second, in any political theory according high value to liberty, paternalistic justifications are themselves to be regarded with suspicion. Criminals are not in the standard classes in society for which paternalistic state intervention is appropriate, such as the severely disordered, the young, or others whose capacity for rational choice is diminished; such a paternalistic theory is suspect on this ground alone. Third, such recasting of punishment in terms of "treatment" for the good of the criminal makes possible a kind of moral blindness that is dangerous in itself. As C. S. Lewis pointed out some years ago, adopting a "humanitarian" conceptualization of punishment makes it easy to inflict treatments and sentences that need bear no relation to the desert of the offender.[45] We may do more to others "for their own good" than we ever allow ourselves to do when we see that it is really for our good that we act.[46]

Retributivism, the final theory used to justify punishment, is the view that punishment is justified by the desert of the offender. The good that is achieved by punishing, in this view, has nothing to do with future states of affairs, such as the prevention of crime or the maintenance of social cohesion. Rather, the good that punishment achieves is that someone who deserves it gets it.

Retributivism is quite distinct from a view that urges that punishment is justified because a majority of citizens feel that offenders should be punished. Rather, retributivism is a species of objectivism in ethics that asserts that there is such a thing as desert and that the presence of such a (real) moral quality in a person justifies punishment of that person.[47] What a populace may think or feel about vengeance on an offender is one thing; what treatment an offender deserves is another. And it is only this last notion that is relevant to retributivism.

Retributivism is also distinct from what is sometimes called "revenge utilitarianism."[48] This is the view that the state must punish because private citizens otherwise will take the law into their own hands and that such private vengeance leads to chaos and disorder. Punishment in such a view is justified by its ability to prevent these bad things. Retributivism has nothing to do with this essentially forward-looking justification. Moreover, this "prevention of private vengeance" theory is to my mind not even a prima facie justifying reason for punishment. The obvious thing to do if citizens are going to violate the law by taking it into their own hands, is to deter those citizens by punishing them, not by punishing someone else. It places retributivism in an unnecessarily bad light to think that it justifies punishment only because of the shadow cast by a threat of illegal violence by vengeful citizens.

The Two Pure Theories of Punishment

It is common to reduce the survivors on this list of prima facie justifications of punishment to two general theories, the utilitarian theory and the retributive theory. To see how this is done, one need only consider the good state of affairs that is to be achieved by incarceration, special deterrence, general deterrence, and rehabilitation (to the extent that it is of the first sort of rehabilitative theory, and not the second). For all four of these rationales for punishment share the prevention of crime as the beneficial end that justifies punishment. In each case, the ultimate justification for inflicting the harm of punishment is that it is outweighed by the good to be achieved, namely, the prevention of future crimes by that offender or by others. This justification of an institution by the social welfare it will enhance make all such theories instances of the utilitartian theory of punishment.

Thus, the denunciation theory of punishment is a second kind of utilitarian theory of punishment, insofar as the good it seeks to achieve is not simply the prevention of crime. To the extent one grants intrinsic value to social cohesion, and does not regard that as a value only because it contributes to the maintenance of public order, the denunciation theory can be distinguished from the other utilitarian theories just considered by the differing social good it seeks to achieve. Nonetheless, it is still a utilitarian theory, since it outweighs the harm that is punishment by some form of net social gain that punishment achieves.

Both crime prevention and the maintenance of social cohesion are types of collective good. The general utilitarian theory of punishment is one that combines these and other forms of collective good that punishment might achieve, and calls them all a "social gain." Whenever the social gain outweighs the harm punishment causes to offenders or their families, such a theory would say that there is a net social gain. Such a vocabulary allows us a succinct definition of any form of utilitarian theory: Punishment is justified if and only if some net social gain is achieved by it.

A retributivist theory is necessarily nonutilitarian in character, for it eschews justifying punishment by its tendency to achieve any form of net social gain. Rather, retributivism asserts that punishment is properly inflicted because, and only because, the person deserves it. That some people deserve punishment in such a theory is both a necessary and a sufficient condition justifying criminal sanctions. A succinct definition of the retributivist theory of punishment, paralleling that given of the utilitarian theory, is that punishment is justified if and only if the persons receiving it deserve it.

The Mixed Theory of Punishment

Once one grants that there are two sorts of prima facie justifications of punishment—effecting a net social gain (utilitarian) and giving just deserts (retributivist)—one can also see that in addition to the two pure theories of punishment there can also be mixed theories. There are two logically possible mixed theories, although only one of these merits any serious attention. There is first of all the popular form of mixed theory that asserts that punishment is justified if and only if it achieves a net social gain *and* is given to offenders who deserve it. Giving just deserts and achieving a net social gain, in such a case, are each individually necessary but only jointly sufficient conditions justifying punishment. The second logically possible mixed theory would be one asserting that punishment is justified if and only if it achieves a net social gain, *or* if it is given to offenders who deserve it. Such a theory has no name, because there is no one, to my knowledge, who has ever adopted it. Such a theory is unnamed and unclaimed because it shares the defects of each of the pure theories, utilitarianism and retributivism.[49] I shall accordingly put this "mixed theory" aside from further consideration.

The first kind of mixed theory itself has two branches. By far the most usual and popular form of the theory asserts that we do not punish people *because* they deserve it. Desert enters in, this theory further asserts, only as a limit on punishment: We punish offenders *because* some net social gain is achieved, such as the prevention of crime, but *only if* such offenders deserve it.[50] It is, in other words, the achieving of a net social gain that justifies punishment, whereas the desert of offenders serves as a limiting condition on punishment but as no part of its justification. The alternative branch of the mixed theory is just the converse: One would urge that we punish *because* offenders deserve it, but *only if* some net social gain is achieved by doing so.[51] In such a case, the roles of net social gain and desert are simply reversed: Giving offenders their just deserts serves as the justification of punishment, and the achieving of a net social gain as the limiting condition.

A cynic might view these two branches of the mixed theory as nothing more than an uncomfortable shuffle by mixed theorists. When accused of barbarism for punishing persons for retributivist reasons, they assert the first branch of the theory (they punish not because some persons deserve it, but because of a collective good that is achieved). When accused of immorality for imposing harsh treatment on someone as a means of making everyone else better off, such theorists shift to the other foot, and claim they do not punish someone to achieve a net social gain, but only to give offenders their just deserts. The cynic has a point here, because there is a sense in which the two branches of the theory are the same, namely, the sense that they justify exactly the same kinds of treatment for all cases. The only difference in theories is in the motivations of those who hold them. And while that may make a difference in our moral judgments of those who hold the different branches of the mixed theory of punishment, it does not make a difference in terms of the actual social institutions and judgments such theories will justify. I shall accordingly lump both of these branches together and call them the mixed theory of punishment.

THE ARGUMENT FOR RETRIBUTIVISM

The Argument Against the Pure Utilitarian Theory

In exploring one's thoughts about punishment, it is perhaps easiest to start with some standard kinds of thought experiments directed against a pure utilitarian theory of punishment. A thought experiment is essentially a device allowing one to sort out one's true reasons for believing that certain propositions are true. To be successful, such a thought experiment need not involve any actual case or state of affairs, nor need the cases envisioned even be very likely; they only need be conceivable in order to test our own thoughts.

It is standard fare in the philosophy of punishment to assert, by way of several thought experiments, counterexamples to the utilitarian thesis that punishment is justified if and only if some net social gain is achieved. I mention only two such counterexamples: scapegoating and preventive detention.[52] With regard to the first, it might be recalled that D. B. Cooper successfully skyjacked an aircraft some years ago, and that this successful, unsolved crime apparently encouraged the mass of skyjackings that have cost so much in terms of dollars, lives, and convenience. Cooper wore large sunglasses in his escapade, and there was accordingly only a very limited description available of him. Imagine that shortly after his skyjacking we had the benefit of the knowledge we now have by hindsight, and we decided that it would be better to punish someone who looked like Cooper (and who had no good alibi) in order to convince others that skyjacking did not pay. For a consistent utilitarian, there is a net social gain that would be achieved by punishing such an innocent person, and there is no a priori reason that the net social gain in such a case might not outweigh the harm that is achieved by punishing an innocent person.

The preventive detention kind of counterexample is very similar: Imagine that a psychiatrist discovers that a patient has extremely dangerous propensities. The patient is also the accused in a criminal trial. It turns out,

The Legal Concept of Insanity

however, that the accused is not guilty of the crime for which he is charged and in fact has committed no crime whatsoever. Should a judge who, we may suppose, is the only one who knows that the man is both dangerous and innocent find the accused guilty? Doing so will prevent the defendant's predicted criminal behavior because he will be incarcerated. In a utilitarian theory, it is difficult to see why such a judgment would not be perfectly appropriate, as long as the prediction is reliable enough, and as long as the crimes predicted are sufficiently serious that the good of their prevention outweighs the harm of punishing that person, even though he has committed no crime as yet.

The general form of the argument arising from these kinds of thought experiments is that of a reductio ad absurdum argument. The argument has three premises:

1. Punishment should be inflicted if and only if doing so achieves a net social gain.
2. A net social gain would be achieved in this case by the infliction of punishment.
3. Punishment should not be inflicted in this case.

Each of these premises corresponds to steps in both of the foregoing thought experiments. The first premise is simply a restatement of the utilitarian theory of punishment. The second premise presupposes that there are some cases where a net social gain can be achieved by punishing an innocent person and asserts that this is such a case. The third premise asserts our intuition that such persons ought not to be punished.

All three premises together yield a contradiction:

4. Punishment should not be inflicted and punishment should be inflicted.

The first two premises have as their joint conclusion that the person should be punished; this conclusion, when conjoined with the third premise, produces the contradictory conclusion.

The strongest possible form of a reductio ad absurdum argument is one that ends in a formal contradiction. To avoid the contradiction, there are only three possibilities, corresponding to each of the three premises. One could give up the third premise and simply admit that in such cases the persons should be punished, despite their innocence. This move is a rather implausible one, inasmuch as it commits one to admitting that one will punish an entirely innocent person.[53] The second possibility is to deny that there will be cases where there will be a net social gain from punishing an innocent person. This move is usually associated with the name of rule utilitarianism[54] and involves the idea that one cannot make a general practice of punishing the innocent, because then the harm of so doing (in terms of demoralization costs in society and the like) will outweigh any possible good to be achieved, even the prevention of skyjacking. The problem with this response, popular as it is, is that it fails to deal fairly with the nature of the thought experiment. That is, suppose there are some risks of detection of punishment of innocent persons, and, thus, some risks of demoralization costs; such risk will only allow utilitarians to say that the number of cases in which punishment of the innocent will maximize utility is somewhat diminished. It does not foreclose as somehow impossible that there are such cases. Such cases are conceivable, and if in them one is still not willing to punish, one thereby shows oneself not to be a utilitarian about punishment.

This brings us to the third possibility: One can simply give up the first premise, that is, one can repudiate the utilitarian theory of punishment. Such thought experiments, I think, when clearly conceived and executed, show almost all of us that we are not pure utilitarians about punishment.

Arguments Against the Mixed Theory of Punishment

The arguments against the pure utilitarian theory of punishment do not by themselves drive one into retributivism. For one can alleviate the injustice of the pure utilitarian theory of punishment by adopting the mixed theory. Since under the mixed theory the desert of the offender is a necessary condition of punishment, it will follow from the mixed theory that in each of the kinds of counterexamples considered (where punishment is not deserved), punishment should not be given. No contradictions will be generated, because the premises are consistent:

1. Punishment should be inflicted if and only if doing so achieves both a net social gain and gives an offender his just deserts.
2. A net social gain would be achieved in this case by the infliction of punishment.
3. It is not the case that punishment would give an offender his just deserts in this case.
4. Punishment should not be inflicted.

From the first three of these premises, the conclusion is deducible that there should be no punishment. This is also what the fourth premise asserts, so that there is no contradiction when one substitutes the mixed theory for the utilitarian theory of punishment.

There is, nonetheless, another sort of thought experiment that tests whether one truly believes the mixed theory, or is in fact a pure retributivist.[55] Such thought experiments are the kind that fill the editorial pages where outrage is expressed at the lightness of sentence in a particular case, or the lightness of sentencing generally in the courts of some communities.

The Legal Concept of Insanity

An example is provided by *State v. Chaney,* wherin the defendant was tried and convicted of two counts of forcible rape and one count of robbery.[56] The defendant and a companion had picked up the prosecutrix at a downtown location in Anchorage. After driving the victim around in their car, the defendant and his companion beat her and forcibly raped her four times, also forcing her to perform an act of fellatio with the defendant's companion. During this same period of time, the victim's money was removed from her purse, and she only then was allowed to leave the vehicle after dire threats of reprisals if she attempted to report the incident to the police.

Despite this horrendous series of events, the trial judge imposed the minimum sentence on the defendant for each of the three counts and went out of his way to remark that he (the trial judge) was "sorry that the (military) regulations would not permit keeping (defendant) in the service if he wanted to stay because it seems to me that is a better setup for everybody concerned than putting him in the penitentiary." The trial judge also mentioned that as far as he was concerned, there would be no problem for the defendant to be paroled on the very first day of his sentence, if the parole board should so decide. The sentence was appealed by the state under a special Alaska procedure, and the attorney general urged the Alaska Supreme Court to disapprove the sentence.

The thought experiment such a case begins to pose for us is as follows: Imagine in such a case that after the rape but before sentencing the defendant has gotten into an accident so that his sexual desires are dampened to such an extent that he presents no further danger of rape; if money is also one of his problems, suppose further that he has inherited a great deal of money, so that he no longer needs to rob. Suppose, because of both of these facts, we are reasonably certain that he does not present a danger of either forcible assault, rape, robbery, or related crimes in the future. Since Chaney is (by hypothesis) not dangerous, he does not need to be incapacitated, specially deterred, or reformed. Suppose further that we could successfully pretend to punish Chaney, instead of actually punishing him, and that no one is at all likely to find out. Our pretending to punish him will thus serve the needs of general deterrence and maintain social cohesion, and the cost to the state will be less than if it actually did punish him. Is there anything in the mixed theory of punishment that would urge that Chaney nonetheless should really be punished? I think not, so that if one's conclusion is that Chaney and people like him nonetheless should be punished, one will have to give up the mixed theory of punishment.

The argument structure is again that of a reductio and is as follows:

1. Punishment should be inflicted if and only if doing so both achieves a net social gain and gives an offender his just deserts.

2. A net social gain would not be achieved in this case by the infliction of punishment.
3. Punishment should be inflicted.

Again, these three premises generate a contradiction:

4. Punishment should not be inflicted and punishment should be inflicted.

From the first two premises, it follows that there should be no punishment; this contradicts the third premise that there nonetheless should be punishment.

One again has the choice of giving up one of the three premises of the argument. To give up the third premise is very unappealing to most people; doing so requires that people like Chaney should not be punished at all. Again, the tempting move is to assert that there will be no cases in which one will be sure enough that the danger is removed, or the ends of general deterrence served, that one can ever successfully assert the second premise. But as in the earlier case, this is simply to misunderstand the nature of the thought experiment. One only need think it conceivable that such dangers could be removed, or such ends of deterrence served, in order to test one's theory of punishment. And nothing in utilitarianism can guarantee that utility is always maximized by the punishment of the guilty. The only other way to avoid the contradiction is to give up the first premise. Yet this means that one would have to give up the mixed theory of punishment.

The Argument for Retributivism

If one follows the predicted paths through these thought experiments, the end result is that one finds oneself, perhaps surprisingly, to be a retributivist. We might call this an argument through the back door for retributivism, because the argument does not assert in any positive way the correctness of retributivism. It only asserts that the two theories of punishment truly competitive with retributivism, namely, the pure utilitarian theory and the mixed theory, are each unacceptable to us. That leaves retributivism as the only remaining theory of punishment we can accept.

It has seemed to some theorists that there is a limited amount of positive argument that can be given in favor of a retributivist theory and still have the theory remain truly retributivist. Hugo Bedau has recently reminded us, for example, that the retributivist faces a familiar dilemma:

> Either he appeals to something else — some good end — that is accomplished by the practice of punishment, in which case he is open to the

criticism that he has nonretributivist, consequentialist justification for the practice of punishment. Or his justification does not appeal to something else, in which case it is open to the criticism that it is circular and futile.[57]

In this respect, however, retributivism is no worse off than any other nonutilitarian theories in ethics, each of which seeks to justify an institution or practice not by the good consequences it may engender, but rather by the inherent rightness of the practice. The justification for any such theories is one that appeals to both our particular judgments and our more general principles, in order to show that the theory fits judgments that on reflection we are sure of, and principles that on reflection we are proud of.[58]

Defining Mental Illness so as to Give Just Deserts

Each of the major theories of punishment would (if accepted) yield quite different theories about excuse in general; each would also yield somewhat different definitions of mental illness and legal insanity. A pure utilitarian theory would seek to define mental illness in such a way as to describe a class that was either nondeterable, nondangerous, or nonreformable by punishment techniques. A pure retributivist theory would seek to define mental illness in the way that best captures the moral principles that make crazy people not deserving of punishment. A mixed punishment theory could have both kinds of definitions, defining mental illness so as to excuse either the class of nondeterable, nondangerous, and nonreformable offenders, *or* those not deserving of punishment.

None of these possible purposes behind giving a definition of mental illness in the criminal law coincide with the possible purposes behind the psychiatric redefinition of the phrase. Psychiatrists may adopt the "trigger for treatment" rationale for their expansive redefinition of mental illness, as we saw in Chapter 5. Even if that is a proper thing to do for psychiatry, such definitional efforts can hardly be relevant to the criminal law's own needs in defining the phrase.

The purpose of giving a criminal law definition of mental illness under any of the three theories of punishment does not make relevant the question of whether psychiatric treatment is or is not more efficacious than punishment for a certain class of offenders. That an offender might be treatable by psychiatrists is thus not the question guiding the legal definition of the phrase, as it might be for psychiatry (although I argued in Chapter 5 that not even psychiatrists should so guide their definitional efforts). Only if one could show the rehabilitative theory (of either branch) to be a viable theory of punishment could one make the case for the relevance of psychiatric conceptualizations for law. Yet, as we have seen, even the nonpaternalistic, utilitarian version of the rehabilitative ideal is, at most, one factor among many justifying punishment or exemption from punishment. And it is only that in the mixed theory; in the retributivist theory, such treatability has no relevance at all.

In the retributivist theory an exemption from punishment must present a moral issue, namely, what class of offenders is not deserving of punishment? Even in the mixed theory the issue is a moral one. For if moral culpability is a necessary condition of punishability, as it is in the mixed theory, then the absence of culpability is a sufficient condition for exemption from punishment. As stated by Bazelon in the *Durham* decision itself,[59] the legal and moral traditions of the Western world have long required that those who are mentally ill are not morally blameworthy and, not being morally blameworthy, cannot be the proper subjects of punishment. The moral nature of the justification for the defense is shown most markedly in those numerous jurisdictions with mandatory commitment statutes, for such statutes commit to hospitals those found not guilty by reason of insanity in order to achieve the utilitarian purposes of incapacitation and reform. Such statutes make clear that for those mentally ill persons who are dangerous, the utilitarian reasons to punish are satisfied; it is only the lack of any moral culpability of the offender that requires that there be an insanity defense. The defense then functions mostly as a morality play, segregating those who will be detained but who cannot fairly be made subject to the moral sanction associated with punishment.

The proper legal definition of mental illness, then, should reflect not medical classifications, nor even utilitarian calculations about the dangerousness, deterrability, or reformability of various types of mentally disturbed defendants. If the issue is a moral one, as it is in the mixed view of punishment (and as it would have to be in the retributivist view), then the legal definition of the phrase should embody those moral principles that underlie the intuitive judgment that mentally ill human beings are not responsible.

The legal definition of mental illness should thus draw on the moral tradition that is the rationale for the defense. What is thus needed is an analysis of that popular moral notion of mental illness. What have people meant by mental illness such that, both on and off juries, they have for centuries excused the otherwise wrongful acts of mentally ill persons?

We have already explored in Chapter 5 the popular understanding of mental illness. To be mentally ill is to be very seriously irrational in the senses of "irrational" explored earlier. Yet why does severely diminished rationality preclude responsibility? It is because our notions of who is eligible to be held morally responsible depend on our ability to make out rather regularly practical syllogisms for actions. One is a moral agent only if one is a rational agent. Only if we can see another being as one who acts to achieve some rational end in light of some rational beliefs will we understand him in the same fundamental way that we understand ourselves and our fellow persons in everyday life. We regard as moral agents only those beings we can understand in this way.

Thus, societies that attribute moral responsibility to natural objects are regarded as primitive, because we are unwilling to accept the primitive animism subscribed to by such societies. If we did believe that natural objects possess beliefs and desires in light of which their movements are to be understood as rational, our misgivings about attributing moral responsibility to such objects would evaporate. Moral responsibility and that mode of explanation I have called practical reasoning go hand in hand.

It is easy to understand the long-standing historical tendency of the criminal law to analogize the mentally ill to infants and animals. For we do not think of these beings as engaging in practical reasoning to the same extent as normal, adult human beings. Only when an infant develops sufficiently that his actions are regularly explicable by rationalizing practical syllogisms do we begin to see him as a moral agent who can justly be held responsible. The same is true of the mentally ill.

The proper definition of legal insanity is one that utilizes this moral criterion. If criminal law is to reflect our shared notions of culpability, an exemption from punishment based on those moral notions ought to utilize those same moral criteria. The only question appropriate to juries is thus one appealing to their moral paradigm of mental illness: Is the accused so irrational as to be nonresponsible? The other definitions of legal insanity all mistakenly transport basic excuses from elsewhere in morals and criminal law to the mentally ill to whom they have only a partial application.

One rather suspects that juries have long applied this criterion, irrespective of the wording of the insanity test. As other observers have also noted: "However much you charge a jury as to the M'Naghten Rules or any other test, the question they would put to themselves when they retire is—'Is this man mad or not?' "[60] The reason they have done so is because they, along with the many lawyers and psychiatrists who have thought "insanity" and "psychosis" to be roughly equivalent,[61] have perceived that madness itself precludes responsibility.

To so define mental illness and legal insanity cabins these concepts severely. Most people who do bad things are bad, not sick, and thus deserve to be punished. Mentally ill they might be, if one defines mental illness so that the phrase can serve as a trigger for psychiatric treatment. But such psychiatric classification, suspect even in psychiatry, can have no relevance to legal and moral responsibility. No amount of attempted "conceptual imperialism" by psychiatry should convince us to draw the line between the sick and the bad any differently than it is drawn by excusing only those who are so irrational that we can accurately describe them as crazy or mad.

III Practical Reason and the Unconscious

7 Does the Unconscious Exist?

The Senses of Unconscious Revisited

AS WE HAVE SEEN, the easiest response for lawyers to the challenges of psychiatry is to deny that such challenges exist at all. The easiest reply to the bloated view of mental illness of post-Freudian psychiatry is to deny that there is such a thing as mental illness. This is the view of Szasz and his legal entourage, which we examined in Chapter 4. Analogously, the easiest response to the challenge presented to the legal view of mind by the idea of the unconscious is to deny that there is any such thing as the unconscious.

Here again, the dispute about the existence of such challenges cannot simply be divided along professional lines. Just as there are "radical psychiatrists" ready to join those lawyers who believe mental illness to be a myth, so there are "radical behaviorists," phenomenologists, and other psychologists and psychologically oriented philosophers who believe the unconscious to be a myth, a metaphor that need not be taken seriously. All such critics, for very different reasons, share Ernst Nagel's sentiment that "the notions of unconscious psychic processes possessing causal efficacies—of unconscious, causally operative motives and wishes that are not somatic dispositions and activities . . . are just nonsense."[1]

The burden of this chapter is to examine these latter claims. As before with mental illness, to assess the claims of the mythicists first requires that we clarify them. This involves separating the various distinguishable arguments having as their common conclusion that the unconscious "does not exist" (to put it very crudely). As I hope to show by the end of the chapter, the unconscious is no myth and the challenge it presents to the legal view of mind is accordingly quite real.

The first thing to be clear about is what one who denies the existence of the unconscious means by "the unconscious." In Chapter 3 we distinguished five meanings attached to that word:

1. The behaviorist unconscious, where the unconscious is a kind of stand-in for earlier factors that have conditioned later responses.
2. The animistic unconscious, where one personalizes the System Ucs by attributing to it causal agency and practical reason.
3. The physiological unconscious, where what is referred to are all those neurophysiological goings-on that underlie intelligent mental processes.
4. The Freudian unconscious, where the unconscious is a theoretical entity in a general theory of human behavior.
5. The pretheoretical unconscious, where the unconscious is a convenient abbreviation for all those mental states of which we are not aware but of which, potentially, we can become aware by our extended memory.

The case for or against there being some thing called the unconscious depends, of course, on which of these meanings one has in mind.

I shall proceed in the following way. Unconscious in its fifth (pretheoretical) sense does not name an entity or thing, be it a "region of the mind," an aggregation of functions, or whatever; unconscious in this sense names a property or quality that mental states possess. The most radical claim of a mythicist is to deny that there are such unconscious mental states. To make out this charge it is not enough to show that Freud's theories are all wrong and that the unconscious, accordingly, cannot name some kind of thing. Rather, a mythicist of this stripe must urge the more radical claim that denies existence to unconsciousness as a property predicable of mental states.

I shall examine this claim first, both because it is most radical and because this is the most important question to be resolved in assessing the impact of the unconscious on the ascription of responsibilities and rights. Rejecting as I shall the mythicists' claims that there can be no unconscious mental states, I shall then proceed to examine the weaker claim that denies existence to something called the unconscious. The second half of this chapter will thus assess whether the unconscious can meaningfully name some kind of thing, be it a mere behavioral construct, an empirical entity in neurophysiology, a theoretical entity in Freud's metapsychology, or even a second person residing within us all.

The Existence of Unconsciousness as a Property

In *The Eternal Husband,* Dostoevsky has Velchaninov muse about an unconscious desire of another character:

Does the Unconscious Exist?

> Had the idea ever entered his head before, if only as a dream in a vindictive moment? He decided that question strangely . . . Pavel Pavlovitch wanted to kill him, but he didn't know he wanted to kill him. It's senseless, but that's the truth, thought Velchaninov.[2]

What we wish to understand in this section is twofold: What tempts Dostoevsky to regard such an unconscious desire to be senseless, and what leads him ultimately to ascribe sense to it nonetheless? As the quotation illustrates, we ask these questions about a usage of unconscious that presupposes nothing about Freudian theory.

There are some notoriously bad arguments leading to the conclusion that the idea of unconscious mental states makes no sense. These should be put aside at the start. One of these stems from Freud's own analogy of unconscious mental states as Kantian kinds of *Ding an sich*, objects that can never be known directly.[3] Such comparisons, if accepted, easily lead to skepticism about the existence of things (unconscious mental states) that are unknowable, in principle, to anyone. Yet such skepticism is unwarranted because the analogy is a poor one to begin with.[4] Although necessarily the holder of an unconscious mental state will not know that he has it, other people (such as his analyst) may well possess such knowledge. Indeed, if therapy is successful, he himself may come to know that fact as well. There is nothing "unknowable in principle" about unconscious mental states.

Also to be ignored here are both radical behaviorist and phenomenological rejections of unconscious mental states. With regard to the first, Skinnerians deny the causal efficacy of unconscious mental states in producing behavior, even if they do not deny the existence of such states themselves. To quote Skinner:

> Freud's contribution [with regard to the unconscious] has been widely misunderstood. The important point was not that the individual was often unable to describe important aspects of his own behavior or identify important causal relationships, but that his ability to describe them was irrelevant to the occurrence of the behavior or to the effectiveness of the causes. . . . We may say that he is conscious of the parts he can describe and unconscious of the rest. But the act of self-description, as of self-observation, plays no part in the determination of action.[5]

Such denials are no more than part of what Michael Scriven once called Skinner's "allergic" reaction to explaining behavior by *any* kind of mental states, conscious or unconscious.[6]

Some phenomenologists, following Merleau-Ponty, have also urged that unconscious mental states are not the terms in which human behavior is to be explained. David Levin urges that "what Freud tries to explain by means of the notion of an unconscious idea or motive, we can now explain solely by reference to the bodily constituted field of phenomena."⁷ What Levin means by the latter phrase is no easy matter to specify. The replacement for Freud that Levin has in mind, he tells us, "is a theory which integrates mind and body by interpreting both in terms of the phenomenological notion of an intentional field of behavior."⁸

In any case, these latter two attacks on there being causally operative (and thus explanatory) unconscious mental states can be put to the side here. For each is hostage to the very general programs in psychology that each represents. These theory-based attacks are *not* the basis for the popular suspicion about unconscious mental states represented by Dostoevsky's Velchaninov. Such suspicions are better captured by those forms of skepticism themselves rooted in the common understanding of mind.

There are two levels at which such popular suspicions are to be captured: at the level of *things,* where the suspicion is that mind is consciousness; and at the level of *words,* where the suspicion is that mind means conscious of. I shall discuss each of these and then close this section with a less general skepticism about unconscious mental states presented by Ernst Nagel.

AN OLD DEBATE: MIND IS CONSCIOUSNESS?

It has often been suggested that unconscious mental states are a conceptual impossibility. This is an argument with a history. The philosophical critics contemporary with Freud often took the view that the nature of mental states required that one be aware of one's own mental states. Moreover, this requirement that one be conscious of one's mental states was not thought to be some incidental feature of mental states, but rather their essence, so that in no sense could a person properly be said to have a mental state if he was not conscious of it. That being so, statements such as Freud's, to the effect that the only point on which unconscious mental states differ from conscious ones "is just in the lack of consciousness in them,"⁹ were thought to be preposterous: "It [Freud's statement] is just like Mr. Churchill's 'cannibals in all respects except the act of devouring the flesh of victims.' "¹⁰ As another contemporary critic more fully spelled out:

> When I reflect on what I mean by a wish or an emotion or a feeling, I can only find that I know and think of them simply as different forms of consciousness. I cannot find any distinguishable element in these experiences which can be called consciousness and separated from the other elements even in thought so as to leave anything determinate behind. And to ask us to think of something which has all the characteristics of a wish or a feeling except that it is not conscious seems to me like asking us to think of something which has all the attributes of red or green except that it is not a colour.¹¹

Does the Unconscious Exist?

Freud was aware that "philosophers find difficulty in accepting the existence of unconscious processes," and that their line of attack was "based on [his] alleged abuse of the word 'conscious.' "[12] Freud's reply to this line of criticism raises an interesting methodological question. He replied that such criticism "sounds like an empty dispute about words";[13] that "it is a matter of convention, of nomenclature," and being such, is "of course, like any other convention, not open to refutation";[14] and that the identification of mind and all its concepts with conscious processes is simply an old prejudice embedded in our language.[15] Freud opposed his critics' logical analysis of language sometimes with the brute fact of his empirical discovery that there are unconscious mental states,[16] and sometimes with his right as a scientist to create a new concept, the only test for which is "whether the convention is so expedient that we are bound to adopt it."[17]

Such replies misconceive the thrust of an analysis into the reference of terms such as wish and motive. If the reference of mental state terms were conscious processes or states, then it indeed makes no sense to speak of unconscious motives, unconscious wishes, and the like. And it is no reply to assert as a matter of fact that one has discovered their existence, for the only criterion of their existence, consciousness, by hypothesis, is not met. If there is no other reference of mental state terms but various forms of conscious experience, there is nothing one can factually discover that entitles one to speak of a mental state once one eschews there being any conscious experience.

Nor would Freud be free to postulate a new theoretical concept and simply call it "unconscious mental state." As a scientist, one may be free to invent any terms one likes, in which event we defer judgment on the utility of their creation until we are in a position to judge the entire scientific system in which they appear. But if one chooses household words like motive or wish as the names of abstract entities that bear no relation to ordinary mental states of motivation or wishing, one can only mislead others as well as oneself about the nature of the claims being made when such concepts are used. Nor in such a view can Freud claim that he has discovered motives and wishes strictly analogous to those of everyday life;[18] and without the latter claim, what is one to make of the imputations of wishes and motives in therapy, which are supposed to make the patient accept responsibility either for the character of which such wishes are a part, or for the actions such motives explain? Such responsibility may follow if one was *motivated* to act, or at least if one's acts express one's wishes, but only if motive and wish here mean what they ordinarily mean. For no one accepts responsibility for his "psychogens" or other inventions of psychological theory.

Although this second of Freud's replies claimed a freedom from the ordinary meaning of motive and wish that he himself did not really want to claim, the philosophical criticisms themselves were not founded on an adequate analysis of mental concepts. Particularly since the work of Ryle and the later Wittgenstein, few philosophers would agree that motive and its related mental states are to be thought of "simply as different forms of consciousness." For one could adopt any nondualistic position in the philosophy of mind and *not* assume that there is "nothing left behind" if consciousness is subtracted. If desire, for example, names a set of dispositions to behavior, or a set of dispositions to further mental states, or a physical state with as yet unknown features, or a functional state, consciousness or the lack of it would simply be an incidental feature. Only if one were a follower of Descartes would one hold that nothing is meant by mental words such as desire but conscious mental experience.

Dualism, the commitment to mental states existing in some kind of special realm, is not a very plausible theory of mind. The two main arguments Ryle deployed against dualism—how a dualist can account for knowledge of others' minds, and how a dualist can conceive of the interaction (or lack of it) between brain and mind—remain serious problems for any dualistic view about minds.[19] More generally, *any* metaphysical dualism, be it of body and mind, fact and value, action and movement, or fact and theory, creates havoc with our basic need for coherence and consistency in our entire system of beliefs.[20] We live in one world, and our task is to understand it in a way that does not leave us speechless on fundamental issues such as how body and mind interact.

Despite this, there is something to the intuition of Laird, Field, and Dostoevsky. There *is* a temptation to deny sense to unconscious mental states. Since I do not think popular thought about mind is inherently dualistic in its presupposed metaphysics, the source of such temptation must be sought elsewhere.

A CONTEMPORARY DEBATE:
MIND MEANS CONSCIOUS OF

The contemporary version of this conceptual impossibility objection follows the linguistic turn of contemporary philosophy by focusing not on what mental states might be, but on certain aspects of the sense (not the reference) of mental words. In modern guise the philosophical objection to Freud's discovery of the unconscious would be that the distinctive feature of mental words lies precisely in the agent's ability to avow (that is, his consciousness of) what it is that he intends, hopes, fears, desires, and so on. First-person, present-tense statements are often said to be mental statements only insofar as they possess this distinctive epistemic feature.

Consider, as an example of this kind of argument, F. A. Siegler's argument about the concept of an intention. Siegler has concluded that it is a mistake to speak of a person's finding out, discovering, detecting or in any way identifying his own intentions. It makes no sense to talk in this way, and so it makes no sense to speak of a person's *failing* to find out, detect, or identify his own intentions. Consequently, it makes no sense to speak of a person's being mistaken in saying "I intend to do X." But this is exactly what Freud requires.[21]

Careful analysis of this conclusion will reveal that Siegler has conflated three distinct epistemic claims. The first is that mental words are asymmetrical with respect to the modes of their verification in their first- and third-person usages. This we earlier (in Chapter 5) called the claim of *privileged access*.[22] If I have knowledge of my desires, intentions, pains, and so forth, that knowledge is acquired in a way distinct from the way in which others come to have the same knowledge of my mental states. I do not observe my own behavior in order to conclude that I am in pain, that I intend to go downtown tomorrow, or that I believe it is raining. Others may use behavioral evidence to make third-person statements about my mental states; I do not perform any acts of observation, inner or outer, to learn my own mental states. If I know them, I know them in a nonobservational way.

Second, some first-person, present-tense mental statements are *incorrigible*. Distinct from the mode-of-verification claim of privileged access is the claim of infallibility in one's judgment about one's own states of mind. The claim of incorrigibility is that, if I say I am in pain, or desire a yacht, and I am sincere about it, then it must be true that I am in pain or desire a yacht at the time I say so.[23] Predictions of my future states of mind, or memories of past states of mind, are fallible; the claim of incorrigibility is that *present*-tense statements in the first person are infallible if sincere.

Third, mental states are often said to be *self-intimating*.[24] This is the converse of the incorrigibility claim, which is that if I think I am in pain, I am in pain. Here what is asserted is this: If I am in pain, I think I am in pain (mutatis mutandis for other mental states). There can be, in this view, no unfelt pains, no unperceived afterimages, no unknown desires.

Siegler, in the passage quoted, begins with a claim of privileged access: We do not "discover" or "detect" our own intentions as we do the intentions of others. As Siegler elsewhere elaborates:

> It is absurd to suggest that I find out what my intentions are by observing my behavior, still less by hearing myself say, "I intend to . . .". Do I then find out on the basis of some "internal" evidence, do I observe what is going on in my mind and infer from that what my intentions are? This sounds equally absurd.[25]

From here Siegler moves to the claim of self-intimation when he concludes that a person cannot *fail* to find out his own intentions. As he puts it elsewhere, "Normally I can come right out and state what my intentions are."[26] The next move is to incorrigibility, Siegler's conclusion that a person cannot be mistaken in his beliefs about his own intentions.

If one is to have any chances of understanding the conceptual impossibility argument, one has to do a better job than this of keeping these three distinct claims separate. For the truth of each of these claims is *not* dependent upon the truth of the others. In particular with regard to Siegler, it will not do to assume that because we have privileged access to our own mental states then we must also be incorrigible about them and such states must be self-intimating to us. As John Wisdom once pointed out: "It is a common mistake to identify the fact that a person has, necessarily has, a way of knowing what's in his own mind which no one else has, with the claim that he can't be mistaken about his own mind. That's a very different matter indeed."[27] We might add that it is an equally common mistake to confuse privileged access to one's own mind with the kind of "perfect" access to one's own mind that self-intimation would give if it were true.

Keeping these epistemic claims separate allows us to state more precisely the alleged conceptual problem with unconscious mental states: For a mental state to be unconscious is to lack just that knowledge held by the claim of self-intimation to be a prerequisite to being in the state in question. Further, such an unconscious mental state would be unaccompanied by the *noninferential* knowledge held by the claim of privileged access to be a prerequisite to being in the state in question. In addition, if one were conscious of some particular mental state, and the incorrigibility thesis were right, that would seem to leave no room for contradiction by the psychoanalytic suggestion of other, unconscious mental states. Thus, from each of these epistemic claims seemingly arises a version of the conceptual impossibility objection. I shall examine each version and each epistemic claim separately.

The Claim of Privileged Access

First, consider the least problematic of the three claims, that of privileged access. On those occasions when we do know what we desire, what we believe, or that we are in pain, do we come to such knowledge in a nonobservational or noninferential way? Rather plainly, it is usually the case that we do. Except to a well-conditioned behaviorist, it is surprising to be asked how we know, for instance, that we want an ice cream cone, that we believe going downtown will get us one, or that our left foot hurts. Yet privileged access to such states in no way renders nonsensical the idea that one may be unconscious of one's desires, beliefs, or other mental states.

To begin with, one might urge that the lack of privileged access to beliefs, desires, and other mental states in no way changes the *meaning* of the words referring to those states. The criteria for belief and desire are not to be confused with the modes of verifying whether those criteria are satisfied. Unless one is a verificationist about meaning (meaning *is* the mode of verification), then the fact that one mode of verification is lacking (because the actor is unaware of it) would not necessarily betoken a change in the meaning of the mental terms used.

Hence, a tempting construction of unconscious wish, unconscious belief, and the like would be to assume that the same criteria are meant as for wish and belief generally, with the proviso that the modes of verification of them are no longer different in first- and third-person usages. This construction is so straightforward that numerous philosophers have given all unconscious mental states such an (inevitably behaviorist) interpretation.[28] In light of the Freudian notion of extended memory, however, such flights to behaviorism seem an unnecessary means of giving sense to the phrase, unconscious mental states.

For I do not believe that there is a difference in the modes of verification between conscious and unconscious mental states. Freud seemed to think that one had what might be called deferred privileged access to one's unconscious mental states, namely, that if one became conscious of such states, one did so noninferentially (through memory). Freud throughout his writings emphasized that the analysand does not become conscious of an unconscious mental state just by looking at the evidence, namely, his own behavior patterns and the authoritative interpretation of his analyst.[29] He has to *remember* it as his motive, to know that it was his motive in a way that surprises him that he did not know it before. One has such a memory because, the theory asserts, in successful therapy one comes to *re*experience the (formerly unconscious) mental states.

Psychoanalytic therapy requires, in short, the same kind of nonobservational knowledge to confirm its interpretations as one has of one's conscious mental states outside analysis. The modes of verification for ascribing a motive to a person are thus still asymmetrical with respect to first- and third-person usages. The only difference a mental state's being unconscious makes is that at the time at which it is unconscious one cannot verify that one has the mental state in the accustomed manner. It may require a good bit of jogging of memory, either by free association, by reexperiencing the emotion via transference, or otherwise, before the subject recognizes the mental state as his. Indeed, for various reasons, he may in many cases never recognize such unconscious mental states. But, in principle, the way in which he comes to know his own mental states is the same, irrespective of whether they were conscious or unconscious.[30] For this reason, even if privileged access is the mark of any state that can truly be called a *mental* state, unconscious mental states are properly so called because of the subject's deferred privileged access to them.

The Claim of Self-Intimation

Unlike the claim of privileged access, the claim of self-intimation, if true, would preclude there being any things properly called unconscious mental states. If mental states must be immediately transparent to their holders (self-intimating) in order to be mental states at all, unconscious mental states would be (in Siegler's words) "incoherent and self-contradictory." We can have unconscious mental states only if the claim of self-intimation is false.

With respect to the causal connections between mental states and behavior there is little or no plausibility to a claim of self-intimation. Many causal connections we readily admit to exist between mental states and behavior are not known to the actor. A pain in my foot may be the cause of my gruffness to a colleague, yet even if the pain itself were a self-intimating state, the causal connection between that state and my behavior is not. I may know I am in pain and I may know that I am being gruff to a colleague; there is not even a hint from ordinary usage that the proper use of the word "pain" requires that I know the causal connection between the two. For belief/desire states the same arguments may be made as were just made for pain states; that is, even if beliefs and desires were self-intimating states, there is nothing to suggest that their causal connection to behavior (as a reason for action or otherwise) need be self-intimating.

Saying this does not, unfortunately, dispose of that part of the conceptual impossibility objection stemming from the claim of self-intimation. Even if the causal connection between belief/desire states and behavior is not self-intimating, if the states themselves are self-intimating, then *unconscious* beliefs or desires would make no sense. One could talk of unconscious reasons, but only in a very limited sense, namely, one where conscious beliefs and desires cause behavior without the actor's being aware of their doing so.

Are beliefs, desires, and other mental states themselves self-intimating? One historically important reason for thinking that they are has been rejected. This was the idea that such states were defined solely by the ability of their possessor to avow that he was in such a state. One would, in other words, be in state S if and only if one had the ability to avow, "I am in state S." This ontologically very spare account (which reduces mind to linguistic competence) does not seem very appealing in light of more substantial theories about what minds are. (Even in a "functionalist" view of mind, mental states are characterized by functions other than that the subject has certain linguistic abilities.)

Another historically important argument with the conclusion that mental states are self-intimating has only partial applicability to mental states. With experiential states, such as pain, one might think that the following two entailments hold: If one is in pain, one *feels* the pain; if one feels the

Does the Unconscious Exist?

pain, one knows (and can avow) that one is in pain. By virtue of such entailments, unconscious pains (or other experiential states of sensation, emotion, or imagination) would make no sense. Desire and beliefs, however, are not experiential states. Although one can experience a strong craving or a passionate desire, or can recite to oneself one's beliefs, such occurrences are incidental to being in the states named by belief and desire. Beliefs and desires are not plausibly interpreted to be occurrences, as philosophy at least since Ryle seems to have recognized. The argument to self-intimation from the immediacy of mental experience is accordingly nonexistent for those mental states connected to reasons for action.

Even for experiential terms such as those like pain that name sensations, the alleged entailments are very problematic, to say the least. Being in pain can entail feeling pain, and feeling pain can entail awareness of the pain, only according to a certain view about meaning that we have encountered before. This theory of meaning freezes our present guides to correct usage as *criteria* in the logical positivists' sense of necessary and sufficient conditions. Since pain as we presently use the word always, when correctly used, is accompanied by painful feelings (and the latter is accompanied by awareness), this view of meaning freezes painful feelings as the meaning of pain. In such a view an unfelt pain is quite literally nonsense (i.e., not in accordance with the *sense*, the criteria, of the word).

The general problem with this theory of meaning is that adverted to before: It cuts off our ordinary understanding from the progressive insights of science. It limits our insights into what pain might be, by a kind of conventional fiat: Whatever aspect of pain we have stumbled across first is all there is to pain. This leaves those psychologists who discover, say, the functions pain may serve in learning, as talking about something else the moment they treat pain as a state more importantly characterized by those learning functions than by the feelings of its subject. Similarly physiologists who wish to characterize pain as a certain form of C-fiber stimulation (even if there are occasionally no painful feelings) would be talking about something else in such an insular view of meaning.

As a last example, consider pain thresholds. Talk of people having different pain thresholds must be nonsense if pain entails feeling and knowing. For what sense could be made of saying that someone had a high pain threshold, i.e., that he neither noticed nor felt pains that others would notice and feel? If he did not notice it and did not feel it, then in the theory of meaning considered here he should not be said to be in pain at all. Nor can such a person be said to "stand more pain" than others – because he has pains only in proportion to what he feels, and if he does not feel much pain, then he does not have much pain. His threshold, in such a case, is mislabeled a pain threshold.

Psychologists cannot be shut out of talking about pain in these ways. It may turn out that persons have pains only when they feel them. If this is the case, however, it will only be because the best scientific theory we are able to muster about what pain really is tells us it is the case. It cannot be shown to be the case by freezing one present guide to usage as a meaning connection, an analytic truth, violation of which is "self-contradictory." The short of it is that the entailments that could justify self-intimation as a characteristic of mental states do not exist even for experiential mental terms.

A different argument for self-intimation focuses on mental terms such as belief and desire, terms that take objects. For such words the most serious argument for self-intimation I take to stem from the nature of Intentional (or intensional) objects. Desires and beliefs, like all mental states taking intensional objects, are individuated in part by those objects. What counts as one desire as opposed to another desire in part depends on the object of that desire. As we examined in Chapter 1, one of the striking facts about mentalistic language is that it is nonextensional; that is, the substitutivity of identicals does not hold for referring terms when part of the objects of mental states. Even if the room referred to by the description "the dirtiest room in the inn" is the very same room as that referred by the designation "Room 10," that identity does not allow one to conclude that Ralph desired the dirtiest room in the inn just because Ralph desired Room 10. A desire for the dirtiest room in the inn is different from a desire for Room 10, even though the things seemingly referred to in the propositional objects of the two desires are in reality one thing.

The upshot of this Intentionality for present purposes is this: Whatever account one gives for what sorts of things mental states are, one must make room for this "essentially linguistic" (see Chapter 1) mode of their individuation. This may seem to require self-intimation, because the most obvious sources for fixing the descriptions of the objects of belief and desire are the descriptions uttered by the person whose beliefs and desires they are. The subject can give such descriptions, the argument concludes, only if he is conscious of what his beliefs and desires are.

The crucial step in this argument for the self-intimation of states of desire and belief requires that some connection exist between the subject's having a certain belief or desire, and his possession of the speech dispositions sufficient to identify it. Requiring such a connection is motivated by the fact that our present abilities to fix the objects of beliefs and desires do depend heavily upon the linguistic abilities of the subject. This is true of our conscious mental states, but is also perhaps true of unconscious ones for which we can invoke extended memory as the means of fixing the relevant objects. Behavior, the most obvious alternative source of evidence here, may only be able to take us so far in pinpointing the object of a belief or a desire. For even if behavior seemingly "pointed to" some object in the world as the goal of the actor, it might not differentiate that object under one description as opposed to another. Yet as the *goal* of the actor, it is so differentiated. This is what the nonsubstitutivity of descriptions of identicals in Intentional contexts means. Without some verbal behavior, one might not, for example, be able to distinguish a desire to occupy Room 10 from a desire to occupy the dirtiest room in the inn, on the basis of behavior of someone's tending to place himself in that room; for there is only one room, and the behavioral tendency is to occupy *that room* (without regard to how it is described).

The essential problem for this step of the argument is the same problem that confronts the claim that *experiential* words are self-intimating: One cannot prevent increasingly better scientific theories about what sort of states beliefs and desires really are by this kind of freezing of present indicators into unassailable entailments (meaning connections, analytic truths, etc.). A theory about what desires are, it is true, must include features not necessary in a theory about pain; it must, that is, include features that account for the linguistic way in which such desire states are individuated. But there is no guarantee that our present best evidence for fixing the objects of a belief or desire, relying on the verbal abilities of the subject, is the only way such individuation can be accomplished. To account for such features, a theory about desires might well include the kind of brain writing we mentioned in Chapter 1, or perhaps some more complicated relation between the content of mental states and brain physiology. Alternatively, a richer behaviorism might indeed allow one to distinguish a desire to occupy Room 10 from a desire to occupy the dirtiest room in the inn and thus to recognize this "essentially linguistic" mode of individuation of desires and beliefs; all that is needed is to recognize there being behavioral dispositions about counterfactual situations, dispositions about what, for example, the actor would do if he believed that Room 10 was not the dirtiest room in the inn. However such physiological or behaviorist theorizing comes out, one cannot rule it irrelevant—as not being about *desires*—simply because it may go counter to our present indicators of the content of such desires; any more than one can rule irrelevant theorizing about pain that does not utilize our present indicator of pain, viz., painful feelings. In short, neither pain nor desire can name self-intimating states because such words are open to revisable scientific theory and are not hostage to a fixed linguistic convention.

Self-intimation cannot thus be made out as a necessary condition of any state's being a *mental* state. Our minds are not transparent to us, and nothing in ordinary usage can bind us to such a view.

The Claim of Incorrigibility

If the incorrigibility claim were true, it would not rule out the possibility of unconscious mental states. For the incorrigibility thesis only concerns the correctness of any beliefs the subject has about his mental states. It does not preclude his having other mental states, even contradictory ones, that are unconscious. Suppose someone, X, thinks he desires to help a friend. The incorrigibility thesis only claims that X must have the desire he thinks he has. It is silent about whether he has other mental states of which he is unaware, including perhaps a desire to hurt (rather than to help) his friend.[31]

The claimed incorrigibility of first-person awareness only becomes a problem for the unconscious with regard to unconscious motives (reasons for action). For with regard to motives, psychoanalysts do need to be able to contradict the actor's beliefs about his motives if they are to have the ability they claim, to divine the "real reasons," the unconscious ones, that motivated an actor to do what he did. The claim of incorrigibility, if true, does seem to stand in the way of there being unconscious motives, and I shall accordingly examine the correctness of this claim with regard to motives.

Richard Peters once advanced a version of this incorrigibility claim against there being unconscious motives. According to Peters, it makes no sense to ascribe unconscious motives to those actions for which we have a perfectly intelligible, conscious motive: "Some actions have such obvious and acceptable reasons that reference to unconscious wishes seems grotesquely out of place."[32] It is only when there is no conscious motive, or when the alleged conscious motive was suspect in some way, that Peters thought that unconscious motives could appropriately be ascribed.

Such a claimed incorrigibility of the subject does not rule out unconscious motives. For sometimes the actions explained by Freud are actions for which the actor is puzzled about his motives. He may even think that he had no motives. A good example of this sort is the obsessive woman who repeatedly rang for her maid for no apparent reason.[33] Her action was intentional, and the action is not intelligible to us as being performed for its own sake: One usually calls for one's maid only in order to get something else. Yet when asked why she performed this ritual, the woman could only answer that she did not know. When Freud suggests an unconscious motive for such an action, we are quite receptive to his suggestions because the action does seem to call out for a reason and the agent has none to give. In such cases where the actor is in such a state of puzzlement, she has no incorrigible knowledge of her motives to be contradicted by a psychoanalyst's discovery of her unconscious motives.

Still, unconscious motive ascriptions both in psychoanalysis and everyday life often do contradict the beliefs of the actor as to his motives. If the claim of incorrigibility were right with respect to our use of motive, then the latter subclass of unconscious motive ascriptions would make no sense. As it turns out, the incorrigibility claim is simply wrong with respect to even this subclass of unconscious motives.

There are a number of avenues to be pursued here. One might start with the observation that most of the motives about which psychoanalysts and laypersons talk are cited to explain *past* behavior. The temptation might be to say that by unconscious motive one means only that one cannot now recall what the motive was, although at the time one performed the action, one did know what it was with certainty. Under such a construction a person could well think he recalls what his motive was and yet be mistaken in his recollection. The apparent incorrigibility of one's expressions of one's own motive would then be no barrier to speaking of unconscious motives, even in situations where one believes one knows one's motive to be different from the unconscious motive suggested by the psychoanalyst.

If unconscious as used by Freud only means that one lacks a *present* ability to recall one's motive, some such construction could be made out. But plainly psychoanalytic explanations are not limited to situations where one was conscious of one's motive when one performed the action, but now has no memory of what one earlier knew. In fact, it is hard even to find an example in psychoanalysis where unconscious motive is so used. Rather, Freud's striking claim is that we perform actions, think with certainty we know why, yet in fact do not know our true motive even as we are acting because of it. Freud challenges, in other words, the incorrigibility of our first-person statements, not just in the past tense where they are clearly open to challenge, but in the present tense as well. The claim is that we do not know what we *are* about, even if we think we do—not just that we cannot correctly recall what we *were* about at some time in the past, even though we think we do recall what it was.

Another avenue that may appear tempting is to grant that present-tense expressions about one's own motives are not subject to contradiction, but to deny that psychoanalysts really contradict them when they cite patients' unconscious motives. One may have both a conscious motive and an unconscious motive in performing a certain action; one can be certain that the former was one's motive, and be correct, and still the latter may also have been one's motive.

Under this construction an unconscious motive, when cited as the explanation of an action for which the actor appears to know his motive, never means *the* (single) motive; it only means one of the *mixed* motives. The conscious and unconscious motives together cause the performance of the action. Citing the unconscious motive as one of the set of mixed motives does not contradict the actor's knowledge that he has conscious reasons as well for doing what he did. Both were his motives for doing it.

There is nothing implausible about this account. We do act for mixed motives, and there is no reason some of them may not be unconscious. Yet neither in psychoanalysis nor in ordinary speech is our use of unconscious motive limited to such situations. The very language we often employ to describe an unconscious motive as "the real motive" reveals our assumption that sometimes we do contradict the actor's apparent certainty about his motives.

The good sense with which we may question the testimony of the agent as to his own motives stems directly from the meaning of motive as a reason for action, discussed in Chapter 1. Unlike pains, future intentions, and imaginings, one does not "have a motive" except in the sense that some action is explicable by reference to it. One may feel pains, imagine things, intend to do various things, and perform no action for which these items may serve as an explanation. By contrast, I cannot have a motive as I *have* a pain or a future intention in the absence of an action; a motive is always given as an explanation of an action.[34]

It is always to the point to ask whether an explanation, of an action or of anything else, is a good one or not. If an agent is citing his motive in the first person, he is explaining his action no less than is a third-person observer who cites his motive in the third-person. In both cases, to be an explanation at all it must have the possibility of being false. It must be possible that the agent's conscious motive is not the cause of his performing a given action, even if he believes that it is.

The moment one uses pain or intention in an explanation of an action, our expressions using these terms also become clearly subject to contradiction. If I attribute my gruffness to a colleague to a pain in my foot, I could easily be said to be mistaken. If I say that I am speaking rapidly because I intend to catch the next bus, I can be mistaken. Intention and the like could only be incorrigible insofar as we do not use them to explain an action. The difference with motive is that it can only be used to explain one's actions. Hence, all uses of motive in the first person allow one to be mistaken about one's motives because all such uses purport to be contingently true explanations.

This last argument, of course, only shows that one is not incorrigible about the causation element in motivational ascriptions (the third criterion of reasons for action), but that one might still be incorrigible with respect to the mental states of desire and belief (the first and second criteria of reasons for action). Yet to make perfectly good sense of there being unconscious motives that contradict the actor's own view as to his motivation, it is not necessary to address the question of the incorrigibility of our usages of desire and belief. Even if one were incorrigible about one's own present desires and beliefs, that knowledge is not contradicted at all by an ascription of unconscious motives to an action. For if the incorrigibly known desires and beliefs are not causally relevant to the action, then the field is open to the analyst to suggest other (unconscious) desires and beliefs as the true motives of the action. Such suggestions in no way contradict the agent's assertions that he does desire q or believe p, only the causal influence of such beliefs and desires, as to which the agent has no special authority. Only if there is something illegitimate about saying there are beliefs and desires of the agent of which he is not conscious would there be a problem here. This would be a problem about the self-intimating nature of the states of belief and desire, a problem that I have argued does not exist.

The upshot of this analysis is that there is nothing suspect about attributing unconscious motives even when the subject believes his motives to be something entirely different. Our ordinary usage reflects this unproblematic character of unconscious motive ascriptions by the idioms of "real reasons" and "deeper reasons." It might be thought that our present use of motive in this way is only due to the "pollution" of the language brought on by the immense popular currency given Freud's ideas about unconscious motives. To some extent our use of real motives probably has expanded since Freud began writing. Yet well before Freud our language admitted a use of motive such that the person whose motive it was was not conscious of it. (Indeed, Freud himself rather charmingly admitted, in reminiscing about his discovery of unconscious processes, that his only claim to discovery was by being ill-read.) George Eliot's novels, for example, are replete with discernment of the hidden motives that activate her characters. Yet no one to my knowledge criticized books such as *Middlemarch* because its characters acted for motives of which they were not aware. We all seem to understand without difficulty that Bulstrode could well act for a reason of which he was not aware, and moreover could even believe with apparent certainty that his motive was something entirely different. Eliot's readers also seemed to understand that well enough, based on their ordinary concept of motive.

Although not strictly necessary to make sense of unconscious mental states, it is perhaps worth noting in closing this section how very suspect the incorrigibility claim is with regard to desires and beliefs themselves (not just, that is, with regard to their causal connection to behavior). Such suspicions are particularly justified about desire. Desire as ordinarily used is a theoretical word tied to satisfaction states, behavioral tendencies, tendencies with regard to other desires and beliefs, and perhaps to physiology as well.[35] One can no more freeze the conscious belief of the subject about what he desires into a sufficient condition of desire (which is what the incorrigibility thesis does) than one could make such belief into a necessary condition (which is what the self-intimation thesis would do). For the same reason there are no analytic truths about desire, only scientific theories about desire. Such fallibility about desire is easily observed in everyday speech, when we say, "He thinks he wants ... [a new car, a new wife, etc.], but he really does not." Such locutions make sense only because things may not be as they seem to the subject, that is, because he is *not* incorrigible about his own desires.

Practical Reason and the Unconscious

On Unconsciously Wishing for the Impossible

Separate from any of the epistemic claims about mental states is Ernst Nagel's conceptual argument toward his earlier quoted conclusion that unconscious wishes and the like are "just nonsense." Nagel reasoned that "there is an important failure of analogy between conscious motives and unconscious mental processes";[36] because of this failure, "It is only by a radical shift in the customary meanings of such words as 'motive' and 'wish' that Freudian theory can be said to offer an explanation of human conduct in terms of motivations and wish-fulfillments."[37] Nagel's charge here is that Freudians can explain behavior by unconscious mental states only if they gerrymander the idea of mental states enough to allow for unconscious mental states.

The crux for any such charge is to see whether there *is* any failure of analogy between ordinary wishes and motives, and unconscious wishes and motives. For Nagel the failure of analogy is to be found in the enduring nature of Freudian wishes:

> These unconscious motives have an enduring character and tenacious attachment to specific objectives that conscious wishes do not exhibit. Indeed, on Freudian theory a thwarted wish of early childhood, directed toward some person, may not completely vanish, but may enjoy a repressed existence in the unconscious, and continue to operate in identical form into the present even though that person has long since died.[38]

It is important at the outset to see that Nagel's kind of argument, even if it succeeded, can only be directed against certain kinds of unconscious mental states; these are the unconscious wishes of childhood so much a part of Freud's developmental metapsychology. *Not* at stake here is the conceptual possibility of there being unconscious motives at all.

In any case, even restricted to the unconscious wishes of childhood of Freud's developmental metapsychology, Nagel's alleged failure of analogy does not have much to do with the kind of states such wishes are. Rather, his point has to do, first, with the degree of attachment Freud says we have to the *objects* of our childhood wishes, and second, with the nature of those *objects* themselves — Freud allows that we may wish for the obviously impossible, as in an Oedipal wish toward a dead parent. Yet neither of these points should convince us that Freud abused the ordinary meaning of wish or motive. Even if these differences in *what* people wished for were large ones, the kind of state that wishing *is* would not differ. And, in any event, these are not really departures from our ordinary pre-Freudian ideas about wishes and their objects. People sometimes at least do orient their lives around some early formed wishes. And they do this even after the original objects of such passions have become impossible of attainment.

Does the Unconscious Exist?

Perhaps this is not very rational (in the sense of rational having to do with mastery of the passions), but it is very human.[39] One need only think of grief, where one wishes a dead person were alive, or guilt, where one may wish one had not done something, to see common examples of this very human tendency.

For my own part I find one of the most attractive features of Freudian theory to be its emphasis on this tragic aspect of human beings. In any case, even if Freud's thesis that our deepest longings are to found in the enduring wishes from childhood is only a tragic picture, aesthetically attractive but literally false, it is *not* a conceptual howler. Freud's developmental metapsychology conceptualized in terms of unconscious wishes enduring from childhood is not suspect on these grounds.

The Existence of the Unconscious as an Entity

That we all possess and act on mental states that are unconscious is a fact that by itself severely challenges the legal view of minds and persons. As we have seen, there are no conceptual shortcuts to getting rid of this challenge, any more than there were to ridding ourselves of the challenge presented by expansive views of health and illness. Even more challenging than the existence of unconscious mental states is the existence of something called the unconscious. As we have seen, the existence of a *property,* the unconsciousness that some mental states possess, does not by itself justify a further ontological commitment to an *entity,* the unconscious. The pretheoretical notion of the unconscious distinguished earlier licenses talk of the unconscious only in an ontologically noncommitting way, as an abbreviation for mental states that are unconscious.[40]

Most of the senses of unconscious have to do with the use of the word to name some ostensible entity. The most challenging (to law) of such entities would be the animistic unconscious. This is the view Freud himself encouraged by his likening of the System Ucs to another person that we infer to be within us on the same grounds as we infer other human beings to have consciousness within them: "All the acts and manifestations which I notice in myself and do not know how to link up with the rest of my mental life must be judged as if they belonged to someone else and are to be explained by the mental life ascribed to that person."[41] The animistic unconscious belongs with ego, id, superego, gatekeepers, censors, and other anthropomorphic subdivisions of self in Freud's metapsychology. I shall discuss the existence of all such "little people" in Part IV, where I shall argue that none of them, including the animistic unconscious, exist.

To understand whether the unconscious exists in any of the remaining three senses of unconscious we have explored is a very complicated question. It is complicated because such a question is bound up with more general issues having to do with the Freudian metapsychology as a scientific theory. A place to begin is Freud's own strident declarations on the reality of the unconscious. Freud complained that Janet "had taken up an attitude of undue reserve" about the unconscious, that he had implied that "the unconscious had been nothing more to him than a form of words, a makeshift, *une façon de parler,* and that he had meant nothing 'real' by it."[42] Such an idea of the unconscious as a kind of fiction Freud rejected out of hand: "If someone objects that here the unconscious is nothing real in a scientific sense, is a mere makeshift, *une façon de parler,* we can only shrug our shoulders resignedly and dismiss what he says as unintelligible. Something not real, which produces effects of such tangible reality as an obsessional action!"[43]

Before we come to what "real" might mean here, let us discuss briefly the conception of the unconscious that Freud brushes aside, the unconscious as merely *une façon de parler.* Perhaps the best modern characterization of this view of the unconscious is what I have called the behaviorist unconscious. Modern behaviorists will treat "the concept of 'the unconscious' as 'an intervening variable'—i.e., as a concept which makes inferences and predictions possible but does not stand for anything whose reality could meaningfully be either asserted or denied. 'The unconscious' would in that case be a concept which intervenes between one set of data and another but does not itself stand for any kind of datum."[44] The data between which the (behaviorist) unconscious intervenes are the childhood events and fantasies, on the one hand, and the adult behavior they explain, on the other.

To deny that the behaviorist unconscious exists is to do one of two things: Either it is to deny that these childhood events for which the unconscious is a stand-in cause adult behavior; or it is to deny that unconscious is the right way to conceptualize this behaviorist thesis of Freud's. The first of these is not a question we can easily resolve. Do we, as adults, react in ways best explicable by the tenets of Freud's developmental (sometimes called "genetic") metapsychology? Do we, that is, fixate at, or regress to, various stages in our sexual or social development? Do we as adults act so as to satisfy Oedipal wishes that events in childhood caused to exist within us? Do we even develop in the stages Freud and later Freudians have described?

Such difficult factual questions fortunately are not our main concern. It is the conceptual question that should most interest us in our inquiry about the challenge the unconscious presents to our concept of a person. Even granting that we develop as the developmental metapsychology says we do, and even granting that such events in early childhood cause us to do what we do as adults (despite the intervention of many other events), the conceptual question remains: Should such hypotheses be cast in terms of the unconscious?

Does the Unconscious Exist?

Ernst Nagel, for one, thought not. One of Nagel's reasons for this we have already explored, namely, the alleged abuse of the word "wish" involved in Freud's developmental thesis. There is, in addition, a quite different objection that Nagel made to the unconscious as a behavioral construct that intervenes between (childhood) stimulus and (adult) response. This is the objection that one need not conceive of there being unconscious *mental* states in order to give Freud's developmental explanations. The unconscious, Nagel tells us, is "a veritable 'ghost in the machine' that does work which a biologically oriented psychology might be expected to assign to the body."[45] This objection does not turn on any alleged failures of analogy or abuse of the meaning of wish and motive; rather, this objection to the behaviorist unconscious is based on a general principle of parsimony in theory construction according to which, to put it colloquially, less is better.

In the present context, at least, this preference for physiology over psychology in theory construction does not amount to much of an objection. For if one grants Freud's developmental thesis that wishes from childhood motivate adult behavior, it is a small step to conceive of those wishes as enduring *psychological* states. Such wishes, like all mental states, undoubtedly are related in some way (identity or otherwise) to underlying physical states. Yet if one grants that such states are wishes in childhood, and that they are wishes when they motivate later adult behavior, parsimonious theory construction might be better secured by conceptualizing these states just as Freud did: as unconscious *wishes*.

A more sophisticated form of this objection is to question whether Freud was correct in conceptualizing the mental states of early childhood as wishes. Jean Schimek, a developmental psychologist, has recently urged that Freud's conception of the unconscious fails at just this point. Unlike Nagel, Schimek urges that "we are no longer limited to Freud's alternatives that the unconscious has to be conceptualized as purely somatic processes or as the mental content of unconscious images."[46] Granting that the unconscious is a "psychological rather than a biological concept" and that (in its behaviorist guise) "it is an inferred construct to account for relationships between observables,"[47] the essential point for Schimek is how these unconscious mental states from childhood are to be conceptualized. What is rejected is Freud's conceptualization of these mental states as *wishes* with *content* (or what Schimek calls "mental representation"). Rather, we are urged to think of such early mental states that cause adult behavior as

> organized action patterns... ways of going at things; tendencies to seek or avoid specific experiences and situations; they do not require any mental representation of past experience as their anticipated goal. They would express the earliest and most basic level of any motive,

> truly unconscious in the sense of not yet being capable of achieving any symbolic representation. The general concept of prerepresentational unconscious organizers of action ... has the same methodological status as Freud's concept of unconscious mental representation.[48]

Schimek's argument that there is no such thing as unconscious mental representations in early childhood rests on the assumption that very young children are incapable of framing the objects (representations) of the wishes that, according to Freud's theory, motivate adults. Post-Piagetian developmental psychology has supposedly shown us that "the earliest forms of thought are sensorimotor actions" and that such thought is at a "prerepresentational" stage in cognitive development.[49] If this is true, the unconscious as Freud's genetic metapsychology conceives it—as containing the unchanging wishes of childhood—could not exist.

Schimek's point is an arresting one. It basically accuses Freud's developmental metapsychology as being static and *non*developmental, positing as it does unchanging wishes in the unconscious. Very young infants surely cannot have wishes whose content requires some sophisticated language capacities even to express. Yet the existence of the unconscious as a behavioral construct does not stand or fall with this last point. The conception of the unconscious does become a more complicated affair because one must treat the states that make it up as developing into unconscious wishes, not starting out as such wishes. Such a "developing unconscious" is precisely what Schimek herself attempts to articulate, in terms of stages in linguistic development.

A more modest kind of skepticism about the existence of the unconscious as an "intervening variable" is that voiced by T. R. Miles[50] and Alisdair MacIntyre.[51] According to Miles and MacIntyre, unconscious wishes are necessary constructs in Freud's developmental theory, but *the unconscious* is not. The link Freud needed between childhood events and adult behavior is supplied by wishes that are unconscious, and nothing, we are told, is gained by positing the unconscious as a thing (even the weak sort of thing that behavioral constructs are supposed to be).

For a behaviorist this last might seem a persuasive objection. Yet the persuasive appearance of the objection really stems from the impoverished view of theoretical concepts that is symptomatic of behaviorism. If theoretical terms in science were only "behavioral constructs," *une façon de parler*, there would be little to choose between fictional *properties* and fictional *entities* in one's developmental hypotheses. Both are only convenient fictions anyway. Neither truly exists to cause behavior. Either will do as a mere redescription (not explanation) of behavior or its stimuli.

This kind of issue—whether one needs the unconscious as well as unconscious wishes—has little significance when one thinks of the unconscious as a mere behavioral construct. Such an issue only makes much sense in light of more substantial conceptions of what theoretical entities in science are. The two remaining senses of unconscious, the physiological and the Freudian, instantiate two more robust ideas of what the entities posited in scientific theory are. They also allow us to move from the unconscious as merely *une façon de parler,* to the unconscious Freud thought to be "something real."

The existence of what I have called the physiological unconscious is very unproblematic as a hypothesis. For it is surely implausible at this date to deny that brain processes in some sense underlie mental processes. Since we are not aware of such goings-on in the brain, the unconscious is an apt enough name for all of them. It is accordingly very difficult to deny that the unconscious exists in this sense, or to deny the causal relevance of neurophysiology to behavior.

It is the Freudian unconscious whose existence is much more in question, because it is the theory in which this concept has a place that is most in question. If the dynamic, economic, topographical, structural, and developmental metapsychologies cannot be welded together to form a defensible theory of human behavior, then the concepts they employ, such as the unconscious, will also be indefensible. If the theory fails, then the Freudian unconscious does not exist. And if all of this is true, then the drastic diminishment in responsibility that the unconscious seems to call for could easily be shown to be unwarranted.

We thus have thrust upon us, unavoidably, the large question of the validity of the metapsychology as a scientific theory. The ontological question, Does the unconscious exist? is only a popular way of stating this larger question. In thinking about the considerable discussion on the validity of the metapsychology that has gone on in recent years, it seems to me that there have been two sorts of criticism of Freud's theory that should be distinguished. One might criticize the metapsychology on the grounds that there is no room in science for any such theory of the mind. Ernst Nagel's earlier quoted criticism, that the metapsychology does the work only a biological theory can do, is representative of this first form of criticism. Alternatively, one might criticize the metapsychology because it, as a *particular* theory of the mind, does not work, admitting that there could be such a thing as a truly scientific theory of the mind. My own criticism of Rapaport at the end of Chapter 1, in terms of his attempt to stipulate connections that must be discovered, is representative of this second kind of criticism.

It is important to separate these two kinds of criticism because I think the first to be wrong. The enterprise Freud attempted was the right enterprise for psychiatry even if he did not pull it off. That he failed has important implications for law (including very practical issues such as how much credence should be given the testimony of dynamic psychiatrists on questions of unconscious compulsions and the like). That it was nonetheless the sort of enterprise Freud should have attempted has important implications for psychiatry. I shall accordingly discuss each kind of criticism in turn.

Representative of the first kind of criticism, that the metapsychology is an impossible enterprise to do at all, is the work of Ilham Dilman.[52] In two papers published over a decade apart, Dilman urged that the unconscious cannot be interpreted as a theoretical term in Freud's general metapsychological theories of human behavior. Dilman's specific argument against what I have called the Freudian unconscious—the unconscious defined by economic, topographical, and dynamic metapsychologies—was a forerunner for what is now a growing chorus of criticism of *all* the concepts of these metapsychologies. The general form of all such arguments is that such concepts fail as theoretical concepts because the theories of which they are a part not only fail, but also were bound to fail given what they were attempting.[53]

Dilman's argument against the Freudian unconscious is based on the epistemic claims about mind that we have already examined. Specifically, it is based on the privileged access we each have to our own mind. As we have seen, Freud's clinical ideal of "making the unconscious conscious" is only attained by the recapture *through memory* of what was previously unconscious. One does not make an inference from a theory to become aware of one's own mental states, conscious or unconscious. Therapy is to prompt the extension of first-person awareness to such states.

Dilman bases two arguments on this clinical ideal of psychoanalysis. The first is that it is a kind of category mistake to think that one could have such privileged access to (direct awareness of) a theoretical entity. As Dilman puts it:

> One cannot talk of seeing an electron (not even as a possibility one might wish to speculate about) without sinning against logic; for if the concept of an electron is theoretical . . . then seeing cannot have a place in statements in which the concept of an electron has a place. . . . While we can talk of observing the effects of electrons, the expression "seeing an electron" is at best a misleading locution. The same would be the case of "making the unconscious conscious" if the concept of the unconscious were a theoretical concept.[54]

Theoretical entities, in this view, must be inferred; they cannot be observed, either by the senses (in the case of electrons) or by introspection (in the case of the unconscious), else the concepts that refer to them are not truly theoretical concepts but are observational concepts. Given the subject's privileged access even to his unconscious mental states, Dilman concludes, the unconscious cannot be a theoretical concept that figures into higher (i.e., nonobservational) levels of explanation. "Statements about a person's unconscious mind are not on a different level from statements about his conscious mind, as they would have to be if the concept of the unconscious were a theoretical concept."[55]

Dilman's second argument is also based on the privileged access we each have to our own mental states. Such privileged access, as we have seen, gives rise to an asymmetry in the modes of verification of first- and third-person statements about minds. Dilman's argument here is that treating the unconscious as a theoretical entity would do away with this asymmetry for unconscious mental states, because then even first-person statements would be verified only by inference from a theory, and not directly from awareness:

> My main objection to the view that the unconscious is a theoretical construct has been that it does not recognize the difference between a person's recognition of his own unconscious feelings and desires and another person's recognition of them. It hinders a proper appreciation of what is involved in what is unconscious becoming conscious.[56]

In making the unconscious conscious, Dilman concludes, "There is no question of anything taking place even remotely describable as the patient accepting a theory."[57]

Dilman's kind of argument has a great deal of appeal among contemporary psychoanalytic theorists. It is to maintain a sharp distinction between psychoanalysis as a therapy (clinical psychoanalysis) and psychoanalysis as a theory (the metapsychology). Clinical psychoanalysis uses only the pretheoretical idea of the unconscious, the unconscious that is not an entity but only a property of mental states that are part of a person because they are recapturable by that person's extended memory. The metapsychological theory posits an entity, the kind of System Ucs we have explored. The crucial step for Dilman and these more contemporary psychoanalysts is to maintain that the metapsychology cannot be a theory about the very same, pretheoretical unconscious that they attempt to bring to consciousness in their clinical practice.

Dilman's two arguments are only two of many arguments seeking to justify this permanent sealing off of the pretheoretical unconscious from a deeper and more general theory that explains it. Unstated in Dilman's argument is the crucial assumption that the unconscious cannot be *both* the recapturable mental states of clinical practice *and* a theoretical entity posited by a theory seeking to explain, among other things, that clinical practice. Yet why cannot it be the case that we could have a theory about things (mental states) that are also the subject of direct awareness?

Dilman's point ultimately comes down to the assertion that one cannot have a theory about the mind. One cannot because then one would have given up the distinctive feature of mind, privileged access. In such a view Freud was closer to the truth than he knew when he proclaimed that "the property of being conscious or not is in the last resort our one beacon-light in the darkness of depth psychology."[58] Consciousness, including the consciousness that can recapture the unconscious, is such a beacon light because without the *potential* for being illuminated by it no state should be thought of as a *mental* state.

Dilman's kind of argument can be constructed no matter what one takes to be the touchstone of mind. Roy Schafer, for example, fastens upon Intentionality—that aspect of language characteristic of our talk about persons, actions, and reasons—as such a touchstone of mind.[59] For Schafer too there can be no metapsychological theory about neurotic symptoms because these symptoms are accurately conceptualized as the actions persons perform for reasons. Because of this "action language" conceptualization of neurotic symptoms, the metapsychology becomes an illegitimate enterprise for Schafer no matter how it is construed. If framed in terms of forces, energies, and drives—the non-Intentional vocabulary of the economic metapsychology—then the theory is not a theory of *mind* because it has left the only vocabulary in terms of which mind can be discussed, what Schafer calls the "action" vocabulary. If framed in terms of little people performing little actions for little reasons, Schafer's complaint is that such (admittedly Intentional) vocabulary is only appropriate for *whole* persons.

In short, for Schafer as for Dilman, Freud's metapsychology is caught in a dilemma: The mentalistic vocabulary of persons in terms of which clinicians prompt patients to recapture unconscious wishes and so on is not a vocabulary in which it makes sense to construct an Intentionalistic metapsychology. But it also is true that any theory constructed in a non-Intentional vocabulary (or one without asymmetry in its modes of verification) cannot be a theory about the *mind,* for these features—Intentionality and privileged access—constitute what is mental.

Dan Dennett summarizes this point of view very nicely in his discussion of the explanation and theories possible for pain.[60] Suppose we seek a theory with which to explain three facts about persons and pains. First, persons can recognize certain sensations as painful; second, persons can locate their pains; and third, persons avoid pain. Dennett explores what kind of theory one can construct about these three observed facts about persons and pains if one restricts oneself to the vocabulary of persons, actions, and mental states. The answer is: no theory at all. To take each of these three facts in order: Persons have no criterion for distinguishing painful sensations from other sensations or mental states. Persons have privileged access to their pains, and noninferentially distinguish them from other sensations. "Pains hurt" is about as much of a theory one gets at the personal level of explanation. Similarly, the ability to locate pains is not something we can break down into subactions that persons do. Persons do

Does the Unconscious Exist?

not frame hypotheses about the locations of their pains, make observations, and the like; they just know where it hurts. And finally, with regard to the third fact about persons and pains:

> What is it about painfulness that prompts us to avoid it, withdraw our hand, attempt to eliminate it? The question is dead because there is nothing *about* painfulness at all; it is an unanalyzable quality. We simply do abhor pain, but not in virtue of anything (but its painfulness).[61]

Dennett's conclusion is that

> When we have said that a person has a sensation of pain, locates it and is prompted to react in a certain way, we have said all there is to say within the scope of this [the personal or mentalistic] vocabulary. We *can* demand further explanation of how a person happens to withdraw his hand from the hot stove, but we cannot demand further explanations in terms of "mental processes."[62]

If we attempt to construct a theory about pain in a different vocabulary — for example, the vocabulary of physiology — it will not be a theory about *pain:*

> When we abandon the personal level in a very real sense we abandon the subject matter of pains as well. When we abandon mental process talk for physical process talk we cannot say that the mental process analysis of *pain* is wrong, for our alternative analysis cannot be an analysis of pain at all, rather of something else — the motions of human bodies or the organization of the nervous system.[63]

It should be apparent that what we have encountered once again is the doctrine of category differences between the extensional, non-Intentional, observation-dependent, mechanistic, causal vocabulary appropriate to explain movements of bodies (including human bodies), on the one hand, and the non-Intentional, intensional, nonobservational, purposive, reason-giving vocabulary appropriate to explain human actions, on the other. The myth of the unconscious, just like the myth of mental illness, depends in part upon the apparent irreducibility of the vocabulary of *persons* to the vocabulary of natural objects. Which aspect of this apparent categorical divide is seized upon by mythicists about the Freudian unconscious does vary. Dilman, as we have seen, seizes upon privileged access whereas Schafer picks Intentionality. Other psychoanalytic theorists latch onto the fuzzier hermeneutic notion of meaning.[64] But the general dilemma for the metapsychology that each of them poses is wholly the same: No theory can be constructed "on the mental side," and although theories are perfectly appropriate "on the physical side," they cannot be theories of *mind*.

This view has to be wrong. Neither supposed ontological divides between modes of being, nor category differences between kinds of concepts, can get in the way of theory construction in the way Dilman, Schafer, and others suppose. It cannot, for example, be the case that one "sins against logic" in talking about seeing an electron. Theoretical entities do not exist in a special realm distinct from empirical entities; theoretical terms do not belong in a separate category from observational terms.[65] If it turns out that we cannot see an electron, it will be because (according to the best theory we have of what electrons *really are*) electrons are not capable of emitting or reflecting electromagnetic radiation within the spectrum of wavelengths of visible light.

It likewise cannot be a sin against logic to come to direct awareness of Freud's theoretical unconscious. How one comes to know a certain fact is an interesting question of epistemology; what one comes to know is an equally interesting but distinct question of ontology. That we have deferred privileged access to our unconscious is no argument at all that it is not the systematically organized set of repressed states obeying nonlogical laws of thought that Freud's theory says it is. We need not, of course, accept such a theory in order to become aware of an unconscious mental state, any more than one need accept the theory that water is H_2O in order to judge that some liquid one is drinking is water. We can be quite ignorant of what things really are (which is what a theory tells us) and still become acquainted with those things in various ways.

The ultimate mistake here is a mistake about meaning. Our pretheoretical, ordinary speech about persons, their actions, and mental states does reflect the distinctions I have telescoped into *the* doctrine of categorical differences. And the pretheoretical unconscious is indeed part of the ordinary vocabulary of persons. Yet the meaning of unconscious (or of any of the other terms of that personal vocabulary) is not to be thought of as a kind of analytic guarantee against there being "merely synthetic" novelties introduced about the unconscious by further scientific discovery. It cannot be the case that "we are talking about something other than pain" when we seek to give physiological accounts of how people can discriminate painful sensations, tell their location, or seek to avoid them. Such physiological theories are theories about what pains really are, just as Freud's metapsychology should be seen as a theory of what the pretheoretical unconscious really is.

There is one last arrow in the quiver of those who would reject the metapsychology as an inherently impossible theory. That is to deny that there is room for a nonphysical theory of the unconscious. We might admit, that is, the possibility of a *physiological* theory of pain, of desire, or of the unconscious. One would, of course, equally admit that our ordinary, *mentalistic* talk of persons, their pains, and desires makes good sense (even if there are no theories to be built in such terms). Denied, however, is that there is some third kind of "medium" in which one can construct the metapsychology. For Freud and his followers have repeatedly stressed that the terms of the metapsychology do not refer to physical things. Since no theory is possible in the ordinary vocabulary of persons and minds, that leaves the metapsychology in some kind of "no-theory's land." This I take to be the point of those who stress critically Freud's borrowing of physical concepts with which to build the metapsychology only to stipulate away their normal (physical) reference. It does indeed leave one wondering what, quite literally, Freud was talking about.

Consider by way of example an aspect of the Freudian unconscious we have not hitherto discussed, the characteristics Freud called "primary process" thinking. The unconscious, Freud thought, has no idea of time; it replaces external with internal reality; terms and concepts have multiple reference, that is, ideas are "condensed"; notions of identity are loosened because the affects attached to one object are "displaced" onto another (which is to say that in the unconscious they are identified as one and the same object); contradiction is acceptable in the unconscious; and negation is unknown there.

These characteristics are not part of our pretheoretical notions of the unconscious. They are not experienced, nor are they recapturable, as *thoughts* a *person* has. Nor are they physical processes, if we take Freud at his word of providing a psychological theory. That leaves one wondering what sorts of entities or processes this aspect of the metapsychological theory of the unconscious can be about.

The answer is that statements describing these six characteristics of primary process thinking are not *about* either the ordinary (personal) states of thinking or *about* some goings-on in the brain. The only *secure* referents of the phrases describing the primary process are functional states Freud hypothesized to exist. Such functional states are like the functional states workers in artificial intelligence devise when they seek to understand intelligent functioning. Such functional states are specified without regard to the kind of physical structure that may realize them. They are not, thus, straightforwardly physical states, nor are they mental states or actions of a person. This last can be grasped by recalling that many such functional states or subroutines are gone through in preprocessing information from the eye, yet we are not inclined in the least to say that the *person* does these things or possesses these as mental states. Such "subpersonal" functional states thus occupy a kind of middle ground between body and mind.

None of this should be taken to mean that there is some "third mode of being" in which functional states exist, or that there is some third kind of category in which their names belong. Rather, such functional states and the concepts that name them are ways of maintaining that we live in one world (a monist metaphysics) even while recognizing that we have different ways of gaining knowledge about it (privileged access) and even if there are distinctive modes of description of it (Intentionality). Such functional states are hypotheses about what kind of physical states must underlie the mental states persons experience or are aware of. One should see primary process thinking (and all concepts of the metapsychology in general) as concepts justified ultimately by their ability to relate brain to mind.

What this means for the concept of primary process thinking is, first of all, that one regards the six characteristics as forming a system. The mathematician, Matte-Blanco, for example, has attempted to weld these six characteristics together into a kind of logic, what he calls a "symmetrical" logic quite different than the "asymmetrical" logic of Frege–Russell–Quine.[66] Such characteristics form a *logic* in the sense that they state the general principles of "valid" inference in the unconscious. The thesis is that even irrationality may draw inferences systematically, that what is irrational need not be chaotic.

Such a systemization of unconscious inference drawing is a theory, a set of hypotheses, that seeks to explain ordinary thinking, the mental states that *persons* possess. Ordinary thinking is not perfectly rational; although we are all fairly good intuitive logicians – in the ordinary sense of "logic" – we are not ideally rational inference drawers. One way of seeking to explain this fact is to see ordinary thinking (the "secondary process") as an output of two subsystems. There is, Eric Rayner hypothesizes, an

> interweaving of symmetrical and asymmetrical logics in the individual's emotional and intellectual life. In extreme emotions infinite experiences and symmetry probably hold sway. But mild, deep, or quiet emotionality is likely to contain thinking which compounds the two logics. In normal states the two logics seem to be in harmony while in pathology they are in discord.[67]

There is no guarantee that this is a fruitful functional organization to give to the subroutines underlying ordinary thinking. There is no guarantee that there are two subsystems in conflict or in harmony, or that if there are, the opposition of ordinary to symmetrical logic is the way to define them. But some sort of states underlie ordinary thinking, and the primary process represents Freud's hypothesis about what sort of states they are. Such a hypothesis is not unverifiable. It must fit not only the (personal) characteristics of ordinary thought, but ultimately it must fit as well the physiology of the brain. Functional states and subroutines do indeed possess the kind of "provisional independence" from physiology we mentioned in Chapter 1. But ultimately some kind of physical structures must realize such functional states if they are truly states that underlie thinking. Subdividing ordinary thinking into subroutines inaccessible to consciousness is a legitimate activity that cognitive psychologists, artificial intelligence specialists, linguists, *and Freudians* can meaningfully engage in. But the functional organizations they arrive at are hypotheses, premised on the assumption that there are physical structures that realize the hypothesized functional divisions.

Does the Unconscious Exist?

Freud at times was quite lucid about this justification of the metapsychology. From the unpublished *Project* of 1895 to the *Outline* of 1940, he first and last saw his task as building a theory to relate body to mind. As he put it in the *Outline:*

> We know two things concerning what we call our psyche or mental life: firstly, its bodily organ and scene of action, the brain (or nervous system), and secondly, our acts of consciousness, which are immediate data and cannot be more fully explained by any kind of description. Everything that lies between these two terminal points is unknown to us.[68]

The metapsychology is Freud's attempt to make known to us what it is that lies "in between" brain and mind. The metapsychology may fail completely in this task, but the task itself is not a logically absurd undertaking. Indeed, it is *the* task that must be undertaken by any theory that would lay claim to being a general psychology.

The second form of criticism is much more difficult to assess. It is easy enough to write off David Rapaport's kind of definitional reductionism, as I argued at the end of Chapter 1. But the metapsychology can be treated as a theory seeking to *discover* the connections between a person's actions and mental states and that person's physical states and processes. When the metapsychology is so construed, then the only question about it is whether it is *true*.

The literature testing the metapsychology is immense. In a thorough and methodologically sophisticated review of that literature, Stephen Morse has concluded that the best that can be said about the metapsychology is the equivalent of the old Scottish verdict, "Not proven." More specifically, Morse concludes:

> The outcome of psychodynamic therapy suggests that it is not uniquely successful and that the theoretically posited variables are not the agents of the therapeutic change that does occur; external, empirical investigations have produced, at best, only equivocal and pallid confirmations of Freud's theory; alternative theories often can explain the results of studies supportive of Freudian theory, and, in any case, psychodynamic theory is only a partial account of reality even in those areas where it may be valid; and a great proportion of Freud's theories, and almost all of the theories of those who have followed him, have never been tested by reasonably scientific means.[69]

Morse's last conclusion is worth dwelling on a bit. The untested nature of much of Freud's theory is in part due to psychoanalysts' unjustified reliance on clinical data as confirming the theory, a mistake for which Morse rightly castigates them.[70] It is also the case, however, that parts of the metapsychology are currently more amenable to test than others. As Morse points out, the tenets of the genetic metapsychology, for example, are more easily tested because of the behavioral correlations they posit. It is not that the rest of the metapsychology is untestable in principle. This old criticism of psychoanalysis has been amply exploded by Adolf Grunbaum in a recent series of papers.[71] Rather, to test those "deepest" parts of the depth psychology calls for more knowledge of brain physiology than we now possess. The primary process hypotheses, for example, are an example of such currently difficult-to-test parts of the theory. That it is "testable in principle" is illustrated by the tests of Freud's dream theory made possible by advances in the physiology of dreaming since 1950.[72]

The result of this partly falsified and largely unproved status of the metapsychology is that the unconscious is itself a very problematic concept. Whether Freud's story about the unconscious in terms of instincts being repressed and of primary process thinking is true is a matter yet to be resolved definitively. Available evidence suggests that most of it is false. Without newer and better evidence, the unconscious unproblematically exists only as a property of mental states; as an entity it is as problematic as the theory that posits its existence.

8 The Nature of Psychoanalytic Explanation in Terms of the Unconscious

IT HAS BECOME something of an orthodoxy in the "philosophy of psychoanalysis" of the past three decades to assert that typical psychoanalytic explanations are motivational in character.[1] This is sometimes put by saying that psychoanalytic explanations give *reasons for actions,* rather than *causes* of mechanical *movements* or processes; that the specific explanations of particular actions in terms of their motives offered in the clinical practice of psychoanalysis are fruitful, but that the "deeper" explanations attempted in psychoanalytic theory are useless; that such particular explanations are framed in terms of ordinary, mentalistic language rather than in the technical language of a theoretical science; or, that psychoanalytic explanations deal with phenomena that themselves have meaning, as opposed to the colorless phenomena with which natural science deals.

Although the title of this chapter might suggest it, it is not my purpose to defend or attack this thesis (not frontally, at least, although I do believe this chapter has some bearing on it). Rather, I wish to examine the purportedly motivational explanations offered by psychoanalytic theory and to ask whether typical psychoanalytic explanations in fact are motivational in character. My conclusion is that, although the idea of there being unconscious motives for our actions makes perfectly good sense (as we examined in Chapter 7), psychoanalytic explanation is rarely motivational in character. As often as not, a deceptively uniform motivational language masks a variety of different kinds of explanations.

I shall not attempt a comprehensive survey of motivational language in all of psychoanalysis. Sufficient to make plausible my thesis, I think, is the set of explanations given in one aspect of the discipline, the theory of dreams. The psychoanalytic theory of dreams is an apt example for a number of reasons. To begin with, it is sufficiently rich in different levels of purportedly motivational explanations to illustrate the variety of types of explanations being offered. Because of this richness, it is sometimes pointed to as the best example of motivational explanation in psychoanalysis. Also, it is one of the most accessible bodies of theory in psychoanalysis, because of its comparative lack of revision after Freud's original theorizing.[2] Thus, one may, with some appropriateness, focus on *Freud's* theory of dreams and ignore more recent developments (which I, in any event, intend to do). Finally, the psychoanalytic theory of dreams may have some intrinsic interest of its own. It is, for example, sometimes well regarded even by critics otherwise quite hostile to psychoanalysis generally.[3] Freud wrote of his dream theory that "insight such as this falls to one's lot but once in a lifetime."[4] The editors of a recent edition of *Daedalus* apparently agreed, including *The Interpretation of Dreams* as one of the classics of the twentieth century.[5] Hence, this often well-regarded and, in any event, historically important example of scientific theorizing in the raw may *ceteris paribus* be preferred to other examples of motivational explanation in psychoanalysis.

I shall proceed by sketching briefly an overview of the psychoanalytic theory of dreams, distinguishing three levels of explanation in the overall theory. I shall then analyze separately each such level, construing each purportedly motivational explanation as more aptly framed in the language of functions or mental causes.

A Sketch of the Psychoanalytic Theory of Dreams

Freud's explanation of dreams presents one of the most strikingly complex explanations in terms of motive and its related terms that one may find in psychoanalysis. The levels of *meanings,* the degree to which motives are given for everything in the content, form, or process of formation of dreams, is matched only by his explanation of neurotic symptoms in the most complex of case histories.

This is to some extent a result of the task Freud set for himself in explaining dreams: He stated that he was going to *interpret* dreams, to find their meaning,[6] the task of the ancient soothsayers. His search was, from the start, for the meaning of dreams, and it should be no surprise that the explanations he found are couched in the language of meaning, that is, in terms of motives, wishes, intentions, and the like.

Freud accused those who dismiss dreams as having no meaning, or who explain dreams solely by reference to physiological or external causes, as abandoning strict, scientific determinism.[7] With such explanations, he thought, one could not explain the content of dreams (why a hen rather than a rabbit, for example).[8] Freud here confused determinism in the sense of "every event has a cause" with his rather animistic version: "Every (mental) event has a meaning." There is nothing unscientific about assuming that dreams are perfectly meaningless and yet are strictly determined by (as yet unknown) causes.[9]

In any event, for good reasons or ill, Freud was committed to finding

The Nature of Psychoanalytic Explanation

meanings for dreams. It is not a task unsuggested by the phenomena, inasmuch as dreams do seem to be expressed in some kind of hidden language. What is surprising is the extent to which all aspects of dream phenomena are found to have meaning by Freud.

The bedrock of Freud's dream interpretations, as everywhere in psychoanalysis, rested on the technique of free association. Freud interpreted each element of the dream as described by the patient and constructed the meaning of the dream from those associations and the elements of the remembered dream. Thus the Freudian attempt to explain dreams rests at least initially on the consciousness of the individual whose behavior (dreaming) is to be explained.

Basic to Freud's explanation of dreams is his distinction between the manifest content of a dream and the latent dream thoughts. The manifest content was defined as what the dreamer could remember of a dream and relate to others: "Whatever the dreamer tells us must count as his dream."[10] In fact, Freud paid very close attention to the precise wording, hesitations, and order of presentation of his patients' remembrances. He recognized that the dreamer's memory of dreams, as of anything else, could be faulty, and that remembering the dream at different times could produce different descriptions of it. Freud decided that since there is no independent check on the patient's memory of what he dreamed, any and all such descriptions should be treated with equal respect and called the manifest content of the dream. The dream as variously described was explicable by reference to the same set of latent dream thoughts, but how the dream was related at different times was itself the subject of motivational analysis. For example, where descriptions of the same dream given at different times differed, Freud believed he had a clue to the sensitive area of the dream. Similarly, for the forgetting of parts of a dream: What we forget, we have a reason for forgetting.[11]

Since dreams as remembered simply do not fit explicitly the pattern of meaning (wish fulfillments) Freud believed they had, or any single pattern for that matter, he felt compelled to invent the notion of the latent dream thoughts. Only by reference to thoughts other than those that we could remember did Freud believe he could justify his discovery of the meaning of dreams without appearing to be obviously wrong.

The latent dream thoughts are "entirely rational" and "have their place among thought processes that have not become conscious – processes from which, after some modification, our conscious thoughts, too, arise."[12] They are not to be conceived of as the forgotten thoughts occurring during a dream; whether remembered or not, those thoughts are all part of the manifest content. If I read Freud correctly, all of those thoughts or images occurring during dreaming that are potentially the subject of recall are the manifest content of the dream. This leaves one to wonder what is left over to be referred to as *latent* dream thoughts, for Freud's distinction between manifest and latent places all recallable contents in the manifest basket, and there seems to be nothing left to put in the one labeled "latent."

One possibility that recurs in Freud's writing is to regard the latent dream thoughts as a set of processes or states that *cause* the manifest dream thoughts to occur. This raises a very general problem about the status of those processes or states that I will discuss later in connection with the dream work. Briefly, to escape the charge of Molière—defining the cause of the manifest dream as "the dream-causing state"—Freud would have to give some independent definition of the latent dream thoughts and of the processes of the dream work that distort them. Since we still know little of the brain physiology involved, latent dream thoughts might be regarded as the name of those functional states (whose physical structure is unknown) that must exist if dreams indeed have the form Freud said they have, *viz.*, wish fulfillments.

An alternative, even more problematical, possibility is to relate the latent dream thoughts to the manifest content of dreams in some logical way, rather than in a causal way. That is, one might regard the latent dream thoughts not as experiential or physiological carriers of the meaning of the dream (and certainly not as Ryle's ghostly nonphysiological carriers) but as that meaning itself. Freud on occasion made this equation himself.[13] So conceived, the latent dream thoughts then become whatever we can infer of the meaning of the dream from its manifest content and from the trains of association produced in psychoanalysis. Assigning them this logical status does not commit one to assuming that there exist processes known as latent dream thoughts measurable in ways independent of the meanings to be inferred in dreams. On the other hand, as we shall see, such a "hermeneutic" interpretation of what the latent dream thoughts are is in danger of trivializing completely Freud's theory of dreams. I shall put aside for now this ambiguity in the status of the latent dream thoughts, since it is resolvable only by considerations raised later in the chapter having to do with the status of the dream work.

The overall hypothesis in Freud's explanation of dreams is that dreaming is a means of staying asleep. The problems we have during the night in remaining asleep are, for Freud, the result of the activities of three potential sleep disturbers: (1) the accidental stimuli occurring during the night, such as a fallen bedcover or a bout of indigestion; (2) continued thoughts from the perceptions or activities of the preceding day; and (3) a repressed, unconscious wish from childhood seeking expression during the night. The last item is the crucial one in Freud's explanation. Such wishes arise during the night because our normal censorship of them is weakened during sleep, presumably in line with the lessened mental activity generally characteristic of the sleeping state.

The Nature of Psychoanalytic Explanation

In any event, in whatever way they arise, such wishful impulses would awaken us if they were directly expressed in thought, since being repressed, they are "unthinkable" for the subject. Hence, such wishes are potential disturbers of sleep. The problem for the subject who wishes to remain asleep is how to defuse them. Our normal form of dealing with such wishes — some form of behavior indirectly expressing the wish — is not available because we are asleep. The only other alternative is fantasy. Hence, the content of the dream represents the repressed wish as satisfied. Freud hypothesized that fantasy relieves the cravings (unconscious wishes) that give rise to it to some extent, a fact somewhat supported perhaps by the phenomenology of daydreams.

Since the unconscious wish is repressed, in Freud's account it cannot even be given direct expression in a dream that fantasizes its fulfillment. Thus, what we dream (the manifest content) is distorted from what, in one sense, we would really like to dream (the latent dream thoughts), namely, that our repressed wish is fulfilled. The processes of the dream work are introduced by Freud as mechanisms by which the dreamer gets the best of both worlds: He is allowed to remain asleep by the fantasized fulfillment of his otherwise disturbing wish, and yet he does not pay the usual cost of recognizing such a wish, because it is so distorted in its fantasized fulfillment that he cannot perceive (except in psychoanalysis) the actual meaning of his dream.

The use of motivational language in this explanation of dreams may be grouped into three levels: (1) Freud explains dreaming as such (as opposed to the particular content of a given dream) as being the result of the overriding wish to sleep; (2) he explains the particular (manifest) content of a dream as being motivated by the fulfillment of a repressed wish; and (3) he further explains certain peculiar aspects of the content of the dream by reference to the processes of the dream work, themselves explicable by reference to motives the dreamer had for distorting his dream. These three levels of explanation together constitute the heart of Freud's theory of dreams.[14] Each of them, it is worth emphasizing, is couched in terms of motives or related terms. I shall next urge that such purportedly motivational explanations are better understood to be functional attributions or explanations, or mental cause explanations, and that motive (understood as the reasons for action of Chapter 1) is an erroneous concept with which to capture Freud's theory of dreams.

Motives for Dreaming

THE WISH TO SLEEP

Freud often spoke of the "double wish fulfillment brought about by dreams."[15] The two wishes to which he was referring are the preconscious wish to sleep and the unconscious wish that is fantasized as fulfilled in the dream. The second is dealt with in the next subsection. The first, Freud thought, is "universal, invariably present, an unchanging wish to sleep." This wish to sleep *"must in every case be reckoned as one of the motives of formation of dreams, and every successful dream is a fulfillment of that wish."*[16]

The notion is that we dream in order to remain asleep. Freud thought that "all dreams are in a sense dreams of convenience: they serve the purpose of prolonging sleep instead of waking up."[17] Dreams serve this purpose by fantasizing the satisfaction of some disturbing impulse, usually a wish in its own right, and by so doing, lessening the demands of such impulses. If we dream of drinking a glass of water when we are thirsty, Freud's thesis is that this helps to relieve the feelings of demand for the water. If we dream of riding a horse when we, in real life, have a painful boil in a position that would make such an action difficult, this potentially sleep-disturbing sensation is diminished by a dream that denies it. "The currently active sensation is woven into a dream *in order to rob it of reality.*"[18]

It should first be noted that this explanation does not, and was not intended to, explain the particular content of individual dreams. It is an explanation of dreaming as an activity in general. It is given in answer to the question, Why do we dream? not to the question, Why did *he* dream *that*? The content of the dream is explained by the wish or some other disturbing impulse (dealt with in the following section); showing why the dreamer lessens the awakening tendency of such impulses by creating a dream at all is the burden of the wish-to-sleep hypothesis. "You dream to avoid having to wake up, because you want to stay asleep."[19]

The nature of the question posed gives a clue to the kind of answer we should expect. To seek an explanation, in *general,* of dreaming should not produce a motivational explanation at all. For our common experience renders highly unlikely that any one motive is always operative for a universal activity such as dreaming. People do not operate from just one motive on all occasions of working or joking or running. One usually has a variety of motives, some operative on certain occasions, and some on others.

One might think that the same should be true of dreaming. On some occasions, we may wish to sleep as a means of getting away from a foreseeably unpleasant morning. Yet this is rare, and there is no reason to think that we *always* dream because we have some such want. Motives are usually assigned only for individual acts of individual persons, not across the board for human processes continually engaged in by us all.

A second clue to the nature of the explanation being given here may be found in the total lack, in all of Freud's work, of a single example where

Freud got the patient to acknowledge the presence of a wish to sleep. In the case studies, and in the theoretical work on dreams, Freud simply postulated the presence of this supposedly preconscious wish.[20] Nowhere did he make the same kind of interpretive effort to recapture the content of this preconscious wish as he made to recapture the unconscious wishes of his patients. There is simply no evidence of a wish to sleep, nor did Freud even bother looking for any.

It is true that we do remain asleep when we dream, and there is thus some "behavioral evidence" of a wish to sleep. But it is also true that we move our eyes when we dream. Do we therefore wish to engage in rapid-eye-movement behavior, and is this a motive for dreaming?

There is, similarly, no evidence of a belief by the dreamer that dreaming will tend to keep him asleep. Freud again simply postulates the existence of the minor premise of the dreamer's supposed practical syllogism: "I am driven to conclude that throughout our whole sleeping state we know just as certainly that we are dreaming as we know that we are sleeping."[21] Freud was driven to such a strange conclusion only because he thought he had to complete a practical syllogism for the dreamer.

What he failed to perceive was that his central insight about dreams could be presented without any talk of a wish, motive, or intention to sleep (Freud used all such terms),[22] nor need he be "driven" to unnecessarily animistic conclusions because of the requirements of a practical syllogism. Freud's explanation of dreaming as an activity simply need not be motivational in character. In this instance, I think it rather clear that what Freud had in mind was an explanation of dreaming in terms of the *function* it served, not the motive dreamers invariably have for dreaming. Indeed, to speak of dreams as serving "the purpose of prolonging sleep" is the language of function, not of motive. Freud occasionally noticed the true nature of his explanation, as in his analogy to dreams of convenience: "The thirst gives rise to a wish to drink and the dream shows me that wish fulfilled. In doing so it is performing a function. . . . If I can succeed in appeasing my thirst by dreaming that I am drinking, then I need not wake up in order to quench it. This, then, is a dream of convenience."[23]

The language of wish and motive in such a case is wholly unnecessary to convey the insight Freud wished to convey. One of the *effects* of dreaming is that we are allowed to continue sleeping. Dreaming is (in those circumstances in which we are subject to disturbing stimuli) a necessary condition of sleeping.

In his transformation of this causal connection between dreaming and sleeping into a functional attribution (the purpose of dreaming is to prolong sleep), Freud is consistent with the requirements examined earlier for significant functional accounts. A general end state (health) is assumed, inasmuch as one may at least plausibly think that sleeping causally contributes to our health.[24] One thus has all the elements of a typical functional attribution: a system (the human organism), a process (dreaming) in the system to be explained, an effect of the process (sleep), and an end state, itself the effect of sleeping (health). One effect (the prolongation of sleep) is emphasized by labeling it as the function of the process, dreaming. Since sleep causally contributes to health, that mode of emphasis is perhaps as justifiable here as elsewhere in medicine, viz., if one is greatly interested in maintaining that particular end state, it is useful to index information by the causal contribution each part or process makes to the maintenance of it.

Beyond the advantages of classification by function, Freud also seems to hypothesize that the system is a self-adjusting one, so that the emphasis on the one effect of the process labeled its function is justified. Despite varying disturbances, dreaming tends to produce the same effect, namely, sleep. This, I think, is all that Freud is attempting to say when he states, in characteristically animistic fashion, that "all through the night the preconscious is concentrated upon the wish to sleep."[25] All that has to mean is that, like other teleological mechanisms, this one tends to produce one effect despite the intervention of varying conditions. Car governors, hearts, and guidance mechanisms in missiles do the same thing.

To translate Freud here as giving a functional account rather than a motivational one eliminates the problems mentioned earlier. There is no peculiarity in assigning *one* function to all occurrences of dreaming as there is in assigning one motive universally present. A "universal, invariably present, unchanging" biological function served by dreaming (namely, the preservation of sleep) is not nearly as implausible as is a psychological wish to sleep with the same characteristics. A functional interpretation also eliminates the difficulty of the lack of evidence of the existence of a wish to sleep. It also eliminates the need to posit beliefs of dreamers about the connection of dreaming and sleeping. One also avoids, with a functional interpretation, the thorny issue of whether a dream is an *action* that can be explained by motives. For as noted before, the range of explanations is broader for function than for motives; any sort of event or process may have a function, whereas only actions are explained by motives.

Construing the theory functionally also eliminates some of the confusions and puzzles of contemporary psychoanalytic dream theory. One need not wonder whether, to be consistent with the wish-to-sleep hypothesis, we should also hypothesize that "every person who is awake wishes to remain awake";[26] in neither case do we *wish* for such states. Nor need one puzzle over the lack of the "dynamic" character of the wish to sleep;[27] construing sleep as a function of dreaming eliminates any necessity of thinking of some dynamic state (a wish) that *causes* dreaming. The dual nature of the wish to sleep – as a psychological wish and as a biological need – is also eliminated in the functional interpretation, for all the theory

The Nature of Psychoanalytic Explanation

need postulate is a biological need to sleep, and thus to dream.[28] In addition, one would hardly herald "the obvious theoretical importance [of the] discovery of the omnipresence in dreams of the wish to sleep,"[29] if one understood that it is omnipresent only because it is the function assigned to all dreaming. Freud did not discover one of our universal wishes, but only an unnoticed but perhaps important characteristic of dreams, namely, that one of their effects is that they tend to preserve sleep.

Whether in fact Freud's hypothesis here is correct is another matter. Does dreaming preserve sleep? The contemporary evidence suggests that it does not.[30] But in any case, translated functionally, the question can be resolved empirically, for one knows how to test an alleged causal connection of dreaming and sleeping. Cast as a wish, however, disconfirmation of the causal connection of dreams to sleep would not disconfirm the "guardian-of-sleep" hypothesis. (For one's wishes may cause one to act, though the action fails to realize the object of the wishes. Indeed, in another context Freud regularly availed himself of this sort of escape hatch from disconfirmation; if the object of a wish is not fulfilled by a dream, "You can say nevertheless that a dream is an *attempt* at the fulfillment of a wish."[31]) Given the total lack of criteria for the "wish" to sleep, those who would test the hypothesis under its wish construction must simply wonder what else they are to test once they have disconfirmed the causal connection.[32]

WISH FULFILLMENT IN DREAMS

Unlike the preceding explanation, Freud's second "motive" in the formation of dreams is not universal, has no one content, and indeed, varies with each action. Freud cannot here be assigning a function to dreams, but must be attempting some more legitimate use of wish and its related terms in his explanation of why it is we dream of certain things. His claim to explain dreams as being fulfillments of wishes rests solely and squarely with this use of wish.

A convenient example with which to begin is Freud's explanation of his dream of a patient's injection. Freud dreamed that he had met his patient, Irma, in a hall with numerous guests. After admonishing her that any pain she still felt was her fault, Freud examined her throat. In doing so he attracted the attention of two other physicians who were Freud's real-life acquaintances. Freud in his dream placed nonsensical diagnoses in the mouths of one of these friends, and accused the other (Otto) of having given the patient an improper injection.

Analyzing the dream phrase by phrase, Freud believed he discovered the motives for such a dream in his desire for revenge against Otto for the latter's real-life reproaches against Freud, and in his desire to be exonerated from any responsibility for the failure of Irma's cure:

> The meaning of the dream was borne in upon me. I became aware of an intention which was carried into effect by the dream and which must have been my motive for dreaming it. The dream fulfilled certain wishes which were started in me by the events of the previous evening (the news given to me by Otto and my writing out of the case history). The conclusion of the dream, that is to say, was that I was not responsible for the persistence of Irma's pains, but that Otto was. Otto had in fact annoyed me by his remarks about Irma's incomplete cure, and the dream gave me revenge by throwing the reproach back on to him. The dream acquitted me of the responsibility for Irma's condition by showing that it was due to other factors—it produced a whole series of reasons. The dream represented a particular state of affairs as I should have wished it to be. *Thus its content was the fulfillment of a wish and its motive was a wish.*[33]

The evidence by which Freud inferred these wishes on his part was by and large limited to his waking thoughts, specifically, the preconscious thoughts produced by free association with each element of the manifest content of the dream. Thus, in deciding that one of his motives for the production of a dream of Irma's injection was revenge on Otto, Freud recalled: "I seemed to remember thinking something of the same kind that afternoon when his words and looks had appeared to show that he was siding against me."[34] As evidence of his "wish to be innocent of Irma's illness," Freud further noted: "I called to mind the obscure disagreeable impression I had when Otto brought me the news of Irma's condition."[35]

It is important to note that Freud did not remember having dreamed that he wished for these things—what he dreamed is just what he remembered and served only as the starting point for his free association. Rather, the phenomenological evidence on which Freud here relies is his memory of consciously thinking of such wishes in his waking life at some time prior to the dream. Neither did Freud have any memory of having dreamed what he dreamed because of such desires. The causal relevance of such wishes to the dream as dreamed is inferred by Freud in the same way Hume says we generally infer causation: We notice a regular concurrence between the two classes of events.

It is also interesting that many of the dreams reported in *The Interpretation of Dreams* are said to be wish fulfillments on precisely the same kind of evidence, that is, rather direct recall of consciously known wishes when the dreamer's memory is prompted by free association. None of them is explained by reference to the repressed unconscious wishes from childhood that Freud consistently throughout his career claimed were necessary to produce a dream.[36] Elsewhere, however, Freud did produce specimens of dreams (not his own) that were explained by a repressed, unconscious wish. It might seem that in such cases the evidence for the existence of

The Nature of Psychoanalytic Explanation

such a wish must be different, but in fact it is not: In all cases the primary evidence for the existence of the wish responsible for the particular content of a particular dream is the dreamer's own subjective recall of what he has wished for in waking life. If the wish is repressed, then presumably the trains of association are less clear in their direction, or cannot be produced at all; but in principle it is the same procedure that ultimately leads to the "motivating wish" of the dream, no matter how deeply such a wish may be repressed.

There is thus in none of Freud's examples or procedures any contradiction of the epistemic peculiarities of mental words, as long as one accepts the notion of deferred privileged access introduced in Chapter 7. Unlike the wish to sleep, there is evidence of the required sort for the existence of the unconscious wish that Freud proposes as the explanation of the content of dreams. Problematic, however, is Freud's claim that this wish is the *motive* the dreamer has for the particular dream.

It strikes me that there are three main candidates for the kind of explanation possible here. First, we could take Freud at his word and try to make out a motivational explanation of an action. Freud's wish to be freed of responsibility for the failure of Irma's cure was his motive for dreaming the particular dream. Second, one might claim that Freud was not really explaining how the particular dream occurred; rather, he was *interpreting* the dream, finding its *meaning,* not discovering its (motivational or nonmotivational) causes. On this account, the rationalizing but noncausal wishes discovered after the dream by free association have nothing to do with producing the dream; they are after-the-fact discoveries made by juxtaposing the manifest content of the dream with the material produced by free association—an interpretive technique that may tell you something about yourself, but nothing at all of what caused your dreams. Finally, one might construe Freud's account as a nonmotivational, causal account of why this dream was produced; its (nonrationalizing) cause was the wish experienced previous to the dream's production. Each of these possibilities deserves separate consideration.

Wish Fulfillments as Motives

There are two related reasons why Freud cannot be giving a motivational explanation with the wish-fulfillment hypothesis in dreams, despite all of the language of motive, intention, and so forth. First, there is no action to be explained by a motive here. Freud did not actively bring about the dream of Irma's injection, not for the motive he claims or for any motive. His dream happened to him in the same way that the death of his father happened to him—in neither case did he bring about the occurrence (which is not to deny, in either case, that he might have had some wishes related to each event). Dreaming is like nondirectional thinking – sudden inspirations, revelations, or images – in that it just happens without the will or agency of the subject. And this does not mean that dreams and nondirectional thinking are chaotic; it means only that *we,* our acting selves, did not give such thoughts the order that they possess. We are not causally responsible for such thoughts or their order. Since motives make sense only when given to explain actions, motive cannot be intended here by Freud.

In making such an objection one must have some criterion for action other than the "existence of a motive" criterion used by some contemporary action theorists. Otherwise, Freudians could simply reply to the foregoing objection that the discovery of unconscious wishes is also the discovery that the seemingly unwilled *events* such wishes cause are really *actions* persons perform. This reply seems to be one of the major points of Roy Schafer's influential, recent book, *A New Language for Psychoanalysis.*[37] Because Schafer believes that "action is human behavior that has a point; it is meaningful human activity; it is intentional or goal-directed performance by people; it is doing things for reasons,"[38] and because Schafer believes that psychoanalysis has shown that (almost) all human thinking and behavior are goal directed, he also conceives of all such thinking and behavior as human action. "Thoughts come and go only as we think them or stop thinking them, or, in others words, . . . thinking is a kind of action engaged in by persons. We are responsible for all our thoughts, including as Freud pointed out, our dreams."[39] To assess the force of this Freudian rejoinder requires a brief excursion into contemporary action theory.

What constitutes an action is still an, at best, partly answered question in the philosophy of action. Much of the earlier work of the past several decades incorrectly interpreted various attributes incidentally true of certain species of *complex* actions as constituting the essence of human action itself. Much may be said about the various features of complex actions. In our action descriptions we may incorporate reference to the consequences of the action,[40] the motive or intention with which the action under another description was done,[41] the circumstances under which it was done, or we may presuppose in our description the rules or conventions surrounding the activity in question, for example, castling a king.[42] Yet these features of action are not what we seek, for the relevant question about dreaming is not whether it is one or the other of these kinds of *complex* actions. Rather, the question necessary for a Freudian to answer is whether dreaming is a *basic* action.

As we examined in Chapter 2, a basic action is an action I do without there being some other action that I do in order to do it.[43] Usually, for example, when I raise my arm, I do not do some (even more basic) action in order to raise my arm; I just raise my arm.[44] Hence, usually raising one's arm is a basic act. If, in contrast, I use wires and pulleys and my foot in

The Nature of Psychoanalytic Explanation

such a way as to raise my arm, the action of raising my arm is a complex action because more basic actions were done (namely, moving my foot) in order to cause my arm to go up.

There are undoubtedly ways in which one can cause oneself to dream and thus make a particular instance of "having a dream"[45] into a complex action. By drinking too little water, for example, one might wish to cause, and succeed in causing, a dream of convenience. Such examples hardly answer the relevant question here, however. Being satisfied with such examples would be like ending an investigation into whether most people can wiggle their ears by finding out that most people can "wiggle their ears" by wiggling them with their hands.

Hence, the relevant question is whether dreaming is a basic act that persons do (or can) perform. And to answer that question requires that we have a criterion of "basic act" that allows us in general to distinguish bodily movements or mental episodes that are our (basic) actions from those that are not. What we seek is an answer to Wittgenstein's famous question, "What is left over if I subtract the fact that my arm goes up from the fact that I raise my arm?"[46]

The answer of some contemporary action theorists has been to explain, in terms of causation of movements by belief/desire sets, the difference between actions I do perform and movements of my body that I do not perform. Alvin Goldman, for example, defines a movement of a person's body as an action of that person if and only if the movement is intentional, and further specifies that a basic act is intentional if and only if that act is caused "in a certain characteristic way" by the agent's beliefs and desires.[47]

If this were an adequate analysis of action, then the objection interposed here would be no objection, for the discovery of unconscious wishes causing dreams (assuming *arguendo* that all elements of a practical syllogism were made out) would necessarily imply that dreams were actions we performed, not mere events that happened to us. Such analyses, however, are not adequate analyses of action.

The problem such accounts run into stems from counterexamples of the following kind: Suppose an actor, Clyde, wishes to kill his pregnant girlfriend, Roberta, and believes that by throwing himself to one side of the rowboat in which they are sitting he will succeed in causing Roberta to drown (she cannot swim, as Clyde well knows). Suppose further that Clyde's desire, together with the belief that his desire could easily be fulfilled, causes him to slip and fall on one side of the boat, capsizing it and drowning Roberta. Clyde had a set of desires and beliefs of the requisite form (set forth in Chapter 1) and that set of mental states caused the event in question. Yet it is possible that the slip by Clyde was just that—a slip—and not an action on his part. It surely is not nonsense for an omniscient novelist to explain Clyde's motion in the foregoing way, and also to tell his readers that the movement of Clyde's body was *not* an action of his. True, we might be very suspicious that Clyde did perform the action of capsizing the boat (as were the police and the psychoanalyst surrogate in Dreiser's novel); but there is at least a factual question to be debated about whether Clyde's movements were an action. If the Goldman account of action were correct, then there would be nothing to argue about once we knew that Clyde's movements were caused by a rationalizing belief/desire set.

What such thought experiments show is that as a criterion of action, "causation by a belief/desire set that also rationalizes an action" is inadequate. What action theorists of Goldman's persuasion must do is refine their criterion of action to exclude counterexamples of the kind just discussed (usually called "deviant causal chains"). Although there is no dearth of such attempts,[48] none thus far seems persuasive. Furthermore, such refinements as are usually offered to exclude these deviant causal chains would be of little comfort to Freudians of Schafer's persuasion. For such refinements usually exclude the unwanted counterexamples from the realm of action by supplementing the criterion of "belief/desire set causing a movement" with further mental states of intention or belief;[49] and for dreams, there is no evidence of the existence of such further states, leaving dreaming still on the "nonaction" side of the line. The end result is the same: One cannot show an event to be a human action just because it is caused by the subject's wishes and beliefs.

None of this is intended to suggest that there is no "conceptual connection" between the concepts of action and motivation. The proper domain for motive explanations is limited to actions. What is denied is that one can show an event to be an action by discovering unconscious motives; rather, one can discover unconscious motives only if what they are cited to explain turns out to be an action.

Although the foregoing discussion is sufficient to dispose of Schafer's kind of rejoinder, a Freudian might try a different line of attack to reach the desired conclusion that dreaming is an action. In the context of urging that we accept moral responsibility for the content of our dreams, Freud thought that we should not be "artificially limited to the metapsychological ego"; that "obviously one must hold oneself responsible for the evil impulses of one's dreams, because such an impulse not only 'is' in me but sometimes 'acts' from out of me as well"; that while it may be true that in the metapsychological sense this bad repressed content does not belong to my ego, but to the id, still "this ego developed out of the id, it forms with it a single biological unit, it is only a specifically modified, peripheral portion of it, [and] it is subject to the influences and obeys the suggestions that arise from the id."[50]

This comes close to saying that we really do perform an action when we

The Nature of Psychoanalytic Explanation

dream, even if that overproud part of ourself Freud calls "ego" did not have a hand in it. Freud seems to be urging, first, that our id performs an action in sending forth a wish to be fantasized as fulfilled in a dream, and second, that we should identify ourselves as much with our id as with our ego.

Yet these assertions presuppose the structural aspect of psychoanalytic theory, not just in the sense in which ego, id, and superego name aggregations of functions. Rather, the structuralism presupposed is the *personalized* version discussed in Chapter 3, according to which the self cannot be analyzed as a unitary agent but only as a series of agents, each of which is capable of performing actions for reasons.

Some regard this fragmentation of the self of Freudian metapsychology as a virtue, and anything that leads to it (such as motives for dreaming) is thus acceptable. It could be the case that some characteristics of human beings force this fragmented view of the self upon us; self-deception is sometimes proposed as a candidate, but recent philosophical analyses of that phenomenon suggest that it does not necessitate the "little people" hypothesis.[51] Unless some such showing is made, it seems to me that stories about motivated actions of subagencies "within" a person differ not at all from the animism of primitive peoples, who might explain the movement of planets as resulting from their love of one another.[52]

In a unitary concept of self, we do not perform an action when we dream.[53] Our impulses (wishes) "arise" from the id—we do not do anything to call them forth; the censorship does metaphorical battle with such impulses, and a dream results. We—our personal selves—have nothing to do with all of these supposed events. In fact, not too surprisingly, *we* sleep through the whole process!

The second reason that the wishes fantasized as fulfilled in a dream are not the motives for dreaming is the lack of any minor premise for the dreamer's practical syllogism. There are no *beliefs* by the dreamer that his "action" of dreaming would be a means to achieving the object of his wish. Freud did not believe that if he dreamed of Otto making an improper injection, then this would give him his desired revenge on Otto, nor did he believe that he could in fact be exonerated from responsibility for Irma's incomplete cure if he dreamed of a host of other factors causing her to remain ill. Freud reports no memory of such a belief, either as part of his dream or as part of his waking belief set. Nor is free association said to produce a memory of such a belief. Yet without such a belief, a crucial element of practical reasoning is missing, which leads one to conclude that the "action" is not to be understood on the model of practical reasoning (motives) at all.

There is a very small minority of dreams for which the requisite beliefs might more plausibly be suggested to be present in the dreamer, namely, counterwish dreams. Freud notes two types: those dreams that are created to demonstrate that he and his theories are wrong; and those he characterizes as mental masochism. To a patient who produced a dream that did not express a fulfilled wish, no matter how interpreted, Freud gave the following explanation: "Thus it was her wish that I might be wrong, and her dream showed that wish fulfilled."[54] To those dreams that appeared only to frustrate, rather than to fulfill, the dreamer's wishes, Freud stated that they fulfilled the wish of the patient to be frustrated, that is, to torture himself by refusing to allow the fantasies of dreaming to assuage his desires.

These are rather suspect formulations, to say the least (in light of the otherwise disconfirming nature of such dreams for Freud's wish-fulfillment hypothesis). They are, however, used here only to illustrate a point about the more typical character of the dreams Freud talks about. Such counterwish dreams do bear the customary means/end relationship to the wish that is given to explain them. The motive in each case—a desire to prove the doctor wrong, or a desire to frustrate oneself—is fulfilled by the doing of the "action," the production of a dream with these contents. The patient does not fantasize in her dreams, "Freud is wrong," either verbally or by depicting a situation in which he is wrong. Rather, the having of the dream itself proves him wrong—that is one of its effects. Counterwish dreams are thus more like normal actions for which we can give motives, because Freud ascribes an actual effect they produce in waking life as the object of the motivating wish. In ordinary dreams, however, it is only the *fantasized* satisfaction of the wish that the dream achieves; the dream itself does not achieve the actual object of the wish.

Because of this feature of all non-counterwish dreams, it becomes very implausible to suggest that the dreamer possesses the required belief that the dream is a means to the actual attainment of the object of the desire. The sort of practical syllogism Freud could plausibly construct for such specimens is at most:

$$D(q)$$
$$\underline{B(p \supset q)}$$
Dreams-that-p

where $D(q)$ means Freud desires that he was not responsible for the failure of Irma's cure; $B(p \supset q)$ means Freud believes that if Otto was responsible for the failure of Irma's cure, then he, Freud, was not responsible for the failure of Irma's cure; and Dreams-that-p means Freud dreams that Otto was responsible for the failure of Irma's cure.

Such a practical syllogism cannot rationalize the "action" it is given to explain, because the logical relationships required do not obtain. More specifically, there is no identity between the antecedent in the content of the belief and the action, that is, the dream. P is not identical in meaning to Dreams-that-p.

The Nature of Psychoanalytic Explanation

To make this schema a practical syllogism requires a second belief. The kind of belief Freud would have to ascribe to his subjects would be a belief in the causal efficacy of fantasy. In the example used, this would be a belief by Freud that if he had the dream about Otto, then Otto would really be responsible for the failure of Irma's cure [B (Dreams-that-$p \supset p$)]. Now it is at least arguable that the required relationships obtain. For if Freud believes $p \supset q$ and he believes Dreams-that-$p \supset p$, then he arguably believes also Dreams-that-$p \supset q$, for the content of the latter belief is implied by the conjunction of the contents of the former two beliefs. It is only arguable because it is very unclear to what extent we are entitled to ascribe a belief to a person simply because the content of such a belief is logically implied by the contents of the beliefs the person clearly has.[55] Assuming nonetheless for the purpose of argument that such a move is legitimate, then Freud would make out a full practical syllogism:

$D(q)$
B (Dreams-that-$p \supset q$)
Dreams-that-p

The logical relationships required now obtain, namely, $q = q$, and dreams-that-p = dreams-that-p. The crux of the matter is to see whether Freud can justifiably posit a belief (during sleep) that fantasy is just as good as reality for the satisfaction of desire, in order to complete the practical syllogism for himself or his patients.

This is, I think, approximately what Freud attempted to do in his "Metapsychological Supplement to the Theory of Dreams," published sixteen years after the first edition of *The Interpretation of Dreams*.[56] For Freud held that the "dream-wish . . . is hallucinated and, as an hallucination meets with belief in the reality of its fulfillment."[57] Freud likened the state of dreaming to amentia, or hallucinatory wish psychosis, and to earliest infancy, when reality testing has not yet deprived us of the tendency to hallucinate the satisfying object whenever we feel the need of it. In all such states, Freud asserted, hallucination brings belief in reality with it.

The question one wants to raise about such a belief is the question of criteria. By no ordinary criterion can Freud be said to have believed that by dreaming the dream he reports, Otto would be made responsible and Freud exonerated. At no point does Freud acknowledge such a belief, nor does he ever seek an acknowledgment from his patients of such a belief (as he does for the companion wish). Rather, Freud gives an elaborate theoretical account of such belief in terms of his topographical metapsychology. Thus, we are told that there is "topographical regression" in the dream work: the dream-instigating unconscious wish enters the preconscious in the guise of a wish-fulfilling fantasy; whereas in ordinary waking life such an impulse would enter consciousness or be "discharged" by motor activity, in dreams the impulse "pursues a retrogressive course through the unconscious, to perception, which forces itself upon consciousness." Since perception (itself a "system" in Chapter 7 of *The Interpretation of Dreams*) is bound up with our beliefs in reality, Freud's thought is that the retrogressive course of this impulse allows it to enter consciousness as real: "When once a thought has followed the path of regression as far back as to the unconscious memory-traces of objects and thence to perception, we accept the perception of it as real."[58]

Whether such speculation by Freud is a good or a bad theory is not a point I need address. The only point important here is that it makes belief a term defined by some such theory, not the name of a familiar mental state that has an assigned place in the scheme of explanation that is the practical syllogism. While one may define theoretical terms as one pleases, and even call them belief if one chooses, one may not substitute such terms to satisfy the demands of an existing schema and claim that the schema is satisfied just because the word "belief" was used. To make out a motivational explanation, Freud needed to discover a belief, not postulate a new theoretical entity labeled belief.

There are thus two reasons for concluding that the wish-fulfillment part of Freudian dream theory is not to be conceptualized as a reason-giving kind of explanation. The first is that dreaming is not an action and thus cannot be an action for reasons; the second is that there is no evidence for the beliefs that would be necessary to make out a full practical syllogism for dreamers, and Freud's theoretical stipulations in this regard are no substitute for the missing evidence.

Each of these reasons has had some attention in the philosophical literature about psychoanalysis. With regard to the first, Anthony Flew noted several decades ago that Freudian explanations in terms of unconscious motives were given for (what Flew called) involuntary behavior as well as for voluntary actions. Although Flew regarded this as a "stretch" of our ordinary concept of reasons for acting, he nonetheless concluded that the concepts in terms of which psychoanalytic explanations were cast were "precisely the notions in terms of which rational agents give accounts of the voluntary and deliberate conduct of themselves and other rational agents," namely, an account in terms of motives or reasons for action.[59]

One cannot be this tolerant and retain a useful concept of reasons for action. Reason-giving explanations as defined in Chapter 1 mark out an important boundary in our understanding of ourselves as persons and in our evaluating our conduct. It is thus important that the distinction between actions we do for reasons, and the involuntary behavior that may nonetheless be caused by our wishes or other emotional states, be maintained. Glossing over this distinction, as Flew does—and behind him Freud and contemporary Freudians such as Roy Schafer—would require some

The Nature of Psychoanalytic Explanation

strong justification for why we should so radically reconceptualize the beings we are. Absent such justification,[60] we have good reason to maintain the distinctions articulated in Chapter 1 between acting for reasons and being caused to behave by wishes.

The lack of the beliefs required for typical Freudian explanations to be of the reason-giving kind has also been noted by a number of philosophers. There are a number of avenues that have been explored by those who nonetheless wish to maintain that psychoanalytic explanations such as the wish-fulfillment hypothesis give reasons for acting. The first such avenue is the most straightforward: to bite the bullet and attribute the required beliefs to dreamers, despite their obvious irrationality. Theodore Mischel, for example, believes that "if we are to understand what the neurotic [or the dreamer] is doing then we must attribute to him (irrational) . . . beliefs of which he is not conscious."[61] Mischel's example is the neurotic behavior of an individual who lunges at lampposts because he hates his father and wants to kill him. The neurotic's behavior is an action for a reason, Mischel assures us, because the neurotic "has (unconsciously) 'identified' lunging at lampposts with killing [his father]."[62] With this unconscious belief, one can make out the further belief that, if he lunges at the lamppost, he will kill his father; and we have a full practical syllogism.

The problem for this approach is that stated immediately before with regard to dreams: There is simply no evidence for such beliefs as there is for the accompanying wish. It does not seem plausible that the neurotic really believes that the lamppost is his father, and Mischel's use of quotation marks around "identified" would seem to betray some hesitancy on his part about this. It is equally implausible to suppose that dreamers believe that if they have a certain dream they will really satisfy some real-life desire of theirs.

The only way to make out a position such as Mischel's is by abandoning the realism about beliefs that I adopted in Chapter 1. As described there, beliefs are states of a person. As such, to make plausible that such states exist requires evidence—evidence beyond merely the existence of behavior that fantasizes the fulfillment of some desire. Such independent evidence for the existence of a belief would not be required if one conceives of beliefs differently. According to some philosophers,[63] there is no fact of the matter about beliefs. In this view, we ascribe beliefs when we are willing to take a certain "stance" about the person: If we are willing to view him as rational, we will attribute the beliefs necessary to complete his practical syllogisms; otherwise, not. Whether we take such a stance depends on whether, like Freud, we have some reason for wanting to widen the circle of behavior that should be conceived of as rational action; such a stance is not determined for us by the existence or nonexistence of the required beliefs.

Yet, as I argued in Chapter 1, this interpretivist tradition has to be wrong about beliefs. No matter how holistic we may be in fixing the objects of a person's beliefs, it remains true that there is a fact of the matter about whether he has the belief or not. As such, there must be evidence for the existence of a belief; ascription cannot be based solely on the stance that we, the observers, adopt.

Another avenue is pursued by those who seek to expand the idea of reasons for acting beyond the belief/desire set analysis given in Chapter 1. J. Balmuth, for example, concedes that Freudian explanations do not require or allow one to conceive of dreaming as an attempt to fulfill the unconscious wish; dreaming for Balmuth would not be the means to securing the object of the dreamer's wish.[64] Nonetheless, Balmuth concludes, such explanations are in terms of (unconscious) reasons for action because such behavior *expresses* the unconscious wish, the tacit premise being that wishes (conscious or unconscious) expressed by behavior operate as reasons for engaging in that behavior.

Such an expanded notion of reasons for action, like Flew's and Schafer's expanded ideas of action, abandon the important distinction marked in Chapter 1 between acting for reasons and having one's body engage in involuntary behavior. Requiring only that the behavior express a wish in no way guarantees that the dreamer acted to achieve the object of that wish.[65] To call such expressive behavior acting for a reason is simply to slur over the systemically important limitations on that important ordinary concept.

Even if one grants the foregoing point, one might be tempted by yet another popular avenue here: Suppose one leaves the wish Freud seemed to think motivated a dream and focused instead on some second-order desire. In the example of Freud's own dream, suppose we ceased speaking of Freud's wish to be exonerated from his responsibility for the failure of Irma's cure, and focused on a wish to relieve the dissatisfactions with himself brought on by the wish to be exonerated from his responsibility for the failure of Irma's cure. If one hypothesizes the existence of this second-order wish, then the beliefs necessary to complete the dreamer's practical syllogism are not as crazy as an identification of fantasized events with reality. The belief required here would be that, if Freud dreamed about Irma's injection, then the dissatisfactions he felt (brought on by his wish not to be responsible) would be relieved.

Freud himself came close to adopting this strategy when he spoke of a wish to discharge the psychic energies attached to the disturbing, unconscious wish that is represented as fulfilled in the dream.[66] The problem with this strategy is that there is even less evidence for the existence of the substituted, second-order set of beliefs and desires than there is for the wish Freud talks about as being fulfilled in the dream. At least with regard to the latter wish, we have good evidence that the dreamer does indeed

The Nature of Psychoanalytic Explanation

possess it; Freud did indeed wish to be exonerated from his real-life failures in effecting a cure in Irma. But what evidence is there that dreamers wish to "relieve their dissatisfactions" or that they wish to discharge the psychic energies attached to their other wishes? Analogously, what evidence is there of any belief in the efficacy of dreaming in either relieving dissatisfactions or in discharging energy? (Such formulations would require that one attribute to dreamers an unconscious belief in the Freudian theory of dreams!) Hypothesizing the existence of a new belief/desire set, for neither part of which there is any evidence, is a peculiar and expensive way of attempting to remedy a lack of evidence for a needed belief. One can hypothesize the existence of a large number of other desires and beliefs that, if the dreamer had them, would render dreaming an action for reasons. But this is a pointless exercise if the wishes one ends up with are even less supported by the evidence than the wishes with which one began.[67]

Pursuit of none of these avenues should convince us that Freud's wish-fulfillment account is a reason-giving explanation. There is no plausible way either to supply the needed beliefs or to show that such beliefs are not really required for a reason-giving account. Puzzling is why Freud and the philosophers who have followed him here should have sought to force dream theory into the reason-giving mold. Surely part of the motivation here stems from the belief that it cannot be a "mere accident" that the dreamer dreams just that dream that (with some distortion) depicts a situation satisfying one of his wishes. Yet, of course, one who rejects the reason-giving conceptualization of the wish-fulfillment hypothesis is not committed to thinking that such a connection between wishes and dreams is some kind of regularly recurring accident or coincidence. There may well be lawlike limitations on the kinds of dreams that can be caused by certain kinds of wishes. Saying that dreams "express" such wishes is one way of drawing attention to such laws. One does *not* have to resort to an intelligent agent plotting out the dream in order to account for such a connection. One only needs mental states to be connected to one another by certain laws of association. Agents who also know of such laws and use them in means/end calculations are wholly unnecessary to account for whatever intelligent (i.e., wish-expressing) pattern dreams may possess.

For two reasons, then, the wishes that Freud tells us are fantasized as fulfilled in dreams cannot explain dreams as motives explain actions performed in waking life. A more difficult question is whether such wishes explain dreams at all.

Wishes and Meanings

One possibility that has gained much favor is to construe Freud's wish-fulfillment hypothesis as nonexplanatory.[68] According to this view, Freud did not set out to explain the content of dreams by their causal antecedents, but merely wished to build an interpretive "map" that would allow him to see the *meaning* of dreams. Support for this view is garnered by Freud's likening his task to that of one who must interpret a picture puzzle,[69] for the meaning one is to find in picture puzzles need not be motivational. Such meaning need only be the observer meaning mentioned in Chapter 1. Construing the wish-fulfillment hypothesis in this way would result in its being a maxim of interpretation, restricting the (observer) meanings to be sought to: (1) fantasized fulfillment of wishes, and (2) those wishes that are unconscious wishes of the interpreter who is also the dreamer. Following such a maxim of interpretation would allow one to exhibit the dream as minimally rational (in the sense of that phrase employed in Chapter 1), because there is a belief/desire set that could have been a motive for dreaming the dream. It would be only minimally rational, because of the irrational belief required (fantasy is reality) in order to complete the practical syllogism. In addition, it does not exhibit the action as rational for the particular dreamer, because only one element of the practical syllogism is a mental state possessed by the dreamer.

Such an interpretation of Freud's theory of dreams has two startling consequences. First, the theory would not be a theory of dreams. It would be a theory about the laws of association, to the effect that if one free associates to elements of one's own dream, one will eventually uncover one's own unconscious wishes. Yet if all one is doing is after-the-fact interpretation — if, that is, the wishes do not *explain* the dream — this law of association would seem to hold for any subject matter relatively rich in suggestive symbols. Free association to the elements of another person's dream, a picture, a cloud formation, and so on would also probably lead to discovery of one's own wishes, even though the starting points for the trains of association were not authored by the interpreter. Hence, the wish-fulfillment hypothesis would be a hypothesis only about what happens when a person free associates; there would be no hypotheses about dreaming as such at all.

Moreover, the wish-fulfillment hypothesis would be only one interpretive maxim among others equally good. To get around the obvious fact that most dreams do not directly express wish fulfillments, Freud hypothesized the distortion of the dream work; most dreams express *in distorted form* the fulfillment of wishes. Yet once one allows the introduction of such secondary interpretive principles to account for all the obvious counterexamples, then seeing a dream as a fulfillment of wishes is only one of many possible interpretive schemata. It is probably true that as many dreams directly express, say, anxiety as directly express wishes as fulfilled. It is also probably true that free association also leads to those anxieties of the subject. As long as one allows the considerable leeway for "distortion" that the dream work allows, the "anxiety maxim" in interpreting dreams is just as good as the wish-fulfillment maxim. Both are merely interpretive maxims heavily qualified by secondary principles of interpretation – the principles of distortion. There might be therapeutic grounds for preferring one to the other, but therapeutic efficacy is hardly to be confused with truth. Telling a patient that his dream is a fantasized fulfillment of his wishes may help him, just as telling a religious patient that God will watch over him may help him; but in both cases the truth of what is told the patient is not supported by the therapeutic efficacy of the statements.

The result of this hermeneutic interpretation of Freud's dream theory is to trivialize it completely. Freud himself was careful to eschew any such interpretation of his work.[70] Although he did see his task as *in part* being interpretation, the interpretation of dreams as fantasized fulfillment of wishes was a therapeutic interpretation only because it was also a true explanation of dreams. He sought, in other words, to explain dreams as well as to interpret them. Since the explanations cannot be motivational, Freud must be taken to provide a kind of causal explanation in terms of wishes.

Wishes as Causes

Freud's intent was pretty clearly to explain dreams as caused by unconscious wishes. Although he may have thought his explanation to be motivational, it is not. Rather, it is the kind of partial practical syllogism I referred to in Chapter 1 as causation without rationalization. Such an explanation depends on two testable hypotheses: Do dreams always express unconscious wishes, which free association to the dreams will reveal? And if so, do such wishes cause the dream to have the manifest content it has?

Whatever might have been Freud's intentions, it may of course turn out that the most his theory can amount to is a set of maxims of interpretation, such as just discussed. Whether that is so depends on whether his explanatory account of dreams is true. One of the striking facts about dreams for a Freudian has to be that most dreams do not, in any straightforward way, express wishes. One need not even resort to counterexamples such as punishment dreams, anxiety dreams, counterwish dreams, or other unpleasant or distressing dreams; dreams with no emotional tone at all also do not express wishes in the straightforward way that many of the dreams of children do. Accordingly, if the wish-fulfillment hypothesis is not to be regarded as obviously false, Freud needed some account of how the unconscious wishes that cause the dream to have the content of a wish fulfillment come to be so unrecognizably distorted. Explaining this was the function of that complicated set of processes Freud called the dream work. This is the last of the three major levels of explanation in the psychoanalytic theory of dreams, to which I now turn.

Practical Reason and the Unconscious

The Processes and Motives of Distortion

"Why is it," Freud asked, "that dreams . . . do not express their meanings undisguised?"[71] Freud's answer came in two parts. First, he purported to discover a series of processes known as the dream work; then he explained why each of the processes occurred by reference to the unconscious motives of the dreamer.

The Dream Work as a Process

How one conceives of the dream work depends on how one conceives of the wish-fulfillment hypothesis. If the latter is only an interpretive maxim to exhibit the dream as minimally rational, then the former need not be thought of as a process at all but only a second interpretive maxim qualifying the first. But if one construes Freud as intending an explanation with the wish-fulfillment hypothesis, then the dream work must be thought of as a set of processes that occur and cause the latent dream thoughts (unconscious wishes) to be transformed into the manifest content of the dream. Consistent with his intent regarding the explanatory nature of wishes, Freud intended the dream work to name a set of processes.

Freud referred to four things by his use of the dream work: condensation, displacement, considerations of representability, and secondary revision. By condensation, Freud meant that one element in the manifest content of a dream could represent many latent dream thoughts, as, for example, one person in a dream appears to represent several people we have known in waking life. Our latent dream thoughts are "condensed" into one image in our dream.

Displacement is an off-centering of these "psychical intensities" of a dream. What is off center is the meaning of the dream: The true meaning is not to be found by implication from the manifest content, but rather it has been displaced in various ways, as by displacing our true feeling for one person onto another about whom we are in waking life indifferent. In such a case, one ends up with an emotion inappropriate to the manifest content of a dream, which is good (but not inevitably present) evidence of a displacement.

By considerations of representability, Freud meant to say that a condition of a dream thought's being expressed is that it doff verbal garb for a pictorial representation. Thinking in dreams is done largely in terms of pictorial images, and Freud takes some pains to deny the apparent counterexamples to that hypothesis: Solving problems, forming judgments, and making arguments in dreams are not in fact done at the time of dreaming but are lifted wholecloth from memory of having done so before in waking life.

Secondary revision is a kind of repiecing of the puzzle. It is, Freud tells

The Nature of Psychoanalytic Explanation

us, the first interpretation of the dream performed while we are yet asleep, a performance that gives the dream a nominal order and a semblance of sanity.

Although displacement is "nothing less than the essential portion of the dream work" and is "one of the chief methods by which ... distortion is achieved,"[72] each of the four parts of the dream work distorts the true meaning of a dream. To condense many dream thoughts into a composite is to disguise each of them. The necessity for transforming thoughts into visual images helps to "explain the appearance of the fantastic absurdity in which dreams are disguised."[73] Secondary revision, while allowing dreams to "appear to have a meaning," in fact "creates a meaning for dreams as far removed as possible from their true significance."[74]

The problem for all of this is that there is no direct evidence for the dream work as a *process* (rather than as an interpretive maxim). We have no phenomenological evidence for the dream work considered as a process; we can remember, sometimes only via analysis, the wish that was the cause of the dream, but we cannot remember the condensation of ideas into one, the displacement of them, the ordering, and so forth. We can only observe: (1) that certain words in dreams, particularly those referring to people, seem via their associations to lead to a rather diverse variety of things; (2) that the inappropriateness of affects to the manifest content of a dream does on occasion strike us as peculiar upon remembering a dream; (3) that dreams are largely cast in visual images; and (4) that dreams often exhibit, not chaos, but a certain insane order, as if they were put together hastily by an idiot.

This kind of phenomenological evidence must have been the basis of Freud's insight into the dream work. Freud does not and cannot, however, label these characteristics of dream memories themselves by the names of the four types of dream work. Rather, he infers from these characteristics the existence of processes taking place during the dream and producing memories, with these characteristics as their corresponding effects. (These processes do not follow one another in time, seriatim, but are conceived by Freud as occurring together throughout the dream. Freud nonetheless believes them to be processes.) So considered, Freud's explanation of the distortion in dreams then becomes an attempted causal explanation: That dreams are remembered in distorted form is caused by the occurrence of these processes.

Since the subcategories of the dream work are not experiential terms—and Freud never claimed that anyone experienced or remembered experiencing these things—there is no obvious way to define the dream work as process. Without some definition independent of that which we would explain—distortion—then the purported explanation is merely tautologous. Perhaps physiology will save the day here by giving such processes some independent definition. Unless and until it does so, however, the dream work as a process is a specification of the functional steps that would have to be performed if the wish-fulfillment hypothesis is true; but the physical realization of those functional steps can only at this stage be speculated upon.

The dream work as a process thus remains a problematical hypothesis. It is at most a research program not yet begun, not an established proposition in a well-tested theory. Without some adequate account of the dream work as a process, Freud's wish-fulfillment hypothesis is equally problematic, for without an adequate explanation of distortion, Freud's theory that every dream represents a fulfillment of a wish is quite obviously false as a causal theory.

If the dream work is as yet only a specification of the functional steps that would have to exist if the wish-fulfillment hypothesis were true, then any *explanation* of the dream work is equally the hostage of successful future research. Still, it is worth examining briefly Freud's account, for it again purports to be a motivational account of why we distort our dreams.

Motives for the Dream Work

Freud gave a variety of specific explanations for each of the processes of the dream work. Condensation, for example, occurs because of the necessity of overdetermination for any latent dream thought to become manifest. What Freud had in mind here was that latent dream thoughts themselves have "psychic intensities." Presumably the most intense find expression in dreams. Yet even the most intense dream thought must "join forces" with others to find its way into the dream; thus they form composite images and we find condensation. To understand the purportedly motivational character of the dream work, however, one must focus on displacement. Freud considered displacement to be "nothing less than the essential portion of the dream work," and one of the "chief methods by which distortion is achieved."

Freud explains displacement (and thus distortion, too) as the means by which the latent dream thoughts escape the censorship imposed by repression. To be expressed in the manifest content of a dream, a latent dream thought must not only be conjoined with other unconscious thoughts (leading to condensation), pictorially represented, and given a semblance of order (by secondary revision), but it must also be distorted so that it may escape undetected the censorship supposedly attached to our repressed desires.

What Freud seems to be saying is that distortion is a form of pain-avoidance behavior. Since certain latent thoughts (namely, those that are repressed) are too abhorrent to be given direct expression, they must be

The Nature of Psychoanalytic Explanation

distorted to find their way into the dream at all. "For what is distressing may not be represented in a dream; nothing in our dream thoughts which is distressing can force an entry into a dream unless it at the same time lends a disguise to the fulfillment of a wish."[75] For example, in the dream about Irma's injection Freud displaced affection onto a colleague for whom it was not appropriate in the context of the dream. "The affection in the dream . . . was calculated to conceal the true interpretation of the dream. . . . Distortion was shown in this case to be deliberate."[76]

Consider also two examples of distortion that are not displacements (and do not fit neatly into the four categories of dream work): (1) The judgment in dreams that this is only a dream "is intended to detract from the importance of what is being dreamt"; and (2) when one dreams that one is dreaming, the wish fulfilled by the dream is one of resistance, to disguise the repressed wish so that it may not be recognized. "The intent is, once again, to detract from the importance of what is being dreamt in the dream, to rob it of its reality."[77]

Despite the considerable language of deliberation, calculation, and intentional action, I do not think Freud could have given a motivational explanation here (the motive for distortion being the avoidance of distressing thoughts), nor need he have tried. He could not have done so, because *none* of the elements of practical reasoning analyzed earlier are even asserted by Freud to be present here. First, we plainly do not perform an action when we distort our dreams via displacement. Indeed, in this case the lack of an action is particularly glaring, since there is not even any behavior of a person here at all, voluntary or involuntary; displacement is an internal process Freud postulated to occur within the organism during sleep. It is thus unlike dreaming itself, slips of the tongue, or neurotic symptoms, since each of these is at least an overt behavior (although often not an action). Freud again resorts to his metapsychological thesis of the fragmented person: The motives for distortion are not assigned to the subject as an integrated person, but to some hypothetical subagency, the censor, who performs the "action" to be explained. "The purpose of which the censorship exercises its offices and brings about the distortion of dreams: it does so *in order to prevent the generation of anxiety or other forms of distressing affect.*"[78] Whatever may be the merits of this early version of Freud's structuralism, in no event is this to say that *we* perform an action, the distortion of the dreams.

Second, as might be expected when *we* do not perform any actions for motives (but our "censors" do), we as persons do not have any first-person knowledge or memory of: (1) a belief that distortion via displacement will conceal from ourselves otherwise distressing thoughts; or (2) a desire or wish not to be distressed. Nor (3) is there any evidence that such a belief and such a desire caused the distortion of the latent dream thoughts. In short, none of the elements of practical reasoning essential to a motive explanation (whether of the conscious or unconscious variety) is present for the nonaction that a hypothetical subagency within ourselves performs.

What Freud could have meant is that distortion has as its *function* the avoidance of pain. Like repression itself, the assertion would be that our thoughts, in dreams as elsewhere, through some as yet unknown mechanisms, avoid direct expression of painful ideas. Since avoidance of pain is thought to be both the effect of a distortion and the cause of a more general end state of well-being, we may emphasize its importance by saying that it is *the* function of distortion.

Stating it in this way, I believe, identifies more precisely what is and what is not being claimed about displacement and distortion. If displacement did not occur, so that dreams would be dreamed and remembered in undistorted form, we would wake up from the disturbing wish that causes us to dream; since we need to sleep in order to remain healthy, displacement (ultimately) is a necessary condition for the general end state of health, because it allows sleep to go on while the fantasized wish fulfillment defuses the otherwise disturbing wish. Such, I think, is the core of Freud's claim here, none of which requires talk of the motives of distortion.[79]

It is worth reemphasizing, of course, that even so construed, the explanation is hostage to some independent definition of displacement as a process. For as it stands, displacement is simply a hypothesis about the kind of process that would be necessary if the contents of dreams are caused by wishes. Only if there really is some process that answers to this hypothesis can one assign to *it* the function of pain avoidance.

Conclusion

The conclusion of this chapter may be simply stated: Despite the motivational regalia in which Freud clothed his various explanations of dreams, none of such explanations are truly motivational in character. I suspect that a similar analysis of other phenomena explained by the theory, such as parapraxes or neurotic symptoms, would reveal similar results, although the explanation of *some* slips and some symptoms are probably genuinely motivational in character because one can legitimately make out an action and the required beliefs.[80]

The importance of this conclusion lies in several directions. First, clarity can be a goal in itself. Freud himself was concerned with "introducing the right abstract ideas whose application to the relevant material of observation will produce order and clarity in it."[81] An interpretive effort such as has been presented in this chapter can be seen as a continuation of Freud's concern for the clearest exposition of his theory. Second, those who would test the theory must know what it is they would test. To look for a function *served by* dreaming is to look for something different from a wish *causing* dreaming; to search for nonrationalizing but causally operative wishes is to search for something other than motives for dreaming.

Third, the interpretation suggested herein may drive a wedge between theory and therapy in psychoanalysis. For if success in therapy depends on getting the patient to accept a dream or slip as a motivated action for which he is responsible, whereas in fact the explanation the theory generates is such that no such implication of responsibility holds, then successful therapeutic suggestions will not be successful because they are also true explanations. We would not be cured because we have come to see the truth about ourselves; rather, we are cured because we have come to accept an account that is not true and a responsibility that is not ours.[82] If such a "wedge" is to be avoided, then successful therapy cannot be seen as getting us to accept responsibility for dreams as motivated actions we perform; rather, therapy would be successful when the patient accepts responsibility for being the sort of person he is, that is, a person who has the wishes his dreams express. If that is all successful therapy requires, then there need be no wedge between theory and therapy, for the latter would only presuppose a form of explanation that the former can deliver.

Fourth, the general thesis with which I began—the chasm that exists between motivational parts of the theory and its supposedly causal accounts—will have to be redrawn. There are, I think, valid distinctions to be made between the particular accounts of specific actions given by psychoanalysts, and the more general accounts attempted by the more abstract parts of the theory. The only point here is that such distinctions may not be so simply drawn as some distinction between motives and causes.

Fifth and finally, the implications of psychoanalytic theory for our assessments of responsibility in morals and law depend on the conclusions reached in the inquiries of this chapter. A psychoanalytic explanation of a dream (or a slip or a symptom) is often thought to show that the person was responsible for the dream, that it was something he did for motives; such an implication seems to hold even if the motives are unconscious. Yet such an implication holds only if psychoanalytic explanations are truly motivational in character. For once we perceive that dreams are not productions we stage for reasons, but are events caused by wishes, then we can be said to be morally responsible for dreams only in the attenuated, Aristotelian sense that we are responsible for the character that includes such wishes. Most of us, the Bible notwithstanding, do not equate responsibility for a wish with that for an action that fulfills it. Hence, to say that our character (which includes our wishes) is revealed by our dreams, is not to say that dreams are motivated actions for which we are responsible. It is to the development of this last point that the succeeding chapter is devoted.

9 The Unconscious as the Source of an Increased Responsibility

IN CHAPTER 3, I noted the paradox that the unconscious is often thought both to *increase* the things for which we are responsible and to *decrease* the scope of our responsibility. We are now in a position to assess the first of these two apparent implications of the unconscious for responsibility. The overall question pursued in this chapter is whether the discovery that there are unconscious mental states should convince us that we are morally responsible for more harms and more attempts than we thought in our pre-Freudian naiveté. (In Chapter 10, I shall pursue the second apparent implication of the discovery of the unconscious, that of a decrease in responsibility.)

To organize the discussion it is helpful to imagine three different cases in which, before Freud, responsibility would be denied. The first is a case in which prima facie, there is no action; the second, in which there is an action but it is not intentional; and the third, in which there is an intentional action but it is not done for some further (bad) intention. Here, then, are the cases:

1. X does something that is not intentional under any description, even a basic one; that is, he does not perform an action. For example, he stumbles and falls through a window, breaking it, thereby chilling the room.

2. X performs an action, but the action is prima facie not intentional under the relevant legal or moral description. For example, X opens the window but does not, consciously at least, have as his purpose the chilling of the room, nor does he know of the likelihood that the room will be chilled by his act. Thus, X does not *intentionally* chill the room, even though he does perform that action.

3. X performs the action of opening the window but does so for no further reason. It is quite warm outside, so that his action of opening the window does not in fact chill the room. X has not, therefore, tried or attempted to chill the room because that was not the reason for which he opened the window.

Increased Responsibility

Suppose in each of these cases that X's behavior is explicable by certain beliefs, desires, or other mental states, even though he was not aware of their existence or of their influence on his actions. Suppose, for example, that he unconsciously desired to offend his guests. What is the effect of this unconscious desire on X's responsibility for chilling the room or for trying to do so? Is X now responsible in all three cases, either because he "really" performed the intentional action of chilling the room or because he at least tried to do so?

An affirmative answer to this inquiry would be based on the following reasoning: The proffered mental state explanation reveals the reason for X's actions. Accordingly, in the third case, X was really trying to chill the room, although he was not aware of it. Such explanation, construed as the real reason for which X acted, also implies that his nominal accident in the first case was really an action he performed; for if X acted for a reason, albeit an unconscious one, he necessarily acted.[1] Similarly, such an explanation also seems to imply that X's nominally unintentional action of chilling the room in the second case was really an intentional action. This is because if X acted for a reason, even an unconscious one, the action for which the reason is given is necessarily an intentional action.[2] Since responsibility, as analyzed in Chapter 2, is determined by these conditions of action, intention, and reasons, X would be responsible for the harm in the first and second cases, and responsible for attempting to bring about the harm in the third case.

The objective of this chapter is to show why the stated conclusion does not follow from this apparently convincing argument. It is helpful to first examine the argument in three parts, corresponding to the three cases just given (which in turn correspond to the concepts of action, intention, and reasons). I shall then consider more generally the effect of this argument on responsibility and conclude with a reminder of certain presuppositions about persons made in this chapter's discussion about responsibility.

Are Accidents Explained by Unconscious Mental States Really Actions?

The three kinds of behavior relied on by Freud as evidence of the unconscious are dreams, parapraxes, and neurotic symptoms. Since we have already considered the Freudian account of dreams in some detail, I shall here consider examples of parapraxes and neurotic symptoms.

Consider first that set of examples of the influence of the unconscious on behavior that comes from what Freud called the "psychopathology of everyday life": slips of the tongue, misreading, forgetting, and awkward movements. A perusal of Freud's work[3] reveals that in many of his examples, such parapraxes are consciously executed actions and not mere movements, even if they are unintentional under some relevant descriptions. Some examples, however, do not seem to be actions at all.

In this latter class are the following examples. (1) While seating himself at his desk, Freud's hand moved in a "remarkably clumsy way" that brushed the cover of an inkstand to the floor where it broke. Freud explained the movement by an unconscious desire to force his sister to keep her promise to buy him a new one. Freud concluded that he had performed "the execution of the condemned inkstand."[4] (2) A Frau X "stumbled on a heap of stones in a street under repair and struck her face against the wall of a house."[5] Once Freud was satisfied that Frau X had an unconscious mental state that explained her stumbling—a desire to punish herself for an abortion—he recharacterized what she did into the language of action: "She used the situation . . . for punishing herself unobtrusively with the help of the heap of stones which seemed suitable for that purpose."[6] (3) At lunch, H, a colleague, was discussing an important position to which he had been appointed but which he had not succeeded in filling, from lack of his own diligence. While describing his failure to pursue the appointment, he dropped the piece of cake that he was lifting to his mouth. Freud concludes that this was an action expressing symbolically something that H was having difficulty relating directly, namely, that he had allowed a very choice morsel to slip from him. Thus, Freud describes the seeming accident in action language: "He let it drop . . . in apparent clumsiness."[7]

From these and other examples, Freud concluded that "falling, stumbling, and slipping need not always be interpreted as purely accidental miscarriages of motor actions."[8] Because such movements are to be explained by unconscious mental states, it is only on the surface that these "make a show of something violent and sweeping, like a spastic-atactic movement."[9] In reality, Freud believed, they are actions one performs.

As an example of a neurotic symptom, consider Dora, the subject of one of Freud's most famous case studies,[10] who developed a hoarseness and a cough in her throat. Nowhere in the case study does Freud claim that she consciously faked her cough and then brought on her throat irritation. Nonetheless, a good part of the analysis is developed to show that Dora had unconscious desires to be ill. Although Freud initially thought that "motives have no share in the formation of symptoms,"[11] he modified that early view and came to believe that symptom formation as well as symptom maintenance (Dora's cough lasted for years) were motivated activities.[12] As with dreams, viewing such symptoms as motivated implies that they are motivated *actions*.

Some contemporary psychoanalytic theorists share Freud's view that the discovery of unconscious mental states expands the category of events one should consider as actions. Thomas Szasz, as we have seen, concludes that mentally ill persons are morally responsible and liable to criminal punishment on the grounds that their behavior is motivated, even though unconsciously.[13] Because "there is method in madness, no less than in sanity,"[14] he concludes that "mentally sick behavior is more akin to *action* than to *happening*."[15] From this it is an easy step to Szasz's explicit conclusion that human beings "are always responsible for their conduct."[16]

Similarly, Roy Schafer's recent work adopts the view that dreams, neurotic symptoms, and slips are really actions one performs, even though one often "disclaims" them; that is, one refuses to recognize them as an action one did.[17] Schafer's views are also based on the Freudian insight that one has unconscious wishes influencing one's behavior.

The tradition in the philosophy of psychoanalysis that (contrary to the last chapter) interprets Freud as having discovered reasons for action[18] is also committed to viewing dreams, slips, and symptoms as actions and not mere happenings. Theodore Mischel, for example, has recently urged that one must not only supply the missing means/ends beliefs I discussed in Chapter 8 in order to make out a reason-giving account in Freudian explanations, but one must also view the *explicanda* as actions and not mere movements. As Mischel also recognizes, symptoms, parapraxes, and dreams must be actions if psychoanalytic explanations are to be understood as providing reasons for actions.

The main problem for Freud, Szasz, Schafer, Mischel, and others lies in the premise from which the thesis that "accidents are really actions" is supposed to follow, namely, that unconscious *reasons* for actions have been discovered. As we explored in Chapter 8, however, most of what passes for unconscious reasons or motives in psychoanalysis are not, in fact, reasons for actions. Accordingly, such explanations cannot logically show that seemingly accidental behavior was really an action that one performed. The study of psychoanalytic explanation done in Chapter 8 was designed to show that most often what are paraded as unconscious reasons fall into three categories of description or explanation quite distinct from that of reasons for actions.

To summarize these categories: First, sometimes such unconscious mental state explanations are not *explanations* at all. In such cases, Freud did not discover the reasons for which people act, but merely the hidden meaning in their behavior. Dream interpretation, when separated from the psychology of dreaming,[19] is not a discovery of the wishes that either motivate or cause dreams; it is simply the divining of wishes *in* the dream. In such an interpretation of Freud, one likens dream interpretation to the interpretation of art or statutes. One looks not for the intention with which the artist painted a picture or the legislature enacted its statute, but rather to the intention to be discovered *in* the painting or *in* the words of the statute. Similarly, to say that slips and neurotic symptoms have a meaning is not necessarily to explain that they occurred because of the actor's belief/desire sets, but only that an observer can perceive such meaning in the slips or symptoms.[20]

Second, sometimes such unconscious mental state explanations are not *mental state* explanations at all, but rather explanations in terms of functions. A prominent example we have already examined from dream theory is Freud's explanation of dreams as due to a "wish" to sleep. Such a wish may explain that dreaming serves the function of preserving sleep, but does not give the dreamer's reason for dreaming. Similarly, Freud's talk of one's wanting to keep painful thoughts from oneself via repression is better understood as saying that one's avoidance of certain thoughts serves a function — the avoidance of pain.[21]

Third, when psychoanalysts do *explain* rather than *interpret* behavior and when they do so in terms of *mental states* rather than *functions*, often they are giving purely causal accounts of the behavior, not the actor's conscious or unconscious reasons for acting. As was discussed in Chapter 1, if one explains a rapid heartbeat as caused by a desire to beat Bobby Fischer at chess, by a belief that there is a prowler in the hall, or by anger at being struck by another, one is not to be understood as giving the actor's *reasons* for increasing the rate of his heartbeat. Rather, his heartbeat is *caused* to accelerate by these mental states of desire, belief, or emotion. Similarly, when Freud explains dreams as being due to an unconscious childhood sexual desire, that wish may *cause* the dream, but it is not the dreamer's reason for dreaming. Because the explanation is not couched in terms of reasons, the dreamer need not be understood as putting on a play for his own entertainment.

Most psychoanalytic explanations fall into these three categories and thus cannot show that seeming accidents are truly actions. Saying this, unfortunately, does not dispose of the issue of whether symptoms, slips, and dreams *are* actions. All that has been said thus far is that one popular reason for saying that these are actions is not a good reason. Left open is the possibility that there are other reasons for concluding that these phenomena constitute human actions. The pivotal question thus becomes whether dreams, parapraxes, and neurotic symptoms can be shown to be actions independent of the irrelevant discovery that unconscious wishes or emotions may be cited to explain them.

Using the personal agency account of action defended in Chapter 2, it should be apparent that to characterize dreams, neurotic symptoms, and parapraxes as actions one would have to say that the actor *knew* he was acting. This does not mean that the actor need know that he is performing some *complex* action in order to be performing that action. He need only know that he is performing some *basic* action; if that basic action constitutes or causes a complex action, he has performed the latter action as well. Consider in this regard a case often regarded as an instance of unconscious action, *Fisher v. Dillingham*.²² In a copyright infringement suit in which the issue was whether the defendant had *copied* the plaintiff's musical score, the judge (Learned Hand) found as a fact that the defendant did not know he was copying the plaintiff's musical score, yet found that the defendant had copied it. This was not, however, an unconscious action because the basic acts involved in the defendant's writing down his score were consciously executed by him. He consciously knew he was doing them, so they were unproblematically basic acts. Because those basic acts, done in the circumstances in which the defendant did them (having earlier read the plaintiff's score), constituted copying, the judge was entitled to say that the defendant performed the circumstantially and causally complex act of copying. No insight about the unconscious is required to reach this conclusion.²³

Unlike the Fisher case, the class of examples we should consider here are those in which the actor does not consciously know he is performing some basic action. In such cases, to show that there is a basic action being performed we would have to say that the actor *unconsciously* knew that he is acting. If we can make sense of the idea of unconscious knowledge, then we can make sense of the idea of unconscious human actions. This would not yet be to say that dreams, parapraxes, and neurotic symptoms *are* unconscious actions; it is to say only that they could be if we can make sense of the idea of unconscious knowledge.

The basic conceptual problem with unconscious knowledge stems from the connection that seems to exist between knowing that some proposition is true and being aware of that proposition. "I knew that" is often taken to mean "I was aware of that," and vice versa. How, accordingly, can we know something of which we are unaware? Moreover, since there is a clear sense in which we might say of some actor, "He did not know he was doing that," contradiction seems inevitable if we are also prepared to say "He did know he was doing that" (because he was *unconsciously* doing it).

Both problems can be resolved by using know in a sense that is not synonymous with aware. Such a sense is available in hypothetical rather than actual awareness. One could say that an actor *consciously* knows he is performing some basic action in the cases where the actor is either thinking of it at the time he is acting, or, much more typically, he could become aware of it if his attention were directed to it.²⁴ An actor *unconsciously* knows he is performing that basic action in the case where he could become aware of it, but only through free association or other psychoanalytic memory-jogging techniques.²⁵

The role of memory is crucial to the idea of unconscious knowledge required here.²⁶ For an individual to unconsciously know that he was acting it is not enough that he could become convinced by the authority of his analyst or by the pattern he perceives in his behavior, that he was acting. Rather, the individual must potentially be able at some later time to remember that he was acting. Without the memory, the individual's later conviction that he had been acting would only show that he could learn this, not that at the earlier time he had already *known* that he was doing something. He needs, as we put it in Chapter 7, deferred privileged access to his unconscious basic actions if they are truly actions by him.

In addition to preserving a distinction between what one already knows and what one can learn, this stress on memory squares closely with the psychoanalytic notion of making the unconscious conscious, the early-acknowledged therapeutic goal of psychoanalysis.[27] The stress on memory also squares with Freud's description of unconscious knowledge. "Where, then, in what field," Freud asked, "can it be that proof has been found that there is knowledge of which the person concerned nevertheless knows nothing?"[28] After recounting Bernheim's demonstration with a hypnotized person who claimed on awakening that he could not remember some fact, but with prodding found that he could, Freud concluded: "Since, however, he knew afterwards what had happened and had learnt nothing about it from anyone else in the interval, we are justified in concluding that he had known it earlier as well. It was merely inaccessible to him; he did not know that he knew it."[29]

The stress on potential recall as the criterion of unconscious knowledge is needed here if one is to show how Freud's insights about the unconscious might expand the domain of events considered to be human actions. Although its precise role has been a matter of dispute at least since Locke,[30] memory is one of the critical ingredients in one's sense of personal identity. If the claim of unconscious knowledge is a claim that one can potentially remember what one knew, such knowledge will expand what one identifies as one's personal self. Specifically, if unconsciously knowing that some event was an act one performed means being able to recapture the experience of having performed that act, then it makes good sense to extend the notion of personal agency to such events. One should see them as unconscious actions done by one's self and not as mere events in which one's body was causally implicated but in which one's personal self had no part.

Before we proceed, we should address a number of grumbles that might be felt toward this account of unconscious actions. One is that such an account is too restrictive because it allows as unconscious actions only those behaviors that were consciously executed as actions but then forgotten. Yet this is not what I conceive an unconscious action to be. Although much that one remembers is what one consciously knew but later forgot, the criterion of potential recall does not involve this sort of memory. The

Increased Responsibility

Freudian claim of extended memory is that one can remember many things one never consciously knew. When one remembers that one was angry, for example, it need not be the case that one was aware at the time that one was angry but then forgot. Rather, if one was unconsciously angry, one experienced the anger without being aware of it. The remembering is of this experience and not of some conscious awareness of it.[31]

One might also be troubled that unconscious knowledge in the sense used here requires that the actor come to know he was acting in a way not based on evidence or inferences from evidence. To reiterate the analysis just completed, for one to be acting unconsciously one must potentially be able to remember that one was acting.

One might argue that this criterionless knowledge is not possible, and that those who "remember" past events as actions are fooling themselves in that what they are really doing is deciding to accept responsibility by owning up to the behavior as an action of theirs. Frank Cioffi, for example, wonders "how much sense we can make of the notion of the belated recognition of noumenal agency detected not inductively but by a subsequent act of introspection?"[32] Yet this noninductive, criterionless feature of the psychoanalytic claim of extended memory is no more problematic than the knowledge that one has of one's own conscious mental states or actions. One comes to know that one wants pie, that one believes it is raining, that one is imagining a sunset, that one feels pain, or that one is acting, without regard to observation or inference. This is usually described by saying that one has privileged access to one's own mind and basic actions. Unconscious knowledge as here conceived requires only that one have deferred privileged access, as well as present privileged access, to one's mental states.

As I discussed in Chapter 7, such privileged access does not mean that one is infallible in one's memory of what was an action; nor does it mean that behavior cannot be an unconscious action unless there is such a recaptured memory. Actual recall is neither a necessary nor a sufficient condition of behavior being an unconscious action, as it would be if the self-intimation or incorrigibility theses were true. To show that some behavior was an action, however, it does seem that psychoanalysts must be committed to saying that the person can *potentially* recall that it was an action. Without such potential recall it is hard to see how we could attribute the behavior to the *personal* agency of the alleged actor.[33]

In deciding whether dreams, parapraxes, or neurotic symptoms are actions, it will thus not do to doubt that these *could* be actions, on some alleged conceptual ground that unconscious actions are not possible. That leaves us with the difficult question of whether there is any *evidence* for the unconscious beliefs necessary to show that these behaviors are actions.

Reverting to the examples discussed earlier: Does one remember, or come to remember, dreams as productions one staged? Or are they simply thoughts with a pattern (wish fulfillments), perhaps caused by wishes, but not a pattern one *gave* to the dreams? Most of the dreams Freud analyzed were not dreams the dreamer remembered, or came to remember via psychoanalysis as productions he had staged. It is only occasionally that the dreamer can recall adopting what Freud called a "supervenient attitude" toward the dream, by which he meant the dreamer's attitude that he is restructuring the dream in certain dimensions to satisfy certain desires. In an anxiety dream, for example, one might recall a loved one being in a situation of danger, and recall the thought, This is not dangerous enough, and then recall that one "replayed" the situation so that the loved one was even in more danger than in the first version of the dream. Undeniably, one sometimes has such attitudes toward one's dreams and remembers having restructured them as one was dreaming. Yet one does not have such a memory for most dreams.

One more typically experiences dreams as events that happen to one and not as productions one stages. Psychoanalysis does not typically produce a recall of such a supervenient attitude, nor does dream interpretation even seem to be aimed at achieving such recall. The thesis that dreams are actions thus stems not from supervenience, which Freud regarded as exceptional, but rather from an inference of the following sort: If dreams are thoughts caused by wishes, then they must be actions.[34] That such an inference is false is the purport of the preceding chapter.

This false inference is even more clearly the basis of Freud's conclusion that parapraxes are actions. Freud inferred that he "executed" the old inkstand from his desire to have a new one. He similarly inferred that Frau X's stumbling was an "infliction" of punishment on herself because she had a reason to punish herself. In neither of these parapraxes did Freud or his patient recall that his slip was an action of his. If he is going to own up to it as his action, the patient must adopt Freud's erroneous theory of action and infer that because his accident was caused by an unconscious wish, it was no accident at all.[35]

Apart from the lack of any memories here (or even of any very serious effort to retrieve such memories), for some parapraxes it is unclear what the required memory could be like. Richard Wollheim, who is sympathetic to Freud's claim that parapraxes are really actions, divides parapraxes into two classes: those that at least "are of a kind that includes actions"; and those "which could never be thought of as actions, or which are of a kind to which no actions belong: for instance, mislaying a book or forgetting a name."[36] Most of us have had the conscious experience of moving our hand so as to smash objects like inkwells; also not unusual is the experience of throwing oneself to the ground. These are basic act types we know how to perform, and thus we can conceive what a memory of such experi-

Increased Responsibility

ences would be like. By contrast, no one forgets a name as a consciously executed action. Although we can "try to think of something else" as the means of forgetting a distressing name, we do not *just* forget a name (as a basic act). Yet if forgetting or mislaying are not types of actions that we have performed, how are we to make out the claim that we nonetheless can *remember* these actions?

Wollheim himself does not regard this as a serious problem but as a mere reflection of the "radical character" of Freud's theory. Yet the example Wollheim gives to show how forgettings or mislayings can be actions unfortunately misses the only interesting point at issue here. Wollheim cites Freud's well-known forgetting of the name "Signorelli" during a conversation he was having with a stranger. Freud explained his forgetting of the name of the painter of the *Last Judgment* as due to his (Freud's) conscious suppression of another thought having to do with a remark he had heard recently. Because of a train of associations not here important, Freud's conscious suppression of his impulse to mention this remark resulted in his forgetting Signorelli's name. As Wollheim describes it:

> Freud... wished to banish from his mind thoughts of death and sexuality. The immediate effect of this was that he checked himself in retailing remarks on this topic; the deferred effect was that he forgot the name of the painter of Orvieto. For an association now connected these thoughts... So we have the stage set for the overall characterization of the case: In trying to forget one thing intentionally, Freud forgot another against his will.[37]

There are several misleading things in this characterization. What Freud did as a basic act was to check his impulse to reveal a remark. He performed this (conscious) act for a reason, perhaps to "banish from his mind thoughts of death and sexuality." If he succeeded at this, we could redescribe his action as a banishing of these thoughts from his mind, a complex action he did by checking his impulse to say the remark. Further, this (if we grant Freud's explanation here) complex act of banishing had a further consequence: Freud could not recall Signorelli's name. We could thus again redescribe the action as a forgetting of Signorelli's name. Yet none of this addresses the only point at issue here: Could Freud (or can anyone) forget a name as a *basic* action? We can all "forget a name" as a complex action—taking drugs might well do the trick. But it requires more than this to show that the unconscious extends the domain of events to be considered actions. We need what seems unintelligible, namely, to imagine that one can simply will the forgetting of a name as one can simply will the movement of an arm.

Turning to the third of the behaviors Freud's unconscious allegedly shows us to be actions: Many neurotic symptoms, like many parapraxes, are conscious actions. Of interest here, however, is that subclass of symptoms, such as Dora's hysterical cough, that nominally are not actions. Freud tells Dora that her cough is an action, although he does so, at least in part, for therapeutic reasons. In addition to his therapeutic concerns, Freud erroneously assumes that because Dora has a set of wishes fulfilled by the cough, the cough is an action. Beyond these ultimately irrelevant considerations, however, Freud also seems to be seeking to have Dora acknowledge from her memory that she was malingering. This requires that she view her hysterical symptom as her act. Moreover, Freud wants Dora to acknowledge this as her action in a noninferential way. Freud's insistence on this matter is consistent with his general insistence that the patient's noninferential knowledge is essential to symptom removal.[38]

If the hypothesis is that Dora would remember that her cough was something she instigated by her own action rather than something she merely suffered, and if the hypothesis is true, then perhaps one can conclude that Dora performed an action in making her throat sore and in causing her cough. For many symptoms such as Dora's, however, there is the same problem as that we just encountered with some parapraxes being actions. (This problem is in addition to the general problem of evidence for the necessary memories.) What would it be like to remember having developed a cough, or a soreness of the throat, as a basic action? Moreover, is effectuating this state of affairs in anyone's repertoire of basic acts, such that one *could* remember doing it? If the claim were that this was a complex act, this problem would not exist. One might cause one's throat to be sore by other basic acts a person *can* perform, such as clearing one's throat constantly and unnecessarily or taking liquids that would make it sore. Yet this cannot be the claim about Dora's having acted if Freud is to make out his claim of extending our concept of action to events to which it was not already commonly applied. Rather, Freud must show that Dora simply made her throat sore; that is, her doing so was a basic action, not a complex one.

Frank Cioffi has questioned the intelligibility of Dora's remembering making her throat sore as a basic action of hers:

> The absurdity of the criterion of retrospective self-intimation often extends beyond the question of evidence to the question of intelligibility. Do we even understand what it would *mean* if Dora, say, retrospectively assured us that on the occasion of Herr K's sexual overtures she had displaced a sensation of pressure from her thigh to her thorax, or that she had transformed the experience of excitation in the genitals into one of disgust at the glottis?[39]

Two aspects of Cioffi's claim of unintelligibility require separation. Did Dora, or does anyone, have the capacity to make herself have sore throats or coughs? Second, even if she could do this, had she ever experienced exercising her capacity so that she knew what it was like to "make a sore

Increased Responsibility

throat"?[40] These questions must be answered affirmatively for it to be possible that Dora knew, either consciously or unconsciously, that she was making her throat sore. Without such a capacity and the prior experience of its exercise, what indeed could it mean for Dora to remember having done these things as actions?

To answer the first question about the capacities for basic actions of persons would require much scientific research. Biofeedback research has shown that people have the capacity to do more basic actions than previously thought. Even granting this, it remains to be shown that anyone can do things like making his own throat sore. In any case, the second aspect of Freud's claim that Dora's throat becoming sore was a basic action of hers is also problematic: Even if people generally have the capacity to simply make their throats sore, could Dora have known, without some training, what it was like to make a sore throat? And if not, how could she remember having done this as an action?

This second point is not to deny that children and adults (at least in a biofeedback laboratory) do learn to perform new basic actions. It is to deny that, before they learn to do a certain kind of basic act, they can be said to be performing it "unconsciously." Suppose someone discovers that he can wiggle his ears. He discovers this capacity when he notices one day that his ears are moving and that he can start and stop them moving. What should we say of his ear movement *before* he discovered that he could move his ears? Was it an action of his, or a mere movement of his body? Using the account of action developed earlier, one should say that it was not his act for he could not, by hypothesis, remember that he was wiggling his ears. He comes to know (1) that his ears were moving, and (2) that he can assume control of their movement once he knows he has such control. However, he does not come to know that *he* moved his ears, unless he makes the false inference from (1) and (2) that such movements must have been acts of his.

Both of these problems in conceptualizing Dora's symptoms as an action by her are serious impediments for the accidents-are-actions thesis. In discussing how hysterics convert mental anxiety into physical symptoms, Freud himself early expressed misgivings about conceptualizing such conversion as an action conversion hysterics perform: "I cannot, I must confess, give any hint of how a conversion of this kind is brought about. *It is obviously not carried out in the same way as an intentional and voluntary action.*"[41] In such moments, Freud too seemed to sense that for a large class of examples the claim that they are actions borders on unintelligibility.

Even bypassing the question of intelligibility, the basic evidentiary question remains: Did Freud's patients, such as Dora, come to remember their symptoms as their own actions, or would they have had they continued treatment? The acknowledgment of the causal influence of some unconscious wish seems to be the much more likely outcome of psychoanalysis than the patients' coming to see that they had performed actions they did not know anyone *could* perform.

It is important in all of these cases to stress how much of Freudian insight can be accommodated in the alternative, nonaction account. Dreams, parapraxes, and neurotic symptoms may all have patterns to them—the fulfillment of certain wishes. All may be caused by certain unconscious mental states. Certain desires of the conversion hysteric, for example, may indeed account for why he cannot move his arm. Yet neither the discovery of the pattern to human behavior, nor the explanation of that pattern by unconscious mental states, requires that one view dreams, parapraxes, or neurotic symptoms as *actions* a person performs, even unconsciously.

Are Accidental Actions Explained by Unconscious Mental States Really Intentional?

The second question posed earlier was whether unconscious mental state explanations can show that nominally accidental actions are actually intentional actions. Unlike the examples in the preceding section, here there is no question that the actor performed some action in which we are interested. The example given earlier was of some actor X opening the window and thereby chilling the room. Those affronted by the cold room may correctly describe the action as "chilling the room," since this is indeed a complex action he performed by performing the simpler action of opening the window. The question to be examined here is whether we may also say X *intentionally* performed the complex action of chilling the room even though he did not consciously know that opening the window would have that effect.

Freud and his followers usually do not distinguish the claim that some accidental actions are really intentional from the claim already examined, namely, that some accidental movements are really actions. Therefore, their arguments for increased responsibility are essentially the same as those just examined. Accordingly, only a brief excursion into further examples and argument is necessary here.

Examples from dreams are rare because dreams are not actions, and therefore the question of whether they are *intentional* actions does not arise. One might consider going to bed to be an action, and if so, then perhaps an example can be found in Freud's notion that going to bed is an "intentional turning away from the external world."[42] Assuming that one does not *consciously* turn away from the world when one goes to sleep, Freud would be saying that an action one does not ordinarily think of as intentional was in fact intentional, because it was caused by the preconscious wish to sleep.

Examples of alleged unconsciously intentional actions abound in Freud's discussions of neurotic symptoms. Consider the obsessive lady who regularly "ran from her room into another neighbouring one, took up a particular position there beside a table that stood in the middle, rang the bell for her housemaid, sent her on some indifferent errand or let her go without one, and then ran back into her own room."[43] All of these are intentional actions of which the lady is aware. Freud purports to show here that in performing this obsessional routine she was also doing another intentional action: She was showing her maid a large spot on the tablecloth. Freud says she wanted to do this because of some vicarious embarrassment for her husband's impotence on their wedding night that he had tried to conceal from the maids by staining the bedsheets with red ink. She was doing something she was not aware of doing, yet because there was some point to what she was doing, Freud suggests that she was doing it intentionally.[44]

The richest field of examples of alleged unconsciously intentional actions comes from parapraxes: slips of the tongue, awkward movements, or misreadings. Although many such slips are not actions at all, as discussed, many others are actions but are nominally unintentional actions. Freud gives the following example:

> There is no sphere in which the view that accidental actions are really intentional will command a more ready belief than that of sexual activity, where the borderline between the two possibilities seems really to be a faint one. A good example from my own experience of a few years ago shows how an apparently clumsy movement can be most cunningly used for sexual purposes. In the house of some friends I met a young girl who was staying there as a guest and who aroused a feeling of pleasure in me which I had long thought was extinct. As a result I was in a jovial, talkative and obliging mood. At the time I also endeavoured to discover how this came about; a year before the same girl had made no impression on me. As the girl's uncle, a very old gentleman, entered the room, we both jumped to our feet to bring him a chair that was standing in the corner. She was nimbler than I was and, I think, nearer to the object; so she took hold of the chair first and carried it in front of her with its back towards her, gripping the sides of the seat with both hands. As I got there later, but still stuck to my intention of carrying the chair, I suddenly found myself standing directly behind her, and throwing my arms round her from behind; and for a moment my hands met in front of her waist. I naturally got out of the situation as rapidly as it had arisen. Nor does it seem to have struck anyone how dexterously I had taken advantage of this clumsy movement.[45]

Although Freud makes no attribution of responsibility, it would seem to follow from the apparent conclusion here that Freud's sexual contact with the girl was intentionally accomplished.

The main problem with Freud's conceptualizing of such cases as intentional actions is the same as for the parallel claim that some nominal accidents are really actions. The problem is that the unconscious mental states typically cited to explain these behaviors are not reasons for action. This being so, the supposed implication of intentionality holds no more than the supposed implication that accidents are actions. Particularly glaring, by way of example, is Freud's reliance upon the wish to sleep as showing sleep to be an intentional turning away from the world. Once this "wish" is seen to be at most a sleep-preserving function served by dreaming, the supposed implication that dreamers intentionally stay asleep drops away.

The examples provided by the obsessional lady who rang for her maid, or Freud's own touching of the girl, are arguably better explained in terms of mental states and not functions. In each case one has the actor's memory of the mental states used to explain the actions. The lady explicitly avowed, under Freud's prodding, that she wished her husband had not been impotent,[46] and Freud was presumably aware of his own sexual attractions. To decide whether these are examples of reason-giving accounts, one must know whether the actors believed their actions were a means to achieve their admitted desires. Without such a belief, to reiterate the earlier discussion in Chapter 8, these explanations are in terms of causally operative desires and not reasons for acting.

This question of the existence of the actor's means/end beliefs in order to make out a reason-giving account is very close to the question one should ask in any case if one wants to find out whether these actions were intentional. The definition of intentional developed in Chapter 2 allowed as a sufficient condition for an action's being intentional that the actor *knows* what he is doing. For example, if Freud knew that he was touching the girl's lap by holding the chair as he did, then his action of touching the girl's lap was intentional. Compare the state of mind necessary to complete a practical syllogism for Freud: To accompany the sexual desire for the girl should be Freud's belief that if he touches her lap, he will enjoy a sexual contact with her. Seemingly, Freud could have had this latter belief (a means/end belief) only if he knew that in holding the chair he was touching the girl's lap. Otherwise, how could he believe that *this touching* would get him what he wanted? Accordingly, the question of whether some of Freud's explanations are truly reason-giving accounts can be collapsed into the ultimate question here, namely, whether the action so explained is intentional. In each case one must carefully examine the beliefs of the actors.

Increased Responsibility

Did the woman who rang for her maid *know* that by summoning the maid she was showing her the spot on the tablecloth? Did Freud *know* that by holding the chair as he did he was touching the girl's lap? Since neither the woman nor Freud consciously knew that they were performing these actions, one might say that they unconsciously knew it; because of such unconscious knowledge, they performed these actions intentionally, albeit unconsciously.

Some philosophers otherwise quite sympathetic to the idea of unconscious mental states have drawn the line at intention. They contend that one cannot be unconscious of one's intentions even if one can be unconscious of other mental states.[47] Usually this is presented as no more than a linguistic intuition of such philosophers, although more systematic arguments have also been made in terms of the epistemic characteristics of first-person avowals of intentions.[48] In any case, such a conceptual claim seems clearly wrong. Once one admits the idea of unconscious knowledge as that knowledge recapturable by extended memory, then one is committed to the idea of unconsciously intentional actions no less than to unconscious actions.

The real question then becomes one of evidence: Would either the woman who summoned her maid or Freud remember having the requisite beliefs in each case? Alternatively, would their memories only recall the actions they did perform, recall the desires in question, and then make the *inference* that the second was the cause of the first? Only in the former case should one say that their actions were intentional; the latter case would only be another instance of mental state causation that does not amount to intentional action for reasons.

In Freud's own example it seems probable that he would indeed remember knowing, at the time, that he was touching the girl's lap by holding the chair as he did. Indeed, this seems to be the point of his anecdote. In such a case one should see this as an instance of an unconsciously intentional action.

The woman who rang for her maid, on the other hand, is a less plausible example. The distinction between these examples exhibits an additional important hurdle that psychoanalysis must cross if it is to show that accidental actions are really intentional.

If the woman's action of showing her maid the spot is to be regarded as intentional, the woman would have had to believe that summoning the maid and standing near the table would draw the maid's attention to the spot. This was, in itself, a rational enough belief to have held; but this belief, however, presupposes an entire range of other beliefs that the woman must also have held. She must have believed, for example, that there was a spot on the table and that the maid's vision was adequate. More pertinently, she also must have believed that if the maid were shown the spot, then the woman's husband would be made less impotent; this is because the desire given by Freud to explain the woman's action was a wish that her husband had not been impotent. To fit the required form of a practical syllogism, the belief the woman necessarily would have to have held would be that this action of showing the maid the spot would achieve the object of her desire. Only with that belief would she have been making a means/end calculation, that is, acting with that desire as her reason, and thus having the knowledge that would make intentional her showing the maid the spot.

Now one can see why a recall of the requisite beliefs was less likely in the woman's case than in Freud's. She would have had to remember having a completely *irrational* belief. It is very unlikely that even her extended memory could have recaptured a belief in something so obviously impossible as making her husband less impotent by showing the maid a spot. There is no evidence for the existence of such a belief, despite the fact that it would be nice for Freudian theory if there were such beliefs because complete practical syllogisms then could be made out.[49]

It is striking how many alleged examples of unconsciously intentional actions in psychoanalytic theory are more like the case of the woman who rang for her maid and less like Freud's own example. When Freud dreamed that his friend Otto had behaved stupidly with regard to Irma, did Freud not only *desire* revenge on Otto but also *believe* that dreaming that dream would actually give him revenge? The implausibility of attributing such a belief to dreamers was discussed in Chapter 8. When a woman who desires a baby misreads "stocks" as "storks," does she also *believe* that reading "storks" rather than "stocks" will conceive a baby?[50] Unless one is theoretically committed to viewing persons as having a dark, subterranean primary process where total irrationality reigns supreme, one does not ordinarily think people have such beliefs. If they do not, then one does not act for reasons in such cases, nor are one's actions to be thought of as consciously or unconsciously intentional.

The way to forget just how limited is the class of examples that can plausibly be thought to be unconsciously intentional actions is to play fast and loose with the concept of knowing. Unconscious knowledge, as I have up to now been using the phrase, names a dispositional state in which one is disposed under certain circumstances to know consciously what it is one knows unconsciously. This is the unconscious knowledge that we have if we have the potential to recall what it is we (unconsciously) knew. Such knowledge is a mental state of ours just because our first-person awareness (privileged access) *can* recapture it, even if often enough we do not.

There are several senses of "knowing" different from this nonbehavioral, dispositional sense I have been using. Three come to mind. Each can be brought out by examining in some detail the actions of Clyde in Theo-

Increased Responsibility

dore Dreiser's novel, *An American Tragedy*.[51] Clyde, the central character in the novel, quite consciously wants to kill his pregnant girlfriend, Roberta, to free himself to marry the rich and beautiful Sondra. He plans Roberta's murder, which is to take place in a rowboat, but finds that he cannot carry it out. When Roberta notices the strange expression on his face and approaches him in the boat, Clyde performs two actions that jointly cause the boat to capsize: He strikes her with a camera, and he then rises to assist her or to apologize. When the boat capsizes because of these two actions, Clyde ignores Roberta's pleas for help, and she drowns. Dreiser's rich description of the incident is worth giving in full:

> And Clyde, as instantly sensing the profoundness of his own failure, his own cowardice or inadequateness for such an occasion, as instantly yielding to a tide of submerged hate, not only for himself, but Roberta—her power—or that of life to restrain him in this way. And yet fearing to act in any way—being unwilling to—being willing only to say that never, never would he marry her—that never, even should she expose him, would he leave here with her to marry her—that he was in love with Sondra and would cling only to her—and yet not being able to say that even. But angry and confused and glowering. And then, as she drew near him, seeking to take his hand in hers and the camera from him in order to put it in the boat, he flinging out at her, but not even then with any intention to do other than free himself of her—her touch—her pleading—consoling sympathy—her presence forever—God!
>
> Yet (the camera still unconsciously held tight) pushing at her with so much vehemence as not only to strike her lips and nose and chin with it, but to throw her back sidewise toward the left wale which caused the boat to careen to the very water's edge. And then he, stirred by her sharp scream, (as much due to the lurch of the boat, as the cut on her nose and lip), rising and reaching half to assist or recapture her and half to apologize for the unintended blow—yet in so doing completely capsizing the boat—himself and Roberta being as instantly thrown into the water. And the left wale of the boat as it turned, striking Roberta on the head as she sank and then rose for the first time, her frantic, contorted face turned to Clyde, who by now had righted himself. For she was stunned, horror-struck, unintelligible with pain and fear—her lifelong fear of water and drowning and the blow he had so accidentally and all *but* unconsciously administered.[52]

Shortly before he is to be executed for Roberta's murder, Clyde and Reverend McMillan attempt to reconstruct his mental state and thus assess his true responsibility. Putting aside Clyde's omission to rescue, the most pertinent question is whether Clyde *intentionally* capsized the boat. He unquestionably performed the complex action of capsizing the boat by performing the two simpler actions: one, of striking Roberta, sending her to the side of the boat and causing the boat itself to tip its edge to the water; and two, of rising and moving toward Roberta, which caused the boat to capsize. Does anything known about Clyde's mental states allow one to conclude that this action of capsizing the boat was *intentional*?

Most of what Clyde avows cuts against such a conclusion. His anger and frustration at being unable to go through with his plan caused him to strike Roberta as hard as he did, and it was in reaction to his having hit her that he rose. "There was also the truth that in rising he was seeking to save her—even in spite of his hate."[53] Notable to McMillan, however, as it had been to the prosecutors and the jury, "was the fact that all through . . . he had been swayed by his obsession for [Sondra], the super motivating force in connection with all of this."[54] Suppose that this desire to be with Sondra caused Clyde to rise when he did. Can one attribute to Clyde a belief that if he capsized the boat, Roberta would die and he could then be with Sondra? If so, and if Clyde rose because of such a belief, as well as because of his corresponding desire, then his capsizing the boat was intentional. (This would have to be true because Clyde would also necessarily have believed that he was capsizing the boat in order to have adopted that action as the means to his desired end.)

Unlike the examples from Freud, the beliefs that must be attributed to Clyde are not irrational or unlikely beliefs. Indeed, if Clyde were asked, while in the boat, whether rising and moving toward Roberta were likely to capsize a boat already tipped to the gunwales, he would probably respond affirmatively. He, like everyone, possesses such general knowledge and beliefs. However, one hesitates to impute such a belief to Clyde here because he did not realize what he knew in general, namely, that this particular action of rising would capsize the boat.

The first sense of knowledge that gets in the way here is what might be called the pure behavioral sense of knowledge. In this sense Clyde "knew" that his rising would capsize the boat, because he did just that act that could cause it. In this sense one might say of any actor who performs a complicated and intelligence-requiring routine, "He must have known what he was doing." Such examples are quite familiar outside of psychoanalytic contexts. Dan Dennett[55] imagines the driver whose "mind is on something else" but who nonetheless successfully negotiates a difficult length of mountain road. He must have known what he was doing, even though his attention was elsewhere.

Further examples abound in the literature of the psychology of perception. Recent work in that field has shown how much intelligent information preprocessing one does before the information is sent up the optic nerve to the brain.[56] Such information processing gives the appearance of being inferences drawn from beliefs that are formed from the stimuli one

Increased Responsibility

receives. However, this does not mean that one really *knows* these inferences. One's personal self does not know these things because the extended memory, the device by which one integrates new beliefs or other mental states into one's personal self, is not operative. This behavioral sense of knowledge or belief treats one as a purely physical system. In this sense, like any other information-processing system with input subsystems, one can be said to perceive and believe all sorts of things.[57]

The law has long been troubled by this behavioral sense of belief. It is one meaning of the notion of objective mental states in the criminal law. This view treats complex and intelligence-requiring behavior not as good *evidence* of the existence of the mental state of knowledge, but rather as the *logically sufficient condition* for saying that such a mental state exists. This is to reject the subjective, personal mental states required for culpability rather than to apply them. This behavioral sense of belief should therefore be ignored when one assesses the impact of the unconscious on Clyde's or anyone else's responsibility; for it cannot show that Clyde *knew* what he was doing, or that he acted intentionally, in the morally relevant sense of those words.

The second sense of knowledge that can get in the way here is that sense often introduced with some versions of the insanity defense. This is particularly true of the M'Naghten version of the defense, where courts have often sought to alleviate the rigors of the M'Naghten test by reading knowledge to require something other than propositional knowing. What is required by such courts is some kind of emotional appreciation by the defendant that what he was doing was wrong.[58] A fighter pilot, it might be said, knows what he is doing when he napalms village schools, in the sense that later he can state what he did. In the sense of "emotionally appreciate," however, he may not know what he has done if he lacks emotional appreciation of the awfulness of his action.

This distinction is one Freud often drew between senses of knowing. Only knowledge that was "emotionally driven home" could effect the removal of symptoms.[59] Freud discussed the various senses of knowing in his Rat-Man case history:

> It must therefore be admitted that in an obsessional neurosis there are two kinds of knowledge, and it is just as reasonable to hold that the patient "knows" his traumas as that he does *not* "know" them. For he knows them in that he has not forgotten them, and he does not know them in that he is unaware of their significance.[60]

(Freud earlier made clear that the "significance" of which he speaks is the *emotional significance* to the patient, whereas what is not forgotten is the "ideational significance," or the object, of that emotion.[61])

Clyde presents an example somewhat the reverse of the fighter pilot in that he *did* emotionally appreciate how awful capsizing the boat and drowning Roberta would be—indeed, he could not bring himself to do it—yet he lacked propositional knowledge that this was what he was doing.

Although Clyde's emotional appreciation of the horror of Roberta's drowning initially would seem to mitigate his responsibility, one might also find that it implies intention on Clyde's part. For it may seem that a necessary ingredient of Clyde's emotional appreciation and repulsion is his knowledge of what it is that he is doing. If this is true, Clyde's action was intentional. Some excuse might be invoked here—perhaps inner compulsion as analyzed in Chapter 10—but if he realized that his rising was capsizing the boat and was horrified at the prospect as he continued to rise, his capsizing the boat was intentional.[62]

Alternatively and much more likely, Clyde's emotional appreciation may simply have repelled him without his being at all clear as to what caused his repulsion. Although emotion words, like most mental words, require intensional objects, it is not necessary for the subject to be aware of those objects. Indeed, a prevalent analysis of the meaning of unconscious emotions is to say that one experiences fear, hatred, or anxiety without knowing *what* one fears, hates, or is anxious about.[63] Viewed this way, Clyde's emotional appreciation does not imply that he knew he was capsizing the boat, even if that was what horrified him.

Thus, although one might say that Clyde knew (emotionally appreciated) what he was doing, this knowledge is no substitute for the knowledge synonymous with intentional. Clyde needed to believe he was capsizing the boat by his actions in order to be said to have capsized the boat intentionally, and no amount of feeling bad on his part can substitute for the required belief.

The third kind of knowledge to be put aside here does not depend on an ambiguity of the word knowledge so much as it depends on some confusion about how we fix the *objects* of belief (and thus of knowledge) states. It is plausible to suppose that Clyde in general knew that rising would capsize a boat already listing to one side, even though he did not know that *this* boat on *this* occasion would capsize if he arose. If one conflates these two different objects of belief, one could say that Clyde "knew" the boat would capsize. Clyde would know this in the same sense in which one says of others that they know the logical implications of propositions they clearly know to be true.[64] Thus, if Clyde knew generally that such an action would have such a result, then he knew that his rising would capsize the boat even though he did not consciously realize any such thing.

Yet one cannot allow this kind of reconstruction of Clyde's beliefs. Clyde's general knowledge, and the inferences drawn from it, cannot be equated with knowing that *this* rowboat would be capsized by his rising. To do so collapses the important distinction between what one actually knew, and what one should have known. This distinction cannot be collapsed, as it sometimes is in the criminal law concept of objective knowledge, because it marks an important moral distinction between harm one does intentionally, and harm one brings about negligently. This sense of knowledge, like the pure behavioral sense, rejects the subjective mental states required for culpability.

The only instance in which we should countenance the equating of these different mental states is when the actor keeps himself from drawing the obvious inference. If Clyde was self-deceived, so that he kept himself from inferring that this rowboat, too, would obviously capsize if he stood up, then, but only then, should we say that Clyde knew his rising would capsize the boat. (In law when such cases approach a conscious purpose not to draw the obvious inference they are called cases of willful blindness.) And even here, it is not so much that Clyde knew as that we hold him responsible just as if he did know, because he possessed the means of knowledge but purposely refused to use them.

In general, we may conclude that although one might say that actors know quite a wide variety of things in these extended senses of know, the knowledge they possess will not show that their actions were intentional. To show that an action was intentional, even unconsciously intentional, requires more than these extended senses of knowledge can deliver. Explicitly putting them aside helps to reveal just how few actions can be shown to be unconsciously intentional by the discovery of unconscious mental states.

Are Intentional Actions Explained by Unconscious Mental States Really Attempts at Unconscious Aims?

As examined in Chapter 2, our ascriptions of responsibility are made when an actor has caused some harm. Sometimes, however, an actor does not succeed in causing the bad result he intended, and in such a case he may be held responsible for *attempting* to achieve such a result. Since in such cases causation of the harm drops out as an element justifying the assignment of responsibility, I shall first sketch briefly the elements of attempt liability prior to assessing the impact of the unconscious in this area.

It is a hornbook rule that the *actus reus* of criminal attempts is conduct going beyond "mere preparation."[65] If, for example, one buys a gun with the intent of using it the next day in a bank robbery, that act is said to be mere preparation and does not satisfy the *actus reus* requirement for attempted bank robbery.

There are actually two separate elements here, each of which is morally important. The first is what might be called the real *actus reus* requirement of an attempt. This is the same act requirement as that necessary to assign responsibility for causing harm; that is, one must have performed some basic act. The second element is the analogue to causing harm (in the case of attempts where there is no harm caused). To hold an actor responsible for an attempt, the basic act must have caused some state of affairs that, although short of the harm, conceptually amounts to an *attempt* to bring about the harm.

This second element is a moral requirement, not just a doctrine peculiar to the criminal law. Morally it is important to distinguish between states of mind that are acted upon and those that are not. States of mind unaccompanied by action are not made punishable in the criminal law, in part because to do so would be unjust.[66] A person who only contemplates what another person does is not seriously culpable, whereas one who attempts to cause some bad result may be just as culpable as one who intentionally accomplishes it.[67] A person whose acts do not amount to an attempt is not as culpable, because he more resembles the person who only contemplates the harm than he resembles the person who tries to accomplish it.

The third element of an attempt is less problematic. In addition to performing some basic act causing some state of affairs close enough to a harm that it amounts to an attempt, one must also so act with the causing of that harm as one's reason. Although the law uses the phrase "specific intent" here, clarity is served by calling it a reason for action. The mental state necessary for an attempt thus requires that a full practical syllogism be made out.

The impact of the unconscious on one's responsibility for attempts should be assessed in light of each of these elements. Because the basic act issue is no different from that previously discussed, only the last two elements need be discussed here. The following two questions thus remain: (1) Does explanation of some action by unconscious mental states supply the "beyond preparation" requirement of an attempt; and (2) does that explanation supply the mental state requirement for an attempt?

An affirmative answer to both of these questions appears to be a central tenet of Freudian theory about the unconscious. Throughout the corpus of Freud's work one finds his patients and others described as *trying* or *attempting* to do various things. Thus, one may be told that Dora was trying to separate her father from his mistress by her hysterical cough. The obsessive woman who repeatedly rang for her maid was trying to make it be the case that her husband had not been impotent on their wedding night. Freud in "executing" his inkwell was attempting to get his sister to buy the new one she had promised. We may even, contemporary Freudians assure us, say that a man struck by lightning may be "deliberately, though unconsciously, trying to get it to strike him."[68]

Sometimes the motives for this sort of talk are less than laudable. For example, to avoid disconfirmation of his wish-fulfillment hypothesis about

Increased Responsibility

dreams, Freud asserted that "you can say nevertheless that a dream is an *attempt* at the fulfillment of a wish."[69] More typically, however, Freud's motives stem from the fact that most of the goals he posits as the objects of people's unconscious desires are not things they actually achieve. Dora did not, for example, succeed in separating her father from his mistress. Indeed, for many of these cases Freud's subjects could not succeed in bringing about the object of their desire.[70] No one can sleep with a mother who is dead. No one can make an event in the past happen differently, even if one fervently wishes that one's husband had not been impotent. Consequently, Freud is led to a description of what his subjects are doing, in terms of what they are *trying* to do. Thus, their symptoms tend to be viewed as attempts at certain ends, not as intentional accomplishments of those ends. Whether Freud is entitled to so view them is the question addressed here.

DISTANT (BUT UNCONSCIOUSLY CLOSE) ATTEMPTS

The first problem with saying that the actions of Dora, Freud, or the obsessive lady are attempts stems from the fact that often the action that is said to be an attempt is so distant from success that it seems odd to call it an attempt at all. In many of Freud's examples, the actions done do not seem to amount to attempts because they are so far removed from the ends toward which they are supposed to be means.

Consider, for example, the obsessive girl of 19 whose compulsive night-time rituals brought her to Freud's attention.[71] Among other things, she regularly took great care to keep the pillow at the head of the bed from touching the back of the wooden bedstead. This Freud explains as follows:

> She wanted—by magic . . . to keep the man and woman apart—that is, to separate her parents from each other, not allow them to have sexual intercourse. In earlier years, before she had established the ceremonial, she had tried to achieve the same aim in a more direct way. She had simulated fear . . . in order that the connecting doors between her parents' bedroom and the nursery should not be shut. . . . Not satisfied with disturbing her parents by this means, she contrived to be allowed from time to time to sleep in her parents' bed between them. . . . Finally, when she was so big that it became physically uncomfortable for her to find room in the bed between her parents, she managed, by a conscious simulation of anxiety, to arrange for her mother to exchange places with her for the night and to leave her own place so that [she] could sleep beside her father.[72]

Although the girl's action of simulating fear when she was young could be described as attempting to separate her parents, the same cannot be said of her bedtime ritual. Arranging her bed seems too remote from the supposed end for it to constitute an attempt to separate her parents.

It should be noted that the discovery of unconscious mental states explaining such cases seems to be irrelevant to the problem discussed here. The objection to calling the girl's activity an attempt concerns the lack of causation of something describable as an attempt, rather than the mental state of the girl. Seemingly, no explanation by reference to mental states can transform buying a gun, for example, into attempting to kill. Indeed, a conscious purpose to kill does not normally make such an action an attempt, for that action is simply too remote. How could an unconscious purpose do more?

Elizabeth Anscombe once imagined a man who moved the handle of a water pump believing that there was water to be pumped and intending to pump that water.[73] If there was no water, then he can be described as "pumping water" only in quotation marks to indicate that he is not really pumping water, but only thinks he is. He can, however, be described as attempting to pump water by his action of moving the handle. This action is an attempt because it is, *under the circumstances as he believes them to be,* the only action he needs to take in order to pump the water.

For some time the law of criminal attempts has been stumbling toward a like result.[74] If one points an unloaded gun at another and, believing it to be loaded, pulls the trigger, one is guilty of attempted murder even though it was impossible in these circumstances to have succeeded in killing anyone. Judged in the circumstances as the actor believed them to be, the act was very close to achieving the prohibited end. Similarly, if one believes (perhaps through some voodoo belief) that the action of buying a gun will somehow kill another, then buying the gun for that reason *is* an attempt to kill.

This analysis applied to psychoanalytic examples of attempts can similarly transform actions with little or no chance of causing some result, into attempts to bring about that result. All that is required is a *belief* by the agent that the circumstances are such that the action will achieve the desired end. If, for example, the 19-year-old girl believes that her father *is* the bedstead and her mother *is* the bolster, then her bedtime ritual of keeping them separate is, given those beliefs, an attempt at keeping her father and mother apart at night. Such a belief is indeed attributed to the girl by Freud: "The pillow, she said, had always been a woman to her and the upright wooden back [of the bedstead] a man."[75]

Hence, what appeared to be a separate problem for unconscious attempts—the lack of any action sufficiently close to success that it could be called an attempt—dissolves into the familiar problem of whether Freud's subjects have the beliefs he says they have. This is the same problem as that involved in his account of the mental state necessary for attempts and will be discussed with it in the following subsection.

Increased Responsibility

UNCONSCIOUSLY AIMING AT BAD RESULTS

As set forth in Chapter 2, to attempt to bring about some state of affairs is to have that state of affairs as one's reason for doing some action. Accordingly, to ask whether unconscious mental state explanations transform apparently innocent actions into attempts at some other result is to ask our already familiar question of whether those explanations give reasons for actions. As argued in Chapter 8 and summarized earlier in this chapter, most unconscious mental state explanations in psychoanalysis do not give reasons for actions. Accordingly, they cannot show that one is attempting to attain a goal of which one is unaware of attempting. To find meanings in dreams, functions served by repression, or unconscious mental states causing slips is not to discover that a person attempted to achieve aims of which he was unaware.

To the extent that psychoanalytic explanations fall into any of these three categories—meanings, functions, or causation—they cannot show that one often attempts to do certain acts of which one is unaware. There are Freudian examples, however, that do not seem to fall into these categories. Perhaps the obsessive girl of 19 is one such example. Her ritual is plainly an action of hers. Freud is attempting to explain it rather than merely interpret its meaning. Moreover, he is not only asserting that the ritual serves the function of keeping the parents apart; Freud also says that the girl wants the parents apart and that this desire explains her actions. Finally, and most crucially, Freud claims that she had the requisite beliefs, although they were unconscious. If all this were true, one would have to say that she was unconsciously attempting to keep her parents apart, that this was what she unconsciously believed she was doing, and that this was what she was *trying* to do.

Freud means this in a stronger sense than when one says of a dog digging in various places, "He is trying to find his bone." For animals, "trying" and other mental words are used only in the weak, behavioral sense. With human subjects, such as the girl, Freud claims something stronger: She is trying because she has beliefs and desires that she can recapture in her memory and that caused her to perform the actions of her ritual.

The problem with the Freudian account is not with the intelligibility of unconsciously attempting or trying, for the concept itself is clear enough, but with the evidence on the basis of which alleged unconscious attempts are verified. In the case of the obsessive 19-year-old-girl, the evidence for the crucial belief state consists of her associations between the parts of the bed and her parents. This is comparatively good evidence for Freud; it is certainly more credible than the universal symbolism Freud sometimes used to "verify" the required beliefs.[76]

Even in her case, however, one should question whether the association of one thing with another (her father with the bedstead) is evidence that the girl believes the two things to be the same. That I associate the smell of fresh croissants with the Charles River in Cambridge is not evidence that I believe the two things are the same. In addition, there is evidence to the contrary; unless she is more than neurotic, she would surely declare that she knows the difference between her father and her bedstead. Given the usual assumption about the consistency of a person's beliefs, there is strong evidence that she does *not* believe that her father and her bedstead are one.

Further, we have expectations about the sort of evidence there should be for a belief that is typically absent in Freudian examples. Any given belief should have systematic connections with the other beliefs of a person, and should also find reflection in other behavior besides the particular slip or symptom for which it is given as an explanation. Yet as Gary Fuller has noted:

> One would expect that in these cases the beliefs in question would manifest themselves at least occasionally in the fantasies and dreams of the individuals, and in fact they never do.... In the bolster-example we might expect that the girl would have anxiety dreams in which a scene in which she omits to separate the bolster from the back of the bed is followed by a scene in which her parents are making love. Or, if it is objected that we should not expect the belief to manifest itself in such an obvious form—since even in dreams the repressive forces are supposed to be partly active, then we can replace the above dream with a dream the first part of which involved her omitting to perform the ritual act and the second part of which involves, say, her father entering a church. But in fact one rarely, if ever, finds in Freud reports of fantasies or dreams which are similar to either of the invented dreams above.[77]

In addition to this evidential objection to viewing wish-fulfilling symptoms as attempts, there is some question of the coherence within Freud's theory of viewing symptoms and the like as attempts. As I shall examine in Chapter 11, Freudian theory is committed to viewing persons as essentially conflicted. Dreams, parapraxes, and neurotic symptoms are all viewed as "compromise formations," that is, as being explained by two or more conflicting mental states. Given this, and given that the repressed, unconscious state cannot be given direct expression, it seems odd to attribute to the patient just that belief that *for him* would make his symptom or dream into just such a direct expression of the forbidden wish. True, patients such as the girl of 19 are said only *unconsciously* to believe that her father and her bolster are one, and thus only *unconsciously* to believe that in separating the bolster from the bedstead she is separating her father from her mother. Yet if the wish to separate the parents is deeply repressed, it is odd to attribute to the person any belief (conscious or unconscious) that would make plain to that person ("at some level of consciousness") what her wish truly was.

J. Balmuth makes essentially this point when he observes that within the Freudian theory of repression

> the relation of behavior to the (unconscious) reason *is the appropriate one of the act expressing – acting out – the desire or wish, but in such a way that it is not the attempt to fulfill the wish*. For it is not accidental but essential to the psychoanalytic explanation that the behavior both express yet be *not* appropriate to the wish ... since it is the claim of the theory that the agent, under tension from the conflict, seeks not merely to express the wish but *also* neither to achieve its normal expression, either in admission or performance, nor reveal that he has such a wish. Thus its expression is disguised so that it will not be recognised and need not be acknowledged, and the action not be performed. For these reasons *neurotic behavior cannot be an attempt, misguided or not, to fulfill the state of affairs described in the wish*.[78]

Neither of these points can, by their nature, conclusively show that in no case are there the beliefs necessary to show us that a patient was attempting to achieve something of which he was unaware. There may be such things as isolated beliefs that are inconsistent with other things one believes, so that our normal evidence for the existence of beliefs is absent. Perhaps the belief of the girl of 19 is such a case. Further, such a belief, so long as it is unconscious, does not make total nonsense of the theory of repression. It will require an amendment of that theory, so that it is a theory of repressed *beliefs* as much as it is a theory of repressed desires.[79] This, in turn, would require one to reconceive of the unconscious and the id as not simply a "seething cauldron" of desire but as much the seat of reasoned beliefs. This, in turn, will be to shift Freud's basic functional organization of the mind. Perhaps one can work out such theoretical implications so that consistency in the theory is maintained. Nonetheless, both the problem of evidential well-foundedness and the problem of theoretical consistency should make one very skeptical about the thesis that the discovery of unconscious wishes is the discovery of unconscious attempts at fulfilling them.

Is One Responsible for Unconsciously Acting Intentionally or for Acting with Certain Unconscious Reasons?

RESPONSIBILITY AND CONSCIOUSNESS

In the preceding discussions the possibility has been left open that some of the phenomena classically cited as manifestations of the unconscious could constitute unconscious actions, unconsciously intentional actions, or unconscious attempts. The examples given that might constitute such actions were (1) those dreams for which the extended memory can recapture the dreamer's supervenient attitude during the dream, that is, the belief that the dreamer was actively creating the dream; (2) those parapraxes, such as Freud's touching the girl, for which the actor's extended memory can recapture the belief necessary to consider the action as intentional; and (3) those neurotic symptoms, such as those of the girl of 19, that can perhaps be viewed as unconscious attempts because perhaps one can discover the belief necessary to complete the actor's practical syllogism. In each case, the main question was one of there being any evidence for the existence of the necessary beliefs.

Assuming for purposes of argument the necessary beliefs do at least sometimes exist, does this have as its consequence that one is responsible for such dreams, parapraxes, or symptoms, in the same manner that one is responsible for conscious actions, intentions, or attempts? Consider the example, discussed by Freud, of the Roman emperor who put to death a man who dreamed that he had assassinated the ruler.[80] Freud's intuition is here probably correct: The punishment was unfair because the man was not responsible for his thought. Yet why not? Assume that punishment is imposed only under those conditions in which fault is fairly ascribed. Specifically, only those thoughts that are actively called forth are punished, and thoughts that just occur to one are not. Assume further that this dreamer could recapture the memory that he had created the scenario in which the emperor was killed. With such assumptions, it might seem that the dreamer could fairly be punished for dreaming the prohibited thought because he has met those conditions under which fault is fairly ascribed.

The implication of responsibility is in fact not this clear. This becomes apparent on reconsideration of the ambiguity of the meaning of know discussed earlier. A person may have unconscious knowledge of a fact and still truthfully assert that he does *not* know that fact. Statements such as "He knew that fact, but did not know that he knew it" make perfectly good sense, as Freud himself recognized. Such expressions make good sense because the speaker has varied the sense of know, using it in differing senses in the same sentence. One sense is synonymous with being aware of, whereas the other is not.

Because the concepts of action, intention, and reasons depend upon the beliefs of the actor, the ambiguity of believe will infect these concepts as well. Showing that an "unintentional forgetting" is intentional, as Freud purports to do,[81] is not to show that it was also not unintentional. If an unconscious intention is discovered, then the action will be both intentional and unintentional. This is not a contradiction; it means that the actor both knew and did not know that he was performing some action.[82]

Increased Responsibility

It is simply a mistake to regard unconscious actions or intentions, even when they are truly discovered, as contradicting commonsense descriptions of nonactions or unintentional actions. Psychoanalytic insight about unconscious intentional actions can supplement one's commonsense descriptions in terms of consciously unintentional accidents, but it cannot force one to withdraw the latter. A forgetting remains unintentional (no awareness) even if it could be shown that that forgetting was also intentional (a belief recapturable by extended memory).

The result is that one is in a moral quandary about responsibility when (if ever) there are the necessary unconscious beliefs. The moral principles under which one ascribes responsibility seem to require *both* that: (1) if a person's movement is an action, and it is intentional, then he is responsible; *and* (2) if it is not an action, or if it is unintentional, then he is not responsible. Yet these movements for which the required unconscious beliefs do exist are both properly described as intentional actions and either as nonactions or as unintentional actions.

To avoid an ambiguity in the term responsibility one needs some way of choosing one sense of knowledge as *the* sense relevant to responsibility assessments. Because one sense of knowledge means being aware of, such a choice squarely raises the question of whether consciousness is required for ascription of responsibility. Do only *conscious* actions, intentions, and reasons count in responsibility assessments? To answer this question requires some additional moral principle, for the principles heretofore relied upon, those requiring actions, intentions, and reasons, allow one to answer either way for this limited class of hypothesized examples.

The moral principle in question might be called a principle of consciousness. It would hold that in order to ascribe fairly responsibility to a person for causing a harm, he must have *consciously* acted intentionally, and to ascribe fairly responsibility to a person for attempting to cause a harm, he must have acted with that harm as his *conscious* reason. Using both ordinary senses of the word conscious, such a principle would have two parts: (1) The person must *have been* conscious in the sense of being awake; and (2) the person must have been conscious *of,* in the sense of being aware of, his acting, his intentions, or his reasons, if he is fairly to be held responsible for causing, or trying to cause, some harm.

One might further sharpen the second part of this principle by eschewing certain senses of conscious of. A principle requiring that the actor *think* of his actions, intentions, or reasons as he acts would be far too narrow. No such stream of consciousness or Joycean sense of conscious of can be at all plausible as a moral requirement, for it would exclude far too many intentional actions or attempts where one is perfectly content to ascribe responsibility. One does not, for example, consciously think or deliberate about going to lunch, yet doing so is an intentional action for which one may justly be held responsible (in those hard-to-imagine circumstances where going to lunch turns out to be a bad thing to do). It is much more plausible to construe the proposed moral principle as using the dispositional sense of conscious of discussed in Chapter 3. In this sense one is conscious of going to lunch if one can state what one is doing when one's attention is turned to the subject. One need not be thinking about some fact to be conscious of it in this sense.

Having stated the moral principle, how does one establish it as correct? There are two ways of noninstrumentally justifying a moral principle: either by a series of particular thought experiments, all of which point to the principle as the best general expression of the intuited results of those particular experiments, or by resort to a more general moral principle from which the principle to be justified is implied. If one's moral sense is fully coherent, the results of the particular thought experiments will match the implications of one's most general moral principles.[83] If the principle to be justified is included in that cohered set of judgments and principles, it will be justified in the only way in which moral principles can or should be justified.

We have already reviewed a set of particular thought experiments with which we may test the validity of the principle of consciousness. In those comparatively few examples of dreams, parapraxes, or symptoms that could possibly be thought to constitute unconscious actions, intentions, and reasons, one need only imagine that the consequence brought about or attempted was morally bad. Freud's example of the traitorous dream will serve as such an experiment, as will his touching the girl. If one imagines the physical separation of the parents of the girl of 19 to be a bad thing, her unconscious attempt to bring it about will also serve to isolate intuitions about responsibility.

Surely one's intuitions in the first of these three cases are the same as Freud's,[84] namely, the dreamer does not deserve to be executed because he is not responsible for the unconsciously produced dream thought of the emperor's death. Of course, one's intuition is to some extent influenced by two extraneous factors: (1) One is reluctant to punish persons for *any* thoughts unaccompanied by physical action, no matter how much such thoughts constitute mental acts and not mere happenings; and (2) one's principles of proportionality are violated even in a moral system that sanctions punishment for mental acts because execution is too severe a penalty for merely thinking of another's death. One removes these extraneous considerations by asking whether the dreamer can fairly be punished at all for his dreams, assuming that one is generally willing to punish persons for mental, as well as for physical, acts. Even so limited, is not one's intuition the same as Freud's?

Similar results are reached in examples such as Freud's sexual advance and the 19-year-old girl's attempt to separate her parents. Neither of them quite literally knew what they were doing. It is true that if one allows that they had the unconscious beliefs Freud claims for them, there is a sense in which they did know what they were doing. But is it not the morally persuasive rejoinder that they did not know that they knew, and that their ignorance should excuse them even in the face of such unconscious knowledge?

Further particular examples may be found in the law in which both parts of the principle of consciousness seem to be clearly established. Unconsciousness, in the sense of a lack of *being conscious,* is a complete defense to both civil and criminal liability. Thus, if one is asleep, dazed by a blow on the head, put out by the shock of being shot in the stomach, or unconscious because of drugs or alcohol involuntarily ingested, one is not held legally liable for the harm one has caused.[85] Sometimes this may be reflective of the fact that the behavior in question is not an action, not even an unconscious one. Yet even if the actor's extended memory could recapture beliefs necessary to make out such behaviors as actions for reasons, he is not legally liable to either tort or criminal sanctions.

Similarly, if a person is conscious (awake) but is not conscious (aware) of his actions, his intentions, or his attempts, he is not subject to punishment or civil damages for those crimes or torts requiring that we act intentionally or for certain reasons. Thus, a person who acts under post-hypnotic suggestion, and is not conscious of his bodily movements as an act he is doing, is not held responsible for any harm that ensues, even if we were willing to say that these were unconscious actions.[86] A person who only subliminally perceives some fact, such as another's copyrighted music, and then intentionally but unconsciously copies that music, is not held liable for *willfully* copying another's copyrighted material because he was not conscious of his intention to do so.[87]

Such examples are presented, not because the law is self-justifying or incapable of incorporating moral mistakes, but because the law is a source of further instances in which one should ask whether the actor could fairly be held responsible. The answers that judges and lawyers have given are at least good evidence of *their* intuitions about the matter: To ascribe responsibility fairly is to require consciousness. If one's own intuitions are similar, one has good reason to subscribe to a similar principle.

The other noninstrumentalist way to justify a moral principle is by resort to more general principles from which the principle in question is implied. H. L. A. Hart once argued that "in most western morality 'ought' implies 'can,' and a person who could not help doing what he did is not morally guilty."[88] John Rawls, following Hart, regards this as *the* principle of responsibility from which more particular principles, such as those requiring actions, intentions, or reasons, may be derived.[89] Whether the latter claim is true is debatable, but the principle, in any case, is one most persons would accept as basic.

The truly debatable point, of course, comes in specifying that the principle *means* in more concrete detail. Using determinist assumptions about the universe, there is a sense of can in which no one can help doing what they do. This, however, cannot be the sense of can employed by Hart, else no one is responsible. Rather, the power or ability referred to is the power to give effect to one's choices. The principle of responsibility is part of a principle of liberty that places a high value on protecting people's choices from the unnecessary interference of moral or legal sanctions.[90]

Whatever else the principle of responsibility might include, it should include the power or ability to appraise the moral worth of one's proposed actions. A person has such ability only if he has moral and factual knowledge of what he is doing and is able to integrate the two to perceive the moral quality of his action.[91] A person who lacks this ability cannot fairly be blamed because, although he is acting intentionally, he does not know that what he is doing is wrong. This requirement is applied in the treatment of children and the insane as nonmoral agents because they have not had a fair opportunity to acquire such moral knowledge.[92]

When the factual knowledge is unconscious, which it is by hypothesis in the class of cases considered here, the ability to perceive the moral nature of one's actions is lacking. One cannot draw the moral conclusion because the factual knowledge necessary to make the inference is unconscious. Only when the factual knowledge is recaptured by one's extended memory does one have the ability to bring one's moral knowledge to bear on the particular action. That such unconscious beliefs can be recaptured only means that one could have, and perhaps should have, recaptured them. Not having done so, however, one did not possess the factual knowledge necessary for responsibility.[93]

There is a sense in which one could have acted otherwise in such cases, and a sense in which one could have drawn the necessary inferences from unconscious beliefs. However, this is the sense in which it is said that a person guilty of a negligent omission *could have* done other than he did. This does not mean that he had the same power to avoid doing evil as someone who consciously knows what he is doing. Rather, it means that he could have placed himself in a position to have had that power if he had paid more attention to himself and to the world around him. Insofar as we all have a duty to know ourselves—and morally if not legally we certainly have such a duty[94]—then we may in some cases be responsible for causing harm. The unconscious, in such a case, does not show us that we are responsible because we acted intentionally and for reasons; rather, the unconscious affects responsibility only in that its existence creates a duty to know it. Failure at such a duty may be a culpably negligent omission that causes others, as well as ourselves, harm. Such responsibility for negligent omission is quite different from the responsibility for positive behavior, the subject of this chapter.

FREUD'S CONCLUSIONS ON RESPONSIBILITY

Do Freudians really want to claim more about an extended responsibility than has been discussed? Some contemporary Freudians plainly do,[95] but Freud's own position is not clear. His intuition about the responsibility of the dreaming traitor suggests he does not. There is, however, a lot of Freudian *talk* about responsibility that seems to point the other way.

For example, Freud concluded for several reasons that a person must assume responsibility for the content of his dreams.[96] First, there is a therapeutic concern: "Obviously one must hold oneself responsible for the evil impulses of one's dreams. What else is one to do with them?"[97] Second, Freud said one has no real choice about accepting responsibility:

> If I were to give way to my moral pride and tried to decree that for purposes of moral valuation I might disregard the evil in the id and need not make my ego responsible for it, what use would that be to me? Experience shows me that *I nevertheless do take that responsibility*, that I am *somehow compelled to do so*. The physician will leave it to the jurist to construct for social purposes a responsibility that is artificially limited to the metapsychological ego.[98]

Third, Freud elsewhere noted that it is "instructive to get to know the much trampled soil from which our virtues proudly spring."[99] Given one's search for such knowledge, "There seems to be no justification for people's reluctance in accepting responsibility for the immorality of their dreams."[100]

Freud's apparent position on one's responsibility for parapraxes is similar. Regarding forgotten appointments, he noted:

> There are two situations in life in which even the layman is aware that forgetting—as far as intentions are concerned—cannot in any way claim to be considered as an elementary phenomenon not further reducible, but entitles him to conclude that there are such things as unavowed motives. What I have in mind are love-relationships and military discipline. A lover who has failed to keep a *rendezvous* will find it useless to make excuses for himself by telling the lady that unfortunately he completely forgot about it. She will not fail to reply: "A year ago you wouldn't have forgotten. You evidently don't care for me any longer." Even if he should seize on the psychological explanation mentioned above . . . and try to excuse his forgetfulness by pleading pressure of business, the only outcome would be that the lady, who will have become as sharp-sighted as a doctor in psychoanalysis, would reply: "How curious that business distractions like

> these never turned up in the past!" The lady is not of course wanting to deny the possibility of forgetting; it is only that she believes, not without reason, that practically the same inference—of there being some reluctance present—can be drawn from unintentional forgetting as from conscious evasion.[101]

The keen-sighted woman, Freud seems to suggest, rightly holds her lover responsible for missing the appointment.

Last, consider Freud's discussion of Dora and her responsibility for her cough:

> I now return to the reproach of malingering which Dora brought against her father.... I was obliged to point out to the patient that her present ill-health was just as much actuated by motives and was just as tendentious as had been Frau K.'s illness. [Frau K. was Dora's father's mistress who faked illness in order to be with the father at a health resort.] There could be no doubt, I said, that she had an aim in view which she hoped to gain by her illness. That aim could be none other than to detach her father from Frau K. She had been unable to achieve this by prayers or arguments; perhaps she hoped to succeed by frightening her father..., or by awakening his pity..., or if all of this was in vain, at least she would be taking her revenge on him.[102]

Freud again seems to be saying that Dora's cough, although nominally not a basic action on her part, was nonetheless something she was doing; that through her cough she was also performing the more complex actions of frightening her father, awakening his pity, and taking her revenge; and that she is just as responsible for these actions as was Frau K., who consciously malingered in order to be with Dora's father. Again, for Freud, all of this seems to follow from the fact that Dora's coughing is to be explained by her unconscious mental states.

Despite all this, Freud was not really committed to such a radical extension of responsibility. His first argument regarding responsibility for dreams invites a confusion between the retrospective and the prospective senses of responsible that I distinguished in Chapter 2. In effect, Freud is saying a person must hold himself responsible for doing something about himself if his dreams reveal wishes that he does not like. This argument is applicable to all of psychoanalytic therapy: One must *accept* responsibility to make oneself better, and one *makes* oneself responsible for that task. Accepting such prospective responsibility, however, does not mean that one is retrospectively responsible for the production of an immoral dream, as one would be for a waking fantasy that one consciously called to mind.

Of course, in therapy the analyst may have to convince the patient that he is retrospectively responsible for some events in his past to get him to accept the task of improving himself in the future. Indeed, that seems to be precisely Freud's strategy with respect to Dora. In this,

Increased Responsibility

however, he may be simply playing on the patient's feelings of guilt for her wishes. As noted in Chapter 2, there is a difference between *feeling* guilty about dreams and *being* guilty for them in the sense of being responsible for their production.[103]

Freud's second argument that we are responsible for our dreams invites this same confusion between being guilty and feeling guilty. Even if Freud is convincing when he says that we are *compelled* by our guilt feeings to accept retrospective responsibility, this does not mean that we *are* responsible. To determine whether we are responsible for dreams, we need to know something other than the psychology of guilt or the therapeutic strategies of analysts. We need to know if events such as dreams, forgotten appointments, or neurotic symptoms are truly intentional actions for which we can fairly be held responsible.

In his own therapy Freud himself on occasion worked against the feelings of responsibility of his patients. In his case study of the Rat-Man, for example, Freud reported his discussion with the Rat-Man regarding the latter's responsibility for the unconscious mental states that were a part of his character, as follows:

> In the further course of our conversation I pointed out to him that he ought logically to consider himself as in no way responsible for any of these traits in his character; for all of these reprehensible impulses originated from his infancy, and were only derivatives of his infantile character surviving in his unconscious; and he must know that moral responsibility could not be applied to children.[104]

On such occasions Freud himself separated the feelings of responsibility (guilt) experienced by his patients from their true responsibility.

Freud's third argument about responsibility for dreams invites a different confusion, this time regarding the *object* for which one is responsible. Freud's insight that one's virtues may spring from unconscious mental states of which one may not be overproud is an insight into one's character. The unconscious wishes expressed in a dream may well show one to be less moral in one's inclinations than one had thought. Insofar as one accepts the Aristotelian notion of being responsible for one's character, one is responsible for such wishes no less than for other aspects of one's character.[105] This is not to say that one is responsible for performing an immoral dream in the same way as one can be responsible for performing an immoral play; the responsibility Freud speaks of here is for character and not for the bad consequences of actions.

The case of the keen-sighted woman, of whose responsibility assessments about her forgetful lover Freud apparently approves, is somewhat different. There are a number of possibilities about what is being claimed by the disappointed woman who holds her lover responsible for having forgotten his appointment with her.[106]

First, she might be playing on her lover's guilt, just as a therapist might use his patient's guilt. She, like the therapist, would not really be claiming that her lover was responsible for an action designed to disappoint her. Her saying that he is responsible, however, triggers his guilt feelings for whatever (presumably nontherapeutic) end she has in mind. As previously stated regarding Freud's claims about one's responsibility for dreams, we must be careful to distinguish guilt (feeling responsible) from responsibility (being responsible).

Second, the woman, as Freud does with dreams, might be confusing prospective with retrospective responsibility; she may want her lover to accept responsibility for not meeting her on this occasion so that in the future he will make himself responsible for meeting her. His prospective responsibility for not forgetting is not to be confused with his having performed some past action for which he is retrospectively responsible.

A third possibility is indicated by Freud's suggestion that the military is as wise as the woman in its insights about responsibility for nominal accidents. Both military and civilian law often hold individuals responsible for phenomena like forgotten appointments because other negligent breaches of duty preceded the event in question. For example, one may be responsible for a car accident caused by one's epileptic seizure while driving; this is not because the epileptic movements are actions, but rather because an epileptic is negligent in driving at all.[107] Analogously, one might hold the lover responsible for not meeting the woman on the grounds that he did certain acts that made it unlikely that he would remember the appointment. For example, he may have gotten drunk. Notice, however, that such an account *does not* succeed because the person had "unavowed motives" transforming his unintentional forgetting into an intentional action that he performed; rather, it succeeds because it finds some earlier action of the actor that causes the harm for which he is held responsible.

The sense in which Freud probably intends to impute responsibility in this case is not adequately characterized by any of the three preceding analyses, for none of these ways in which responsibility might be attributed makes use of the most likely explanation for the lover's forgetting. This would be that the lover no longer loves the woman and, even though he may not realize this, the absence of emotion causes him to forget the appointment. To discover the kind of responsibility intended by Freud, it is important to see that the woman's frustration, disappointment, and anger at her lover do not arise from his supposed unavowed motives nor do they depend upon characterizing his forgetting as intentional. Rather, the woman is angry because her lover does not care for her anymore. His failure to arrive at the appointed time shows that he does not care, not that he adopted his behavior as a means to show the woman that he no longer cares. His emotion, or lack of it, explains his behavior, but does not mean that he chose, even unconsciously, that specific behavior as the means of achieving some particular desire.

Consider the following analogous example: One raises one's voice *because* one is angry. Explaining one's behavior in this manner might be taken to mean that one raised one's voice to show anger, in which case the raising of the voice was an intentional action, done for reasons. Much more often, however, the proffered explanation is the following non-reason-giving account: One's anger caused one's voice to become louder, just as it may have caused one's heart to beat faster. One did not perform an action for reasons; these occurrences—the raised voice and the faster heartbeat—were simply caused by one's emotional state.

The nature of the lover's responsibility for missing the appointment can thus not be the responsibility we have for our intentional actions. One might say that the angry person and the lover are responsible for the behavior in question (shouting or not showing up) because they are responsible for their character, which includes certain emotions (or lack thereof in the case of the fickle lover). As stated earlier, everyone may be somewhat responsible for his own character. This includes the character of one's wishes and emotional states. In this attenuated sense one might then hold the lover responsible for the forgotten appointment, not because he did so intentionally or for reasons, but because his forgetting was an expression of a character for which he is responsible.

In neither law nor morals is this kind of responsibility for a harm to be equated with the responsibility that we have when that harm is caused by our intentional actions. Neither the expression of anger and desire nor the lack of emotion is an intentional action that we perform. They are events that happen to us, even though we may have had some choice in the past as to whether such events would be "in character." We may well shun the friendship or the company of those with bad character, but we should not blame them in the way that we blame those who intentionally cause harm or try to do so.

We should note that these distinctions dispose equally well of Freud's arguments to Dora that she was responsible for her symptoms and for trying to separate her father from his mistress. The responsibility need only be Dora's prospective responsibility to improve herself, based on her acceptance of responsibility as part of Freud's therapeutic strategy. Also, the therapeutic strategy is furthered if she feels responsible (guilty) for causing her father suffering and anxiety.

We may thus be said to be responsible for dreams, slips, and symptoms in a variety of ways, all of them different from the way in which we are responsible for intentional actions and attempts. Perhaps not all of Freud's conclusions about responsibility can be fairly reinterpreted in this way, but enough of them can be to raise serious questions about whether Freud himself really believed that his "discovery of the unconscious" compelled the extended responsibility discussed throughout this chapter.

Persons, the Unconscious, and the Body

In closing this chapter it is worth remarking on the concept of a person presupposed throughout it. The idea of a person relied on here (and throughout this part of the book) might be called the Lockean conception of a person. It is Lockean in that it shares Locke's idea that consciousness and memory are essential ingredients in any coherent theory of what persons are. Such a conception of the person surfaced earlier in Chapter 7, where I distinguished "subpersonal" states from mental states truly part of the person, on the basis of a person's privileged access to those states. Such a conception resurfaces here, mostly by the assertion that for any behavior to be an action by the person that person must have privileged access (or deferred privileged access) to the fact that he was acting.

One might wish to attack the conclusions on responsibility of this chapter by attacking this Lockean conception of a person. More specifically, one might urge that the concept of a person should be expanded to include states and events in a person's body that are neither consciously experienced nor recapturable by extended memory. Are not, for example, subliminal perceptions, perceptions by the *person*? Are not the inferences drawn in preprocessing of perceptual information the person's inferences, and is not the drawing of them an action by the person? Indeed, in some sense is not Roy Schafer correct in saying that "all thinking [is] an action"?[108]

Utilizing this concept of a person presupposed throughout this chapter, the correct answer to such questions is a straightforward denial. And the answer to the inevitable rejoinder, "Whose actions or mental states are they, then?" is: "No one's."

It must be understood, however, that we do talk of persons in an alternative way that does allow us to answer these questions differently. Being six feet tall is a state a *person* can be said to be in; having his knee jerk in response to being hit with a hammer is a reflex a *person* can be said to have.[109] This is not the same concept of person, however, that has been presupposed throughout this chapter. The difference can be seen in such sentences as "He did not know that he was six feet tall." "His body" would be an appropriate substitute for the second use of "he," but not for the first because the latter use would suggest that his body knew things that he did not.

As I discussed in Chapter 2, when person is used to refer to the physical body of some member of the human species, it becomes very easy to talk of dreams, slips, and symptoms as the actions of the person. Like any physical object, we can animize talk of event causation by attributing agency to the human body and talk in terms of that body's "actions." Such

Increased Responsibility

actions, however, are actions of a person only in the sense in which water seeking its own level is an action by the water.

One of the deepest aspects of our metaphysics is that we have this bifurcated notion of who we are. We regard ourselves both as physical systems and as personal selves. We even possess, as discussed in Chapter 1, a (provisionally) independent vocabulary with which to discuss ourselves, separate from the vocabulary in terms of which we describe and explain natural objects. When we use the vocabulary of actions, reasons, and intentions, it is clear which concept of a person we have in mind in attributing such events and states. It is not the concept of a person as a physical system. (This can be seen by attempting to substitute "his body," or any other phrase conceptualizing the person as a physical system, for the grammatical subject in mental or action sentences.) Rather, it is the Lockean concept of a person presupposed in this chapter; it is the person who performs actions, and who possesses both conscious and unconscious mental states, that is meant.

The metaphysical concept of one's self is matched by the concept of a person presupposed by our moral principles. The principle of responsibility discussed earlier will serve for illustration. The point this principle illustrates is who the person is who could or could not choose otherwise. Conceptualizing persons as physical systems makes moral nonsense of the principle, for such conceptualization leads to the hard determinist position that no one is responsible for anything. This is because the only sense of "could have done otherwise" relevant to the "actions" of a physical system seems to be the contracausal sense, and in that sense no person could have done otherwise, given the probable existence of sufficient causes for all brain states and physical movements. So construing person also makes metaphysical nonsense of the principle, for there is no room for the concept of choice among the concepts appropriate to regarding one's self as a physical system. Choice belongs to the category of concepts appropriate to describe and explain the actions of persons in the Lockean sense of persons. To speak of a person's body choosing makes as little sense as speaking of a heavenly body choosing to be near the sun.

Hence, whatever scientific usefulness there might be in conceptualizing one's self exclusively as a physical system, one's moral concept of oneself requires eschewing the broader notion of person. Even if one can think of one's self simply as a physical system,[110] with the kind of agency attributed to natural objects such as water and acid, and with the kind of mental states found useful to attribute to computers, such a concept of self will not match the concept of person used to describe and explain behavior and with which we ascribe moral rights and responsibilities. That being so, the extended or physical self, with its metaphorical actions and mental states, cannot be the basis of a claim of extended responsibility.

10 The Unconscious as the Source of a Decreased Responsibility

IN CONTRAST to the kind of examples considered in Chapter 9, the examples to be considered here are those where the individual by our normal criteria has performed an intentional action or an attempt, yet his responsibility is in question because that action is explained by unconscious mental states. In such cases unconscious mental states seem to diminish responsibility rather than increase it.

It will be helpful in bringing out various arguments for decreased responsibility to use a detailed example. Consider the case of *Pollard v. United States*.[1] Francis Pollard was a Detroit police officer who attempted to rob several banks and grocery stores. He was singularly ineffective in his attempts. In the first bank he was nearly captured on his way out because he had his hostage behind him; the hostage grabbed Pollard, who dropped the money and ran. In his second attempt a bank employee raised an alarm, and Pollard again fled. His third attempt was likewise unsuccessful; he was arrested after returning to the scene of an attempted grocery store robbery to pick up his car. He then confessed to eleven other robberies or attempted robberies.

When Pollard was apprehended he confessed the robberies and explained why he had committed them in seemingly comprehensible terms:

> On May 21, 1958, I was reflecting about the hard life that my first wife and I had led in attempting to achieve financial security. Inasmuch as I was about to marry my second wife, I decided that I would not lead the same type of financially insecure life that I led with my first wife. I needed about $5,000 in order to buy a house. My only purpose in deciding to rob a bank was to obtain $5,000, and, if I obtained the money, I did not intend to continue robbing.[2]

The testimony given by the psychiatrists in the case as to Pollard's true purposes for the robberies was quite different, however. The psychiatrists testified that Pollard really robbed the banks and stores out of an unconscious desire to be punished. Such a desire arose from Pollard's guilt about the brutal death of his first wife and child at the hands of a drunken neighbor two years before. The psychiatrists testified that Pollard felt guilty because he was away from home at the time of their deaths. On the basis of this testimony as to Pollard's unconscious motivation, a divided court of appeals held, as a matter of law, that Pollard was not responsible for his robberies.[3]

If one accepts the proffered explanation in terms of unconscious guilt and a consequent unconscious desire to be punished, is Pollard responsible for his robberies and attempted robberies? That the unconscious mental state explanation now seems to decrease rather than to increase the actor's responsibility stems from four separable considerations: (1) that the unconscious mental state *caused* Pollard's robberies, and thus the argument is that they were not his *actions;* (2) that such a state shows Pollard's actions not to have been *intentional;* (3) that such a state shows that Pollard was not as *rational* as he seemed; and (4) that Pollard was *compelled* by his unconscious mental state to commit the robberies.[4] The first two of these considerations—no action because of causation, or lack of intention—rebut those conditions necessary to hold an actor even prima facie responsible. The last two considerations—irrationality and compulsion—invoke traditional excuses to the prima facie responsibility that one has for one's intentional actions. Each factor thus seems to negate responsibility in some way. Each will be considered separately.

Do Unconscious Mental States Diminish Responsibility Simply Because They Are Causes of Behavior?

Dynamically oriented psychiatrists believe that unconscious mental state explanations excuse behavior because they think such unconscious mental states *cause* the bad behavior and that causation is an excuse. The testimony in *Pollard* suggests this in saying that Pollard was "governed by unconscious drives"[5] that exempt him from responsibility.

The problem with such a view of excuse is that of a reductio: If Pollard is to be excused simply because his behavior was caused by unconscious mental states, why are all actions not similarly excused? If all conscious mental life is determined by unconscious mental states, as many psychoanalysts believe, why is everyone not excused for all of his actions, seemingly the product of his conscious decisions but in fact determined by his unconscious mental states?

Some accept this conclusion, not as an absurd implication of a therefore unacceptable premise, but as an important insight about human beings. John Hospers, for example, believes psychoanalysis to have shown that one's "conscious will is only an instrument, a slave, in the hands of a deep unconscious motivation which determines his action."[6] In Hospers's view, one is much like a "puppet whose motions are manipulated from behind by invisible wires, or better still, by springs inside."[7] The effect on responsibility is sweeping. "Criminal actions in general are not actions for which their agents are responsible; the agents are passive, not active—they are victims."[8]

The proper way to view this supposed vitiation of responsibility by the discovery of the unconscious is as part of a general philosophical position known as hard determinism. Determinism is the doctrine that every event (including every human action) has a cause; there are no "free" (in the sense of uncaused) events, in a deterministic world view. *Hard* determinism is the view that moral responsibility for an action cannot be justified if that action is caused. Hard determinism interprets Hart's principle of responsibility (mentioned in Chapter 9) to require contracausal freedom for persons before they can fairly be blamed for their actions, for how "could one have acted otherwise" if one's actions were fully determined?[9]

Psychiatrists, and dynamic psychiatrists in particular, are among the most vehement of hard determinists. Freudians especially believe that at last we have a theory bringing human behavior under the universal, causal laws distinctive of science: "For the first time in history," Karl Menninger assures us, "we have a logical and systematic theory of personality, an explanation of what human nature is and how behavior is determined and modified."[10] Given the prominence of unconscious forces in such a theory, free action (in the sense of uncaused action) is merely an illusion:

> Freud, in 1904, brilliantly demonstrated by analysis of slips of the tongue, forgetting and trains of association that what we call free will or voluntary choice is merely the conscious rationalization of a chain of unconsciously determined processes. Each act of will, each choice presumably made on a random basis, turns out to be as rigidly determined as any other physiological process of the human body.[11]

And without free action, it is further assumed, how can there be any moral responsibility?

Many psychiatrists, to be sure, attempt to escape the hard determinist conclusion that (to quote Hospers) "criminal actions in general are not actions for which their agents are responsible." Yet the escape routes they have proposed end in puzzles that are at least as bad as the puzzle about responsibility that they would escape. Consider four such routes.

The most popular is to take free action as a kind of "first postulate" of both responsibility in law and responsibility in therapy. An example of such a view of therapy is provided by Louisell and Diamond, who assure us that

> it is a mistake to assume that the Freudian psychoanalyst with his emphasis on the specific psychodynamic determinants of behavior abrogates all concept of individual responsibility. Actually, it is an essen-

tial part of the value system of psychoanalytic therapy that the individual be willing to accept more responsibility for himself and his behavior than society ordinarily assigns. The psychoanalyst insists that the individual must accept responsibility for his own unconscious as well as for his conscious thinking.[12]

An example of such a view of moral and legal responsibility is the view of Alexander and Staub that "we may for practical purposes hold the individual responsible for his acts; that is to say, we assume an attitude as if the conscious Ego actually possessed the power to do what it wishes. Such an attitude has no theoretical foundation, but it has a practical, or still better, a tactical justification."[13]

Lawyers have been very sympathetic with this last "reconciliation" of the deterministic viewpoint of psychiatry with the moral responsibility necessary for law to exact a just punishment. Lawyers are apt to be apologetic and are likely to think that the psychiatrists are right about the inability to do other than one's unconscious causes one to do. In such apologetic moments, lawyers talk of *positing* free human actions while admitting that scientifically there could, of course, be no room for such freedom. For example, Judge Levin, the trial judge in *Pollard,* perceived the deterministic assumptions of the psychiatric testimony before him and responded in this typical way:

> Psychiatry and law approach the problem of human behavior from different philosophical perspectives. Psychiatry purports to be scientific and takes a deterministic position with regard to behavior. "Its view of human nature is expressed in terms of drives and dispositions which, like mechanical forces, operate in accordance with universal laws of causation...." Criminal law is, however, "a practical, rational, normative science which, although it draws upon theoretical science, also is concerned to pass judgment on human conduct. Its views of human nature asserts the reality of free choice and rejects the thesis that the conduct of normal adults is a mere expression of imperious psychological necessity. Given the additional purpose to evaluate conduct, some degree of autonomy is a necessary postulate."[14]

This kind of "reconciliation by fiat" cannot possibly work. The law demands more (and so does therapy if it is to avoid being mere propaganda and indoctrination) than that we can *pretend* that people are free and thus hold them responsible *as if* they were. A just legal system (and a nonpropagandistic therapy) requires that people really *be* responsible. Nor will it do to say that people are free because there is a system of thought (law, morals, or therapy) that makes no sense unless they are free; for the whole point of the hard determinist is that such systems of thought indeed make no sense in light of the scientific truth of determinism. If the hard determinist is right about there being no free action, it cannot be the case that we can nonetheless found our moral system on some supposed "postulate" of free action *that we believe, as a matter of scientific fact, to be false!* Our moral beliefs cannot be "sealed off" from our scientific beliefs in this way. If our moral beliefs require that we be free, and if determinism shows that we are not, then we cannot be responsible. Attempting to escape that dilemma by simply swallowing a known contradiction is a peculiarly expensive strategy (for what one then gives up is logic itself).

In fairness to the proponents of this view, what they could have in mind is a kind of Kantian dualism about persons: We are "noumenal" beings free of the laws of causation, and we are empirical objects subject to the usual causal laws to which all objects are subject. There is no contradiction, in such a view, because we are free only in one mode of being and determined only in another. The more modern version of this kind of dualism follows the "linguistic turn" of twentieth-century philosophy, talking not about how things are, but rather, about our talk about how things are. According to the more modern "linguistic dualism" there is a category difference between the concepts of intention, choice, and action on the one hand, and the concepts of motion and mechanistic cause, on the other. We have, in this last view, two quite different ways of conceptualizing our selves: as intelligent persons, or as complicated bits of dumb clockwork. Conceptualized as clockwork, we are fully determined; but conceptualized as intelligent agents who make choices, we are free from determinism—free in the sense that it becomes a kind of "category mistake" to say that our actions are caused. Again, there is no contradiction in saying both that we are free and that we are not, because the system of thought in which free is true is different from the system of thought in which determined is true. The completion of this kind of argument would be to say that law and morality view persons in one system of thought (intelligent agents) and psychiatry views persons in the other (a kind of driven clockwork).

The problem with any such attempt to allow us to have both free will and determinism and yet not contradict ourselves, is that there is no categorical barrier to talking of actions being caused. We fully attribute causation of actions to sets of beliefs and desires, when we explain actions by reasons; to mental causes, such as emotions; to environmental stimuli, such as childhood experiences; and to physiological events, when we know them. As we saw in Chapter 4 with regard to Thomas Szasz's extreme use of the doctrine of category difference, there is simply no reason to deny that causal relations exist between Intentionally characterized states, such as actions, and non-Intentionally characterized states, such as physiology.

Even though there are systematic regularities in our usage of the vocabulary of persons that allow us to grant provisional independence

Decreased Responsibility

(Chapter 1) to this vocabulary from that of natural science, such categorical differences do not prevent scientific discoveries about what causes our various actions. There is thus no separate system of thought—set of categories—in which we are necessarily free. We cannot "have our cake and eat it too," free of contradiction; we are either free or we are not, but we are not both free and not-free because we and our doings can be described in two different categories.

As unsatisfactory is a second strategy sometimes adopted to avoid the rigors of hard determinism. "Not all psychiatrists are dogmatic in their determinism," Wilber Katz advises us.[15] Such psychiatrists conceive of the possibility of there being "a little bit" of determinism. Sheldon Glueck, for example, finds it helpful to "imagine a simple chart which shows the freedom/determinism proportions of a feeble-minded person, an extreme psychotic, an average 'sociopathic' or psychopathic personality," and others.[16] We might then, Glueck tells us, speculate that the feeble-minded person's freedom/determinism mix "will consist of, say, 10 percent . . . endowed intelligent free-choosing capacity, and 90 percent . . . predetermined blocking of freedom of conscious, purposive choice and control."[17] By contrast, the "chart of the psychopath or sociopath, will consist of, say, 30 percent to 45 percent . . . amount of free choice capacity, the balance rigidly controlled."[18]

Human actions, on this view, can sensibly be said to be more or less determined. Causation, in such a view, is more like baldness than it is like pregnancy: One can be more or less bald (depending on the number of hairs on one's head), but it is difficult to imagine being "a little bit" pregnant.

Such a view, if it could be made out, might be the basis of avoiding a complete collapse of responsibility. For one might hold that only those persons who are "strongly caused" to act are not responsible, but that those who are "weakly caused" to act are responsible. Psychiatrists, in such a case, would separate the responsible from the nonresponsible on the basis of the strength of the unconscious determinants.

Stephen Morse has examined this view in psychiatry recently and has given it the apt name of "selective determinism."[19] It is not, as Morse notes, an exclusively psychiatric view, but has at least partial support in commonsense intuitions about responsibility: "Philosophically impure common sense consistently rejects the philosophically pure view [of the irrelevance of causation to responsibility] by assuming that the behavior of all persons is subject to various causes and that these causes vary in their salience and strength."[20] One might, for example, believe that a slum environment is a "strong and salient" cause of criminal behavior in one person, while believing that an emotionally deprived (but materially well-off) childhood is only a weak cause of criminal behavior in another. Popular judgment of a liberal sort might distinguish such cases, urging that the second can fairly be held responsible but the first not.[21]

The stunning problem for both psychiatry and common sense here is that there is no sense to the idea of a "little bit" of either causation or of freedom. It makes sense to say that we are determined or that we are free, but to speak of being partly determined or partly free makes as much sense as speaking of being partly pregnant. There are, to be sure, comparative judgments we make about when one cause is more important than another in producing behavior. There is, indeed, quite a literature on the criteria we use in preferring some causally relevant conditions to others in various contexts.[22] But none of this literature can make sense of the quite different comparative judgment we must make here; this is not a comparison of the relative importance of different causes, but rather, a comparison of the importance of *all* causes, on the one hand, and freedom, on the other. How much causation was there? has to be a sensible question to ask, in this view; the problem is that such a question seems to make no sense at all.

Stephen Morse points out that psychiatrists might attempt to work out the needed idea of "degrees of causation" with the idea of *predisposing causation*, that is, causation that only predisposes (makes more likely) bad behavior and that does not operate as a sufficient condition for that behavior.[23] With such a concept, psychiatrists can urge that unconscious forces that are "strongly predisposing" excuse from responsibility without being driven to admitting that no one is responsible. Strongly predisposing here would mean "renders the bad behavior highly likely." It is an essentially probabilistic notion; when certain factors make the probabilities of bad behavior high enough (strongly predisposed), responsibility is said to evaporate.

Morse himself goes on to argue that the unconscious mental state explanations typically proffered by psychiatrists are at most "weakly predisposing"; thus, even by their own criterion psychiatrists have not shown that the unconscious excuses.[24] There is, however, a more fundamental objection here. This is to question whether talking of strongly or weakly predisposing causes can make any sense of the ideas of more causation or of less freedom.

There is no doubt that there are such things as predisposing causes. To give explanations in terms of probabilistic laws—what Carl Hempel calls inductive-statistical explanations[25]—is an unquestioned feature of both natural and social science. It is also undoubtedly true that the probability of bad behavior following various factors varies greatly among such factors; in short, various correlations make bad behavior variously probable. Much more problematic is the assumption, however, that psychiatric explanations are *irreducibly* probabilistic in character.

356

Decreased Responsibility

It may well be that the psychiatric explanations currently available cite factors that only make bad behavior probable; the factors psychiatrists cite as the causes of crime are not sufficient to produce it. Yet this may reflect only our ignorance about *all* the factors truly sufficient to produce the behavior in question. It is a very controversial matter to assert that *there is no such set of sufficient conditions* for human behavior, and that the best one will ever be able to do is to give probabilistic explanations. Imagine a similar claim about the explanations available to explain the pattern of heads/tails landings of a coin that has been flipped repeatedly. The only explanation we might well have for a roughly 50/50 pattern of heads/tails is a probabilistic one. That does not rule out, however, an explanation of each of the coin's landings (and thus of the overall pattern of landings) in terms of a set of sufficient conditions. One might well think that the physical laws governing matter in motion would explain those events if only we knew enough about the original force exerted on the coin each time, about the coin's physical features, the motion of the air, the features of the landing surface, and so forth.

To be sure, in subatomic physics a plausible case has been made for the claim that events are *only* explainable in terms of probabilistic laws. But no similar case has yet been made showing that explanations (psychiatric or otherwise) of the behavior of human beings must be limited to the probabilistic kind. Yet unless such a case is made, the thesis that there are strongly predisposing or weakly predisposing causes is not a metaphysical thesis about there being degrees of freedom from causation, but rather, a thesis having to do with the degree of our present ignorance. Psychiatrists must thus defend the dubious metaphysical position that human behavior, like the behavior of subatomic particles, cannot be explained by sets of sufficient conditions. Those psychiatrists reluctant to defend any such position cannot make sense of the idea of there being degrees of causation via the idea of "predisposing cause."[26] Rather, the latter group of psychiatrists is committed to a robust determinism (with its supposedly dramatic implications for responsibility).

A third purported escape from the rigors of hard determinism is slightly different from that just explored. It is to admit that human behavior, like other events, is fully determined. In this view, it makes no sense to think of there being a "little bit" of causation. Yet one might urge that our responsibility is affected, not by the degree to which we *are* caused to act, but rather by the degree to which we *have knowledge* of such causes.

If studies show us, for example, that 80 percent of kids from a certain environment commit crimes, we would in this view excuse them from responsibility. If there were no such studies, so that we were ignorant of this probabilistic correlation, then those same individuals would be fully responsible. Since our present knowledge about the causes of human behavior is scant, most people would remain responsible. Only where psychiatrists or others could show us strongly predisposing causes would we excuse. In some such way psychiatrists might seek to avoid the abolition of responsibility yet retain the relevance of unconscious mental state causation to it.

Yet it is wildly inconsistent with our other basic beliefs to think that we attribute responsibility based on the fortuity of our present state of knowledge. If we truly believe that behavior is fully determined and that fully caused behavior is not the responsibility of the person whose behavior it is, it is immoral to say that we will nonetheless hold most people responsible because *we* are ignorant of what causes them to behave as they do. *Our* ignorance of a causation that we think universally exists surely can make no difference to another's responsibility. To say otherwise would be like excusing only those who we know have some *particular* excuse, and holding all others responsible because we are ignorant of what excuse they have, even though we believe that all of those others have some valid excuse but we just do not know which one. If causation excuses, it excuses everyone for determinists. There can fairly be no selection based on a fortuity such as how much of the causal story we may happen to know at any particular time.

It may well be that what Morse calls "philosophically impure common sense" here joins psychiatry in urging either the second or the third purported escape route from the rigors of hard determinism. Many people undeniably soften their judgments about responsibility the more they know of the causal story behind any person's bad behavior. *Tout comprendre c'est tout pardonner* does indeed reflect such persons' judgments on responsibility. Yet such philosophically impure common sense should not survive these insights into its philosophical impurity. If common sense believes that there can be a little bit of causation, then it is wrong—wrong because this is inconsistent with our more basic metaphysical ideas of what kinds of causal relations exist. If common sense believes that the degree of a person's responsibility can depend on the degree of our ignorance about a universally present, excusing condition, then common sense is wrong—wrong because this is inconsistent with our more basic moral belief that such fortuitous factors unconnected to the actor have anything to do with his responsibility. Such inconsistencies cannot protect themselves under the mantle of common sense.

As a fourth and last possibility, one might reason in the following way so as to avoid any of the foregoing pitfalls: One would grant that behavior is fully determined, that causation itself, and not our knowledge of it, excuses; but deny that *all* causes excuse. In such a view, only some kinds of causes excuse; if these are not universally present causes of human behavior, then not everyone is excused by determinism.

Decreased Responsibility

In their attempt to show that expert testimony about the causation of behavior by unconscious mental states is relevant in criminal trials, Bonnie and Slobogin appear to adopt this view.[27] In order to make out such a view, a morally compelling case must be made to show why some unconscious mental states excuse but others do not. As Stephen Morse has pointed out,[28] totally lacking in the Bonnie and Slobogin view is any such case. They seem to assume that "abnormal intrapsychic forces" of the unconscious excuse,[29] but no case is made for why causation by abnormal forces is an excuse when causation by normal unconscious forces is not. Abnormality itself may preclude responsibility; if abnormal is taken to mean madness, then that is indeed the case. But that in no way advances the argument that unconscious mental state causation excuses. Crazy defendants may be held nonresponsible, but that is because they are crazy, not because they suffer from some peculiar form of causation (Chapter 6).

An alternative possibility would be to urge that unconscious mental state causation always excuses, but to deny that all of our behavior is caused by unconscious mental states (even if it is caused by some set of sufficient factors). This is not, of course, an argument a Freudian psychiatrist can make, given the Freudian's theoretical commitment to a universally operating unconscious that underlies *all* of our conscious thinking and action.

Still, a psychiatrist might claim that Freud was wrong here, and that only some behavior is caused by unconscious mental states. The burden on such a psychiatrist is to show why causation by unconscious mental states excuses when causation by other factors (e.g., the environment, physiology) does not. Prima facie, as we saw in Chapter 3, the pretheoretical unconscious recapturable by extended memory would seem to *expand* responsibility, not contract it.

It might be argued that causation by unconscious mental states is different from the causation of behaviorism or physicalism because the structuralism in psychoanalytic theory posits the interaction of separate agencies "within" each person as the source of unconscious mental state causation. Thus, psychoanalytic causal hypotheses are not about familiar, "dumb" causation; rather, the theory is that we are caused to act by the id, the superego, or the unconscious. We might liken such causation to coercion of the self by our "other selves."

This tack is flatly inconsistent with Freud's assertion that we are responsible for unconsciously governed activities because we are identical with the unconscious id as much as the conscious ego.[30] In any case, this task fails even if one grants the animistic concept of subagencies within the self, because mere causation (not amounting to coercion) of some action by that "other person" is irrelevant to one's responsibility. Suppose one person, X, knows another, Y, to have a limited repertoire of jokes that he will tell audiences on the proper occasion. Although X can probably *cause* Y to tell the jokes simply by saying something that jogs Y's memory—for example, the first line of one of the jokes—Y's responsibility for telling a bad joke is still his. It is his free, uncoerced action even though caused by another.[31]

With regard to all four of these purported escape routes, the short of it is that psychiatrists are stuck with a genuine dilemma about the determinism of their theory and the responsibility presupposed by both the law and their own therapy. Psychiatrists cannot consistently believe (1) that all behavior is determined by the unconscious; (2) that causation by the unconscious is inconsistent with responsibility; and (3) that persons are morally responsible, not only in morals and law but also in the clinical practice of psychiatry. None of the four strategies we have examined gives any room to psychiatrists to hang on to all three of these beliefs.

In the face of this unavoidable dilemma psychiatrists are prone to eliminating (3), the belief that anyone is really responsible for anything. This is the hard determinist position. In such a case they will think that law and morality make distinctions (between the responsible and the nonresponsible) that are inherently arbitrary. If they participate in the legal system at all, such psychiatrists do so with the sense that they should manipulate whatever archaic formulas the lawyers are these days using, so as to excuse the maximal number of defendants.[32] Lawyers, on the other hand, tend to adopt the strategy of William James, who, believing there to be an irreconcilable conflict between determinism and responsibility, chose to give up determinism (the first belief discussed).[33] Much of the lawyer's talk of law being premised on free will is designed to deny that determinism is applicable to human action.

Neither lawyers nor psychiatrists very often perceive that they need not make such extreme choices. They need not throw out the window that entire sphere of experience we call our moral life, on the grounds that it rests on an illusion; nor need they, in order to validate that moral experience, engage in a bit of speculative metaphysics of a highly dubious sort. The obvious alternative to either of these extreme views is to deny that there is any inconsistency between determinism and responsibility. (One, in other words, gives up the second of the three beliefs just outlined.)

This alternative is not the same as the supposed middle ground explored earlier. For each of those four alternatives assumed that causation was relevant to responsibility, but tried to avoid hard determinism by notions of degrees of causation, inconsistent but nonetheless assertable first postulates, and the like. The present alternative avoids the need of any such notions because causation itself, in any "degree," is simply irrelevant to responsibility. We are fully responsible no matter what causes may exist for our behavior, be they physiological, behavioristic, or psychoanalytic.

Decreased Responsibility

To make the case for this position—"soft determinism" or "compatibilism"—is by and large to show the irrelevance of causation to the elements of responsibility.[34] Put another way: It is to show that nowhere in the elements under which responsibility is justly attributed to a person is there any presupposition that the person is *free* (where free means free from being caused to act). There are two elements of responsibility with which causation is commonly confused: action and compulsion. I shall discuss each briefly.

John Hospers's earlier quoted, "puppeteer" view of human beings clearly assumes that causation is relevant to the question of whether there has been an action performed. More specifically, Hospers assumes that causation by external forces precludes there having been an action. With such assumptions, his next step is to liken the unconscious to an external force: "Between an unconscious that willy-nilly determines your actions, and an external force which pushes you, there is little if anything to choose."[35] There *is*, however, something to choose here. In the case of the external force—someone else grabbing X's arm, the wind blowing it, getting hit by an avalanche, or being carried out to sea—X does not act. The notion of action is independent of any notion of causation. As set forth in Chapter 2, a basic act is performed only when the actor knows that he is performing it. Presumably the choice to act, and the action, are always determined by various factors, such as chemical balances in the brain, early environment, or character, but the fact that one acts is completely independent of there being, or not being, causes for the action.

This point is unfortunately confused by certain contemporary philosophical accounts of action that urge that a caused action is inconceivable.[36] These accounts assume that if the wind caused X's arm to move, therefore X did not move it. This is simply a mistake. X did not move his arm because X did not know, consciously or unconsciously, that he was moving it. Whether there was a cause, either external or internal, or whether X knew about it, is irrelevant to whether X moved his arm on some occasion. If the wind caused X's arm to move through pressure, or by causing X to shiver involuntarily, then X did not move his arm. If it caused his arm to move because X, made cold by the wind, put on his jacket, then X did move his arm. Causation by the wind is no guarantee that X does not perform the action of moving his arm. Whether X moves his arm depends on the presence or absence of his nonobservational knowledge, including his memory, that he has moved it.

There is, to be sure, a sense in which the concept of a basic action presupposes a view of persons as autonomous. Yet autonomy here does not mean free of causation. As set forth in Chapter 2, the autonomous person presupposed by our practices in blaming is first and foremost a being with causal powers over his own body. Such autonomy does not mean that persons must be "uncaused causers." Causal power of a person is not inconsistent with the exercise of those powers being fully determined by other factors. That we are both autonomous agents and fully determined is not a contradiction.

It is true, there can be no *reduction* of the causal agency of a person to event or state causation, as I argued in Chapter 2. But because we cannot *reduce* personal agency to event or state causation does not mean that a person's acts must be uncaused by those states or events. That the concept of basic action does not have as its criterion, causation by certain states of belief or desire, for example, does not rule out the possibility that basic acts are caused by such states of belief or desire. Indeed, as I pointed out earlier, commonly most basic acts are caused by various belief/desire sets, either conscious or unconscious, and they remain basic acts nonetheless.

There is, thus, nothing in the idea of a basic act (nor in the autonomy or causal power a person must have to perform basic acts) that presupposes persons to be free of the laws of causation. The other kind of autonomy presupposed by the concept of a *complex* action also does not require that we view persons as exempt from the laws of the universe. Autonomy in the sense that we have the causal power not only to move our bodies but to do so in such a way as to change external features of the world is similarly uncontaminated by any presuppositions of freedom. Our capacities to reason practically and to perform complex actions is a power we have to change things in the world to suit our wants. Again, the exercise of such capacities on particular occasions can be as determined as one likes; the truth that we have such capacities remains untouched by the truth of determinism. For our basic acts to cause other events to occur in the world does not require that those basic acts themselves be uncaused.

Persons thus need not stand outside the causal order in order to perform human actions. The other element with which causation is commonly confused is compulsion. Compulsion, as we have seen in Chapter 2, is a well-accepted excuse or partial excuse from responsibility. Yet it no more than the concept of action has anything to do with causation. The factors that may quite properly be said to compel us may (often or always) be causes of the behavior they compel. We would properly describe a threat, natural necessity, high emotional states, or addictions as causes. Yet it is not because such factors are causes that they excuse as compulsions. Such factors excuse as compulsions because they make the choice to do what is required very difficult.

It has been a commonplace at least since the writings of Moritz Schlick[37] and A. J. Ayer[38] that causation does not "make us" do certain things in the way in which a gunman makes us do them. Causation analyzed in terms of regularity of sequence is one way of describing the order we find in nature. As Schlick admonishes:

Decreased Responsibility

> The laws of nature must not be thought of as supernatural powers forcing nature into a certain behavior ... but simply as abbreviated expressions of the order in which events do follow each other.[39]

As Schlick elsewhere elaborates:

> Since natural laws are only descriptions of what happens, there can be in regard to them no talk of "compulsion." The laws of celestial mechanics do not prescribe to the planets how they have to move, as though the planets would actually like to move quite otherwise, and are only forced by the burdensome laws of Kepler to move in orderly paths; no, these laws do not in any way "compel" the planets, but express only what in fact planets actually do.[40]

Compulsion, as we saw in Chapter 2, essentially involves interference with practical reasoning. To be compelled is to have one's normal capacities to reason practically interfered with, either by the constraint on means imposed by threats or natural necessity, or by the constraint on ends posed by internal cravings and emotions.

Most causes of behavior do not operate as such constraints. Simply because we are caused to act by our beliefs and desires, for example, can hardly show that we are compelled. That I am caused to go downtown by my desire to get a haircut is hardly a case of compulsion. This is my uncompelled act, the product of my undisturbed practical reasoning.

Similarly, if I am caused to engage in sharp practices by my greedy character, this is not to say I am compelled. My greed is my characteristic way of unconstrainedly dealing with others in financial matters. It does not constrain my powers of practical reasoning so much as describe how I decide when I am unconstrained.[41]

Similarly, there are doubtlessly large numbers of physiological states and events necessary for each of us to engage in various kinds of basic acts. There may even be certain physiological conditions characteristic of what used to be called volitions or acts of will.[42] Such causes hardly disturb our practical reasonings; rather, they are the conditions that make possible the execution of our desires in action.

Consider last the environmental causes that behaviorists tell us can alone be made into sufficient conditions with which to explain adult behavior. Here, one might think, causation *is* compulsion, because with this species of causation our choices are severely constrained. John Hospers, for example, exercises this familiar argument along the way to showing that the unconscious makes none of us responsible:

> Everyone has been moulded by influences which in large measure at least determine his present behavior; he is literally the product of these influences, stemming from periods prior to his "years of discretion," giving him a host of character traits that he cannot change even if he would ... An act is free when it is determined by the man's character,

say moralists; but what if the most decisive aspects of his character were already irrevocably acquired before he could do anything to mould them? . . . What are we to say of this kind of "freedom"? Is it not rather like the freedom of the machine to stamp labels on cans when it has been devised for just that purpose?[43]

Hospers's last question is not as rhetorical as he seems to think. The freedom essential to responsibility is the freedom to reason practically without the kind of gross disturbances true compulsions represent. Machines have no such freedom because they have no practical reasoning capacities to begin with and so can hardly be disturbed in the exercise of those capacities. Persons, on the other hand, do have such capacities, and simply because what a person desires or believes is caused by his environment in no way makes the exercise of those capacities difficult.

Causation as such is not the same as compulsion. If one wants to show that some causally relevant factor mitigates responsibility, one can do so only by bringing it within some true moral or legal excuse. A deprived childhood, for example, may cause one to be psychotic, in which event one is not responsible because one's general capacities to reason practically are disturbed. Alternatively, such a childhood may cause one to become addicted to drugs or to have certain compulsive cravings. Such addiction or cravings may operate as a partial excuse because they disturb an agent's ability to do what is required in certain circumstances. In any of such cases, however, it is the disturbance of practical reasoning that excuses, *not* the fact that such disturbance was caused.

The upshot of this is very simple. One can grant as true Freud's entire metapsychological story—about events in childhood combining with instinctual drives to cause adult behavior via the intermediate mechanisms of forces and energies operating in the unconscious—and yet reject any supposed implication for responsibility. That adult behavior is caused in this way is no more relevant to responsibility than are the competing causal stories of behaviorism or physiological psychology. One should thus reject out of hand conclusions such as that of David Rapaport's, that "motivated behaviors are those which we cannot help doing,"[44] reached because (for Rapaport) motivations are drives or drive derivatives and thus are causes of behavior. Such psychoanalytic hard determinism is no more sustainable than is any other form of this philosophically indefensible doctrine.

Given the hard determinism of many psychiatrists, their testimony about the effect of the unconscious on responsibility is of dubious value.[45] The psychiatric report in *Pollard,* for example, read in pertinent part:

During that period a dissociative state may have existed and his actions may not have been consciously activated.

"It is therefore our opinion that during the period in question, Pollard, while intellectually capable of knowing right from wrong,

> may have been governed by unconscious drives which made it impossible for him to adhere to the right. It is our belief that this unconscious motivation, which could only be positively identified by prolonged analysis, might have been related to guilt feelings in connection with the death of his wife and child, which compelled subsequent acts that would certainly lead to apprehension and punishment.[46]

If the psychiatrists here meant that Pollard's unconscious mental states acted as a compulsion, all well and good. We shall examine shortly when such a case can plausibly be made out. What one suspects, however, is that these psychiatrists drew no distinction between compulsion and causation, that their idea of being compelled is simply to be "governed by unconscious drives," that their idea of impossibility is not that of a hard choice but of a supposed causal necessity. If this latter interpretation of the testimony is correct, then the testimony is irrelevant to any concern of morality or the criminal law.

Can Unconscious Mental States Show an Apparently Intentional Action to be Unintentional?

It is, of course, paradoxical for psychiatrists to assert that unconscious mental state explanations can show both that what was taken to be an accident was actually an intentional action (the claim examined in Chapter 9), *and* that what was taken to be an intentional action was actually an accident (the claim to be examined here). Two senses in which the latter claim is sometimes articulated can be easily dismissed. The first invokes the mechanistic part of psychoanalytic theory just discussed. The claim is that because of one's instinctual drives one does not really perform any actions intentionally; that is, acting on intentions is just part of the illusion of freedom. This claim fails even more dramatically than the parallel claim about actions; people act intentionally despite being caused to act. Whether there are instinctual drives that cause people to act as they do is as irrelevant to their actions being intentional, as are the questions of whether environment or physiology causes persons to act as they do.

The other sense in which it is sometimes said that an actor failed to act intentionally despite his seeming knowledge of what he was doing is illustrated by the kind of testimony courts receive under the diminished capacity and insanity defenses. As argued in Chapter 6 and examined in the next subsection, one diminishes the responsibility of an accused by showing his irrationality and, as we saw in Chapter 2, rationality and intentionality are closely connected. Yet psychiatric insights in this area speak to a *general* incapacity for rational action and not to the intentional nature of some *particular* action. Such insights can negate intention only in the extreme cases, that is, when an *agent* is so fundamentally nonrational or irrational that he is not so regularly the proper subject of the action/intention predicates typically employed to describe behavior. Unconscious mental states may show an actor to be less rational than previously thought and thereby influence one's *general* willingness to apply the action/intention predicates to him. However, this need have little to do with some particular action being unintentional.[47]

There are two other possibilities that are not so quickly dismissed. The first is to invoke the excuses of mistake or ignorance by claiming that unconscious mental state explanations show that such excuses existed even though the conscious knowledge of the agent would ordinarily preclude either of them. The second is to alter the description of the action that must be intentional if the actor is to be culpable, and to argue both that psychoanalytic insights show that such an expanded description of the action must be used, and that under the new description, the action may *not* be intentional. Each of these requires more elaborate treatment, and each is considered in turn.

UNCONSCIOUS MISTAKES OR IGNORANCE

If we apply the analysis of ignorance and mistake developed in Chapter 2 to a case such as Pollard's, to say that Pollard was mistaken about some fact would be to say that he believed some proposition p to be true when it was false. For example, suppose Pollard had believed that the gun in his hand was a toy. If armed robbery is worse than unarmed robbery, then a person who knows he is robbing someone at gunpoint is more culpable than someone who believes he is using a toy gun. Only if Pollard believed he held a real gun would he be said to be intentionally robbing another *with a gun*.

Ignorance, in contrast to mistake, is where the actor has no belief one way or the other about the relevant fact. Suppose Pollard did not know whether the gun in his pocket was real and yet carried out the robbery. His ignorance would also mean that he did not intentionally rob another with a gun.

The actual testimony in *Pollard* indicated that the only thing of which Pollard was ignorant, or about which he was mistaken, was his motivation. Yet that ignorance or that mistake was surely irrelevant to the question of whether his actions of robbing the banks were intentional. If he did not rob the banks to secure funds to buy a house, but did so for some other reason, such as a desire to be punished, he still robbed the banks intentionally.

One must create some imaginary testimony about Pollard's unconscious if one is to find an instance where it is even arguable that Pollard did not intentionally rob the banks. Suppose that Pollard unconsciously identified

Decreased Responsibility

banks with wombs and pistols with penises. Would this, if true, mean that he did not believe he was committing armed robbery of a bank, even though that is what he said he was doing? The answer plainly seems to be in the negative. At most, such testimony would show that Pollard believed inconsistent things; he seemingly believed both that he was robbing a bank, and that he, as one example, was returning to his mother's womb. Here the difference between mistake and ignorance becomes crucial: His mistaken beliefs simply do not imply that he does not also have the beliefs that he says he has. The latter conscious beliefs mean that he was intentionally robbing the bank, even if the former *unconscious* beliefs mean that he was unconsciously albeit intentionally doing something else at the same time. Rather than denying that Pollard believed he was robbing a bank, such psychiatric insight should lead us to abandon our general assumption that a person's beliefs are consistent.

There is one situation in which it might be said the actor does not have the belief he claims to have in light of our discovery of another inconsistent belief. This is the situation envisioned by the Model Penal Code's definition of willful blindness.[48] Even if an actor knows to a high probability some proposition p, if he also believes that p is not the case, then he is excused. The actor is excused in such cases because the clear existence of the mistaken belief causes one to question one's initially uncertain assumption that the actor believed p to begin with. Pollard, for example, might believe that he has his real gun because he remembers that he fired it yesterday at the firing range, and that he then put it in the pocket of the coat he is now wearing; yet if it is discovered that he also believes that it is not a real gun—just before going into the bank he takes it out of his pocket and finds "Revell Toys" stamped on the handle—he is excused. His first belief is the result of an inference he makes from evidence that on reflection still seems unshakable. His second belief, however, is also based on unshakable evidence of a more direct and more recent nature. Pollard's state of mind might be described as saying to himself, This must be a real gun, but how can it be? In such circumstances our confidence that he knows the gun is real evaporates.[49]

The hypothesized psychoanalytic insight that Pollard was mistaken about the presence of the real gun cannot, however, fit itself into this special situation. The mistaken belief to which it points is unconscious and does not therefore shake one's confidence in the conscious, contradictory belief. One belief being conscious, the other unconscious, it is easy to say that the actor has both beliefs even though their contents contradict each other.[50]

Suppose, however, that psychiatric testimony is in terms of ignorance and not mistake; that is, the claim is that Pollard did not know he was wielding a real gun in his robberies. The problem, of course, is that faced earlier: Pollard in some sense plainly *did* know he was using a real gun, so that to make the imagined insight comprehensible, one must distinguish senses of know.[51] The most plausible thing to say is that Pollard knew the gun was real only in the sense of propositional knowledge; he could describe what he was doing as using a real gun, but he did not know the gun was real in the sense that he did not emotionally appreciate that he was endangering innocent lives by using a real gun. Unconscious mental states could explain why he was "emotionally ignorant" of his use of a real gun. Self-deception is one possibility, but other unconscious mental state explanations would also be possible. Whether such emotional ignorance in the face of propositional knowledge excuses is a matter of degree; one must inquire how "dissociated" was the individual? One can imagine war-hardened fighter pilots who do not appreciate the horror they know they cause not being excused in the least. On the other hand, such pilots may have such unconscious feelings of guilt so that they cannot let themselves emotionally appreciate what they are really doing. In this case there might be some mitigation of their responsibility. Unconscious mental states have at least this potential for excuse.

This would, however, be a matter of affirmative excuse. It would not convince one that the action in question was unintentional. Pollard intentionally committed armed robbery if he knew (could state) that robbery was what he was doing, even if he did not know (emotionally appreciate) the moral nature of what he was doing. The result is that no explanation of his action by unconscious mental states can induce one to withdraw the description of the action as intentional. Even if unconscious mistaken beliefs are discovered, or if other unconscious mental states are discovered that prove plausible ignorance of some sort, the actor acted intentionally.

THE EFFECT OF UNCONSCIOUS MENTAL STATES ON THE DESCRIPTION OF THE PROHIBITED ACTION

Pollard intentionally robbed some of the banks and attempted to rob the others. Nothing about his unconscious mental states can show otherwise, given his clear knowledge of what he was doing and his purpose in doing it. If psychoanalytic insight about the unconscious is to show that he did not act intentionally, it will have to be along avenues quite different from the traditional excuses of mistake and ignorance. The avenue that suggests itself is to leave the *criteria* of intentional, which seem satisfied no matter what unconsciously mistaken beliefs are supposed, and talk about the *object* of the intention.

This avenue is suggested by the *Pollard* case because of the way in which Pollard went about his robberies. His methods were singularly ineffective. Suppose it were true, as the psychiatrists testified, that he unconsciously wanted to get caught in order to expiate his unconscious guilt

Decreased Responsibility

about his wife and child. That would mean that he did not really intend to rob the banks *and get away with it*; rather, he intended to go to jail. Does this affect his culpability?

For purposes of ascribing moral responsibility, one asks whether an action was intentional under that description of it that renders the action morally bad. A change in the description may change the answer to the question, Was the action intentional? Suppose, first, that "robbing the bank" is the relevant description. Suppose further that an accused quite consciously wants to go to jail, gives notice to the police that he will rob a certain bank at a certain time, and then does so. If such a person had confederates, they might well conclude that he did not really intend to rob the bank. One might say that their idea of robbing a bank includes getting away with the money.

This, however, would be a mistaken line of analysis. The confederates have expectations beyond those generated from the meaning of robbing a bank. Success may be a part of their plan, but it is not part of the meaning of robbing a bank. Rather, one should say of the man who wants to go to jail that he robbed the bank in order to go to jail. His intentional robbing of the bank is his adopted means of getting something he wants, but it is a good means only if he truly does rob the bank. Otherwise, he will not go to jail.

Because of this, psychiatric testimony cannot show that people like Pollard do not intentionally rob banks. If the psychiatric insight about Pollard is to be relevant to his culpability, one has to urge that it is because it changes the morally relevant description of his action. Such insight might refine the categories of culpable acts by suggesting the possibility that an action thought to be quite bad (robbing a bank) can be less bad if done with no intention of getting away. One might then expand the description of the bad action to "robbing the bank *and keeping the money.*" If this is the object of the intention or of the attempt, then Pollard and the individual who wants to go to prison were not trying to do this and did not intend to accomplish this.

Pollard is, of course, a bit different from the hypothetical bank robber who planned to go to jail. The latter had no conflicting reasons for robbing the bank. Pollard, in contrast, probably thought that the reason for which he robbed the bank was exactly what he said: to get enough money to buy a house. To say of Pollard that he did not intend to rob the bank and keep the money, it would be necessary not only to show that he had unconscious reasons to the contrary, but also to deny that his conscious reasons were reasons for his action at all.

As we saw from the analysis in Chapter 7, psychoanalysis may do both of these things. An actor may be quite confident that he knows the reason for which he is acting and be completely wrong about it. Psychoanalytic insight does not simply add to the conscious reason an unconscious reason for which one also acts; in many cases the unconscious reason *supplants* entirely the conscious reason as an explanation of the action. The practice, long before Freud, of novelists and historians finding "the real reasons" for actions illustrates the intuitive sense that psychoanalytic explanations have in this regard.

In Chapter 7 we examined the contrary view of Richard Peters on this point. Peters attempted to show first that "there are a large number of cases . . . which have such an obvious and acceptable explanation in terms of conscious reasons that it seems absurd to look around for unconscious motives" at all;[52] and second that "if the stated reason for an action is not implausible as an explanation of it . . . it would be odd to discount the conscious reason because there was *also* a plausible explanation in terms of an unconscious wish."[53] The court of appeals in *Pollard* also implicitly adopted this view, for it felt obliged to discount Pollard's conscious motivation in order to make room for the unconscious mental state explanation proposed by the psychiatrists:

> The claimed motivation [money] seems pointless. Pollard, during his first marriage, had been receiving the regular salary of a policeman with promotions . . . His second wife, at the time of her marriage to him, had money of her own—enough to pay her own bills, and take care of her daughter with the money which was paid for support by her former husband . . . Pollard's financial condition could not be considered a reasonable motivation for his attempted bank robberies. As far as income went, he was much better off than most other policemen and if such a financial condition could be considered a reasonable motivation for Pollard's attempted robberies, every other policeman in the department would have had twice the motivation to commit such crimes as Pollard had.[54]

The problem with this view is the one stated in Chapter 7: The sets of beliefs and desires that *caused* Pollard's robberies cannot be decided upon in some *a priori* way. No matter how plausible or implausible his conscious motivation may have been, it is quite possible that his unconscious guilt and desire to be punished were his only motives. Although one's expectations about a person's actions may be better satisfied by some motivational accounts than others, such pragmatic considerations about the explanation have no effect on its truth.

As a consequence, Pollard may not have intended to get away with the money even though he thought he did. His real reason for robbing the banks may indeed have been to get punished. If this is true, then Pollard is only guilty of intentionally robbing a bank, and not of intentionally robbing a bank with the intent of keeping the money. If there is a difference morally, then Pollard's culpability is correspondingly less.

Decreased Responsibility

It may seem that however much psychoanalytic insight might generate such refinements in moral descriptions, it is irrelevant to legal liability for punishment. One might think that the trial judge in *Pollard*, for example, was stuck with one description of the prohibited action, namely, bank robbery, and that therefore Pollard's liability cannot be altered even if his responsibility is diminished. To some extent this is true; laws do spell out those categories of actions that constitute not only the *actus reus* of an offense but also the object of the prohibited intention. However, judges cannot rest content with only the statutory description of the object of an intention, or any other mental state.[55] They must include other descriptions, and their only criterion for doing so can be their assessment of the relative culpability of those who act with those differently described objects of intention. They thus have considerable latitude to alter the descriptions, perhaps as much as any moralist.

UNCONSCIOUSLY IMPOSSIBLE "ATTEMPTS"

Implicit in the foregoing discussion of *Pollard* is the possibility that for the attempted bank robberies, although not for the completed robberies, testimony about unconscious mental states might show that the specific intent required for conviction is not present. It will be recalled that to be guilty of a general intent crime such as murder the accused need only know that his action is substantially certain to cause the death of another; he need not have death as his purpose. Yet to be guilty of a specific intent crime such as *attempted* murder, the accused must have performed some act with the death of another as his purpose. The reasons with which he acted, in other words, must have included a desire to kill.

Because psychoanalytic insight may show that the reasons for which a person thought he acted are not the reasons for which he acted at all, it is possible that what the actor himself thinks is an attempt to kill, for example, in reality is not. What he is really trying to accomplish may be something else entirely, although he is unaware of it.

Accordingly, the psychiatric testimony in *Pollard could have been* such that one should not convict him of attempted bank robbery. Suppose the testimony was that Pollard entered the banks because unconsciously he wanted to scare the female tellers. He thought at the time, and thinks now, that the reason for which he entered the banks was to rob them, yet he always found some pretext not to rob them, as indeed he did in many of his actual "foiled" attempts. Suppose the psychiatric testimony explains this failure as being consistent with his true motivations in entering the banks. In such a case one should say that Pollard did not attempt to rob the banks, even though he thought he did.

There is a related case that should also be mentioned here. Suppose

Pollard had conflicting mental states when he entered the bank with a gun; he wanted to rob the bank, but his moral beliefs were such that he did not want to rob the bank. His entering the bank with the gun is truthfully explained by his desire to rob the bank; his failure to rob the bank is explained, not by the beliefs he thinks explain it—that the teller has pressed an alarm—but by his unconsciously executed moral beliefs. One might excuse Pollard in such a case, but not because he did not attempt to rob the bank. Assuming his entering with the gun goes beyond mere preparation, he did attempt to rob the bank because he did an act with that as his reason. If he is to be excused in this latter case, it would be because of some affirmative defense of "internal control." Such a defense has in fact been proposed although not adopted. Alan Dershowitz once urged the defense on utilitarian grounds—the nondangerousness of self-frustrating attempters—rather than on grounds of diminished culpability.[56] To make an argument on the latter ground might be analogous to the affirmative defense of withdrawal.

If one fractionates the self as does Freud's topographical and structural metapsychologies, it becomes problematic for both these cases whether the actor should be held not guilty of an attempt. Pollard consciously thinks he is entering the bank to rob it; he is attempting to rob the bank. He (his consciousness) might be thus likened to the bank robber whose attempts are, unknown to him, factually impossible. The only difference is that in this situation he cannot succeed because "another part of him" either wants something else not requiring the robbery of the bank (the first case), or wants not to do the robbery (the second case). Yet if one takes seriously the split between Pollard's System Csc. and his System Usc., *he* (Csc.) deserves to be punished like any other whose attempts are factually impossible. This is another reason (in addition to those adduced in Chapter 11) to talk, not of personified subagencies, but of whole persons with conflicting or competing mental states. Doing so gives credit where credit is due, namely, to Pollard for the complete set of his mental states.

Although each of these two kinds of unconsciously impossible attempts is conceptually possible, surely they are quite rare in real life. Most bank robbers are like Pollard; they may have unconscious mental states causing them to act as they do, but the kinds of unconscious mental states they have (not being unconscious *reasons* for action—see Chap. 8) do not in the least affect their status as intentional or attempted robbers of banks.

The Unconscious and Rationality

The second way unconscious mental states might reduce responsibility for otherwise intentional actions is by showing the actor to be less rational than he seems. As set forth in Chapter 2, a basic moral requirement for

Decreased Responsibility

holding an agent responsible *for* some harm or some attempted harm is that the agent *be* a responsible (i.e., a rational) agent. This is because human beings who are seriously irrational or nonrational lack an essential attribute of personhood. Beings must possess rationality, the essential feature of our shared humanity, to be the proper subjects of praise or blame. Beings who lack this feature to some serious degree, such as animals, young children, and very crazy adults, cannot fairly be held responsible for some particular harm because they are not responsible (accountable) at all.

Lawyers often confuse this requirement that the agent be rational with the determinist thesis discussed earlier. It is often said that the mentally ill do not have free will, using free to refer not to lack of compulsion but rather, lack of causation. Although this is true, in that sense of free nobody has any free will. Unless one can make sense of something like Glueck's sliding scale of degrees of freedom, to excuse the mentally ill because their behavior is caused requires that all of us be similarly excused (since our behavior is similarly caused).

The responsibility of the mentally ill thus turns on their lack of rationality, not on their lack of freedom from causation that all of us in fact lack. Since an agent's serious irrationality by itself reduces or eliminates his responsibility, one can readily see how insights about the unconscious may contribute to that reduction. If the unconscious mental states that truly explain an agent's actions over time are irrational desires or beliefs, then he is irrational. If, for example, such unconscious mental states conflict with other things he wants very much, such an agent is irrational because he frustrates himself with his actions. Indeed, this possibility of conflicting desires would seem to be the typical consequence of many unconscious desires. By hypothesis, an actor is not aware of unconscious desires in a way that allows him to integrate them into an ordered set of wants that he can then maximally satisfy.[57] This is true even if an actor such as Pollard seems to be normally rational with respect to both his criminal act and his acts in general. For seemingly quite rational actors, however, such as Pollard, one may be more suspicious of the *truth* of the psychoanalytic explanations in terms of their unconscious mental states. One should particularly be suspicious of such explanations if they follow from the deterministic assumptions of the metapsychology rather than from the detailed clinical observations of the individual necessary to discover his unconscious mental states. Still, it is possible that individuals such as Pollard act from irrational desires or beliefs, and not for the seemingly intelligible and rational reasons for which they think they act. If one believes the psychoanalytic explanations in terms of such states, and enough of Pollard's behavior over time is so explained, then his behavior could be excused because it is so irrational as to be mad. The actual testimony in the case was not broad enough to establish this because it did not show Pollard to be in that small class of grossly irrational human beings we call mad or crazy.

Unconscious Mental States as Compulsions

The third and final way in which unconscious mental states may reduce responsibility is by *compelling* actions. Although I argued in Chapter 6 that compulsion is not the reason for which one excuses the mentally ill, it is a well-established excuse in its own right. Moreover, some unconscious mental states do seem to have the potential at least to operate as compulsions. One must carefully delineate when this is the case, however. If the blunderbuss approach of those who identify all causation as compulsion is to be avoided, a careful account of the relation of unconscious mental states to the excuse of compulsion is required.

Discovery of an actor's unconscious mental states has often been thought to show that an intentional action by that actor was compelled on either of the two models of compulsion distinguished in Chapter 2. The first such model was one in which an external constraint—either a threat or natural necessity—artificially constrains the means to an end that the actor legitimately wants. As an example of where the unconscious might involve this kind of compulsion, consider one of Freud's obsessional neurotics, the Rat-Man.[58] One of the Rat-Man's symptoms was a bizarre series of thoughts and actions focused on the repayment of a small debt. The Rat-Man, while on maneuvers in the military, had ordered a new pince-nez. It had been sent "payment on delivery" and the female post office clerk paid for it out of her own pocket. Although the Rat-Man had been told this, his captain subsequently told him that a certain Lieutenant A had paid for the pince-nez, and it was to him that the Rat-Man owed the money.

The Rat-Man became obsessed with repaying Lieutenant A. However, A told the Rat-Man that he had not paid for the pince-nez. The Rat-Man therefore planned a complicated maneuver in which he was to take Lieutenant A and another to the post office to which the pince-nez had been delivered and to have A repay the clerk so that the Rat-Man could then keep his vow to "repay" A.

The Rat-Man on one particular occasion was undecided about carrying out his extraordinary plan and found himself on the train going *away* from the town in which A was located. At each stop of the train the Rat-Man found himself unable to get off and do as he had resolved to do, namely, go to A and take him to the post office to repay the debt. If we assume that nonpayment of the debt was wrong of the Rat-Man, should his failure to do so be characterized as compelled?

Freud offers the following explanation for the Rat-Man's inability to repay the debt. Through a series of puns on the German word for rats

Decreased Responsibility

(*ratten*) and the patient's associations, Freud concluded that the Rat-Man had come to believe that if he repaid the loan, his father and a close female friend would be subject to the "rat-punishment." The rat-punishment, which had been described to the Rat-Man by the same captain who had said Lieutenant A had paid for the pince-nez, consisted of rats feeding at the anus of the victim. Freud further explained the patient's peculiar mode of repayment (involving A, who was owed nothing) as due to a vow that he had made to himself: "Now you must really pay back the money to A." Such a vow, impossible to fulfill, was a kind of punishment the patient had imposed on himself for a fantasy he had had about his lady friend and his father having children (which neither could do).

The crucial item in assessing the Rat-Man's responsibility for not paying back the money is his belief. If the Rat-Man in some sense believed that he had to refrain from repaying the money to protect his father and the lady from the rat punishment, then he was compelled in the first sense of compulsion analyzed in Chapter 2. Both his father, who was deceased at the time, and his lady were dear to him; he was consciously horrified at the thought of the rat punishment being inflicted on them. His belief left him "no real choice": He could not repay the money, at least not directly.

The Rat-Man did not consciously believe this. Thus, Freud's explanation once again (as in Chapters 8 and 9) depends on his supplying evidence for the hypothesized unconscious belief. The evidence Freud mainly relied on here was the patient's recollections of two different occasions. The first was when the patient first heard of the rat punishment. "At that moment," the Rat-Man told Freud, "the idea flashed through my mind that this was happening to a person who was very dear to me."[59] Freud then obtained from the patient the admission that there was not one person but two, and that they were his lady friend and his father. The second crucial occasion remembered by the patient was later in the same evening when the same captain handed the Rat-Man the packet containing the pince-nez. "At that instant," Freud relates, "a 'sanction' had taken shape in his mind, namely, *that he was not to pay back the money* or it would happen – (that is, the phantasy about the rats would come true as regards his father and the lady)."[60] It was then, the patient also recalled, that he made the vow to himself to repay the money to A and not to the post office clerk to whom he knew it was truly owed.

One problem with ascribing to the Rat-Man the belief that his father would be punished was the fact that the latter had long before died. Freud, however, produced a complicated story about how, in a sense, the patient never really believed this: During his childhood the patient had unconsciously hated his father and unconsciously wished for him to die; this gave rise to unconscious guilt feelings, which in turn caused the patient to deny that his father was dead. As evidence of such denial, Freud noted:

> For a long time he had not realized the fact of his father's death. It had constantly happened that, when he heard a good joke, he would say to himself: "I must tell Father that." His imagination, too, had been occupied with his father, so that often, when there was a knock at the door, he would think: "Here comes Father," and when he walked into a room he would expect to find his father in it.[61]

Even crediting all of this, do we want to say that the Rat-Man believed that if he paid back the money the rat punishment would really be visited upon his lady friend and upon his long-dead father? If the patient were asked, he doubtlessly would deny that he believed any such thing. But that might only show that his conscious beliefs contradicted his unconscious beliefs, not a surprising fact to a Freudian. The fantasies recalled by the patient are comparatively good evidence for the belief in question, but even here one should ask whether conscious fantasies necessarily evidence unconscious beliefs.

Even if we grant in such cases the existence of the problematic belief, there is another problem with making out compulsion here. That is in saying that the Rat-Man used this belief in his practical reasonings about not getting off the train and repaying his debt. The Rat-Man deliberated at each stop about getting off the train, yet among his conscious practical reasonings there appears none that include his desire not to punish his friend and his father and the belief that if he repaid the debt, he would subject them to the rat punishment. So to say that he made this calculation, one must say that he did so unconsciously.

And now we face the problem raised in Chapters 8 and 9 about Freud's explanations: Does the unconscious belief operate here only as a *cause* of why the patient decided to stay on the train, or does it, in conjunction with a desire, operate as a reason? If only the former, then we cannot say that the patient's practical reasoning was disturbed or was artificially constrained—the first model of compulsion—because there was no practical reasoning to be constrained. Only if Freud can show that the Rat-Man's unconscious belief operated as part of an unconscious reason for action can he show the Rat-Man to have been compelled.

These are serious problems for a Freudian in making out the Rat-Man, or other instances of obsessional neuroses, as fitting the first model of compulsion. Needed is what Freud rarely if ever seems to be able to give us: unconscious reasons for action.[62] Despite that, my own intuition is that a strong case can be made for obsessional neurotics such as the Rat-Man being compelled to some degree. This, I think, is because they may fit the second model of compulsion, which does not require that the unconscious belief figure into a reason-giving explanation.

If we were to pursue the Rat-Man case study further along these lines, we would cease talking of unconscious *beliefs* and begin emphasizing the

Decreased Responsibility

patient's unconscious *emotions*. (Indeed, Freud talks of the Rat-Man's "great obsessive fear" more than his obsessive beliefs.[63]) Still, I shall return to the simpler example of Francis Pollard as an illustration of when unconscious mental states might plausibly be taken to establish that an intentional action was compelled.

Pollard was tried under the version of the insanity defense that explicitly raises the issue of compulsion: Was the accused "irresistibly impelled" to do what he did? Putting aside the concept of drives that is simply the causal theory of the instinct and economic metapsychology, one might still discern some compulsion in Pollard's situation by examining the explanation given by the psychiatrists.

Suppose Pollard did unconsciously feel guilty about the death of his first wife and child. He may have felt guilty because he had not been there; alternatively, he may have felt guilty because he had unconsciously wished to kill them himself.[64] In either case, could such unconscious guilt *compel* Pollard to do an act for which he would be punished? If one can discover unconscious emotions, seemingly cases such as Pollard's might sometimes fit into the second model of compulsion distinguished in Chapter 2.

How can one experience a *feeling* of guilt and not know it? More generally, how can one *feel* compelled to act in certain ways so as to expiate such guilt, and yield to such compulsion, without being aware of the feeling or the yielding? This problem revives the epistemic puzzles we examined in Chapter 7, about how one can sensibly use experiential terms without the person whose experience it is being aware of it.

Contrary to what philosophers contemporary with Freud may have thought,[65] Freud was aware of this conceptual problem. In discussing unconscious emotions generally, Freud wrote, "It is surely of the essence of an emotion that we should be aware of it, i.e. that it should become known to consciousness. Thus the possibility of the attribute of unconsciousness would be completely excluded as far as emotions, feelings and affects are concerned."[66] Nonetheless, Freud continued, "In psycho-analytic practice we are accustomed to speak of unconscious love, hate, anger."[67] The meaning Freud attached to such expressions was that the *idea* attached to the emotion can be unconscious even if the feeling that *is* the emotion cannot. Although Freud expressed this in the paramechanistic language of his economic metapsychology,[68] his thought can be explained without this theoretical baggage.

As we have seen in Chapter 1, mental words require intensional objects. Thus, one believes *something* and does not believe or desire in the abstract; one hates something, fears something, or loves something. Thus, to say that one is conscious of a desire or an emotion is to say that one can state what the object of that desire or emotion is. One's privileged access in knowing one's mental experiences usually includes immediate knowledge of the intensional objects and not just of the kind of state one possesses.

The psychiatric claim about an unconscious emotion such as Pollard's unconscious guilt can be understood as the claim that an actor does consciously experience or feel something, but does not know the object of his emotion.[69] One may feel angry or afraid without knowing the object of such anger or fear; one may experience the uneasy and tensed craving characteristic of compulsive desires without knowing what one craves. A further example is Freud's idea of "free-floating anxiety," a felt anxiety without the subject's knowing what he is feeling anxious about. If Freud's "idea" is defined as the intensional object of an emotion, then one can say with Freud that the affect is conscious but its idea is unconscious.

The sense in which we can speak of the actor yielding to such unconscious but passionately felt desires should be evident. Kleptomaniacs feel compelled and know that they yield to compulsion when they steal; yet they do not know the object of their passionate desires. They know only that they feel that they must steal. They are compelled by an indefinite craving for some unknown object or objective. A few thefts readily tell them it is not the stolen objects themselves.[70]

Pollard presents a less convincing example of compulsion than does the kleptomaniac or the obsessional neurotic, probably because one is less inclined to believe the explanation proposed for his behavior. Unlike the obsessive lady discussed in Chapter 9 who called her maid for no apparent reason, Pollard had a perfectly intelligible, conscious motive for acting. In such circumstances one is often more reluctant to accept as a factual matter that some unconscious emotion really explains his behavior. But if one does believe the psychiatrists in this case, then Pollard's action of robbing the banks may also be compelled to some degree. If his unconscious guilt and consequent need to be punished truly explain his action of robbing the banks, then it may have been very difficult for him to act in any way but to alleviate this guilt feeling.

This does not mean, however, that persons such as Pollard are necessarily excused. Compulsion is a matter of degree. One can be more or less compelled, depending on the severity of the constraints on choice or the strength of the emotions on which one acts. The more serious is the legal offense charged, the greater the compulsion necessary for exculpation. The compulsion sufficient to excuse will be difficult to determine since it is a matter of degree and relative to the gravity of the offense. This will be particularly true where a jury must ascertain whether the accused acted from certain unconscious beliefs or unconscious emotions. In the standard cases of compulsion discussed in Chapter 2 the evidence is better. If there is a threat to an actor or some objective circumstances that create a "natural necessity," there is good evidence that the actor believed himself to be

Decreased Responsibility

acting under the duress of threat or natural circumstance. Even in the case of provocation, which depends on the existence in the actor of a passionate emotion, one can draw from a fund of common experience to ascertain whether one would be enraged at whatever constitutes the provoking circumstances. One uses this fund to infer whether the actor was in fact enraged.

On this second kind of compulsion the law may get some help from psychiatry. If it is shown, for example, that a kleptomaniac's thefts are tied to strong sexual feelings, one can begin to understand what it would be like to experience what kleptomaniacs experience before and as they steal. Sexual tension is an emotion with which most people are familiar. If the urge to steal is similar to a sexual urge, then there is a fund of experience on which to draw in determining whether the choice was hard enough to mitigate or excuse the actor from responsibility.

It may seem that the unconscious provides an excuse of compulsion much more often than the limited circumstances allowed so far. One might think that unconscious desires *always* compel the behavior they cause. Consider, in this regard, an argument along these lines by David Blumenfeld:

> As long as we are aware of conflicts, we are free to determine what most we want and to act accordingly. But once we accept the notion that our desires may be repressed, conflict assumes a different status. For repression makes it psychologically impossible for a person to become aware of at least one of his conflicting desires and the possibility of taking that desire into account in his decisions is closed. If I desire both to do X and not to do X and I am rendered incapable of making myself aware of the conflict, I cannot deliberate effectively about which desire to act on, for my deliberation must lack essential data. I cannot bring to bear my powers of consideration, rational faculties, power of review or whatever we wish to call the agency of conscious control, upon some aspect of my mental makeup that is unknown to me. And this seems to me a paradigm of the limitation of freedom. The desires I am unable to assess consciously continue to affect me without my having access to them or control over them. They influence my decisions, although my decisions are not *based* upon them.[71]

If one accepts such an argument, and accepts the idea that all thoughts and actions are ultimately caused by unconscious mental states, then anyone's responsibility for anything quickly disappears.

Compulsion can be given no such extended reading. Blumenfeld's mistake is to think that lack of information about my own desires *compels* me to do whatever I do under the influence of such desires. Yet lack of information generally is an odd candidate for being a compulsion. If another person withholds information from me that is crucial to some decision, I may claim ignorance as an excuse but not compulsion. (And about desires, ignorance is never an excuse because the existence of a desire is never the object of a prohibited intention.)

Still, Blumenfeld seeks to make a special case for ignorance of one's own desires as a compulsion in the following way. Without knowing all of one's component desires, one cannot form the overall ("all things considered") wants on which one acts. And, to pursue his argument, we should see such interference with the formation of the major premises of our practical syllogisms as no less an interference with our practical reasoning than is to be found in the two standard models of compulsion. If we can be compelled by a threat (which constrains the means to the fulfillment of something we legitimately want a great deal) or by craving (which interferes with our ability to act on our normal desire to behave morally), why are we not compelled whenever we cannot even form the want on which we would act?

Plausible as this may sound, it ignores an important limitation built into our concept of compulsion. We are compelled only when our *existing* desires are made more difficult to satisfy. We are not compelled by being unable to *form* certain desires. Compulsion as an excuse takes people as they are, with the desires they have, and excuses those whose already existing (and legitimate) desires are made very difficult to satisfy. The overall wants discussed by Blumenfeld are, as he admits, not in existence when the actor acts; rather, "it is the resulting evaluation which itself *constitutes* what a man most wants."[72]

If we were to regard as compulsions all of the factors that prevent people from forming new desires (on which they *would* act if they formed such desires), we would quickly collapse compulsion into hard determinism. For it is surely the case that if certain events in our past had happened differently than they did, we would have desires different than we do. To avoid this reductio, we must adhere to the line marked by our existing excuse of compulsion: We are compelled only by factors that make difficult the satisfaction of desires we actually have, not by factors that prevent us from having different desires. Such a line is not some arbitrary convention we have adopted. It marks our respect for persons as they are actually constituted, with the character and the desires they actually have. That they might have been different people if their genes or environment had been different is no doubt true but irrelevant to our assessment of *these* persons' responsibility.

Of course, there is one desire in the cases we are considering here that does by hypothesis exist: the "component," unconscious desire itself. Moreover, one might develop the argument of Chapter 8 to say that such desire (because unconscious) cannot be acted on as a reason, even if it may causally influence behavior. In such a case a desire that does exist cannot serve as the major premise of the actor's reasoning, and one might conclude that such a disturbance of practical inference should count as an excuse as much as do the standard cases of compulsion.

One can grant all of this and yet deny that unconscious desires, just because they are unconscious, act as compulsions. Compulsion is an excuse because of disturbed practical reasoning that actually takes place. In the argument just given, no practical reasoning actually takes place, although it would have if the desire had been conscious rather than unconscious. There is thus no practical reasoning (involving the unconscious desire) to disturb, and thus no compulsion. If the unconscious desire operates as a craving or other emotion, then it disturbs some existing practical reasoning the agent went through, involving his desires to do what is morally required. *Then* one might invoke the second model of compulsion: a limited use of the excuse that does not collapse all unconscious mental states into excusing compulsions.

Conclusion

Psychoanalytic theory is not the first theory of human behavior that purports to contradict ordinary attributions of responsibility. Two views of humankind, one in an ancient and one in a modern version of the Orestes legend, make even more radical claims. Aeschylus's version diminishes personal responsibility to the vanishing point because of the uncontrollable influences of fate. Sartre's version extends a person's responsibility to all that happens. Each thus more radically extends each of the claims of psychoanalysis about our responsibility that we have examined in this and the preceding chapter.

Psychoanalytic theory is perhaps unique in its claim that its insights compel a reassessment of responsibility that both generally diminishes and generally increases the items for which each person is responsible. The burden of this and the preceding chapter has been to argue that although psychoanalysts may show that each person's responsibility on *particular occasions* is greater or lesser than common sense would allow, they may not make both of these claims at the level of generality at which they are made. Particularly they may not do this as an implication from what is supposed to be the very same insight, namely, that there are unconscious mental states.

These inconsistent implications for responsibility are symptomatic of a kind of conceptual schizophrenia from which psychoanalytic psychiatry suffers. Unlike behaviorism, which purports at least to eschew the Intentional vocabulary of persons entirely, psychoanalysis attempts to retain that vocabulary and yet build a theory about persons in non-Intentional terms. The result is a discipline fundamentally bifurcated between its clinical accounts of particular actions using an Intentional vocabulary. and its metapsychological viewpoints, which use a paramechanistic, non-Intentional vocabulary.[73] The more discerning critics of the theory have long noticed this split. Paul Ricoeur, for example, divides the theory between its "hermeneutics" and its "energetics";[74] Antony Flew distinguishes between motives and causes;[75] Herbert Fingarette draws the line between Freud's "meaning-reorganization" views and his "hidden reality" views.[76]

When Freud talked to his patients in his clinical practice, or explained slips or dreams in particular cases, he used the Intentional vocabulary in the same way as do historians, ordinary persons, novelists, and lawyers. Freud himself often pointed this out: "All the categories which we employ to describe conscious mental acts, such as ideas, purposes, resolutions, and so on, can be applied [to unconscious mental acts]. Indeed, we are obliged to say of some of these latent states that the only respect in which they differ from conscious ones is precisely in the absence of consciousness."[77] In looking back on his development of the theory of the unconscious, Freud also said, "Everywhere I seemed to discern motives and tendencies analogous to those of everyday life."[78]

There is a good reason for this commitment of pyschoanalytic therapy to the mentalistic vocabulary of ordinary speech. Psychoanalysts want to say something about their patients' responsibility, in some meaningful sense of responsibility. If an analyst were, for example, to tell the lover who missed the appointment that he was responsible for doing so because of some "psychogen," the lover would also miss the point. Any argument about the lover's responsibility must not stipulate some new theoretical terms, but must show the patient that he *wanted*, in the ordinary sense of want, to miss the appointment. Therapy otherwise becomes as irrelevant to self-assessment as behaviorism.

On the other hand, when Freud came to theorize about the etiology of dreams, slips, and symptoms, he attempted to conceptualize their origins in the non-Intentional terms of the dynamic and economic metapsychologies. As I argued in Chapter 7, there was nothing illegitimate about such theorizing about persons simply because the non-Intentional vocabulary of energy and instincts was used. But because the concepts employed in the metapsychology are different from those employed in therapy, psychoanalysts are inclined both ways on responsibility for actions explained by unconscious mental states. At the level of individual explanations in case studies and therapy, psychoanalysts use desire the same way everyone uses the term: either as the motive of an intentional action, or as a mental cause of behavior. At the theoretical level, however, and when they carry their theoretical perspective into court, they use desire as if they were talking of some of the basic, mechanistic springs of human action. Given this sometimes mechanistic and sometimes Intentional interpretation of the unconscious, it is not surprising that the discovery of the unconscious should lead them to view human beings as both more and less responsible than was commonly thought.

The main burden of Chapters 9 and 10 has been to demonstrate that the insights of psychiatry into the unconscious compel neither of these views on responsibility. One is not made *more* responsible for nominal accidents explained by unconscious mental states. Whether an accident can be shown to be an action, an intentional action, or an attempt, depends in each instance on what the actor believed: Did he know that he was acting at all, did he know *what* action he was performing, and did he believe circumstances to be such that he could achieve certain effects? Although one can make sense of the idea of an unconscious belief, and thus of unconscious actions, unconscious intentions, and unconscious attempts, few if any of the psychoanalytic examples forming the classical data of the unconscious turn out to be unconscious actions, intentions, or attempts. Furthermore, even for those that do, there is nothing unscientific or irrational about a moral system that attributes responsibility only to behavior involving conscious knowledge.

Nor are persons less responsible when their actions are explained by unconscious mental states. Even if the economic and dynamic metapsychologies give us at long last a unified account of the mechanistic causes of action, such an account is irrelevant to responsibility. One may be less responsible only if the unconscious mental states discovered either rebut the prima facie intentional nature of the action, call into question the rationality of the agent, or show his action to have been compelled. Since only fundamentally irrational agents or seriously compelled choices are excused, and since few prima facie intentional actions may be shown to be unintentional in this way, the range of cases where responsibility is diminished because of the unconscious is small. Most people are not excused by such factors, as the theory of drives would have us believe.

Freud calls upon us to be considerably more subtle in the ascriptions of responsibility that we make in particular cases. His insights about the unconscious do not, however, generally require one to alter the legal view of persons as autonomous and rational beings who may justly be held responsible for their consciously intentional actions.

IV Legal Persons and Psychiatric Subagents

11 The Unity of the Self

AS WE NOTED in Chapter 3, the most dramatic challenge to the legal view of persons comes from those aspects of psychiatric theory suggesting that each of us is in reality possessed of (by?) several selves. I shall again use psychoanalytic theory as my stalking horse, since Freud's theory most strongly suggests disunity of self. I shall proceed, first, by analyzing the case to be made for disunity of self. This involves retracing Freud's steps through data having to do with conflict, functional organization of the mind, and the unconscious, and sifting such data for what it is that suggests that each of us is something of a corporation. Having restated the psychoanalytic case for disunity, I shall then analyze the sense(s) of disunity in which the facts about functional organization, conflict, and the unconscious can show us we are not one, unified self. My conclusion here is that the senses in which psychoanalysis may show us to be disunified are not the senses that could seriously challenge the legal view of persons as unified agents. I shall, third, conclude the chapter by questioning the utility of the topographical or structural metapsychologies as fruitful conceptualizations within psychiatry itself. If, as I hope to show, such conceptions have no proper place in a well-constructed psychiatric theory, then their apparent challenge to the law's view of persons as unified is wholly dissolved.

The Psychoanalytic Challenge to the Unity of the Self

A useful analytic device that separates the various factors suggesting disunity of the self is to begin with a very simple example and add other factors one by one. This is done in this section, the ordering principle being my own intuitions that as the list progresses we are increasingly tempted to speak of more than one person per body. These factors are initially stated in a way most favorable to the multiple selves thesis; as will be discussed subsequently, the actual discoveries of psychoanalytic theory vary significantly from this idealization. Nonetheless, I proceed to state the ideal psychoanalytic case for multiple selves in order to understand what in the theory and in the phenomena that generated the theory at least suggests such a thesis.

Very generally, three discoveries of Freud's suggest that there is more than one person within us all: first, that we have conflicting mental states, and experience them as conflicting; second, that mental states can be given a functional organization; and third, that part of our mental life is unconscious. I shall pursue each of these in the ensuing sections.

DISCOVERY OF CONFLICT IN A PERSON'S
MENTAL STATES

The Discovery of Simple Conflict

One should start where Freud himself began, with the fundamental insight that people have conflicting mental states. It is useful to begin with an example from outside psychoanalytic theory so as not to overload the mere fact of conflict with premature theoretical baggage. Consider the recognizable portrait of conflict drawn by Thomas Schelling, a game theoretician and an economist interested in the rational consumer:

> People behave sometimes as if they had two selves, one who wants clean lungs and long life and another who adores tobacco or one who wants a lean body and another who wants dessert, or one who yearns to improve himself by reading *The Public Interest* and another who would rather watch an old movie on television. The two are in continual contest for control....
>
> How should we conceptualize this rational consumer whom all of us know and who some of us are, who in self disgust grinds his cigarettes down the disposal swearing this time he means never again to risk orphaning his children with lung cancer and is on the street three hours later looking for a store that is still open to buy some cigarettes; who eats a high calorie lunch knowing that he will regret it, does regret it, cannot understand how he lost control, resolves to compensate with a low calorie dinner, eats a high calorie dinner knowing he will regret it, and does regret it; who sits glued to the TV knowing that again tomorrow he'll wake early in a cold sweat unprepared for that morning meeting on which so much of his career depends; who spoils a trip to Disneyland by losing his temper when his children do what he knew they were going to do when he resolved not to lose his temper when they did it?[1]

The temptation to regard ourselves as consisting of several selves starts, as Schelling recognizes, with this basic fact that each of us at least sometimes

The Unity of the Self

possesses mental states that are in conflict. We may have inconsistent beliefs, conflicting wants, opposing emotions.

It is surprisingly difficult to give an adequate philosophical characterization of this "simple fact" of conflict. Given *de dicto* and *de re* ambiguities regarding the contents of mental states, such conflict is not even clear with respect to beliefs, for which the notion of logical contradiction seems most readily available. And the matter is even muddier with respect to desires and emotions, between which conflict does not seem so amenable to characterization in terms of the logical contradiction between the contents of such mental states.[2]

In any case, assuming that some philosophically respectable account can be given of conflict, one needs to say how second-agent temptations begin with this not-so-simple fact. Surely some kinds of conflicts do *not* tempt us in the way Schelling suggests. The world being as it is, we will often, for example, have general desires that conflict in particular circumstances: One cannot satisfy both a general desire to relax and a desire to do well at one's job when the means available to satisfying the one (watching TV) will prevent the satisfaction of the other (being prepared the next day). Such conflict, inevitable simply because we are creatures with more than one general desire, should not generate any second-agent temptations.

The kind of conflicting desires (ignoring emotions and beliefs) that do generate such temptations are those unresolved conflicts between desires that will *necessarily* conflict on individual occasions. Given the causation of obesity by desserts and lung cancer by smoking, a person who maintains each of Schelling's conflicting desires—long life versus smoking, lean body versus desserts—may seem somewhat irrational in his failure to combine his desires into a consistent preference order. Such failure is irrational because it is unnecessarily frustrating to act on such unresolved conflicts.

The way in which this leads to second-agent temptations is by our assumption of rationality for persons. If we expect rational persons to order their mental states into consistent preference orders, belief systems, and emotional responses, then unresolved conflict itself will lead us to at least think of separate selves, each of whom is more rational (i.e., consistent) than is the whole person with her conflicts. Still, isolated conflicts between particular mental states are only the beginning of this temptation; other discoveries about such conflict must be made before the temptation to talk of multiple selves can be very strong.

Discovery that Certain Types of Conflicts are Recurring

One way to organize this potential chaos of conflicting states is by aggregating those states by virtue of their instantiating recurring *types* of conflicts. If, for example, the desires to smoke, for dessert, or to watch TV typically conflict, not with each other but with the desires to prolong life, to promote a lean body, and spiritual improvement, respectively, these might be organized into two groups of conflicting desires. This is, indeed, one of Freud's principal concerns in his definition of ego, id, and superego: One assigns mental states to these structures on the principle of best exhibiting the conflicts that recur within each person.[3] Ego, id, and superego are thus not evidence of mental conflict, but are themselves aggregations of mental states constructed so as to best exhibit the recurring types of conflict already discovered to exist.

The discovery that mental states do not conflict in a random manner increases the temptation to talk of multiple selves, because it betokens an enduring nature to mental conflict. The temptation to think of "structures" is more natural if there is a consistent pattern of the mental states in conflict to be assigned to such structures.

Discovery that the Types of Conflicting Mental States Instantiate Intelligible Characters

Suppose we now discover that the conflicting mental states aggregated by their instantiation of types of recurring conflicts are just like people we know. For example, suppose our previous principle of organization aggregates the mental states of Schelling's not so rational consumer by putting the desire for dessert, tobacco, and TV in one system, and the desire for a lean body, long life, and spiritual improvement in another system. These, suitably enriched, might instantiate patterns of character that are intelligible to us as a character a person in our culture might hold. We might think of gluttons, on the one hand, and ascetics on the other.

It is important to see that not every pattern of mental states, nor even most such patterns, will instantiate characters that are for us intelligible. Only certain patterns of mental states will be recognizable to us as a potential character structure of a person. These will satisfy two requirements: First, the patterns will have exceeded some threshold of coherence that we expect of any person; and second, these patterns will have within them desires that are intelligible to us as reasons for action, beliefs that are intelligible to us in light of the prevailing beliefs of our culture, and emotions that are appropriate in kind and in intensity to their objects.[4]

Because of these cultural limitations on types of intelligible characters, it is a distinct organizing principle to aggregate mental states by their instantiation of intelligible characters. There is no guarantee that mental states aggregated by types of recurring conflict will be like the intelligible characters of whole persons. Nonetheless, if one were to believe this with

The Unity of the Self

respect to the structural metapsychology, one might then *characterize* the ego, id, and superego as persons we know: "Psychoanalytic theory suggests that man is essentially a battlefield, he is a dark cellar in which a maiden aunt and a sex-crazed monkey are locked in mortal combat, the affair being refereed by a rather nervous bank clerk."[5]

Discovery that One Set of the Recurring Types of Mental States in Conflict Is Experienced as Alien

Loaded into Schelling's portrait is yet another factor: In some sense we might say that Schelling's individual *most wants* to remain healthy, long lived, self-improving, and patient with his children. He is not deceived about these desires; he might well say, without deception, that he is conflicted but that he most wants the objects of the "noble" set. Nonetheless, he frustrates this set of desires, manifesting what philosophers since Aristotle might call *akrasia*, or weakness of will.

For present purposes it is not so important to dissolve the air of paradox surrounding the idea that a person with eyes open can fail to do what he most wants to do. The important point here is how the akratic regards some of his own desires, namely, the ones to which he yields. He may typically regard them as less a part of himself than the "higher" desires that oppose them. If so, this aspect of *akrasia* is but a special case of that general phenomena that formed one of the important bases for Freud's concept of the id. As Morris Eagle has pointed out, some mental states are experienced as "ego-alien," as not belonging to *me* but to an "it."[6] In such cases, one experiences one set of conflicting mental states as outside the self. If these ego-alien mental states instantiate one of the types of states that regularly conflict, and these ego-alien states themselves form a pattern intelligible as the character of a person, second-agent temptations become considerably strengthened. This will particularly be so in the special case of *akrasia*, because the actions one dislikes can be attributed to "someone else."

ORGANIZATION OF MENTAL STATES BY THE FUNCTIONS THEY SERVE

A second major organizing principle with which Freud was much concerned is the aggregation of mental states in terms of the functions served by such states. Thus, for example, the ego is assigned the function of self-preservation and the functions governing motor control, and the id is assigned those mental functions representative of the sexual instinct. Although Freud (as examined shortly) believed that mental states sorted by this organizing principle would be the same as those sorted by the previous principle of best exhibiting types of recurring conflict, the principles themselves are quite distinct, as can be seen from an analysis of how functions might be assigned to mental states.

Freud and his followers, together with many contemporary philosophers of mind and researchers in artificial intelligence, analogize the mind to the physical body in the sense that each is given a functional organization. As we saw in Chapter 1, what this means for physical medicine is that one assumes certain end states (homeostatic balances) toward which a healthy body tends despite disturbing conditions; with regard to the mental states that are the subject of psychiatry, one likewise assumes some end state of (mental) health toward which various mental states contribute. One in each case indexes a great deal of information about the causal contribution mental or physical states make to the maintenance of the general end state of health, by assigning functions to such physical parts or mental states. That the function of the heart is to circulate the blood is just to say that one of the consequences of the heart's beating is that the blood circulates, and that this consequence itself contributes to the maintenance of that end state with which physical medicine is concerned, physical health. Analogously, to assign to the ego self-preservation as one of its functions is to say that the mental states designated as being part of the ego serve the function of preserving the organism, itself a state that contributes in an obvious way to the overall end state of the health of the organism.

It is important to note that when one aggregates mental states by the functional organization attributed to a person, one assigns them to such functionally defined components universally, that is, to all human beings. Such assignment of mental states to various aggregate functions is not (for Freud at least) peculiar to each person; rather, Freud assumes the existence of universal tendencies, and thus the functional organization of a person should be the same despite differing characteristics of that person's mental states.

There is very little in a functional organization of the mind that should by itself incline one to a multiple-self thesis. If psychologists study perception, for example, and subdivide the perceiving that a person does into discrete, functionally defined subroutines that take place when the person perceives, it is the crudest anthropomorphism to posit separate persons as the performers of each subroutine. Rather, a functionalist about minds such as Dan Dennett,[7] will talk of the "subpersonal" level of description explicitly to avoid the suggestion that his functional subdivisions are to be confused with a *person's* actions or mental states. That there are various stages of information preprocessing in visual perception, for example, is not to say that the person (or any little person) is doing any of the things described at the subpersonal level.

The Unity of the Self

It is only because Freud thought a functional organization of the mind would aggregate mental states in the same way as do the conflict principles that second-agent temptations come into being. For if one set of typically conflicting, intelligibly characterized yet ego-alien mental states are just those mental states serving certain universal functions but not others, one may be tempted to think that such a set of mental states is more than just a set, but is itself a "structure" in the mind and, with the hoped-for function/structure correlation, in the brain as well.

DISCOVERY OF THE UNCONSCIOUS

Unconscious is ambiguous: It can mean that a person is unconscious, in the sense of not being awake; or it can mean that, although the person is awake, he is unaware of certain of his own mental states. Freud exploited both senses of the word, emphasizing the first in his earlier theorizing and the second in his later statement of the theory. I have accordingly separated the discovery of the unconscious into two principles of aggregation: (1) by the characteristics of a mental state being unconscious; and (2) by the characteristics of a mental state being experienced or acted upon while the agent is unconscious.

Discovery of Unconscious Mental States

Discovery that Some Aggregates of Conflicting Mental States Are Unconscious: A fundamental organizing principle for Freud was based on the discovery that some mental states are conscious and others unconscious. This was the organizing principle he most relied on in the topographical metapsychology of the "systems" conscious-preconscious and unconscious that preceded (and then uncomfortably coexisted with) the structural metapsychology of ego, superego, and id. One might discover, to revert once again to Schelling's example, that the desires for dessert, for tobacco, and to watch TV were all unconscious desires. If conflicting mental states were sorted by all three principles into the same aggregation, the suggestion of such separate selves, one of whom is conscious and the other of whom is unconscious, becomes that much stronger.

Discovery that Some Unconscious Mental States Appear to Serve as the Rational Motivation for Behavior: Suppose now that the unconscious mental states one has discovered not only exist, but also sometimes "win" over their conscious opposites. That is, they win in the sense that such unconscious mental states causally influence behavior. Moreover, they influence that behavior in the particular way that delineates the fundamental sense of rationality. An action is rational in this fundamental sense if it fulfills the object of the desire that is given to explain it. For example, one may unconsciously wish to be an artist, and this could cause one to do almost anything, such as cut off an ear. Even if the existence of such a mental state and its causal connection to behavior were substantiated, however, this would not explain the action as rational because the action cannot be seen as a means to fulfillment of the object of that desire.

As we have seen, Freud's discovery that the unconscious was causally active has not been presented as just the discovery that sometimes unconscious mental states influence behavior; Freud also thought he had discovered that the unconscious acts in the way in which rational agents typically act, adopting means to the ends they desire. Of course, in most of Freud's examples, some symbolic transformation must take place before one can even entertain the hypothesis that the dreams, parapraxes, or neurotic symptoms of Freud's patients are means to the attainment of unconscious ends. For example, one might find oneself sucking a pen rather than eating the dessert one truly desires; or one might call out for just deserts as the sublimated form of one's unconscious desire for dessert. Although some of the claims are more tenuous than others, a basic claim of Freud's is that sometimes the unconscious mental states look for all the world like the use of an action to achieve, in a somewhat attenuated way, the object of an unconscious desire.

The way in which second-agent temptations are increased by this discovery should be obvious. First, that one set of the conflicting mental states—say, the more gluttonous desires of Schelling's conflicted individual—causes behavior tempts one to posit an agency with causal powers. Since these states are unconscious, the personal agency we all possess may seem inappropriate; hence, the second agent. Second, if one perceives a pattern of behavior that adjusts itself to serve just those ends that are unconscious, one will be tempted to attribute that behavior to a personlike agent, because the behavior and the mental states that explain it seem to possess an essentially human characteristic, namely, rationality. Morris Eagle recognizes this in his recent paper on psychoanalytic disunity:

> This formulation complicates and deepens the challenge to concepts of unity of the self because in this account all aspects of the complex story are purposive in nature and are occurring simultaneously within the same person. According to the Freudian view, occurring simultaneously are purposive mental maneuvers we normally believe can only be consciously carried out by a person—including strivings for gratification, avoidance of displeasure, and reaching of compromises—which are now claimed to be carried out unconsciously and are attributed to partial components constituent of the person.[8]

One in short *personifies* such partial components by attributing to them causal agency and practical reason.

The Unity of the Self

Discovery of Self-Deception: Self-deception is often pointed to as one of the crucial facts suggesting a multiplicity of selves within any person. Morris Eagle, for example, relies upon an analysis of self-deception as "the decisive aspect which threatens unity of personality."[9] Essentially, the idea of self-deception amounts to the discovery that there are unconscious mental states that are causally active and rational, only twice over. That is, when one is self-deceived not only does one have unconscious mental states that causally influence action in a seemingly rational way, but there are second-order, unconscious mental states that are also causally active and rational, and what *they* cause is the first-order unconscious mental states to be unconscious. One may, for example, not only unconsciously desire dessert, but one may perform certain maneuvers just to prevent oneself from knowing or learning that one has the unconscious desire for dessert.

Self-deception seems to increase the temptation to talk of multiple selves because of its notion that there is both someone who is deceived and someone who is the deceiver. Deception is a lie, not a mistake, and the difference is that the person who lies knows that what he is saying or implying is false. Someone who is deceived, on the other hand, does not know what he is deceived about, else he would not be deceived. Thus, the temptation: One way of reconciling the person who knows and yet does not know is to say that there are two persons, one of whom knows and the other of whom is ignorant.

Discovery of the Repressed Nature of the Unconscious: Suppose now that one explains why an individual's desires may be unconscious, and why he may be deceiving himself about them. Suppose the explanation is itself in terms of an activity engaged in by "someone" who does what he does for an understandable reason. Schelling's consumer, for example, may have *repressed* certain of his desires because of their connection to painful memories from his childhood. Moreover, he may continue to repress them for the same reasons. Since he does not view himself as performing an action called "instituting repression," yet since it too appears to be an activity engaged in for reasons, the temptation is to talk of other agents doing so. Remarkable in Freud's corpus is the number of such repressing second agents, variously termed censors, gatekeepers, or part of the ego. Such second agents may seem required here in part for reasons already explained in connection with self-deception and the simpler cases of unconscious mental states; repression adds, however, one additional factor. Repression is unlike neurotic symptoms or the slips of the tongue and the like that formed most of the classic evidence for the unconscious in that instituting repression is not a recognized kind of action that persons perform. Repression is much like the processes Freud postulates as part of the dreamwork in that none of these inner processes seems to be within the act repertoire of a person. This is true no matter how intensive psychoanalysis might be or how frequently he may visit a biofeedback laboratory to increase that repertoire. Because of this, "little agents" seem necessary if one is to make sense of the talk of *actions* by someone in such cases.

Discovery of Mental States and Behavior Engaged in While Unconscious

Long before Freud one might speak not only of unconscious mental states, but also of persons being unconscious in the sense of not being fully awake. A distinct Freudian claim has to do with the explanation of behavior engaged in by the person when he is unconscious (not just when the person is conscious but his behavior is influenced by unconscious mental states). The claim is that the mental states that are either expressed in behavior while unconscious, or that influence dreams while asleep, are just those (unconscious) mental states that explain waking behavior. To revert to Schelling's example once again, suppose that when the individual is dazed by a blow to the head, is rendered unconscious by the nervous shock of being shot in the stomach, is put into a hypnotic trance, or is simply asleep, then out pops the very same mental states thought to exist as unconscious mental states when the person is awake. Thus, for example, he either when asleep engages in somnambulism and walks to the refrigerator, takes out the dessert, eats it, and lights up while he turns on the TV, or if he does not actually engage in these behaviors, he nonetheless dreams of doing them. In such a case, the temptation to posit a second intelligent self within the selfsame body may increase, first, because there is a sense in which we certainly say that *we* (referring to a self) are asleep or otherwise unconscious. Yet surely *someone* is doing all these things. And second, such repeated appearance of one set of mental states when we are in an altered state of consciousness may also make us think that there is more conflict than we had thought. It may, that is, lead one to Freud's early views that such unconscious desires are always present in us, waiting for expression whenever we relax our state of vigilance (by being unconscious or in an altered state of consciousness). This is the "loaded spring" or oozing notion of the unconscious:

> He that has eyes to see and ears to hear may convince himself that no mortal can keep a secret. If his eyes are silent, he chatters with his finger-tips; betrayal oozes out of him at every pore.[10]

MORE PATHOLOGICAL CONDITIONS

The previous three factors exhaust what I take to be those aspects of psychoanalytic theory, and of the data on which the theory was con-

The Unity of the Self

structed, most strongly suggesting separate selves within one and the same human being. Certain particular pathological conditions, namely, multiple personalities, and some of the recent research on split brains, may even more strongly suggest reconceptualizing a person as separate selves. Such data are included here because this information is sometimes referred to as buttressing the Freudian subdivisions of self, even though it does not form part of the general data for Freud's topographical or structural metapsychology. It is important to see at the outset that such phenomena could not constitute strong support for the universal subdivisions Freud thought to exist in all of us, because all of us do not have multiple personalities or brains whose hemispheres have been severed.

Discovery that Behavior Over Time Manifests Several Different Intelligible Characters

Suppose we alter Schelling's not so rational consumer with the following additional facts: Not only are his mental states in systematic, intelligibly characterizable conflict, organized along certain functional principles, and aggregated according to their being conscious or unconscious, but the person's behavior *over time* also matches the aggregations of mental states previously achieved by these three principles. That is, suppose the gluttonous person "takes charge" for a period of time, and then is supplanted by the ascetic or spiritual individual, who also reigns for a time. If one suspends the agency attributions, what this comes to is the claim that the conflicting mental states previously organized by their instantiation in intelligible characters will also find expression in aggregates of behavior that are temporally continuous. It looks as if the person is more than one person because he acts so "in character" for periods of time, yet the character he is in changes abruptly from period to period. If one adds the fact of partial memory loss over time, we have an instance of that phenomenon known as multiple personalities.[11]

Discovery that Each Such Character Has Physical Location in the Brain

Now suppose as a further fact that we discover that the gluttonous character previously discovered to be a character apparently taking charge of aggregates of behavior also has physical location in the brain. One might think of the glutton being in the right hemisphere, and the more spiritual character in the left. To the extent that our intuitions of what it is to be a person are in part based on being embodied "in" some physical structure, this discovery of the separate, autonomous, intelligible functioning of the two hemispheres of the brain may seem to increase the temptation to speak of separate persons.

If one goes beyond contemporary split brain research to posit the possibility of separating all physical functions that feed into one hemisphere from those that feed into another, so that there are two separately embodied hemispheres of the brain, the temptation to speak of persons seems to be increased. For now not only is there physical location of the mental states previously characterized in separate regions of the same brain, but there also is not even a shared physical unity of a body that those two hemispheres at least share. (If one is bothered by such recherché philosophical thought experiments, one might think of such splinter bodies as the limiting case of Siamese twins.)

The last factor that might be eliminated is the developmental unity that artificially created splinter bodies would have; that is, they at least have been formed as one physical unit. If one were to discover that such splinter persons were a naturally occurring phenomenon, the temptation to regard them as separate persons, given the lack of any developmental unity, would be overwhelming. The limiting case of such splinter persons is, of course, simply two persons with separately developing and fully functioning bodies.

The Psychoanalytic Challenge to the Unity of the Self Reconsidered

THE UNITY OF THE SELF 1: ONE PERSON PER HUMAN BEING

Each of these factors may increase our temptation to speak of a disunified self. Before reassessing these data to judge whether this temptation is warranted, one needs to be clear about what one means by the unity of the self. The first and most obvious sense is one utilizing the notion of numerical identity of a person. (This I shall henceforth call the question of personal identity, following relatively standard philosophical usage.) This most basic sense of the unity of the self may be defined as the doctrine that there is one person per body, and disunity, accordingly, as there being two or more persons per body. Such a view of the unity of the self need take no position on the metaphysics of the mind/body relationship and explicitly is not committed to any form of identity theory that urges that a person is identical with his or her body. Rather, the claim of the unity of the self in this sense is only that persons are individuated by their bodies, even though not necessarily identical with them.

A natural contrast to talking of the numerical identity of persons is to talk of the qualitative identity of persons. There is only a limited range of phenomena for which such talk could make sense, if one believed in the unity of the self in the first sense just identified, namely, that there is one and only one numerically distinct person per body; for given such a belief, one could not hold that at any given time there was more than one kind of person in that body. (One could not hold this because Leibniz's law states that if two nominally distinct things are in reality one and the same thing, then anything predicable of the one must be predicable of the other, and vice versa.) Accordingly, at any one time, if there is unity of the self in the sense of numerical identity, there must also be unity of the self in the sense of qualitative identity.

Where this will not be true is for the identity of persons over time. In this context, we often do say of a (numerically distinct) person that he is not the "same person" as he was at some earlier point in time. What we mean when we say this is not that he is not the same person that we knew before; rather, such language is simply a dramatic form of saying that he is not the same *kind* of person as he was.

The unity of the self that this notion of qualitative identity would define would simply be the doctrine that over time persons remain the same kind of persons as they were previously, and disunity would be the denial of this claim. There is nothing very problematic about this sense of the unity of the self, nor is any disunity discovered in this sense very troublesome to the basic assumptions of metaphysics or morals discussed in Chapter 3. Hence, it is worth distinguishing this other sense of personal identity mostly to put it aside from further consideration.

If psychoanalytic theory could make out the idealized case recreated around Schelling's consumer, buttressed perhaps by the findings of multiple personality or split brain research, would it show us a disunity of the self in the sense just set forth, viz., more than one person per body? My inclination is to say that it could. If one discovered that certain types of mental states are regularly present and in recurring conflict with one another; that each of these aggregates of mental states in conflict were coherent enough and intelligible enough to constitute characters of a person; that the mental states composing at least one of these aggregates were experienced as belonging to another (if they were conscious at all); that these aggregates of mental states are just the aggregations one would achieve if one sorted such states by the functions they served; that these aggregations of mental states are also just those aggregations one would achieve if one sorted such states by their being conscious or unconscious, or by their being manifested when the agent is conscious or unconscious; that the unconscious mental states included full practical syllogisms causing actions by some agent; that such actions included deceiving one's consciousness; and that such actions included activities, such as repression, that no consciousness is aware of or becomes, even after psychoanalysis, aware of — if one discovered all of this, I suspect that we might embrace Freud's conclusion that "we are not masters in our own house"[12] but that "someone else" — id, unconscious — is.

Legal Persons and Psychiatric Subagents

One could only decide this question by having ready at hand some successful analysis of personal identity that could be defended against the extended thought experiments in the philosophy of personal identity. Since such thought experiments seem to present counterexamples to taking any of the three leading candidates of personal identity—spatiotemporal continuity, consciousness and memory, or coherence and consistency of character structure—as the criterion of personal identity,[13] I shall take a different tack, which will be to reexamine the Freudian case.

The presentation of the Freudian case for disunity has been idealized. It is now time to ask whether Freud actually made out all or even most of his idealized case for disunity of the self. To begin with, there is good reason to believe that Freud's three major principles for aggregating mental states will not in fact sort them into the same sets. Freud himself conceded part of this point when he defined the System Ucs, not in terms of the property of being unconscious, but rather in terms of the common functional role of mental states part of that system.[14] Freud was even more explicit about the lack of overlap between consciousness and function when he shifted from the topographical metapsychology to the structural; "part of" the ego was unconscious, he thought, namely that part that does the repressing.[15] One accordingly cannot assume that mental states functionally assigned to the ego are conscious (nor, one might add, is there any reason to believe that all mental states having to do with sex are unconscious). Likewise, the conscious/unconscious principle does not seem to map onto the conflict principle. Many conflicts, even of a recurring nature, are between mental states both of which are quite conscious; analogously (at least if one believes many parts of the Freudian theory) many conflicts of a recurring nature are between unconscious mental states. Conflict is not necessarily between mental states allocated to different topographical systems.

Less often noticed is the lack of fit between the conflict principle and the functional principle. If one aggregates mental states because of a functional organization of the mind, one will do so universally, for all persons. Yet conflicts seemingly vary greatly for different people. The conflicting emotions Dora felt for the gentleman who propositioned her seem to have little resemblance to the conflicting intentions Freud used to explain slips of the tongue. Only by relying on an extraordinarily reductionist notion about mental states, such as an instinct theory that reduces them to either sex or aggression, can one make such differing conflicts in fact be of a more general, universal type. Without such a (highly suspect) reduction, the mental states sorted by the highly individualized conflict principle will not be sorted into the same sets as is done by a function-based assignment.

Even within the general aggregating principles considered by themselves, the differing strands of each of those principles will not sort mental states into the same sets. With regard to the unconscious subprinciples:

The Unity of the Self

Only with some extraordinary transformation can one discover that dreams are the "royal road" into those unconscious mental states that explain conscious behavior. The mental states people unproblematically have when they dream (the manifest content) are not the same as the mental states Freud uses to explain neurotic symptoms. Similarly, the mental states one experiences or acts upon in hypnosis may include some of those unconscious mental states on which one acts when fully awake, but seemingly many of the states that are experienced while under hypnosis are the same *conscious* desires, beliefs, and emotions on which one acts while fully awake.

With regard to the subprinciples of conflict: There is no reason to believe that the mental states aggregated upon the subprinciples of best exhibiting recurring types of conflicts and of being experienced as ego-alien, on the one hand, will instantiate intelligible character structures. Indeed, the parody of the superego, id, and ego as the maiden aunt, the sex-craved monkey, and the nervous bank clerk betrays the fact that these are not intelligible characters in the way that multiple-personality persons have different, intelligible characters within them. Rather, these are caricatures. One can see this by pressing the kinds of questions Irving Thalberg has asked regarding Freud's mini-agents. Consider, Thalberg advises, the ego's wish to sleep, one of the two main motives for dreaming in Freudian theory:

> For whose sleep does it yearn? Mine? Just its own? Who is the owner of the "free attention" which is on duty? Whose waking may the attentive "guard" consider "more advisable" than a continuation of sleep? His own? Mine? When we hear of the sleeping "townsman," we should raise further questions. On his overall view of human motivation, can Freud suppose that any "watchman" is "conscientious" enough to care about his fellow townsmen? Does he call them from sleep just to help him put down rowdy instincts? What harm can the most licentious instincts do him? If Freud were talking about ordinary sentinals and sleeping townsmen, we would be able to answer.[16]

We would be able to answer because whole people have characters that allow us to decide whether, for example, an altruistic response is in character or not. Ego, id, or superego—or their subagents of censors, watchmen, and so on—are insufficiently rich in character to answer such questions.

Aside from the lack of fit between the different organizing principles and subprinciples, there are more serious problems with the idealized case for disunity of self. To begin with the fundamental fact of conflict: In reading psychoanalytic theory one is struck by how often conflict is posited for reasons of theoretical neatness, rather than being a datum that is discovered and need be accounted for by the theory. An example is Freud's theory of dreams (where conflict does not naturally suggest itself as it does in some parapraxes and many neurotic symptoms): Freud simply posits a wish to sleep conflicting with the unconscious wish from childhood seeking expression in a dream. He does so because he wished to maintain the parallel he thought ought to exist between dreams and neurotic symptoms. Both, he thought, should be viewed as compromise formations between mental states belonging to different topographical systems. Although one undoubted fact of mental life is that there are conflicts, assessing how much conflict there is, and whether it fits a certain pattern, is not aided by a theory that posits just those mental states necessary for there to be conflict of the right pattern.

With regard to the discoveries about the unconscious, there are several points to be made. The first is a quibble about the amount of our mental life that is unconscious. If one has in mind by the unconscious what I called in Chapter 3 the pretheoretical unconscious—the name for those mental states not presently known to their possessor but recapturable by extended memory—then unconscious mental states do not appear everywhere; they are manifested in dreams and some behavior. Only if Freud's dynamic and economic metapsychologies succeed can one plausibly maintain that *all* of our conscious thinking or action is determined by our unconscious mental states.

Second, there is in psychoanalytic theory an enormous extension of action language to behavior caused by unconscious mental states. This is true not only of Freud's own theorizing, but also of the recent reconceptualization of the theory by Roy Schafer.[17] Such Freudians assume that if one discovers an unconscious desire, for example, that causes a dream, therefore dreaming is an action. As I argued in Chapter 8, this connection need not hold. Dreams could be wish fulfillments in that their contents fantasize situations in which the dreamer's wishes are fulfilled, and dreams could be caused by such wishes; even so, they need not be actions. The less dreams, parapraxes, or symptoms are conceptualized as human actions, the less, of course, there is a need to find an agent whose actions they are.

Third, with regard to repression and the other mechanisms of defense, one should systematically reconceptualize Freud's mini-agent stories from purported tales of actions for reasons into functionally characterized subroutines requiring no personal agents, however small. Repression, for example, not being an action persons engage in (or even recapture with extended memory that they have engaged in) should be seen as the process that must take place if some mental states are significantly harder to recapture than others (i.e., are unconscious rather than preconscious). This recommendation parallels that made in Chapter 8, to the effect that stories about little agents engaged in displacement, condensation, pictorial representation, and secondary revision (the four categories of the dream work

The Unity of the Self

that distort the manifest content of the dream) are better retold as functionally characterized subroutines that must go on if dreaming is caused by unconscious wishes that cannot be given direct expression.

Self-deception may not be as easily dealt with as this, for it and certain other phenomena, such as resistance to therapy, may be genuine instances of unconscious actions. That is, one may well not be able to reconceptualize such phenomena as either processes serving functions or as (nonactive) behavior caused by wishes, for either of such reconstruals seems to leave out an important part of the Freudian claim: The person is acting to deceive himself, or to resist treatment, and will (in principle) come to see noninferentially that these were indeed actions by him.

Granting that all of this may be true about self-deception and resistance does not strengthen the case for disunity of the self. Rather, the opposite would seem to be the effect of so regarding these phenomena. The (single) person deceives himself and unconsciously resists a recovery he himself desires. The semantic puzzle about self-deception mentioned earlier—the apparent contradiction of knowing and not knowing—can be dealt with in ways less costly than positing two persons. One should vary the senses of know along the lines suggested in Chapters 9 and 10; if one does this, a (single) person may without contradiction be said to know something to be the case and yet not know it. He may know that some proposition is false, for example, in the sense that he can recapture with his extended memory such a belief and find it reflected in his behavior, and he may not know that the proposition is false in the sense that he was not aware (conscious) of it.

In these ways, one can grant Freud's insights about the unconscious without giving rise to any second-agent temptations. What of the more recent phenomena of split brains or multiple personalities? Although the multiple-personality cases require more extended discussion, which I shall pursue in the succeeding section, one can be more abbreviated with split brains. Nothing about such phenomena should convince us of there being two or more persons per human body; after all, the fact that there are anatomically isolatable centers of autonomous, intelligent functioning should come as no surprise. Presumably any information-processing system will have correlations between the functional subroutines necessary for the system to process information intelligently, and the structural characteristics of that system. If we had not discovered such function/structure correlations between crude anatomy and mental functions, we should surely have discovered such correlations in more complex and sophisticated electrochemical terms. There is thus, ultimately, nothing remarkable or particularly challenging about the fact that the left hemisphere and the right hemisphere of the brain can function relatively autonomously of one another once the connecting tissue has been severed. Such could be true of any functionally defined "centers," no matter what their structural characteristics turned out to be.

I conclude that psychoanalysis has not made its case for disunity of the self in the fundamental sense of more than one person per body. Although Freud clearly and continuously talks in a way that seems to presuppose disunity in this most fundamental sense, none of the data on which he has relied in fact justifies such talk. To talk of ego, id, superego, censors, watchmen, guardians, systems unconscious, and the like performing actions for reasons, intentionally, with their own mental states, awareness, character structure, and responsibility, is simply an anthropomorphic mistake. Nothing is gained by personalizing these functional subdivisons of the mind, and a great deal, in terms of our moral, legal, and metaphysical needs, is lost.

THE UNITY OF THE SELF 2: ONE PERSONALITY PER PERSON

A second sense of the unity of the self distinct from the fundamental sense just explored is found by ceasing to speak of persons and moving to speaking of personalities in the sense of character structures. There may be problems about speaking of the *identity* of personalities, because of the problems in regarding personalities (or characters) as particulars. Personalities are particulars only in what Bernard Williams calls a "weak sense,"[18] as can be seen by the fact that for personalities there is no real separation of qualitative from numerical identity. If, *within the same person,* two personalities are qualitatively identical, then they will also be numerically identical. (Thus, for the personalities of any given person, the other part of Leibniz's thought, commonly called the identity of indiscernibles, will be true, although it is not generally true.) Because of this, one may want to think of personalities as universals so that talk of different characters within one person is just talk about that person and his (differing) mental states and behavior.

In any case, if one can regard personalities as particulars, the second sense of unity of self will be defined as one personality (intelligible character structure) per person, and disunity as two or more personalities per person. This will, again, not be to say that persons are identical with their personalities, but only that if there is unity of the self in this second sense, there will be at most one personality per person.

It is an interesting question how the phenomenon usually referred to as multiple personalities should be conceptualized. Surely in some sense the phenomenon suggests disunity of self, but the question is, in what sense? There seem to be three possibilities. First, one might take such phenomena to challenge the unity of self in its most basic sense, that is, one person per body.[19] One might thus think of multiple-personality persons as really being separate persons, even though acting through the same body. Alternatively, one might utilize the second sense of the unity of the self just defined and talk of there being more than one personality (as a particular) per person. Third, one might simply talk of such persons as manifesting different characters over time; they are not, that is, the same kind of person at different times.

The phenomenon of multiple personalities does not seem adequately conceptualized in the third of these ways. For the third, using the idea of qualitative identity of a person over time, fails to capture several salient features of the multiple-personality cases. First, there seems to be a dramatic difference between normal people who act out of character and those with multiple personalities who act out of character for one self but in character for different selves. The difference seems to lie in the coherence and the intelligibility of the character formed by aggregating the mental states out of character for the multiple-personality person. Such sharp breaks between different, intelligible characters may incline us toward regarding such personalities as particulars and not as universals. Second, multiple-personality persons not only possess different characters, they also appear to experience themselves as being different "characters" (now in the literary sense). The data seem to be that only sometimes do the personalities "know" each other; that when they do, they may regard each other as separate; that they think of self-interest in terms consistent with the character adopted by that personality, not by some overall self-interest; and that there is a good deal of amnesia with regard to the mental states and behavior taking place when other personalities are in charge, at least with respect to emotion-laden issues.[20] All of this suggests a disunity much more radical than that described as "not being the same kind of person" at all times. Third, multiple-personality persons appear to have different characters that are coconscious and not just appearing at different times.[21] Qualitative identity *over time* cannot capture this disunity *at a particular time*.

Whether multiple personalities should be thought of as being disunified in the first sense distinguished earlier is a more difficult question. Certainly some of the basic assumptions we make about persons (outlined in Chapter 3) are challenged by this phenomenon: Locke's claim that our experience is of one self, the presupposition of an atomic rather than a molecular self-interest of an egoistic moral theory, and perhaps even the unity of self presupposed by our responsibility assessments are sufficiently threatened that one might think that here at least there is disunity in its most fundamental sense, namely, more than one person per body. On the other hand, certain of our basic metaphysical and moral assumptions about persons are not shaken by the multiple-personality phenomenon. There is still but one physical body to be acted through, and but one physical brain to which mental states may be related in some nondualistic way. Likewise, our assignment of rights, by theories of distributive justice or of property, still seems applicable to persons as individuated by bodies. The phenomenon of multiple personalities at best suggests a standoff on the unity of the self in its most basic sense; for pitted against the fact of a single physical embodiment are the facts of radically disunified character and discontinuous conscious experience, and pitted against the unity suggested by our assignment of rights to such persons is the disunity suggested by our absolving them of responsibility.

One way of resolving this apparent standoff would be to defend either the spatiotemporal continuity criterion of personhood or the experiential and characterological criteria, and to come out accordingly for or against unity of self (in its most basic sense) for multiple personalities. Alternatively, one might view such persons in the same way as we regard others who are mentally ill, as having "suspended personhood." There are entities that we recognize are not (fully) persons even though they (the *same* entities) may in the future become persons, namely, young children and the mentally ill. The suspended personhood of such entities is recognized most dramatically in the legal and moral spheres: They are not accorded the full panoply of rights held by sane adults, not held to be proper subjects of responsibility, and not held to be able to calculate their own self-interest. Such suspension of personhood is also reflected in the lack of another basic attribute of being a person, rationality.

Multiple-personality persons should be regarded as but a special case of suspended personhood. There was but one person originally, and (if therapy is successful) there will be but one person again.[22] During the time that intervenes, the only answer to the question, How many persons? may be none.

In any case, however one comes out on conceptualizing multiple personalities, such phenomena are comparatively rare and cannot be the basis for the general psychology that psychoanalytic theory purports to be. They are not universal characteristics of persons, but only pathological conditions applicable to a limited class of human beings.

The more universal phenomena described earlier as the data of psychoanalysis do not show a disunity of self in anything like the sense(s) in which multiple-personality persons do, for two reasons. First, once one leaves the phenomenon of multiple personalities, one leaves behind the crucial fact of there being temporally continuous behavior manifesting the different personalities posited to exist within the single person. That is, neither Freud nor anyone else would claim that for the different "characters" of the id, ego, superego, for the System Ucs, or for their subagents, there is behavior over time manifesting just those characters. One does not have an "id character" as one who has multiple personalities might have a gluttonous character.

The Unity of the Self

Rather, the characters of the id, ego, and superego are manifested in behavior only in the sense that certain bits of behavior may be said to be due to them, rather there is no large aggregation of behavior that can be said to be *exclusively* due to them; rather, aggregations of behavior are to be explained as being due to a mix of all three such characters.

The importance of this difference is this: Without the temporally continuous behavior manifesting these different characters, there will be no unique or correct determination of what sorts of characters one may possess. Psychoanalysis will join other interpretative schemes relying on "ideal types" and will share with them one of their most serious problems of method, namely, the seeming total lack of any criterion of correctness for selection of the pure ("ideal") types. What, for example, is to prevent a Nietzschean psychologist from positing Dionysian and Apollonian characters, neither of which "takes charge" for any aggregates of behavior, but each of which influences every piece of behavior in which one engages? Once one is free to explain all bits of behavior as mixes of these character types, there seems to be nothing but aesthetics as a ground on which to prefer one interpretative scheme to another. Although one may posit behavior to manifest ego, id, and superego, one may equally well posit it to manifest Dionysian and Apollonian characters, and there seems to be no room for intelligent debate.

The second reason the data of psychoanalysis do not show a disunity of self, even in the sense of more than one personality per person, has already been mentioned: Ego, id, and superego are all very "flat" characters, not the kind of "round," or well-developed, characters we find in good fiction and real life. True multiple personalities, by way of contrast, are much more like character structures of whole persons in their richness and intelligibility.

THE UNITY OF THE SELF 3: ONE (INTEGRATED, CONGRUENT) SELF PER PERSON

The foregoing discussion, I think, disposes of any serious threat to the kind of unity of self presupposed by the moral, legal, or metaphysical needs outlined in Chapter 3. The Freudian case for multiple persons, or even personalities, is (despite its initial appearances) quite weak. Having said all of this, however, there remains the nagging suspicion that one has avoided some sense of unity of self such that one can talk of disunified selves. After all, the temptation to talk of disunity is not limited to Freud, as the Schelling article indicates. Indeed, phenomena such as "standing back from oneself" (self-consciousness), or forming second-order desires about one's own first-order desires, join Schelling's battle for self-control as the kind of common, everyday experience that suggests separate selves.

The temptation for philosophers discussing personal identity is to regard the unity of the self in one of the just explored two senses because they employ the familiar notions of identity in relation to particulars. This allows one to talk about personal identity in a philosophically familiar way. Much of the discussion of personal identity in psychoanalytic theory, or psychology in general, cannot be reduced to a discussion in terms of real identities between real entities (particulars). One can see this because of two characteristics of such talk by psychoanalysts and others. First, the notion of self-identity employed by psychoanalysts must be about a "scalar" phenomenon, that is, a matter of degree. The unity of the self is often regarded as an achievable state, something that a person who is successful in psychoanalytic therapy reaches.[23] Saying this about the unity of the self means that one is discussing a scalar phenomenon in the sense that the identity presupposed by the unity of the self is something at which one can be more or less successful. It will be a matter of degree, not the all or nothing kind of question true identities between entities will raise. Second, the self-identity commonly discussed by psychoanalysts is rather clearly tied to psychological experience. The unity of the self discussed is not a relation between entities; rather, it seems to be a *sense* of self-identity that a person possesses. One can talk of there being a *sense* of self-identity without making Locke's further inference to the reality of self-identity. The sense of self-identity requires no ontological commitments to real entities.

Each of these characteristics suggests that further senses of the unity of the self are necessary if one is to capture what psychoanalysts commonly discuss under that rubric. The first such additional sense of the concept is what I shall call the sense of self-identity, and the second, the congruence between the mental states one includes as part of oneself and those that form part of one's total personality.[24] I shall discuss each briefly in turn.

The Sense of Self-identity

This is the sense one has when one has crossed some threshold in the coherence of one's mental states. One does not, that is, regard oneself as the possessor of a *chaotic* pattern of mental states, but rather as having a relatively well-ordered set, a preference order, a relatively consistent set of beliefs, and a relatively nonconflicting set of emotional attachments.

The opposite of someone who is unified in this sense is not someone who experiences multiple selves, but rather loses his sense of self entirely. If one believes R. D. Laing on the phenomenology of schizophrenia, schizophrenics often lose just this sense of I, even losing their ability to differentiate themselves from their external environment.[25] Heinz Kohut, in his recent restructuring of psychoanalytic theory around this idea of the self, tells us that what he calls narcissistic personality disorders and borderline conditions also give rise to this experience of an unintegrated, noncohesive self.[26]

The Unity of the Self

The unity of the self in its third sense should be defined as the achievement of a certain threshold of coherence of mental states, and disunity of self as a failure at that essential task for any person.

Some of the data of psychoanalysis do indeed show a lack of unity of self in this sense; some persons do have a diminished *sense* of self-identity. However, one should remember that these are a limited class of cases, not a claim across the board to show that all of us have disunity in this sense. And second, one should also recall that the disunity that is the opposite of unity is not that there is more than one self in any sense; rather the opposite is that one lacks a sense of (a whole, integrated) self at all. The experience of being more than one self really only comes in the multiple-personality cases with memory discontinuities. More typical disavowed or ego-alien mental states are not themselves cohered into a sense of second self; they are simply alienated as being "not me."

For both these reasons, the lack of a unified sense of oneself, although an important phenomenon for certain pathological conditions, is not and cannot constitute a general challenge to the unity of self presupposed by our moral, legal, and metaphysical needs.

Congruence of the Sense of Self and the Total Personality

The last sense of the unity of the self is once again dependent upon the phenomenology of self-identity, that is, upon the sense of self-identity a person achieves. Here, however, the unity of the self is not to be defined as the coherence or nonconflicting nature of one's mental states. Rather, assume that one has a strong sense of self; the mental states one consciously affirms as part of the self are relatively conflict-free, coherent, and so on. Nonetheless, there may be lack of unity of the self in the sense that the mental states thus affirmed as part of the self do not include significant portions of the total personality of the person. Unity of the self in this fourth and distinct sense will thus be defined as a congruence between the mental states and traits of character identified as oneself, and those traits of character and mental states that are parts of one's total personality. Disunity, accordingly, is a lack of congruence between one's actual mental states and those that one affirms as constituting oneself.

If one believes the data of psychoanalytic theory, all of us suffer from some form of this disunity. Indeed, the entire notion of "mechanisms of defense" is a charting of the various ways in which we exclude from our sense of self-identity those aspects of our total personality which are painful, threatening, or in some way unpleasant. One of the most important ways of defending one's sense of self from these threatening mental states is to render them unconscious. This is Freud's notion of repression, a process by which those mental states of which the person is ashamed, unable to affirm, and the like are kept from consciousness and thus from one's sense of oneself. Similarly, even if one does not render the mental states unconscious, one may experience them as being ego alien. That is, certain thoughts may occur to one which one says are "not me," not part of myself, but seem to come from someone else. The thoughts are not unconscious, but just disassociated as not being part of one's conscious sense of self. A third maneuver ("displacement") is to rob one's own mental states of their true emotional significance; as before, such defensive maneuvers do not render the mental states unconscious, but only make them seem unimportant because the emotional significance they do possess for the person is not consciously experienced by that person.

If certain mental states are unconscious, or disavowed in some other way, one will have a sense of self divorced from the total personality, and thus, disunity of the self in this fourth sense. Such disunity is true of all of us to some degree, the degree depending upon how well we have integrated the mental states constituting our total personality into our conscious sense of self. But as before, the opposite of unity here is not that there are several selves but only that a person has not successfully integrated parts of himself into his sense of self. Only in multiple personalities do we get any second agent temptations, that is, that we have a sense that the mental states or traits of character excluded from the sense of self themselves form or are to be regarded as, or experienced as, a second self. There is thus no serious challenge to our basic needs for the unity of the self by a showing of disunity in this last sense.

The Disunities of Self and Psychoanalytic Structuralism

To the extent that the data of psychoanalysis, or related matters, show us that there are significant disunities of self, to what extent are the topographical or structural subdivisions of the Freudian metapsychology an appropriate way to conceptualize those disunities? I shall take each of the four senses of disunity of self just distinguished in turn. Freud at times seemed to have assumed that he had shown disunity of the self in its first and most fundamental sense; that is, that there is more than one person per body, given the degree to which he attributed states attributable only to persons to the subagencies of ego, id, and superego. However, as argued, the data do not support such a claim, and there is thus no point to asking whether such "disunity" should be conceptualized in these terms, for the simple fact is there is no such disunity to be so conceptualized.

Although there are disunities in the sense put aside earlier—the sense in which we might say of a person that he is not the same *kind* of person he was the day before—these are not disunities that in any way track into the

The Unity of the Self

topographical or structural subdivisions of self. One would have to change the developmental part of psychoanalytic theory considerably before one came to a notion of development such that a person was at one stage of his development pure ego, at another time pure id, and so forth. Since neither Freud nor anyone else makes such a move, nor is it very tempting independent of its history, conceptualizing this sort of disunity as ego, id, superego requires no further discussion.

Disunity in its second sense, as being more than one personality per person, is, as discussed before, largely limited to the situation described earlier as multiple personalities (if there). This phenomenon also does not track into the functionally organized, conflict-reproducing distinctions of ego, id, or superego, or into those distinctions in terms of conscious, preconscious, and unconscious. These are different sets of distinctions because the kinds of personalities a multiple-personality person has are not the same as the "personality" the ego, id, superego, or the conscious and unconscious components might be said to have. The fact that this disunity may exist for a limited class of persons is no justification for the metapsychologies in question. Freud never claimed to the contrary, so this sense of disunity also is not to be conceptualized in terms of the topographical or structural metapsychology.

The third sense of disunity of self, having to do with the lack of cohesion of those conscious mental states one affirms as part of one's self, is more arguably to be conceptualized in terms of either the topographical or structural metapsychology. Indeed, it is common for psychoanalysts to discuss this phenomenon as a "splitting of the ego." The first question one wants to raise about such a way of talking about this phenomenon is the simple matter of clarity. We have a pretheoretical, ordinary, and comprehensible way of discussing it in terms of a lack of a sense of self. One has to ask whether anything is gained by taking a language we already understand and replacing it with a language we do not antecedently understand, particularly if the new language is simply the provision of a set of synonyms for the old (i.e., we talk of ego rather than self, and a splitting of some "thing" rather than a lack of a sense of self-identity). Prima facie, such needless multiplication of vocabulary is less (rather than more) clear because of its seeming ontological commitment, and its seeming (but illusory) increased precision.

If, of course, "ego" does good theoretical work, the clarity of a commonsense description cannot stand in the way of a more advanced, theoretical understanding. Yet it is far from clear that the ego named by the structural metapsychology is the same thing as the ego that is "split" when one experiences a loss in one's sense of self-identity. For when one aggregates mental states by their functional contribution to the overall functioning of the organism, one will seemingly have given a different definition of ego, different in the sense that the mental states includable within it will not be the same as the mental states includable when one talks of it as a synonym for the sense of self-identity. This will be true because of the fact adverted to earlier: The sense of self-identity will vary with each individual; indeed, it would have to, since it is an achievable state, something at which some people are more successful than others. By way of contrast, the ego defined by the functional organization of persons would universally include that fixed set of mental states sharing the functional roles definitive of states of the ego and will not be variable between persons. There is no reason to expect, and every reason *not* to expect, that these two ways of aggregating mental states will aggregate just the same states. A sense of self peculiar to each person will seemingly sometimes match, and as often not match, the ego defined by the functional aggregation of mental states. Simply put, the sense of self-identity is unique to each person, whereas the functional organization of persons is not.

This same problem will infect a conceptualization of disunity in its fourth sense in terms of the topographical or structural metapsychologies. It will be recalled that the sense of disunity in its fourth sense is the lack of congruence between one's sense of self-identity, and those mental states truly a part of one's total personality. Thus, if the id is to be conceptualized as all those mental states which a person, via the mechanisms of defense, disavows, or represses in some way, then we have simply provided a synonym for the disavowed part of the total personality. As before, little seems to be gained by adding a technical-sounding word for what we already understand; namely, there are mental states that are experienced as not being part of oneself but which are nonetheless part of one's total personality.

As before with ego, id could be a theoretical term forming part of the explanation for why some persons experience a lack of congruence between their sense of self and their total personality. Again, however, the *universal,* functional definition of the id will simply get in the way of the *personally variable* parts of the total personality that each person disavows and represses. It simply will not be the case universally, for example, that a person's sexual wishes will either be repressed or disavowed in some other way. Sometimes that will be the case and sometimes it will not. Thus, when id is used as a synonym for that part of the total personality not affirmed as part of oneself, sometimes such sexual wishes will be included in the id, and sometimes they will be excluded. The problem lies in the fact that this highly individualized mode of aggregating the mental states belonging to the id will not match the universal attribution of those sex drives of any person to the id demanded by Freud's functional organization of the person. As is well known, basic to the drives functionally assigned to the id are those of sex. This lack of congruence between the id defined as the excluded total personality and the id defined by its functional organizing principle will result in two senses of id, just as it will two senses of ego. The result of such two quite different things being named by the same name is confusion, not theoretical advancement.

The very features that blunt any serious challenge to the unity of the self also throw into question the topographical or structural theories as fruitful modes of conceptualizing what disunities there are. The ideal case for disunity constructed before depends on the congruence between Freud's three sorting principles, functional assignment, conflict, and lack of awareness. As we have seen, such congruence is not very likely, given the difference in these three sorting principles.

In retrospect it is perhaps easier to see the implausibility of thinking that there would be such a congruence. Today, with the emergence of cognitive psychology and artificial intelligence research, it is particularly implausible to think that there would be a congruence between the conflict principle and the functional organization principle. From beginning to end, Freud was concerned that his functional subdividing of mind be a fruitful way of solving the mind/body problem. This is not the commonly made point that Freud simply transported the physiological speculations of the unpublished *Project*[27] into his economic metapsychology — he did. Rather, it is the point that what he hoped to achieve by such transfer was a theory that, Janus-like, faced both the psychological experiences of his patients and the physiology of their brains. At the beginning of the *Outline*, his last work, he reaffirmed this role for his theory:

> We know two things concerning what we call our psyche or mental life: firstly, its bodily organ and scene of action, the brain (or nervous system), and secondly, our acts of consciousness, which are immediate data and cannot be more fully explained by any kind of description. Everything that lies between these two terminal points is unknown to us and, so far as we are aware, there is no direct relation between them.[28]

Freud's theory, including the functional subdivisions of mind of the topographical and structural metapsychologies, was intended to bridge this unknown chasm, to chart the *in*direct relations between brain and mind.

There is no reason to think that a functional subdivision of mind that will be fruitful for understanding the relation of mind to brain will utilize just those subdivisions experienced by conflict-ridden neurotics. Such functional subdivisions, as in perception, need not be (and are not) *experienced* by anyone, not as conflict and not as anything. Such states are subpersonal, that is, beyond awareness and extended memory.

By attempting to lump these two different aggregating principles together, Freud distorted both of them and thus, his resulting theory. He tried to force the variability and richness of the conflict experienced by persons into the rigid mold of his instinct theories and the defenses; he warped his functional subdivisions in the direction of experienced conflict. The result is a theory whose subdivisions neither capture the phenomenology of conflict nor appear fruitful in exploring the relation of mind to brain.

Freed of this forced marriage, psychoanalytic theory could construct subdivisions of mind more faithful to each of these different tasks. Indeed, much of "ego psychology" should be seen as a movement toward the first of these tasks. In Fairbairn, for example, there is explicit recognition of the distorting influence Freud's functional organization had on ego, id, and superego.[29] Fairbairn accordingly attempted to restate such subdivisions "within the ego" itself, that is, without regard to the physiologically tied id.

The second task, giving a functional organization to the mind, could also proceed better unhampered by the distraction of having to subdivide the mind so that experienced conflict can be had between the subdivisions. For as it stands, ego, id, and superego are little better than Plato's tripartite scheme of the psyche; both are very general functional subdivisions unlikely to be fruitful in finding correlations with physiology. What is needed is a much finer-grained functional subdivision than either Freud or Plato gave us.

Consider by way of comparison the current artificial intelligence approach to functionally subdividing mental operations. As described by Dan Dennett:

> AI program designers work backwards on the same task behaviorists work forwards on.... The AI researcher starts with an intentionally characterized problem (e.g., how can I get a computer to *understand* questions of English?), breaks it down into subproblems that are also intentionally characterized (e.g., how do I get the computer to *recognize* questions, *distinguish* subjects from predicates, *ignore* irrelevant parsings?) and then breaks these problems down still further until finally he reaches problem or task descriptions that are obviously mechanistic. Here is a way of looking at the process. The AI programmer begins with an intentionally characterized problem, and thus frankly views the computer anthropomorphically: if he *solves* the problem he will say he has designed a computer that can understand questions in English. His first and highest level of design breaks the computer down into subsystems, each of which is given intentionally characterized tasks; he composes a flow chart of evaluators, rememberers, discriminators, overseers and the like. These are *homunculi* with a vengeance; the highest level design breaks the computer down into a committee or army of intelligent homunculi with purposes, information and strategies. Each homunculus in turn is analysed into *smaller* homunculi, but, more important, into *less clever* homunculi.

The Unity of the Self

When the level is reached where the homunculi are no more than adders and subtractors, by the time they need only the intelligence to pick the larger of two numbers when directed to, they have been reduced to functionaries "who can be replaced by a machine." The aid to comprehension of anthropomorphizing the elements just about lapses at this point, and a mechanistic view of the proceedings becomes workable and comprehensible.[30]

The problem for Freud was that his subdivisions are much too large to be fruitful. The functions assigned to the ego in particular make it almost like a whole mind, with a full panoply of functions. This is no "army" of "less clever" homunculi, but one much-too-smart general. Freed of the need to reproduce conflicts persons can experience, the needed, finer-grained subdivisions become possible, for psychoanalytic theory as for any theory claiming to be a general psychology.

If psychiatry pursued both of these suggestions, it is doubtful that the result would look much like the topographical or structural metapsychologies. Rather, we might have something like Kohut's psychology of self, attempting to be faithful to the phenomenology of conflict, and something like the artificial intelligence picture of mind, attempting to get at the relation of mind and brain. The two different subdivisions of mind that these two tasks would probably produce would have little to do with each other. Neither would be an *unpacking* of ego, id, and superego so much as a *replacement* of these notions. And with the disappearance of the topographical or structural metapsychologies would go the last vestiges of any challenge to the commonsense view of persons as unitary. Persons are conflict-ridden, functionally organized, and partly unaware of their own mental states—but unified nonetheless.

Conclusion: Toward a Philosophical Rethinking of Law and Psychiatry

IT IS TIME to return to the methodological and substantive theses with which we began: Lawyers and psychiatrists need to know more philosophy if they are to progress in understanding one another (the methodological thesis), and such deeper understanding should center on a shared view of persons as rational and autonomous agents (the substantive thesis). I shall deal with each in turn.

The Methodological Thesis: The Need for Philosophy in Law and Psychiatry

Hopefully this book has illustrated (but not exhausted) the kinds of payoffs available to lawyers and psychiatrists if they would be more philosophical. It is perhaps worth reiterating in closing what some of those payoffs are. They may be grouped into three classes: those with respect to psychiatry itself, those with respect to law itself, and those having to do with the relationship between law and psychiatry. I shall discuss each of these.

THE NEED FOR A PHILOSOPHICAL UNDERSTANDING OF PSYCHIATRY

In light of the widely acknowledged failures of the grand theoretical edifices erected by psychiatrists, such as Freud, there is today in psychiatry a temptation to retreat to *a*theoretical work. The kind of work to which psychiatrists have currently retreated has been one of two kinds. One is a return to the diagnostic categories of mental illness with a kind of empiricist vengeance. An example of this tendency is the response prompted by an early version of Chapter 5. That paper was delivered by me at an annual meeting of the American Psychopathological Association and was met in some quarters with a plea that psychiatrists should ignore such "new scholaticism" and should instead direct their efforts at empirical research on the cause and

Conclusion

etiology of particular syndromes.¹ Such a plea illustrates the turn of mind that fears theory building in psychiatry and seeks to return to the safer task of improving the psychiatric nosology. Such a task is "safer" not only because it does not present the dangers of speculative flights or arid scholasticism, but also because the development of such a taxonomy of diseases has been a central focus of medicine generally since Sydenham. And psychiatrists very much want to be "real doctors" again.

Similarly motivated is the second kind of work done by those who are part of the current psychiatric flight from theory. This is the faith being placed by psychiatrists in drugs and drug-based therapies. The large strides made in the psychopharmacology of the last two decades have encouraged psychiatrists to return to the nineteenth-century hope that mental disease will be found to be brain disease. Again, this hope is partly motivated by the desire of psychiatrists to return to the medical fold. And again, this hope encourages psychiatrists to engage in an empirical kind of research, here, research into the effects of various drugs in altering the symptoms of the various mental diseases. The ultimate effect again is to abandon the search for an adequate general theory of human behavior in favor of a much less speculative, narrower, seemingly atheoretical concern with particular causal connections.

One of the intended payoffs of this book is to convince readers that this psychiatric flight from theory is neither necessary nor possible. It is not necessary, because there *are* answers to be found to the difficult questions of how mental illness as such should be defined, how our conscious mental processes are to be explained in terms of our unconscious, and how the facts of conflict, functional organization, and partial awareness are to be integrated into an overall theory of the person. Indeed, this book seeks to defend my answers to those questions (answers on which, no doubt, considerable improvement is possible, but only by more theoretical work, not by less).

In any case, whatever one thinks of my answers to these large questions, psychiatrists cannot avoid the questions themselves. The questions do not go away because one limits one's research and therapeutic energies to drugs or to the diagnostic categories. Indeed, either of these contemporary concerns of psychiatrists involves them, like it or not, in theory building.

In the case of drugs, it is something of an article of faith, given the present state of our knowledge, to think that all the syndromes classified as mental diseases must be caused by some condition of the brain amenable to correction by drugs. But even accepting such an article of faith, it would not follow that psychiatrists need not concern themselves with the general nature of mental illness or with the psychological machinery that underlies conscious thought. The successes of psychopharmacology do not compete with these theoretical concerns; rather, they are part of our developing

Conclusion

answer to when a person is mentally ill and what underlies our conscious thoughts. Knowing something about the neurotransmitters in the amine pathways of the brain and the effect of the level of those transmitters on affect and mood, for example, tells us more about the physical machinery underlying the emotions. It does not eliminate the need to "philosophize" about what the emotions are, how they are individuated, whether they or their objects can be unconscious, whether certain emotions are functionally isolatable from others because they recur together or jointly cause certain effects, and so on. We need such psychological and philosophical theorizing as much as we need the chemistry of the emotions, if we are to progress toward a systematic, unified account of the emotions.

Suppose, by way of a second example, that it were discovered that homosexual tendencies are caused by some chemical present in all and only those with such tendencies. Suppose further that this chemical "imbalance" could be reversed by a simple drug therapy. Neither of these facts would tell psychiatrists whether they should classify homosexuality as a mental disease or not. To answer this question requires that one take a position on the issues raised in Chapter 5 as to the purposes that should lie behind psychiatric definitions of mental disease. Only then can one answer whether including homosexuality serves those purposes or not. Again, knowledge of physical causation and of reversibility may help one in classifying homosexuality, but only if one answers the antecedent, philosophical questions in certain ways but not others.

There is equally no possibility of maintaining a "theory-free" stance about psychiatric nosology. The disorders classified in the second and third editions of the American Psychiatric Association's *Diagnostic and Statistical Manual* may look like simple, inductively established aggregations of symptoms, but they are not. As I have argued in the preceding chapters there is implicit in such classifying efforts causal hypotheses about the hidden natures of such diseases. It is this presupposition of a hidden nature that makes sense of the provisional status of any given symptom in the search for tighter and tighter syndromes.

Such implicit causal hypotheses involve one in asking very theoretical questions about the psychological and physical machinery that underlies the mental or behavioral symptoms. If one wants to get at the hidden nature of paranoia, for example, one can do so only through a psychological theory about the nature of beliefs in general and of delusional beliefs in particular; this in turn should involve one in answering an instantiation of the mind/body problem, namely, how belief states are related to certain brain states. There can be no avoidance, ultimately, of these theoretical questions if one wants to place paranoia securely in some nosology of diseases.

Similarly, if one wants to know whether paranoia *is* a mental disease, knowledge of its symptoms (and of its causes) will be part of one's answer,

Conclusion

but only part. Even after the regularities in symptom development are inductively established, and even after the psychological and physical nature of those symptoms is understood, one cannot say paranoia is a mental illness. To reach this conclusion, one must also ask and answer the theoretical questions of what separates the normal from the diseased, or, in terms of paranoid beliefs, what distinguishes an irrational belief from one that is merely false. Knowing only that a belief is delusional, or that it is caused in a certain way, tells us something about whether the subject is or is not mentally ill only in some theory about persons (viz., that they are rational beings) and about rationality with respect to beliefs. In these ways a taxonomy ultimately begs for an answer to the question, What is it a taxonomy of? Giving a label—mental illness—is a start, but one needs to say a great deal more about what the label names, an unapologetically theoretical task.

One cannot help but have noticed throughout the body of this book the preeminent place given to Freud in the field of psychiatry. If this book were written thirty years ago, in the heyday of psychoanalysis in Great Britain and the United States, such emphasis would not have seemed unusual. But today such emphasis requires explanation. The explanation should be apparent from the foregoing defense of theory in psychiatry. Despite all of the limitations of the metapsychological theories that Freud invented, he understood one thing very clearly: Psychiatry only makes sense in the context of some more general psychological theory. One cannot study abnormal functioning except in the context of some background theory about normal functioning. This is as true of physical medicine with its roots in biology and anatomy as it is of psychiatry with its roots in psychology (including physiological psychology).

Psychiatrists thus cannot help but work out an image of humankind—a theory of the person—as they go about their more mundane tasks. Their choice is thus to philosophize about persons badly or well, unconsciously or consciously; there is no ostrichlike choice of not philosophizing about persons at all.

It is no doubt somewhat dangerous to extend an invitation to theorizing about minds and persons to psychiatrists, in light of the past history of the profession, where many have brought it off so badly. The plea, however, is for a philosophically sophisticated psychiatric theorizing, not for a return to the often pretentious and usually ill-read versions we have seen in psychiatry's recent past.

THE NEED FOR A PHILOSOPHICAL UNDERSTANDING OF LAW

The legal profession too has its own flight from theory. Although there is a well-established place for philosophical work in contemporary legal schol-

Conclusion

arship, there is also a tradition of legal scholarship that shuns such theoretical work in favor of more doctrinal or empirical concerns. As in psychiatry, we can distinguish two dimensions to this tradition. The first is the analogue to the contemporary psychiatric concern with the diagnostic categories; in law, this is a concern with legal doctrine. In this vein of legal scholarship there is an attempt to limit ourselves to the least problematic of the standards we think of as law, namely statutory texts, constitutional texts, and judge-made rules (the latter being either interpretations of texts or common law rules). "Knowing the law," in this narrow, positivistic idea of law, amounts to a knowing of a bunch of rules that have been authoritatively laid down by someone in the past. A lawyer, even an academic lawyer, is accordingly someone who knows a lot of this kind of institutional history.

Sometimes opposed to this concern with doctrine (although sometimes thought compatible with it) is the second kind of atheoretical legal scholarship. This is the empiricist concern with law. Here the proper enterprise of an academic lawyer is thought to be either the study of the historical or psychological *causes* of existing doctrines having been accepted or the study of the social *effects* of those doctrines having been enacted into law. One in such a case does doctrinal history, explaining changes in law by factors operating in the society as a whole; or one does "impact studies," detailing what effects various statutes or decisions have had on people's behavior.

Although there is nothing wrong with such approaches to law, they cannot be made exclusive of the more theoretical approach to law taken by this book. One may begin to understand the criminal law, for example, by learning the various doctrines that define the elements of particular crimes – the legal equivalent of psychiatry's taxonomic concerns. Yet such knowledge of doctrine can only be the beginning of understanding, even when supplemented by historical explanations and impact studies. The next step is to master those *general* doctrines that cut across all crimes, that state or modify the elements of all crimes. These doctrines, such as that requiring the simultaneous presence of *actus reus, mens rea,* and causation, are usually termed the "general part" of criminal law just to mark them off from the "special part," which deals with the elements of particular crimes. The general part, although still at the level of doctrine (cases, statutes), is already a theory-laden organization of the otherwise varied and chaotic doctrines of the special part.

We still have not understood the criminal law when we have mastered the doctrines of both the special and the general part. In addition, what is needed is a mastery, first, of a moral theory that spells out when fault is fairly ascribed to a person, and, second, a metaphysical theory that describes what sort of a being persons are such that fault can fairly be

Conclusion

ascribed to them. I have laid out in Chapter 2 my understanding of these moral and metaphysical theories.

Although we can distinguish such moral and metaphysical theories from the legal doctrines they underlie, it would be a mistake to regard them as extraneous to "the law," properly understood. The law—or here, the criminal law—must include such theories, and not as peripheral, but as central features. In an emerging natural law tradition,[2] such moral and metaphysical theories are law in the sense that they are among those standards judges do, should, and cannot help but take into account in deciding cases. Such theories enter in necessarily as judges formulate common law rules or principles and as they interpret statutory or constitutional texts. They are thus not some dispensable features of our concept of law but are central to our understanding of that concept, as that understanding is revealed by our practices as lawyers.

The upshot is that no one can pretend to understand the law simply by eschewing theoretical work and focusing exclusively on legal doctrine. Lawyers who wish to understand the insanity defense, for example, cannot rest content with regurgitating the differing doctrinal tests we examined at the beginning of Chapter 6. Rather, they must organize those tests by the moral and metaphysical theses about persons that the tests embody. Only then do they have any idea of what the tests are about or how they should be applied.

Lawyers, thus, no more than psychiatrists, can ignore the philosophical basis of their own discipline. This, as I next propose to show, is equally true of those lawyers or psychiatrists interested in understanding the relationship between law and psychiatry.

THE NEED FOR A PHILOSOPHICAL FORENSIC PSYCHIATRY

If a person stays at the doctrinal surface of law and at the taxonomic surface of psychiatry, he will also remain at a superficial level in his relating of law and psychiatry. He will mechanically juxtapose legal doctrines with psychiatric dogmas on a topic-by-topic basis. When the two approaches appear to be similar, he will talk of "interdisciplinary interfaces"; when they appear to disagree, he will talk of the "incommensurability" of the two points of view, each starting with opposed basic premises. An example of the first is the psychosis/insanity parallel noted by many psychiatrists and lawyers; an example of the second is the free will versus determinism perspectives supposedly distinctive of law and psychiatry, respectively.

This kind of interdisciplinary work—a topic-by-topic juxtaposition of unquestioned doctrine—leads to a kind of role playing by both lawyers

Conclusion

and psychiatrists. The lawyers can contribute "the legal point of view" on some topic while the psychiatrists can contribute "the psychiatric viewpoint." Each group can in this way "contribute" to the discussions while: (a) eschewing any responsibility to say which (if either) view is *true;* and (b) insulating their own contributions from extradisciplinary criticism. Like all role playing, this kind of interdisciplinary role playing serves the dual functions of limiting the horizon of things that need be considered while insulating the subject from criticism about results (or the lack of them).

Lawyers and psychiatrists have to do better than this if any true dialogue is to be commenced between the disciplines. For the problems they each face are no respecters of the jurisdictional boundaries that mark the separate disciplines. The problem of giving a legal definition of insanity that is not psychiatrically naive, for example, will not yield itself to those who simply juxtapose legal doctrine with unexamined psychiatric dogma; one cannot, for example, slant legal "irresistible impulse" formulations to match psychiatric talk of instinctual drives "compelling" actions. Instead, one must penetrate the legal doctrine to examine its moral point and metaphysical assumptions *and then* assess the psychiatric theory for its ability either to show that the moral requirements of a just punishment are met or to show that such requirements cannot be met because the metaphysical assumptions of such a moral theory are false.

At the ultimate level of their respective metaphysical views about minds and persons law and psychiatry can and must join issue. Here there is no room for trivial coincidence or incommensurable disagreement. For here the theories are theories about the same thing: What are persons like in their most fundamental respects? Here there can be no room for peaceful coexistence; if the theories of minds and persons disagree, one of them is true and the other false (or both are false and some third theory is true).

The upshot is that law and psychiatry as a field also must be philosophical in the broad sense in which that term is used here. We cannot put off forever questions such as the difference between health and goodness, or between illness and badness, no more than we can ignore the role of the unconscious in our theories of minds or morals and no more than we can defer the question of how the facts of conflict, functional subsystems, and partial awareness fit in with our ideas of self. These questions cannot be put off because the answers to them determine how we should come out on very practical issues in forensic psychiatry, such as the proper definition of legal insanity, the admissibility of expert testimony about the unconscious, and how we should deal with multiple personalities. Yet these basic questions cannot be answered by the surface approaches of doctrinal lawyers or "zoological" psychiatrists. Needed is the philosophical approach to the problems of law and psychiatry that this book is intended to illustrate.

Conclusion

Lest all of this should seem like a plea for added employment opportunities for professional philosophers, I shall append a word about the kind of philosophy needed here. In my view the philosophy of mind and the philosophy of science merge imperceptibly into psychology and thus psychiatry. Similarly, there is no clear line to be drawn between law, on the one hand, and political theory, ethics, or the philosophy of law, on the other. The philosophies of law or of psychiatry are simply the disciplines themselves, carried on at somewhat higher levels of abstraction than those employed by typical practitioners in each. To draw lines here would be like trying to separate philosophical theories about perception from psychological theories of perception.[3]

The methodological thesis thus does not have as its implication the unemployment of lawyers and psychiatrists and their replacement by professional philosophers. To work in this field philosophers need to know as much about law and psychiatry as lawyers and psychiatrists need to know about philosophy. True interdisciplinary work here requires the ability to work comfortably in all three areas. Indeed, ultimately one's professional pedigree should become irrelevant. There are only problems to be solved and questions to be answered, and what academic authority licensed one to hunt them down should be relegated to the scrapbook of one's intellectual biography. It should not be used as an excuse from seeking answers that one is prepared to defend as true (and not just "true from the psychiatric perspective," and so forth).

The Substantive Thesis: The Shared View of Persons in Law and Psychiatry

The overall substantive thesis of the book is that a properly regimented law and a properly regimented[4] psychiatry will not reveal a view of human nature that conflicts in any fundamental way. If one plumbs beneath the various legal doctrines that assign rights and liabilities to the moral theories that underlie them, and if one then asks, What must beings be like to have assigned to them these rights and responsibilities? the answer will be the theory of the person developed in Chapter 2. Such a philosophical plumbing of the moral and metaphysical presuppositions of law reveals the view that persons are rational and autonomous agents. One of the payoffs of this philosophically reconstructed theory of persons is the ridding of law of the common myths attributed to it by psychiatrists. Nothing in the law, or in the morality that underlies it, presupposes that people act outside the laws of causation ("free will"). Autonomy, as I argued in Chapters 2 and 10, only means that persons are agents with causal powers, not that the exercise of those powers is uncaused. Nor does much in the law require

Conclusion

the strong sense of autonomy having to do with the shaping of one's own character. Limited areas of law presuppose some of this kind of autonomy, but not much. Similarly, nothing in the law presupposes that people are rational in any problematically strong sense of the word. The bloodless, emotionless type of rationality that psychiatrists are fond of attributing to the law's view of persons is not the kind of rationality generally presupposed by the law. In each case the law presupposes versions of rationality and autonomy weaker than those attributed to it by psychiatrists bent on showing the difference (usually to the detriment of law) between the legal and psychiatric views of persons.

A philosophical regimentation of psychiatry also shapes that discipline so that the conflict between the legal and the psychiatric views of persons is more apparent than real. To be sure, psychiatrists who worry only about the discipline's taxonomic scheme *say* that all sorts of conditions are mental disorders; further, they say that so classifying a condition in a medical context has implications for responsibility in law and morals. Again, however, one cannot take such statements at face value. If one asks why psychiatrists wish to define what mental illness is, and if one then limits the definition of mental illness so as to achieve those purposes, the definitions proposed will not encompass all conditions psychiatrists treat, as I argued in Chapter 5. Further, if one asks whether those psychiatric purposes are the same as the purposes that lie behind the law's definition of mental illness, it may turn out (as I argued in Chapter 6) that psychiatric definitions do *not* have the implications about responsibility that some psychiatrists think they have.

Similarly, one cannot allow psychiatrists to be the final authority on what they mean by unconscious or how the unconscious ought to be conceptualized. In order to be faithful to the very phenomena they wish to describe with that concept, one should deanimize the notion. One does this by ignoring all the talk about subpersonal agents acting for reasons. Such a reconstrual of our mental topography eliminates any purported, radical disunities of self, as I argued in Chapter 11. One must also go beneath what psychiatrists say they are providing us with when they give explanations of behavior in terms of the unconscious; one must ascertain for oneself what sort of explanation is truly being given (Chapter 8). One must do such theoretical restructuring of psychiatry if one is to have any chance to get at the question of whether law and psychiatry, in their deepest and most systematic expression, really disagree in their views on human nature.

The substantive thesis is that they do not, once each is restructured in the ways suggested. Psychiatry and law both view persons as agents with irreducible causal powers who act for reasons, that is, as autonomous and rational agents. (This does not mean that either discipline is committed to viewing all behavior as an action or to viewing all mental state explana-

Conclusion

tions as reason-giving explanations; as we have seen in Chapter 8, one of the mistakes of some psychoanalytic theorists is to overextend those concepts.) This *is* to say that both law and psychiatry by and large remain in the Intentional vocabulary of persons. They remain, that is, in the vocabulary that can tell us something about our *selves* — even if that something is not that we acted for a reason but that one of our wishes caused us to behave in certain ways.

The true challenge to *both* law and psychiatry comes from those who would replace the Intentional vocabulary of persons with other ways of thinking about human beings. Such views are distinct from Freud's enterprise, which was to explain the Intentionally characterized states of minds and persons by reference to subpersonal states (the primary process) and ultimately, by reference to the non-Intentional states of neurophysiology. To explain is not to explain away, so that the metapsychology should not be seen (as I argued in Chapter 7) as an instance of this kind of wholesale discarding of our most basic views of our selves (in Intentional terms) as rational and autonomous agents. A better example of the true challenge to both law and psychiatry is that presented by B. F. Skinner's radical behaviorism. What must be abolished, Skinner has proclaimed, is "the autonomous man — the inner man, the homunculus, the possessing demon, the man defended by the literature of freedom and dignity."[5] Skinnerian behaviorism would urge us to abandon the Intentional idioms of persons, to abandon the concepts of rationality and autonomy, knowing full well that this entails abandoning the moral theories ("freedom and dignity") presupposing this view of human beings.

More generally, as science progresses in its understanding of the relationship between genetic background, environmental influences, the brain, and behavior, the view of persons as rational and autonomous agents will be increasingly threatened. For it will become increasingly tempting to bypass the difficult question that haunted Freud of how mind and brain are related. It will become increasingly tempting to recast actions in the non-Intentional language of bodily motions and to recast explanations of those movements in the non-Intentional language of neurophysiology and environmental stimuli. There will be more — and better — books urging us to lay aside the Intentional idioms of minds and persons and to move beyond the accompanying moral vocabulary of freedom and dignity. Advances in genetic research, brain physiology, sociobiology, information theory, and artificial intelligence will increasingly seem to many to provide the basis for a complete replacement of our present Intentional conceptualization of persons. In this fight about a radical rethinking of who we are, both law and psychiatry are on the same side in defending an Intentional conceptualization of persons as rational and autonomous agents. On this issue both, to my way of thinking, are on the side of the angels.

Notes

Introduction

1. For one influential expression of this view of law and psychiatry, see Jerome Hall, *General Principles of Criminal Law,* 2d ed. (New York: Bobbs-Merrill, 1960), p. 455: "The most important fact in the current polemics regarding psychiatry and criminal responsibility is the clash of elementary philosophical perspectives. Every science rests upon distinctive axioms or postulates that are accepted by the scientists as 'given,' while philosophers remain curious about them. Without describing the postulates of current psychiatry, we can perceive the general perspective that it, especially psychoanalysis, draws from them. It purports to be rigorously scientific and therefore takes a determinist position. Its view of human nature is expressed in terms of drives and dispositions which, like mechanical forces, operate in accordance with universal laws of causation.

   On the other hand, criminal law, while it is also a science in a wide sense of the term, is not a theoretical science whose sole concern is to understand and describe what goes on. It is, instead, a practical normative science which, while it draws upon the empirical sciences, is also concerned to pass judgment on human conduct, entailing serious consequences for both individuals and the community. Its view of human nature asserts the reality of a 'significant' degree of free choice, and that is incompatible with the thesis that the conduct of normal adults is merely a manifestation of imperious psychological necessity. Given the scientific purpose to understand conduct, determinism is a necessary, although by no means the only helpful, postulate. Given the additional purpose to evaluate conduct, some degree of autonomy is a necessary postulate."
2. Indeed, the concept of mind is often thought to collapse into the concept of a person. See Gilbert Ryle, *The Concept of Mind* (London: Hutchinson & Co., 1949), and P. F. Strawson, *Individuals* (London: Methuen & Co., 1959), for two philosophical attempts to reduce the problems of mind to problems about persons.

1. Practical Reason and Explanation

1. For two philosophical analyses of reasons for actions sympathetic to that

done in the text, see Donald Davidson, *Actions and Events,* (Oxford: Oxford University Press, 1980), particularly pp. 3–19; and Daniel C. Dennett, *Brainstorms* (Montgomery, Vt.: Bradford Books, 1978), particularly chaps. 1 and 12.

2. This was the position of the older action theorists who argued that reasons could not be the causes of actions. This literature is cited in n. 5 this chapter, and discussed in the subsection on hermeneutic interpretation.

3. One can transform practical syllogisms into the valid inference patterns of standard deductive logic with the addition of the two premises discussed in chaps. 4 and 10.

4. These difficulties have to do with what is later described in this chapter (see the subsection on hermeneutic interpretation) as the "essentially linguistic" nature of the objects of mental states. More specifically, the difficulties in characterizing the p, p and q, q relationships as those of propositional identity stem from two controversial assumptions: first, that the objects of mental states are propositions (and not, say, sentences); and second, that some coherent account can be given of propositional identity. The difficulties in characterizing the p, q relationship in the second premise of a practical syllogism stem from the non-truth-functional relationship that holds between p, q and $p \supset q$ when the latter is enclosed within the scope of a belief operator. Also, it is undoubtedly the case that the means/end belief of a rational agent is not that the action is a sufficient condition for the bringing about of his desired end, but only that it is possible that it is.

5. A sampling: Gilbert Ryle, *The Concept of Mind* (London: Hutchinson, 1949), chap. 4; Richard Peters, *The Concept of Motivation* (London: Routledge & Kegan Paul, 1958); Peter Winch, *The Idea of a Social Science* (London: Routledge & Kegan Paul, 1958); A. I. Melden, *Free Action* (London: Routledge & Kegan Paul, 1961); G. E. M. Anscombe, *Intention,* 2d ed. (Ithaca, N.Y.: Cornell University Press, 1963); Richard Taylor, *Action and Purpose* (Englewood Cliffs, N.J.: Prentice-Hall, 1966).

6. D. Davidson, *Actions and Events.*

7. A. R. Louch, *Explanation and Human Action* (Berkeley: University of California Press, 1966).

8. Ernest Jones, "Rationalization in Everyday Life," *Journal of Abnormal Psychology,* vol. 3(1908): 161–9.

9. See, e.g., Brian Fay, "Practical Reasoning, Rationality, and the Explanation of Intentional Action," *Journal of the Theory of Social Behavior,* vol. 8(1977): 77–101. Fay's kind of argument for this causal notion of reasons is discussed shortly; see this chapter, subsection on mental state causation.

10. These kinds of examples are discussed by D. C. Dennett, *Brainstorms,* chap. 12.

11. George Hendrik Von Wright appears to conflate these two in *Explanation and Understanding* (Ithaca, N.Y.: Cornell University Press, 1973). Fay, in "Practical Reasoning," nicely untangles the two, as does Joseph Raz in his introduction to J. Raz (ed.), *Practical Reasoning* (Oxford: Oxford University Press, 1978), p. 4.

12. It is not at all clear what Aristotle meant by practical reasoning and practical syllogisms in the scattered writings in which he used these phrases. For a defense of the view that he used it in the manner suggested in the text, where the premises of a practical inference are just the contents of a belief/desire set, see Martha Nussbaum, "Practical Syllogisms and Practical Science," in her *Aristotle's De Moto Animalum* (Princeton, N.J.: Princeton University Press, 1977).
13. As far as I know, the phrase "mental cause" originates with Elizabeth Anscombe's *Intention*, sec. 11. Anscombe, however, defined a mental cause as being "what someone would describe if he were asked the specific question: what produced this action or thought or feeling on your part: what did you see or hear or feel, or what ideas or images cropped up in your mind, and led up to it?" By my use of the phrase I intend no such tie of mental causes to the first-person avowal of the person whose mental states they are. Rather, mental cause is my catchbasket for any mental state that causes behavior but is not a reason for action.
14. This causal theory of action is discussed in chap. 2.
15. This possibility is easily overlooked, as in J. Goslin, "Mental Causes and Fear," *Mind,* vol. 71(1962): 289–306, who on p. 299 appears to believe that mental causes explain only bodily movements but not human actions.
16. See Fay, "Practical Reasoning."
17. It was weakness of will that induced Davidson to abandon his earlier position about the necessary validity of practical reasoning in reason-giving explanations. See Davidson, *Actions and Events,* pp. xii and 21–42.
18. This shifting of questions yielding different answers is what Alan Garfinkel calls explanatory relativity. *Forms of Explanation* (New Haven, Conn.: Yale University Press, 1980).
19. This is Freud's move in his attempt to make out a practical syllogism for dreamers, as I discuss in chap. 9.
20. See, e.g., Peter Winch, *Idea of a Social Science.*
21. This sense of meaning is what Grice called the natural sense (as opposed to the nonnatural sense involved in communication). H. P. Grice, "Meaning," *Philosophical Review,* vol. 66(1957): 377–88.
22. The phrase possible motive comes from the law of evidence. See H. Wigmore, *Evidence,* vol. 1, 3d ed. (Boston: Little, Brown, 1940), sec. 118. Possible motives for an action are motives one has just because one is in a situation whereby one stands to gain an intelligible advantage from such an act. Evidence of possible motives, or the lack thereof, is relevant evidence admissible in a criminal trial; the prosecution may show that the accused had a possible motive for the crime as circumstantial evidence that he did the criminal act, and the accused may show that he had no possible motive for doing it as circumstantial evidence to the contrary. Such motives are *possible* motives precisely because they are not true mental states at all. A person "has" such "motives" simply because he is in a certain situation; that he has such possible motives says nothing about his desires, his beliefs, or any of his mental states at all. Compare the philosophical notion of there being good reasons

for acting in a certain way; there being such reasons is totally independent of the actor's having acted on them as his reasons. See G. R. Grice, "Motive and Reason," in J. Raz (ed.), pp. 168–77.
23. For a beginning at least on the difficult idea of rational belief, see R. J. Ackermann, *Belief and Knowledge* (Garden City, N.Y.: Doubleday [Anchor Books], 1972), chap. 3.
24. On the intelligibility of desires, see G. E. M. Anscombe, *Intention;* A. J. Watt, "The Intelligibility of Wants," *Mind,* vol. 81(1972): 553–61; Richard Peters, *Concept of Motivation;* and Anthony Kenny, *Action, Emotion, and Will* (London: Routledge & Kegan Paul, 1963), pp. 94–8. The distinction between unintelligible and morally bad desires is an important one, for it forms one of the distinctions between mental illness and socially deviant behavior. See chap. 7.
25. This is the sense of "rational" Carl Hempel discussed in "Rational Action," in N. S. Care and C. Landesman (eds.), *Readings in the Theory of Action,* (Bloomington: Indiana University Press, 1968), pp. 281–305.
26. See text at n. 7, this chapter.
27. L. Wittgenstein, *Philosophical Investigations,* 2d ed. (Oxford: Blackwell Publishers, 1958).
28. Richard Peters, *Concept of Motivation.*
29. A. I. Melden, "Action," *Philosophical Review,* vol. 65(1956): 529–41.
30. Peter Winch, *Idea of a Social Science.*
31. Thomas Szasz, for example, was influenced by this approach to social science early on, as I discuss in chap. 4.
32. Winch, *Idea of a Social Science,* p. 30.
33. Ibid., p. 31.
34. Michael Oakeshott, *Experience and its Modes* (Cambridge: Cambridge University Press, 1933).
35. William Dray, *Laws and Explanation in History* (Oxford: Oxford University Press, 1957).
36. Carl Hempel, *Aspects of Scientific Explanation* (New York: Free Press, 1965).
37. R. G. Collingwood, *The Idea of History* (Oxford: Oxford University Press, 1946). For a sympathetic relating of Collingwood to the issues of contemporary action theory, see Rex Martin, *Historical Explanation: Re-enactment and Practical Inference* (Ithaca, N.Y.: Cornell University Press, 1977).
38. For a brief discussion of the *verstehen* tradition in German history and sociology, see G. H. Von Wright, *Explanation and Understanding,* pp. 4–7. The logical links between this tradition and the neo-Wittgensteinian tradition of Melden-Winch-Peters are nicely summarized in K. O. Apel, "The Erklären-verstehen Controversy in the Philosophy of the Natural and Human Sciences," in G. Fløistad (ed.), *Contemporary Philosophy: A New Survey* (The Hague: Martinus Nijhoff, 1982), pp. 19–50.
39. This is a tentative strategy put forward by Dennett in "Intentional Systems," *Journal of Philosophy,* vol. 68(1971): 87–106. By his "The Conditions of Personhood," in A. O. Rorty (ed.), *The Identities of Persons* (Berkeley: Uni-

versity of California Press, 1976), the tentativeness is gone, as Dennett concludes that "there is no objectively satisfiable sufficient condition for an entity's *really* having beliefs . . ." (p. 193). Both essays are reprinted in Dennett, *Brainstorms*.

40. See the helpful summary of the claims of the hermeneutic tradition in Josef Bleicher, *Contemporary Hermeneutics* (London: Routledge & Kegan Paul, 1980).
41. G. H. Von Wright, *Explanation and Understanding*.
42. Richard Rorty, *Philosophy as the Mirror of Nature* (Princeton, N.J.: Princeton University Press, 1979).
43. Von Wright, *Explanation and Understanding*, p. 115.
44. Ibid., p. 117.
45. Ibid., pp. 117–18.
46. The word "Intentional" is capitalized to distinguish this characteristic from the more familiar intention or intentional of ordinary speech. Brentano, one of Freud's early teachers, held that "every mental phenomenon is characterized by what the scholastics of the Middle Ages called the Intentional Inexistence of an object and which we would call . . . the reference to a content, a direction upon an object." F. Brentano, *Psychologie vom Empirischen Standpunkt* (Leipzig: 1874). Selection translated in R. Chisholm (ed.), *Realism and the Background of Phenomenology* (Glencoe, Ill.: Free Press, 1960).
47. Roderick Chisholm's explication of the concept is in terms of three criteria: (1) A sentence is Intentional if it uses a name or description in such a way that neither the sentence nor its contradictory implies either that there is or is not anything to which the name or expression truly applies. "I hope for a 60-foot sailboat," for example, does not imply that there is a 60-foot sailboat. (2) A sentence is Intentional if it contains a propositional clause whose truth or falsity is not implied by the sentence as a whole, or its contradictory. "I hope that it will rain," for example, does not imply that "It will rain" is true or false. (3) A sentence is Intentional if co-designative names or descriptions cannot be substituted and preserve truth. I may, for example, order the largest room in some inn. Even if the largest room is identical with the dirtiest room in the inn, one cannot substitute the second description for the first; I did not order the dirtiest room in the inn. R. Chisholm, *Perceiving: A Philosophical Study* (Ithaca, N.Y.: Cornell University Press, 1957), pp. 120–71. Many have urged that Intentionality is *the* distinguishing mark of our talk about minds.
48. These last two characteristics – lack of a truth-functional relation and lack of truth-preserving substitutivity of identicals – mean that descriptions of mental states create intensional and not extensional contexts. An extensional language is one of which two things (at least) must be true; its logical connectives must be truth functional, and one must be able to substitute numerical identicals without change of truth value. Such are thought to be necessary requirements for a scientific language, because they allow scientific laws to be formulated without regard to varying descriptions of the particular things covered. Whatever can be truthfully said of the morning star can also truthfully be said of the evening star, because they are one and the same thing,

Venus. This substitution-preserving truth is not possible for the mental predicates we use for describing and explaining the actions of persons. Such vocabulary is accordingly said to be intensional, in that substitution-preserving truth now depends on sameness of meaning (intension) of descriptions. If we are not talking about the evening star itself, but about George's *beliefs* about the evening star, the fact that "evening star" and "morning star" name the same thing is no guarantee that the one description may be substituted for the other and still preserve truth. For the classic treatment of this, see Willard Van Orman Quine, "Reference and Modality," in his *From a Logical Point of View* (Cambridge, Mass.: Harvard University Press, 1953), pp. 139–59. As one may have noticed, to say that a language is Intentional is to say that it is not extensional. See James Cornman, "Intentionality and Intensionality," *Philosophical Quarterly*, vol. 12(1962): 44–52.
49. Donald Davidson (despite his staunch adherence to a causal view of reasons) is led to what he calls "the necessarily holistic character of interpretations of propositional attitudes" by this motivation. See Davidson, *Actions and Events*, pp. 238–9.
50. Davidson, ibid., who sees this analogy, believes that to say what the utterance *meant* is to infuse one's own (observer) concepts into the interpretation of the utterance. Yet Davidson would not dispute that there existed a particular act of speech at a particular time, even if that act of speech requires interpretation to be understood.
51. Whether there is anything that could be called a "language of the brain" is a hotly contested matter. For an introductory, if skeptical, treatment of the issues involved, see Dennett, "Brain Writing and Mind Reading," in his *Brainstorms*, pp. 39–50. Compare Jerry Fodor, *The Language of Thought* (New York: Crowell, 1975).
52. See Jonathan Cohen, "Teleological Explanation," *Proceedings of the Aristotelian Society*, vol. 51(1955): 255–92.
53. This example is that of Carl Hempel, "The Logic of Functional Analysis," in Hempel, *Aspects of Scientific Explanation*, pp. 297–330.
54. In the recent philosophical literature on functions it is commonly claimed that function statements do more than simply describe the causal contributions parts or processes make to the attainment of various goals. Such function statements are said to constitute some kind of *explanation* as well as a mere description of the phenomenon in question. In some senses of explanation this claim is harmless enough because it asserts no more than is asserted by saying that function statements describe relations within a system. In this vein is John Canfield's claim that function statements *explain* what an item is there for, what it does, or how it contributes to certain goals (J. Canfield, "Teleological Explanations in Biology," *British Journal for the Philosophy of Science*, vol. 13 [1963]: 285–95). Equally compatible with my descriptivist thesis is Christopher Boorse's observation that often function statements give what he calls "operational explanations," explanations that answer the question, How does some system S work? (C. Boorse, "Wright on Functions," *Philosophical Review*, vol. 85 [1976]: 70–86.)

More troublesome is a stronger claim about the explanatory force of function statements, namely, that functions explain the existence of the part or process given the function. (See notably L. Wright, "Functions," *Philosophical Review*, vol. 82 [1973]: 139–68; see generally A. Rosenberg, "Causation and Teleology in Contemporary Philosophy of Science," in G. Fløistad [ed.], pp. 51–86, for a good summary of the post–World War II literature on this topic.) According to such a view, to say that the function of the heart's beating is to circulate the blood is to say that the circulation of blood's being a consequence of the heart's beating explains why there are hearts. This quickly involves function statements into hidden assertions about the genesis of various parts or processes within a system, either evolutionary or intentionalistic hypotheses about how the system in question originated. The problem for such a view is that forcefully articulated by Boorse ("Wright on Functions"): The view commits one to linking the meaning of function statements to the history of the system under consideration, so that two systems identical to each other in structure and performance might yet have different functional organizations if they have different histories. Preferable is Boorse's general view (ibid., p. 77) that "functions are, purely and simply, contributions to goals" (or what I call end states). For Boorse and for me, functions have to do with the relations between parts or processes within systems, not with the history of how those systems came to have the organization they possess.

55. Peters, *Concept of Motivation*, p. 21.
56. Ernst Nagel, *The Structure of Science* (New York: Harcourt Brace & World, 1961), p. 73.
57. This literature is discussed briefly in chap. 10.
58. Alan Garfinkel, *Forms of Explanation*, p. 49.
59. Norman Malcolm, *Problems of Mind* (New York: Harper & Row, 1971), p. 63.
60. Hilary Putnam has collected many of his functionalist papers into *Mind, Language and Reality* (Cambridge: Cambridge University Press, 1975).
61. Garfinkel, *Forms of Explanation*, p. 62.
62. See Ryle, Peters, Winch, Melden, Anscombe, and Taylor, n. 5, this chpater; Louch, n. 7; and Kenny, n. 24, for various attempts to show a "categorical difference" between talk of minds and talk of brains or bodies. A more sophisticated antireductionism stems from the Intentional nature of mentalistic language; many have thought that on this ground alone there could be no *reduction* of the (Intentional) mentalistic language to the (extensional) physicalistic language and no *identity* between mental states and physical states. See, e.g., Daniel Dennett, *Content and Consciousness* (London: Routledge & Kegan Paul, 1969), chap. 2; and Donald Davidson, *Actions and Events*.
63. Sigmund Freud, "On Narcissism," in vol. 4 of *Collected Papers* (New York: Basic Books, 1959), p. 36.
64. David Rapaport, "On the Psychoanalytic Theory of Motivation," in 1960 *Nebraska Symposium on Motivation* (Lincoln: University of Nebraska Press, 1960), p. 183.

65. Eventually published as vol. 1 of *The Standard Edition of the Complete Psychological Works of Sigmund Freud* (London: Hogarth Press, 1971).
66. For the separation of methodological from philosophical behaviorism, see Michael Martin, "Interpreting Skinner," *Behaviorism*, vol. 6(1978): 129–38.
67. Norman Malcolm (with a good deal of textual support) construes Skinner to be a reductionist about mental terms. Malcolm, "Behaviorism as a Philosophy of Psychology," in T. W. Wann (ed.), *Behaviorism and Phenomenology* (Chicago: University of Chicago Press, 1964), pp. 141–54. In her attempt to construe Skinner in such a way as to immunize him from the defects of philosophical behaviorism, Brenda Mapel makes the case for Skinner as a nonreductionist. Brenda M. Mapel, "Philosophical Criticism of Behaviorism: An Analysis," *Behaviorism*, vol. 5(1977): 17–32. Dan Dennett, in *Brainstorms*, nicely separates Skinner's various arguments against mentalist language and rightly concludes that Skinner has never even seen that he has to take a position on this issue: "It is unfathomable how Skinner can be so sloppy on this score, for reflection should reveal to him, as it will to us, that this vacilation is over an absolutely central point in his argument" (p. 63).
68. Rudolph Carnap, "Psychology in Physical Language," in A. J. Ayer (ed.), *Logical Positivism* (New York: Free Press, 1959), p. 165.
69. Clark Hull, *Principles of Behavior* (New York: Appleton-Century-Crofts, 1966), p. 25.
70. See the citations in Malcolm and Dennett, n. 67, this chapter.
71. Ryle, *Concept of Mind*.
72. Malcolm, "Behaviorism."
73. Peters, *Concept of Motivation*.
74. W. V. Quine, *Word and Object* (Cambridge, Mass.: MIT Press, 1960). Quine admits that "there is no breaking out of the intentional vocabulary by explaining its members in other terms" (p. 220).
75. Michael Moore, "The Semantics of Judging," *Southern California Law Review*, vol. 54(1981): 151–294. (See particularly pp. 208–10.)
76. See Mapel, "Philosophical Criticism of Behaviorism."
77. See the discussion and citations in Charles Taylor, *The Explanation of Behavior* (New York: Humanities Press, 1964), pp. 236–7, 259–60.
78. Rapaport, "Psychoanalytic Theory."
79. Ibid., p. 200.
80. Ibid., pp. 202–3.
81. Ibid.
82. Ibid.
83. Ibid., p. 187 (emphasis in original).
84. Ibid.
85. Ibid., p. 198.
86. Ibid., p. 187.
87. Ibid., p. 188.
88. Ibid., p. 198.
89. Ibid., p. 213.
90. Ibid., p. 212.

91. Freud's mechanistic tendencies found an early expression in chap. 7 of *The Interpretation of Dreams*, vols. 4 and 5 of *The Standard Edition*.
92. See particularly the work of Heinz Hartmann, cited and summarized in his "Psychoanalysis as a Scientific Theory," in S. Hook (ed.), *Psychoanalysis, Scientific Method, and Philosophy* (New York: New York University Press, 1959), pp. 3–37; and Otto Fenichel, *The Psychoanalytic Theory of Neurosis* (New York: Norton, 1945).
93. Ernst Nagel, "Methodological Issues in Psychoanalytic Theory," in S. Hook (ed.), pp. 38–56; Roy Schafer, *A New Language for Psychoanalysis* (New Haven, Conn.: Yale University Press, 1976).
94. Rapaport, "Psychoanalytic Theory," p. 186.
95. Ibid., p. 189.
96. Ibid., p. 211.

2. The Legal View of Persons

1. John Locke, *An Essay Concerning Human Understanding* (New York: Dover, 1959), book 2, chap. 27.
2. W. Hohfeld, *Fundamental Legal Conceptions* (New Haven, Conn.: Yale University Press, 1923), pp. 27–31. See also Alf Ross, "Tu-Tu," *Harvard Law Review*, vol. 70(1957): 812–25.
3. For a discussion of genuine cases of ambiguity in legal uses of words, see Michael Moore, "The Semantics of Judging," *Southern California Law Review*, vol. 54(1981): 151–294, especially pp. 181–8.
4. These are the two illocutionary speech acts judges perform in using a legal concept to decide cases. Insofar as judges bring about those legal consequences in so using the concept, they are also performing a perlocutionary speech act. The *locus classicus* of speech-act analysis is J. L. Austin, *How to Do Things With Words* (Cambridge, Mass.: Harvard University Press, 1961).
5. Compare Daniel Dennett, "The Conditions of Personhood," in A. Rorty (ed.), *The Identities of Persons* (Berkeley: University of California Press, 1976), pp. 175–96. Dennett urges that we have two different concepts of a person, "the moral notion and the metaphysical notion" (p. 176). That different speech acts are performed with person is no argument that the word is ambiguous.
6. H. L. A. Hart, "The Ascription of Responsibility and Rights," *Proceedings of the Aristotelian Society*, vol. 49(1949): 171–94. Hart later came to repudiate his ascriptivism.
7. George Fletcher, *Rethinking Criminal Law* (Boston: Little, Brown, 1978), p. 397.
8. John Dewey, *Human Nature and Conduct* (New York: Holt, Rinehart and Winston, 1922), pp. 120–1.
9. 248 N.Y. 339, 162 N.E. 99 (1928).
10. Ibid., 354, 162 N.E. at 104.
11. Stanley Ingber, Book Review, *UCLA Law Review*, vol. 27(1980): 822–4.
12. This Szaszian argument will be explored in chap. 4.
13. For some history, see William Twining, *Karl Llewellyn and The Realist Movement* (London: Weidenfeld and Nicholson, 1973); Bruce Ackerman,

"Law and the Modern Mind," *Daedalus,* vol. 103(1974): 119–30; G. White, *Patterns of American Legal Thought* (Indianapolis: Bobbs-Merrill, 1978).
14. Felix Cohen, "Transcendental Nonsense and the Functional Approach," *Columbia Law Review,* vol. 35(1935): 809–49.
15. E.g., C. L. Stevenson, *Ethics and Language* (New Haven, Conn.: Yale University Press, 1944); R. M. Hare, *The Language of Morals* (Oxford: Oxford University Press [Clarendon Press], 1952). For a helpful summary of the early forms of emotivism in ethics, see J. O. Urmson, *The Emotive Theory of Ethics* (Oxford: Oxford University Press, 1968).
16. Christopher Stone, "Corporate Accountability in Law and Morals," in J. Houck and O. Williams (eds.), *The Judaeo-Christian Vision and the Modern Business Corporation* (Notre Dame, Ind.: University of Notre Dame Press, 1982), p. 284 (emphasis in original).
17. Ibid., p. 285.
18. Ibid., p. 285.
19. Moore, "Semantics of Judging"; Moore, "Moral Reality," *Wisconsin Law Review* (1982): 1061–1156.
20. Such a view is defended in Charles Fried, *Contract as Promise* (Cambridge, Mass.: Harvard University Press, 1981).
21. For an introduction to some of the literature, see Robert Rabin (ed.), *Perspectives on Tort Law* (Boston: Little, Brown, 1976).
22. For a comparison, see Frank Michaelman, "Property, Utility and Fairness; Comments on the Ethical Foundations of 'Just Compensation' Law," *Harvard Law Review,* vol. 80(1967): 1165–1258; for a natural rights view of property rights, see Margaret Jane Radin, "Property and Personhood," *Stanford Law Review,* vol. 34(1982): 957–1015.
23. These theories of punishment are contrasted in Moore, "Closet Retributivism," *Cites* (spring-summer, 1982): 5–15.
24. H. L. A. Hart, *Punishment and Responsibility* (Oxford: Oxford University Press, 1968), p. 211. In addition to Hart's own analysis of these senses of responsible, see Kurt Baier, "Action and Responsibility," in M. Brand (ed.), *The Nature of Human Action* (Glenview, Ill.: Scott, Foresman, 1970), pp. 100–16.
25. Liability to moral sanctions is the *normal* consequence of being morally culpable. This need not always be so, however. John Stuart Mill gives one instance of this: Although we may morally disapprove of actions another does that harm himself, we are not justified in publicly blaming him any more than we are legally sanctioning him. Mill, *On Liberty* (Arlington Heights, Ill.: AHM Publishing, 1947). (First published London: J. W. Parker & Son, 1859.)
26. See the discussion, text, at nn. 153 and 154, this chapter.
27. Friedrich Nietzsche, *On the Genealogy of Morals,* trans. W. Kaufmann (New York: Random House, 1967).
28. Discussed in Herbert Morris, "Moral and Non-Moral Guilt." Unpublished manuscript, 1980.
29. Donald Davidson, *Actions and Events* (Oxford: Oxford University Press, 1980).
30. Ibid., p. 52.

31. Richard Taylor, *Action and Purpose* (Englewood Cliffs, N.J.: Prentice-Hall, 1966).
32. Ibid., p. 17.
33. For a taxonomy of such tests, see Morton White, *Foundations of Historical Knowledge* (New York: Harper & Row, 1965), chap. 4.
34. This argument is more fully drawn out in the discussion of negligence, text at nn. 107–110, this chapter.
35. H. L. A. Hart and A. M. Honore, *Causation in the Law* (Oxford: Oxford University Press, 1959).
36. Ibid., pp. 40, 70.
37. *Palsgraf*, n. 9, this chapter.
38. Lon Fuller, *The Morality of Law*, 2d ed. (New Haven, Conn.: Yale University Press, 1969).
39. Theodore Benditt, *Law as Rule and Principle* (Stanford, Calif.: Stanford University Press, 1978).
40. Ronald Dworkin, *Taking Rights Seriously* (Cambridge, Mass.: Harvard University Press, 1978).
41. Moore, "Moral Reality."
42. Fuller, *Morality of Law*, p. 162.
43. Oliver Wendell Holmes, Jr., *The Common Law*, ed. Mark deWolfe Howe (Boston: Little, Brown, 1963).
44. Ibid., p. 9.
45. Ibid., p. 12.
46. This is the Legal Realist or functionalist approach to moral language discussed earlier.
47. John Ladd, "Morality and the Ideal of Rationality in Formal Organizations," *Monist*, vol. 54(1970): 500.
48. Peter French, "The Corporation as a Moral Person," *American Philosophical Quarterly*, vol. 16(1979): 207–15.
49. W. F. LaFave and A. W. Scott, *Criminal Law* (St. Paul: West, 1972), p. 351.
50. Year Books of Edward II, *Year Book Series*, vol. 5, W. C. Bolland, F. W. Maitland, and L. W. V. Harcourt (London: Selden Society, 1909).
51. LaFave and Scott, *Criminal Law*, p. 352.
52. A. Platt and B. Diamond, "The Origins of the 'Right and Wrong' Test of Criminal Responsibility and Its Subsequent Development in the United States: An Historical Survey," *California Law Review*, vol. 54(1966): 1227–60.
53. J. Briggs, *The Guilty Mind* (New York: Harcourt Brace, 1955), p. 311.
54. I. Epstein (ed.), *Babylonian Talmud, Baba Kamma* (London: Soncino Press, 1935).
55. L. E. Becker, "Durham Revisited," *Psychiatric Annals*, vol. 3(1973): 16–49.
56. M. Hale, *Select Pleas of the Crown*, vol. 1 (London: Selden Society, 1887), p. 30.
57. See Platt and Diamond, "The 'Right and Wrong' Test."
58. See Briggs, *The Guilty Mind*, p. 82.
59. *Beverly's Case*, 4 Coke 1236, 1246 (1603).
60. *Rex v. Arnold*, 17 How. St. Tr. 695, 764 (1724).

61. Mike Royko, as reported in *Kansas City Star*, June 22, 1975.
62. See Arthur Danto, "Basic Action," *American Philosophical Quarterly*, vol. 2(1965): 141–8; D. F. Pears, "The Appropriate Causation of Intentional Basic Actions," *Critica*, vol. 7(1975): 39–69.
63. Danto, "Basic Actions." For further discussion of this, see also A. I. Melden, *Free Action* (London: Routledge & Kegan Paul, 1961), pp. 56–65.
64. Ludwig Wittgenstein, *Philosophical Investigations*, 2d ed. (Oxford: Blackwell Publisher, 1958), p. 161.
65. For further argument and example, see Richard Taylor, *Action and Purpose*, p. 59.
66. American Law Institute, Model Penal Code, sec. 1.13(2), Proposed Official Draft (Philadelphia: 1962).
67. Holmes, *Common Law*, pp. 45–6.
68. Model Penal Code, sec. 2.01(1).
69. Ibid., sec. 2.01(2) (d).
70. John Stuart Mill, *A System of Logic* (London: Longman Group, 1965), p. 35. (First published London: J. W. Parker & Son, 1843.)
71. John Austin, *Lectures on Jurisprudence* (London: J. Murray, 1869), p. 427.
72. J. L. Mackie, "The Grounds of Responsibility," in P. M. S. Hacker and J. Raz (eds.), *Law Morality and Society* (Oxford: Oxford University Press, 1977), pp. 175–88.
73. H. L. A. Hart, *Punishment and Responsibility*, pp. 90–112.
74. Mackie, "Grounds of Responsibility," p. 179.
75. Alvin Goldman, *A Theory of Human Action* (Englewood Cliffs, N.J.: Prentice-Hall, 1970).
76. See Roderick Chisholm, "The Descriptive Element in the Concept of Action," *Journal of Philosophy*, vol. 61(1964): 613–25; C. Peacocke, "Deviant Causal Chains," *Midwest Studies in Philosophy*, vol. 4(1979): 123–55.
77. Goldman, *Theory of Human Action*, p. 61 (emphasis in original).
78. Ibid., p. 62.
79. Donald Davidson reviews Goldman's and other causal theorists' attempts to provide a criterion for actions and concludes that one must "despair of spelling out . . . the way in which attitudes must cause actions if they are to rationalize the action." Davidson, *Actions and Events*, p. 79.
80. *People v. Newton*, 8 Cal. App.3d 359, 87 Cal. Rptr. 394 (1970); *Fain v. Commonwealth*, 78 Ky. 183 (1879); *Hill v. Baxter*, [1958-1] Q.B. 277.
81. Model Penal Code, sec. 2.01(2)(b).
82. Glanville Williams, *Criminal Law: The General Part*, 2d ed. (London: Stevens and Sons, 1961), pp. 36–8.
83. Arthur Danto, "What We Can Do," *Journal of Philosophy*, vol. 60(1963): 435–45.
84. This is not, of course, to say that an actor need know that he is performing a *complex* action in order to perform that action. To be said to have *killed* another, for example, it is enough that the actor knew he performed some basic act, and the basic act causes a death; the actor need not know that he is killing someone.

85. Wittgenstein, *Philosophical Investigations*, p. 162.
86. Such examples must be reconsidered when the possibility of unconscious knowledge (and thus unconscious actions) is raised, which is done in chap. 9.
87. Richard Peters, *The Concept of Motivation* (London: Routledge & Kegan Paul, 1958), p. 4.
88. A similar taxonomy of action types is developed in Goldman, *Theory of Human Action*, chap. 2.
89. Peters, *Concept of Motivation*, p. 12.
90. A. I. Melden, "Action," in M. Brand (ed.), *The Nature of Human Action* (Glenview, Ill.: Scott, Foresman, 1970), p. 96.
91. G. E. M. Anscombe, *Intention*, 2d ed. (Ithaca, N.Y.: Cornell University Press, 1963), p. 87.
92. ibid., p. 1.
93. Jeremy Bentham, *An Introduction to the Principles of Morals and Legislation* (New York: Hafner Press, 1948), p. 83. (First published Oxford: Clarendon Press, 1876.)
94. See e.g., Goldman, *Theory of Human Action*, chap. 3; Pears, "Appropriate Causation."
95. See Anthony Kenny, "Intention and Purpose," *Journal of Philosophy*, vol. 63(1966): 642–51; D. Locke, "Intention and Intentional Action," in J. J. MacIntosh and S. Coval (eds.), *The Business of Reason* (New York: Humanities Press, 1969), pp. 129–49; Anscombe, *Intention*, sec. 25; B. Fleming, "On Intention," *Philosophical Review*, vol. 73(1964): 301–20, for expressions of the purposive theory of intention.
96. Bentham, *Morals and Legislation*, pp. 82–8. See also J. W. Meiland, *The Nature of Intention* (London: Methuen & Co., 1970), pp. 7–14; and Stuart Hampshire, *Thought and Action* (New York: Viking Press, 1960), p. 145, who agree with Bentham that there may be oblique or "nonpurposive" intentions.
97. Hart, *Punishment and Responsibility*, p. 121.
98. Something, of course, that purposive theorists such as Anscombe explicitly deny. See Anscombe, *Intention*.
99. On intensional vagueness, see Moore, "Semantics of Judging," pp. 193–200.
100. In particular by Kenny, "Intention and Purpose," and by Charles Fried, "Right and Wrong: Preliminary Considerations," *Journal of Legal Studies*, vol. 5(1976): 165–200. See also Lord Hailsham's interesting espousal of the contrary position in *Hyam v. Director of Public Prosecutions* [1975] A. C. 55 (1974).
101. See generally William Prosser, *Handbook of the Law of Torts*, 4th ed. (St. Paul: West, 1971), sec. 8.
102. LaFave and Scott, *Criminal Law*, sec. 28.
103. This last discussion should help to distinguish between two sorts of accidents. If one says that X killed a donkey *accidentally*, this means that X performed no basic action, but that his bodily movements caused the donkey to be killed (e.g., X's finger slipped on the trigger of his gun). Alternatively, it may mean that X did perform some basic action but this particular, causally complex

redescription of his action was not performed intentionally. An example of the latter case is where X intentionally shot at a tree near the donkey but the wind carried the bullet to the donkey instead. It is easier to understand psychoanalytic claims that nominal accidents are intentional actions if these two senses of "accident" are kept distinct.
104. Anscombe, *Intention*.
105. LaFave and Scott, *Criminal Law*, p. 202.
106. 169 F.2d 169 (2d Cir. 1947).
107. See the materials collected in W. Bishin and C. Stone, *Law, Language and Ethics* (Mineola, N.Y.: Foundation Press, 1972), pp. 428–31.
108. Hart, *Punishment and Responsibility*, p. 152.
109. Ibid.
110. Consistency would urge that the severely mentally ill should also be excused from the objective standard, as Holmes recognized long ago. Holmes, *Common Law*, pp. 87–8. Aside from "suddenly arising insanities," however, tort law holds the insane to the objective standard of the reasonable person despite their lack of the practically reasoning capacity that would make that a fair thing to do.
111. Fletcher, *Rethinking Criminal Law*, p. 759.
112. Aristotle, *Nicomachean Ethics*, book 3, chap. 1, in R. McKeon (ed.), *Introduction to Aristotle* (Chicago: University of Chicago Press, 1973).
113. External negation might be represented as $\sim xB(p)$, internal negation, as $xB(\sim p)$, where p is the proposition to be believed, B is the belief operator, $\sim$ represents the logical connective "not," and x denotes the person who holds the belief.
114. See, e.g., the Comments to the Model Penal Code, sec. 2.04, dealing with mistake and ignorance: "The rule relating to mistake is not a new rule; and the law could be stated equally well without reference to mistake." American Law Institute, Comments to Tentative Draft No. 4, 1955. The drafters of the Code thought no new rule was required for mistake because they assumed a mistake was necessarily the negation of knowledge, so that a rule requiring the *mens rea* of knowledge was all one really needed.
115. Knowledge, $xB(p)$, is contradicted by ignorance, $\sim xB(p)$.
116. Knowledge, $xB(p)$, is not contradicted by mistake, $xB(\sim p)$. x could both believe p and believe not-p if he is inconsistent in his beliefs.
117. The deduction is:

1.	$\sim [xB(\sim p) \cdot xB(p)]$	Premise of consistency of x's beliefs
2.	$xB(\sim p)$	Premise that x has made a mistake
3.	$\sim xB(\sim p) \vee \sim xB(p)$	1, De Morgan's laws
4.	$xB(\sim p) \supset \sim xB(p)$	3, Equivalence for material conditional
5.	$\sim xB(p)$	2, 4, *Modus Ponens*

118. Model Penal Code, sec. 2.02(7) (Proposed Official Draft, 1962): "When knowledge of the existence of a particular fact is an element of an offense, such knowledge is established if a person is aware of a high probability of its existence, unless he actually believes that it does not exist."

If one equates "awareness of a high probability" of the truth of some proposition p with a belief that p, the Model Penal Code thus envisions the situation where someone both believes that p and that not-p, symbolized as: $xB(p) \cdot xB(\sim p)$.

119. Aristotle, *Nicomachean Ethics*, Bk. III, chap. 1.
120. Fletcher, *Rethinking Criminal Law*, pp. 352–3.
121. Robert Audi also has two models of compulsion, although they differ somewhat from those distinguished in the text. See R. Audi, "Moral Responsibility, Freedom and Compulsion," *American Philosophical Quarterly*, vol. 11(1974): 1–14.
122. The idea of constraints upon choices is not as straightforward as it may sound. For example, in the context of that kind of compulsion known as duress, one must distinguish between the constraints posed by threats and the inducements offered by promises. See H. Frankfurt, "Coercion and Moral Responsibility," in T. Honderich (ed.), *Essays in Freedom of Action* (London: Routledge & Kegan Paul, 1973), pp. 65–86; and Robert Nozick, "Coercion," in S. Morgenbesser, P. Suppes, and M. White (eds.), *Philosophy, Science and Method*, (New York: St. Martin's Press, 1969), pp. 440–72.
123. What is meant here is the distinction Gary Watson has drawn between that part of an actor's character one might call the "evaluational system" and that appetitive part one might call the "motivational system." Watson, "Free Agency," *Journal of Philosophy*, vol. 72(1975): 205–20. That part of our character that is appetitive may compel us, but one could say this of the evaluational system only at the cost of giving up the possibility of free actions entirely.
124. The sense of "character" meant here is the appetitive character just discussed, n. 123, this chapter.
125. On these two uses of emotion words, see Anthony Kenny, *Action, Emotion, and Will* (London: Routledge & Kegan Paul, 1963), p. 35; Richard Peters, "Motivation, Emotion, and Schemes of Common Sense," in T. Mischel (ed.), *Human Action* (New York: Academic Press, 1969), pp. 135–63; Richard Peters, "More About Motives," *Mind*, vol. 76(1967): 92–7.
126. French, "The Corporation," p. 208.
127. Bentham, *Morals and Legislation*, p. 224, n. 1 (emphasis in original).
128. H. L. A. Hart, "Definition and Theory in Jurisprudence," *Law Quarterly Review*, vol. 70(1954): 49.
129. Stanley Benn, "Rights," in P. Edwards (ed.), *The Encyclopedia of Philosophy*, vol. 7 (New York: Macmillan, 1957), p. 196.
130. This discussion follows generally the analysis of liberty and equality put forward by S. Benn and R. Peters, *Social Principles and Democratic State* (London: Allen & Unwin, 1959). See particularly chaps. 5 and 10.
131. Benn, "Rights," p. 198.
132. The phrase is from Alan Gewirth, who attempts to *derive* a right to liberty from our practical reasoning capacity. Gewirth, "The Basis and Content of Human Rights," in J. R. Pennock and J. W. Chapman (eds.), "Human Rights," *Nomos*, vol. 23(1981): 119–47. My own claim is not this strong; it

is that a right to liberty *presupposes* practical reasoning capacities in persons, not that such capacities justify the right to liberty by themselves.
133. Mill, *On Liberty*. n. 25.
134. Hare's argument, in *Freedom and Reason* (Oxford: Oxford University Press, 1963).
135. A. I. Melden, *Rights and Persons* (Berkeley: University of California Press, 1977), p. 192.
136. Ibid., p. 193.
137. Ibid., p. 199.
138. Ibid.
139. G. Calabresi and A. D. Melamed, "Property Rules, Liability Rules, and Inalienability: One View of the Cathedral," *Harvard Law Review*, vol. 85(1972): 1089–1128.
140. John Locke, *Two Treatises of Government* (New York: Hafner Press, 1956), pp. 133–46; Robert Nozick, *Anarchy, State and Utopia* (New York: Basic Books, 1974), esp. pp. 174–82; Richard Epstein, "Possession as the Root of All Title," *Georgia Law Review*, vol. 12(1979): 1221-43. Compare Radin, "Property and Personhood," for a different connection of property rights and personhood.
141. Locke, *Two Treaties of Government*, p. 143.
142. See H. P. Grice, "Meaning," *Philosophical Review*, vol. 66(1957): 377–88.
143. Hart, *Punishment and Responsibility*, p. 34.
144. The example is examined in A. J. Watt, "The Intelligibility of Wants," *Mind*, vol. 81(1972): 553–61.
145. The example is from G. E. M. Anscombe, *Intention*.
146. H. Wigmore, *Evidence*, vol. 1, 3d ed. (Boston: Little, Brown, 1940).
147. Robert Cooter, in his "Justice and Mathematics: Two Simple Ideas," in R. Skurski (ed.), *New Directions in Economic Justice* (South Bend, Ind.: University of Notre Dame Press, 1983), nicely explores the differences between transitivity of preferences and consistency of norms.
148. I explore objectivity in ethics in Moore, "Moral Reality." Compare Richard Brandt, *A Theory of the Good and the Right* (Oxford: Oxford University Press [Clarendon Press], 1979), who on p. 114 seeks to develop a procedural notion of rational desire in terms of the survivability of that desire despite "careful cognitive psychotherapy."
149. Model Penal Code, sec. 3.02.
150. For development of an idea of coherence of beliefs that is stronger than freedom from contradiction, see Michael Williams, *Groundless Belief* (Princeton, N.J.: Princeton University Press, 1977).
151. For suggestions about our norms of appropriateness about emotions and their objects, and the tie of appropriateness to rationality of the emotions, see Ronald de Sousa, "The Rationality of Emotions," in A. Rorty (ed.), *Explaining Emotions* (Berkeley: University of California Press, 1980), pp. 127–51; see also R. Scruton, "Emotion, Practical Knowledge and the Common Culture," in A Rorty (ed.), *Explaining Emotions*, pp. 519–36. David Sachs examines Freud's treatment of the emotions and concludes that implicitly

Freud too thought that even in the unconscious the norms of appropriateness (of feelings to their objects) are obeyed. Sachs, "On Freud's Doctrine of the Emotions," in R. Wollheim (ed.), *Freud: A Collection of Critical Essays* (Garden City, N.Y.: Doubleday [Anchor Press], 1974).

152. Any moral theory that takes emotional experience to be relevant to moral insight will not regard all moral experience as equally the harbinger of moral insight. Rather, the theory will be turned back onto the experience itself to judge some as correct and some as misleading. See Moore, "Moral Reality"; Ronald Dworkin, "Lord Devlin and the Enforcement of Morals," *Yale Law Journal*, vol. 75(1966): 986–1005; Bernard Williams, "Morality and the Emotions," in Williams, *Problems of the Self* (Cambridge: Cambridge University Press, 1973); G. Kerner, "Passions and the Cognitive Foundations of Ethics," *Philosophy and Phenomenological Research*, vol. 31(1970): 177–92.

153. As Heidegger puts it, with uncharacteristic clarity, "Because Dasein is in each case essentially its own possibility, it *can*, in its very Being, 'choose' itself and win itself." *Being and Time*, trans. J. Macquarrie and E. Robinson (New York: Harper & Row, 1962), p. 68.

154. Aristotle, *Nicomachean Ethics*. Charles Taylor, "Responsibility for Self," in A. Rorty (ed.), pp. 281–99, nicely articulates and defends this Artistotelian view of autonomous persons.

155. See Harry Frankfurt, "Freedom of the Will and the Concept of a Person," *Journal of Philosophy*, vol. 68(1971): 5–20.

156. A. P. Herbert, *Uncommon Law*, 7th ed. (London: Methuen & Co., 1952), pp. 2–3.

3. The Challenge of Psychiatry

1. Sigmund Freud, "The Unconscious," in vol. 4 of *Collected Papers* (New York: Basic Books, 1959), p. 101.
2. Ibid.
3. It is clear, for example, that general determinist notions largely motivate Karl Menninger's lifelong effort to merge badness into sickness. See, e.g., K. Menninger, *The Crime of Punishment* (New York: Viking Press, 1968). Similarly, Philip Roche reaches the conclusion that "Criminals differ from mentally ill people only in the manner we choose to deal with them," largely because of his assumption that the behavior of both is determined by unconscious forces: "From the standpoint that the individual reverts to a magical orientation in social adaptation, the distinction between the criminal and the mentally ill is arbitrary. Every criminal is such by reason of unconscious forces within him just as every mentally ill person is so dominated by unconscious forces, and the so-called 'normal' people operate in their lives with margins not far from either." Roche, *The Criminal Mind* (New York: Wiley, 1958), p. 29. More generally, Antony Flew notes this motivation of psychiatrists in chap. 3 of *Crime or Disease?* (London: Macmillan Press, 1973).
4. See, e.g., Seymour Halleck, *Psychiatry and the Dilemmas of Crime* (Berkeley: University of California Press, 1971), pp. 46–50. For further citations, see Flew, *Crime or Disease?* pp. 9–10.

5. Christopher Boorse, "On the Distinction Between Disease and Illness," *Philosophy and Public Affairs*, vol. 5(1975): 49. There are actually two kinds of conceptual claims in Boorse's psychiatric turn: one, the replacement of moral terminology with medical terminology—what I later call the "medicalization of morals." The other claim is the replacement of medical terminology by moral terminology—what might be called the "moralization of medicine." If one believes that there is some strong meaning connection between the language of morals and the language of medicine, one is free to *reduce* one to the other.

   Although in chap. 4 I deal with Szasz's kind of moralization of medicine, my main concern in part II will be the medicalization of morals. Despite the language quoted in the text, Boorse's main concern in the article cited is with the reduction of medical language to morals, not vice versa.
6. J. L. Austin, "A Plea for Excuses," *Proceedings of the Aristotelian Society*, vol. 57(1956): 17–18.
7. Such considerations led G. H. Von Wright to distinguish two senses of health, a positive sense and a privative sense. The privative sense is merely the absence of disease, whereas positive health is to be understood independently of illness. Von Wright, *The Varieties of Goodness* (London: Routledge & Kegan Paul, 1963), pp. 54–5. A third possibility, different from the two mentioned in the text, is to regard health and illness as having little to do with each other, so that neither term can be defined as the negation of the other. For an attempt in this direction, see Caroline Whiteback, "A Theory of Health," in A. L. Caplan, H. T. Engelhardt, and J. J. McCartney (eds.), *Concepts of Health and Disease* (Reading, Mass.: Addison-Wesley, 1981), pp. 611–26.
8. Plato, *Republic*, 444E, in E. Hamilton and H. Cairns (eds.), *The Collected Dialogues of Plato* (Princeton, N.J.: Princeton University Press, 1961), p. 687.
9. Ibid.
10. Flew discusses what he takes to be the affinities between Plato and modern psychiatry's extended view of madness. See Flew, *Crime or Disease?* pp. 10–25. See also Anthony Kenny, "Mental Health in Plato's Republic," in *Proceedings of the British Academy*, vol. 55(1969): 229–53.
11. Aristotle, *Nicomachean Ethics*, book 1, chap. 7, 1097b, in Richard McKeon (ed.), *Introduction to Aristotle* (Chicago: University of Chicago Press, 1973), p. 335.
12. Ibid., p. 356.
13. Ibid., p. 366.
14. Aristotle thought that there were two elements in the psyche, one rational but the other irrational. Part of what he meant by the latter element sounds much like Freud's unconscious, being unseen and opposed to the rational element in the psyche. See ibid., pp. 367–8.
15. Erich Fromm, *Man for Himself: An Enquiry into the Psychology of Ethics* (New York: Fawcett, 1947), p. 32.
16. Ibid., pp. 176–7.

17. Ibid., p. 29 (emphasis in original).
18. Ibid., p. 45. See also Fromm's *The Sane Society* (New York: Fawcett, 1951), where he defines mental health in terms that he there recognizes have the effect of identifying health with virtue: "Mental health is characterized by the ability to have and to create, by the emergence from incestuous ties to clan and soil, by a sense of identity based on one's experience of self as the subject and agent of one's powers, by the grasp of reality inside and outside of ourselves; that is, by the development of objectivity and reason" (p. 69).
19. Ibid., p. 227.
20. Ibid., p. 221. Fromm qualifies this last move by a concession to the conventions giving neurosis its meaning: "Lack of integration and productiveness does not *always* lead to neurosis. As a matter of fact, if this were the case, we would have to consider the vast majority of people as neurotic." Ibid., p. 222. Such a concession is only minimal, however, since Fromm shortly introduces the concept of "defect" to cover nonneurotic failures to attain his ideal of health: "It seems to be useful at this point to differentiate between two concepts: that of defect, and that of neurosis. If a person fails to attain maturity, spontaneity, and a genuine experience of self, he may be considered to have a severe defect, provided we assume that freedom and spontaneity are the objective goals to be attained by every human being." Ibid., p. 222–3.
21. Abraham Maslow and Bela Mittelmann, *Principles of Abnormal Psychiatry: The Dynamics of Psychic Illness*, rev. ed. (New York: Harper & Row, 1951), p. 15. "Adequate life goals" are defined as those that are achievable and realistic and that "include some good to society."
22. Ibid.
23. Ibid. "This [adequate self-evaluation] includes adequate self-esteem—a feeling of value proportionate to one's individuality and achievements," and it includes "an adequate feeling of worth-whileness—feeling morally sound, with the feeling of no severe guilt."
24. Ibid. Adequate spontaneity and emotionality are defined as "the ability to form strong and lasting emotional ties, such as friendships and love relations; the ability to give adequate expression to resentment without losing control; the ability to understand and to share other people's emotions; the ability to enjoy oneself and laugh." Maslow and Mittelmann go on to note that "everyone is unhappy at times, but this must have valid reasons[!]"
25. Ibid.
26. Ibid.
27. Rollo May, "The Work and Training of the Psychological Therapist," in M. H. Krout (ed.), *Psychology, Psychiatry and the Public Interest* (Minneapolis: University of Minnesota Press, 1956), pp. 161–85.
28. For summary and citations, see C. Buhler, *Values in Psychotherapy* (New York: Free Press, 1962). See generally Frank Goble, *The Third Force* (New York: Grossman, 1970).
29. F. C. Redlich, "The Concept of Health in Psychiatry," in A. H. Leighton, J. A. Clausen, and R. N. Wilson (eds.), *Explorations in Social Psychiatry* (New York: Basic Books, 1957), p. 144.

30. Such temptation was tentatively explored in Heinz Hartmann, "Psychoanalysis and the Concept of Health," *International Journal of Psychoanalysis*, vol. 20(1939): 308–21. The identification of health with the therapeutic goals of psychoanalysis—particularly "making the unconscious conscious"—is put forth much more boldly in Lawrence Kubie, *Practical and Theoretical Aspects of Psychoanalysis* (New York: International Universities Press, 1950), pp. 13–20, 133–4. Freudian political theorists have also adopted Freud's therapeutic goals as political ideals for a healthy society. The two most notable examples are Norman Brown, *Life Against Death* (Middletown, Conn.: Wesleyan University Press, 1959), and Herbert Marcuse, *Eros and Civilization* (Boston: Beacon Press, 1955).
31. Redlich, "Concept of Health in Psychiatry," in Leighton et al. (eds.), p. 158.
32. Marie Jahoda, *Current Concepts of Positive Mental Health* (New York: Basic Books, 1958), p. 13.
33. Hartmann, "Psychoanalysis."
34. Karl Menninger, *The Human Mind* (New York: Knopf, 1961), p. 1. The rest of Menninger's definition is that mental health is "not just efficiency, or just contentment, or the grace of obeying the rules of the game cheerfully. It is all of these together. It is the ability to maintain an even temper, an alert intelligence, socially considerate behavior, and a happy disposition. This I think is a healthy mind."
35. An excerpt from the Constitution is reprinted in Caplan et al. (eds.), *Concepts of Health and Disease*, pp. 83–4.
36. The classical argument against naturalism in ethics is to be found in G. E. Moore's *Principia Ethica* (Cambridge: Cambridge University Press, 1903). Emotivists and prescriptivists adapted Moore's arguments to their own theories of meaning about "ethical words." See A. J. Ayer, *Language Truth and Logic*, 2d ed. (New York: Dover, 1952), chap. 4; and R. M. Hare, *The Language of Morals* (Oxford: Oxford University Press [Clarendon Press], 1952).
37. Michael Moore, "Moral Reality," *Wisconsin Law Review* (1982): 1061–1156.
38. See Moore, "Moral Reality," for a discussion of ethical relativism as one form of moral skepticism.
39. Ruth Benedict, *Patterns of Culture*, 2d ed. (Boston: Houghton Mifflin, 1959), p. 257.
40. Thomas Scheff, *Being Mentally Ill: A Sociological Theory* (Chicago: Aldine, 1966), p. 33. The considerable literature of labeling theory that arose after Scheff's book is reviewed in W. R. Gove (ed.), *Deviance and Mental Illness* (Beverly Hills, Calif.: Sage, 1982).
41. Philip Roche, *The Criminal Mind*, p. 15.
42. Karl Menninger, *The Human Mind*.
43. Menninger, *The Crime of Punishment*.
44. Karl Menninger, Martin Mayer, and Paul Pruyser, *The Vital Balance: The Life Process in Mental Health and Illness* (New York: Viking Press, 1967).
45. Ibid., p. 66.

46. Ibid., p. 148.
47. Ibid., p. 77.
48. Ibid.
49. Ibid., p. 5.
50. Ibid., p. 228.
51. Ibid., p. 229.
52. Ibid., p. 234.
53. Menninger at one point, at least, perceived that his was *not* a thesis about the intertranslatability of moral and medical terminology, but rather was a thesis aimed at *divesting* moral and legal terms of their customary application and their replacement by the language of medicine: "According to the prevalent understanding of the words, crime is *not* a disease. Neither is it an illness, although I think it *should* be. It *should* be treated, and it could be; but it mostly isn't." *The Crime of Punishment*, p. 254.
54. Donald Klein, "A Proposed Definition of Mental Illness," in R. L. Spitzer and D. F. Klein (eds.), *Critical Issues in Psychiatric Diagnosis* (New York: Raven Press, 1978), p. 69. The criticism I voiced at the 1977 annual meeting of the American Psychopathological Association, at which Klein's paper was presented, was that psychiatric definitions of mental illness could not have this "marked social impact." As Klein subsequently made clear, however, such was precisely his intent: "As for Dr. Moore, I think he accused me of academic imperialism. . . . I think it is an obligation on the part of the psychiatric profession to try to come up with definitions that will tell the ill from the bad." Ibid., pp. 105–6.
55. Talcott Parsons, *The Social System* (New York: Free Press, 1951), pp. 428–79. This kind of literature is discussed in Robert M. Veatch, "The Medical Model: Its Nature and Problems," in Caplan et al. (eds.), pp. 523–44. Veatch notes that "it seems clear that one of the primary functions of the medical model is to remove culpability," although Veatch himself is critical of this use. Ibid., p. 530.
56. See, e.g., Boorse, "Disease and Illness." Antony Flew, in *Crime or Disease?* also adopts the idea that "the core of illness is victimization" (p. 74) and, because of this, exempts the sick from responsibility. Samuel Butler, in *Erewhon* (London: Trübener, 1872), assumes that the Erewhonian practice of punishing the ill is absurd.
57. See E. Jellinek, *The Disease Concept of Alcoholism* (New Brunswick, N.J.: Rutgers Center of Alcohol Studies Publications, 1960).
58. Henry A. Davidson, "The Psychiatrist's Role in the Administration of Criminal Justice," in R. W. Nice (ed.), *Criminal Psychology* (New York: Philosophical Library, 1962), p. 16.
59. *Robinson v. California*, 370 U.S. 660, 666–667 (1962).
60. *Powell v. Texas*, 392 U.S. 514, 561 (1968).
61. A familiar exponent of this view is Barbara Wootton, *Social Science and Social Pathology* (New York: Macmillan, 1959).
62. The compatibility of libertarian political theory with an objectivist metaethical position about moral judgments is explored in Moore, "Moral Reality."

63. This dispositional sense of conscious of is explored in T. W. Smyth, "Unconscious Desires and the Meaning of 'Desire,'" *Monist*, vol. 56(1972): 413–26.
64. A point Gilbert Ryle defended at length about his analogous concept of heed, in *The Concept of Mind* (London: Hutchinson, 1949).
65. Freud discussed his usages of unconscious at numerous points in his work. See "A Note on the Unconscious in Psychoanalysis," written in 1912 and printed in vol. 4 of *Collected Papers*, pp. 22–9; "The Unconscious," first published in 1915 and printed in vol. 4 of *Collected Papers*, pp. 98–136; lectures 7, 18, and 19 of the *Introductory Lectures on Psychoanalysis*, written and delivered in 1915 and 1917, first translated and published in America as *A General Introduction to Psychoanalysis* (New York: Washington Square Press, 1952); chap. 1 of *The Ego and the Id* (New York: Norton, 1960) (first published in 1923); and lecture 31 of the *New Introductory Lectures on Psychoanalysis*, trans. and ed. James Strachey (New York: Norton, 1965) (first published New York: Norton, 1933. Translated by W. J. H. Sprout). At various places and times in these works he spoke sometimes of two senses of unconscious, and elsewhere of three. The primary distinction he consistently marked, however, was between mental states that were only descriptively unconscious and those that were dynamically so. The topographical use of the unconscious he seemed to regard as a necessary corollary of the dynamic use: What was repressed was in the System Ucs. Thus, for example, he spoke of "repression" as denoting "a purely psychological process" that "would be even better described as topographical, by which we mean that it has to do with . . . the structure of the mental apparatus out of separate psychical systems." *General Introduction to Psychoanalysis*, p. 351. Summaries of Freud's use of unconscious may be found in James Strachey's introduction to *The Ego and the Id*, pp. ix–xiii, and in Samuel Abrams, "The Psychoanalytic Unconscious," in M. Kanzel (ed.), *The Unconscious Today* (New York: International Universities Press, 1971), pp. 196–210.
66. Freud, *The Ego and the Id*, pp. 3–4.
67. Freud, "A Note on the Unconscious in Psychoanalysis," in vol. 4 of *Collected Papers*, p. 23.
68. Freud, *New Introductory Lectures*, p. 70.
69. Freud, *General Introduction to Psychoanalysis*, p. 120.
70. *The Ego and the Id*, p. 4.
71. *New Introductory Lectures*, pp. 70–1.
72. "The Unconscious," in vol. 4 of *Collected Papers*, p. 103. Freud was not very consistent on this last point. See his analogy of the unconscious to the minds of others. Ibid., pp. 101–2.
73. This I shall discuss in part IV.
74. *General Introduction to Psychoanalysis*, pp. 443–4.
75. Ibid., pp. 292–3.
76. Ordinary language is open-ended to further scientific discovery in just the way mentioned in the text. We *refer* to the same thing by our term "whale" as the Greeks did by their term for whales, even if the theories we have about whales (that they are warm-blooded mammals, etc.) differ considerably from

the theory the Greeks had about whales (they thought they were fish). One should not, accordingly, think that the Greeks used their term for whale in a different *sense* than we use ours. What they meant by their word for whale we mean by "whale," namely, to refer to *those things*, whatever their true nature should turn out to be. (For an explication of meaning along these lines, see Hilary Putnam, "The Meaning of 'Meaning,'" in his *Mind, Language and Reality* [Cambridge: Cambridge University Press, 1975], pp. 215–71.) The different conceptions of the unconscious mentioned in the text should not, accordingly, be thought of as different *senses* of the word unconscious. The dynamic and topographical conceptions are part of Freud's theory about what unconsciousness really is.

77. For a general statement to this effect, see Freud, "Repression," in vol. 4 of *Collected Papers*, p. 89.
78. Ibid., p. 92: "The motive and purpose of repression was simply the avoidance of 'pain.'" As will be discussed at length in chap. 9, such motivational language of Freud must be reconstrued into the functional reformulation of the text.
79. Ibid., p. 86.
80. Thus, in "Instincts and their Vicissitudes," in vol. 4 of *Collected Papers*, pp. 60–83, Freud conceives of instincts first "from the side of physiology" and later, "as a borderline concept between the mental and the physical" which, as the *mental*, was "the mental representative of the stimuli emanating from within the organism and penetrating to the mind" (p. 64).
81. Freud, "A Note on the Unconscious in Psychoanalysis," in vol. 4 of *Collected Papers*, p. 29.
82. See T. R. Miles, *Eliminating the Unconscious* (London: Pergamon Press, 1966), particularly pp. 75–89; I. Dilman, "The Unconscious," *Mind*, vol. 68(1959): 446–73; Dilman, "Is the Unconscious a Theoretical Construct?" *Monist*, vol. 56(1972): 313–42; Antony Flew, "Psychoanalytic Explanation," *Analysis*, vol. 10(1950): 8–15; Flew, "Motives and the Unconscious," in H. Feigl and M. Scriven (eds.), *The Foundations of Science and the Concepts of Psychology and Psychoanalysis*, Minnesota Studies in the Philosophy of Science, vol. 1 (Minneapolis: University of Minnesota Press, 1956), pp. 155–73, particularly pp. 159–60; Alisdair MacIntyre, *The Unconscious* (London: Routledge & Kegan Paul, 1958).
83. See, e.g., Elbert Ellis, "An Operational Reformulation of Some of the Basic Principles of Psychoanalysis," in Feigl and Scriven (eds.), pp. 131–54. T. R. Miles, *Eliminating the Unconscious*, is another example of such attempted behaviorist interpretations of the unconscious, starting with Ryle more than with Skinner.
84. See R. L. Gregory, *Eye and Brain* (New York: McGraw-Hill, 1966).
85. To say this is not to fall into the error against which Freud constantly cautions us, that of identifying what is mental with what is unconscious. It is to say that there is a prima facie difference between the concepts in terms of which we talk of a person's body, including his brain, and the concepts in terms of which we discuss the person himself and his mental states. Dan

Dennett introduces the term "subpersonal" to denote those concepts we use to describe those physiological goings-on that must underlie a person's mental states. See Dennett, *Content and Consciousness* (London: Routledge & Kegan Paul, 1969), pp. 90–6.
86. Noam Chomsky, "Language and Unconscious Knowledge," in his *Rules and Representations* (New York: Columbia University Press, 1980), pp. 217–54.
87. Richard Peters, in *The Concepts of Motivation* (London: Routledge & Kegan Paul, 1958), has a nice discussion of this, pp. 52–61, even if he overstates the case against an omnipresent unconscious.
88. Freud, "The Unconscious," in vol. 4 of *Collected Papers*, p. 98.
89. *The Ego and the Id*, pp. 7–8.
90. See, e.g., MacIntyre, *"The Unconscious"*: "Freud's whole recognition of unconscious purposes is a discovery that men are more, and not less, rational than we thought they were" (p. 93).
91. 44 N.J. 453, 210 A.2d 193 (1965).
92. 44 N.J. at 477, 210 A.2d at 206.
93. 44 N.J. at 477–8 210 A.2d at 206.
94. 44 N.J. at 475–6, 210 A.2d at 205.
95. 44 N.J. at 477, 210 A.2d at 206.
96. Norman Brown, *Love's Body* (New York: Random House [Vintage Books], 1968), p. 147.
97. Joan Riviere, "The Unconscious Phantasy of an Inner World," in M. Klein, P. Heimann, and R. E. Money-Kyrle (eds.), *New Directions in Psychoanalysis* (New York: Basic Books, 1955), pp. 358–9.
98. Freud, "My Contact with Josef Popper-Lynkeus," in vol. 5 of *Collected Papers*, p. 297.
99. *Republic*, 436B, in *Collected Dialogues*, p. 678.
100. *Republic*, 439D, in *Collected Dialogues*, p. 681.
101. Freud, *New Introductory Lectures*, p. 76.
102. Ibid., p. 74.
103. Jacob Arlow and Charles Brenner, *Psychoanalytic Concepts and the Structural Theory* (New York: International Universities Press, 1964), p. 39.
104. *New Introductory Lectures*, p. 66.
105. *The Ego and the Id*, p. 15.
106. Freud, "A Case of Successful Treatment by Hypnotism," in vol. 1 of *The Standard Edition of the Complete Psychological Works of Sigmund Freud* (London: Hogarth Press, 1953), pp. 122–8.
107. Freud, "A Difficulty in the Path of Psycho-Analysis," in vol. 17 of *The Standard Edition*, p. 141.
108. *The Ego and the Id*, p. 15.
109. *New Introductory Lectures*, p. 77.
110. Ibid, p. 60.
111. Ibid., p. 68.
112. *The Ego and the Id*, p. 48.
113. *New Introductory Lectures*, p. 69.
114. Freud, *The Problem of Anxiety* (New York: Norton, 1963), p. 28.

115. Freud, *An Outline of Psychoanalysis* (New York: Norton, 1949), p. 122.
116. Freud, "A Difficulty," in vol. 17 of *The Standard Edition,* p. 141.
117. Freud, "Moral Responsibility for Dreams," in vol. 5 of *Collected Papers,* pp. 154–7.
118. *New Introductory Lectures,* p. 77.
119. Heinz Hartmann, "Psychoanalysis as a Scientific Theory," in S. Hook (ed.), *Psychoanalysis, Scientific Method, and Philosophy* (New York: New York University Press, 1959), p. 29.
120. Ibid.
121. See, e.g., Skinner's apology for use of mentalist language in "casual discourse" in his *About Behaviorism* (New York: Knopf, 1974), pp. 19–20.
122. Irving Thalberg, "Freud's Anatomies of the Self," in R. Wollheim (ed.), *Freud: A Collection of Critical Essays* (Garden City, N.Y.: Doubleday [Anchor Books], 1974), p. 151.
123. The view of metaphor that sees its essential function as being to nudge us to see some underlying similarity is developed in Michael Moore, "The Semantics of Judging," *Southern California Law Review,* vol. 54(1981): 151–294, esp. pp. 188–92.
124. *Introductory Lectures on Psychoanalysis,* vol. 16 of *The Standard Edition,* p. 296.
125. It is true, as was pointed out in chap. 1, that a kind of explanation can be constructed by reference to a function being served. These explanations, however, are limited to showing that a *particular* heart's beating is to be expected in light of the *general* characteristic of the self-regulating mechanism that is the human body to tend to keep the blood circulating. The function, in such a case (of circulating the blood), does not explain the heart's beating by reference to some *cause* of that process.
126. Ernst Nagel, "Methodological Issues in Psychoanalytic Theory," in S. Hook (ed.), p. 46.
127. Ibid., pp. 46–7.
128. See Ronald de Sousa, "Rational Homunculi," in A. Rorty (ed.), *The Identities of Persons* (Berkeley: University of California Press, 1976), pp. 217–38, who argues against a disunified-self account of weakness of will on the ground that mental states would be needlessly multiplied in this way.
129. Identity theorists might try to hang onto the multiple selves thesis by giving up the individuation of mental states by persons. They might, that is, say that different persons could have the same mental state token. That, interestingly enough, commits one who believes in multiple selves also believing in *group minds.*
130. Ryle, *The Concept of Mind.*
131. For a fine-grained approach, see Alvin Goldman, *A Theory of Human Action* (Englewood Cliffs, N. J.: Prentice-Hall, 1970): for a more coarse-grained view, see Donald Davidson, *Actions and Events* (Oxford: Oxford University Press, 1980). For a comparison of the two approaches, see Baruch Brody, *Identity and Essence* (Princeton, N.J.: Princeton University Press, 1980).
132. Spelling out this relation is one of the basic questions in both the philosophy of

action and the philosophy of law, as discussed in chap. 2. Since Wittgenstein's *Philosophical Investigations* (2d ed. Oxford: Blackwell Publisher, 1958) it has seemed difficult to urge that the relation is simply one of identity.
133. *Philosophical Investigations*, p. 161.
134. A good thought experiment to test this is to ask how many basic acts are performed when Siamese twins move a shared body part. I think our intuitions are that we do not know what to say about such cases, because our individuation by movements suggests that there is one basic act whereas our individuation by persons (or by persons' "willings" or "volitions") suggests that there are two. The point of the text is simply that multiple selves within the same body will generate such puzzles about *all* basic acts.
135. For a nice summary of this, see David Wiggins, *Sameness and Substance* (Cambridge, Mass.: Harvard University Press, 1980), pp. 149–89.
136. Indeed, Freud often speaks of threats being directed against the ego by the superego and the id, and of the ego being *compelled* to act as it does by these other two agencies; e.g., *The Problem of Anxiety*, p. 28; *The Ego and the Id*, p. 15.

4. Does Madness Exist?

1. *Blocker v. United States*, 229 F. 2d 853, 859 (D.C. Cir. 1961) (concurring opinion of Warren Burger, present chief justice of the United States Supreme Court, quoting Philip Roche).
2. B. M. Braginsky, O. D. Braginsky, and K. Ring, *Methods of Madness: The Mental Hospital as Last Resort* (New York: Holt, Rinehart and Winston, 1969), p. 164 (the authors are here speaking of schizophrenia).
3. W. V. Quine, "Speaking of Objects," in *Ontological Relativity and Other Essays* (New York: Columbia University Press, 1969), p. 1.
4. T. Szasz, *The Myth of Mental Illness* (New York: Harper & Row, 1961), p. 1.
5. David Michael Levin, "The Concept of Mental Illness: Working Through the Myths," *Inquiry*, vol. 19(1976): 362.
6. Ibid.
7. L. S. King, "What Is Disease?" *Philosophy of Science*, vol. 21(1954): 199. King recognizes that "the problem . . . is the ontological status of a relationship," not the existence of concrete objects such as witches. Thus Szasz's scornful, "Mental illness thus exists or is real in exactly the same sense in which witches existed or were real" (*Ideology and Insanity: Essays on the Psychiatric Dehumanization of Man* [Garden City, N.Y.: Doubleday, 1970], p. 21) completely misses the only ontological point at issue.
8. G. Frege, "Über Sinn und Bedeutung," *Zeitschrift für Philosophie und Philosophische Kritik*, vol. 100(1892): 25–50. Translated and reprinted in H. Feigl and W. Sellers (eds.), *Readings in Philosophical Analysis* (New York: Appleton-Century-Crofts, 1949), pp. 85–102, and in P. T. Geach and M. Black (eds.), *The Philosophical Writings of Gottlob Frege* (Oxford: Blackwell Publisher, 1960), pp. 56–78.

9. W. V. Quine, "On What There Is," in *From a Logical Point of View* (Cambridge, Mass.: Harvard University Press, 1953), pp. 9 and 11.
10. See the examples by Quine in his "Speaking of Objects," in *Ontological Relativity and Other Essays*, pp. 14–15; see also his *Philosophy of Logic* (Englewood Cliffs, N.J.: Prentice-Hall, 1970), pp. 68–9.
11. Quine, "Existence and Quantification," in *Ontological Relativity and Other Essays*, p. 100. Quine goes on to observe that "many of our causal remarks in the there are form would want dusting up when our thoughts turn seriously ontological."
12. Thomas Szasz, "The Concept of Mental Illness: Explanation or Justification?" in H. T. Engelhardt and S. F. Spicker (eds.), *Mental Health: Philosophical Perspectives* (Dordrecht: Reidel, 1978). Reprinted in A. L. Caplan, H. T. Engelhardt, and J. J. McCartney (eds.), *Concepts of Health and Disease* (Reading, Mass.: Addison-Wesley, 1981), pp. 459–73, quotation on p. 468.
13. Szasz, "The Concept of Mental Illness," in Caplan et al. (eds.), p. 473.
14. Szasz, *The Myth of Mental Illness*, pp. 1–2.
15. Levin, "The Concept of Mental Illness," p. 361.
16. T. Szasz, *The Manufacture of Madness* (New York: Harper & Row, 1970), p. 123.
17. Braginsky et al., *Methods of Madness*, p. 171 (emphasis in original).
18. Ibid., p. 171.
19. Szasz, *The Myth of Mental Illness*, pp. 142–3 (emphasis in original). Alan Stone has some fun exposing other aspects of the illogic of this passage in "Psychiatry Kills: A Critical Evaluation of Dr. Thomas Szasz," *Journal of Psychiatry and Law*, vol. 1(1973): 23–37.
20. A. Kenny, *Action, Emotion, and Will* (London: Routledge & Kegan Paul, 1963), p. 108. A more complete discussion of the "epistemic interdependence of belief attributions and goal attributions" will be found in Carl Hempel's "Rational Action," *Proceedings and Addresses of the American Philosophical Association*, vol. 35(1962): 5–23. Reprinted in N. S. Care and C. Landesman (eds.), *Readings in the Theory of Action* (Bloomington: Indiana University Press, 1968), pp. 281–305.
21. For a critique of Szasz along these lines, see A. R. Louch, *Explanation and Human Action* (Berkeley: University of California Press, 1969), chap. 9.
22. Extended memory, as discussed in chap. 3, should be included here so as to make room for unconscious beliefs and desires. Yet Szasz abandons even this limitation in attempting to find strategies or goals pursued by hysterics. In addition, it is worth pointing out that such unconscious motive explanations as do satisfy this limitation do not typically render the behavior they explain *fully* rational even if they render it *minimally* rational. See P. Alexander, "Rational Behaviour and Psychoanalytic Explanation," *Mind*, vol. 71(1962): 326–41; T. Mischel, "Concerning Rational Behaviour and Psychoanalytic Explanation," *Mind*, vol. 74(1965): 71–8; H. Mullane, "Psychoanalytic Explanation and Rationality," *Journal of Philosophy*, vol. 68(1971): 413–26.
23. R. D. Laing, *The Politics of Experience* (New York: Ballantine Books, 1967), pp. 114–15 (emphasis in original). Laing here relies on Esterson and Laing,

Sanity, Madness and the Family, 2d ed. (Harmondsworth: Penguin Books, 1970), where on p. 26 they disavow any use of unconscious motives or beliefs to make out this thesis.
24. Esterson and Laing, *Sanity, Madness and the Family,* pp. 75, 131.
25. R. D. Laing, *The Divided Self* (London: Tavistock, 1960), chap. 10, pp. 191–2. The case was originally reported in M. Hayward and J. E. Taylor, "A Schizophrenic Patient Describes the Action of Intensive Psychotherapy," *Psychiatric Quarterly,* vol. 30(1956): 211–48.
26. *The Divided Self,* p. 191.
27. Ibid., p. 191.
28. R. J. Ackermann, *Belief and Knowledge* (Garden City, N.Y.: Doubleday [Anchor Books], 1972), p. 33. See generally chap. 3, "Rational Belief."
29. G. Ryle, *The Concept of Mind* (London: Hutchinson, 1949), chap. 1.
30. Ibid., p. 22.
31. T. Szasz, *Law, Liberty, and Psychiatry* (New York: Macmillan, 1968), p. 11, quoting Ryle, *The Concept of Mind,* p. 8. See also *The Myth of Mental Illness,* pp. 88, 93–4, where Szasz gains further theoretical support from the notion of a category mistake. In a generally perceptive review of Szasz's work, Ronald de Sousa concludes that "the basis of the contention that mental illness is a myth ... is the philosophical doctrine of category difference between intentional behavior and natural events in the causal order of the physical sciences." de Sousa, "The Politics of Mental Illness," *Inquiry,* vol. 15(1972): 187–201. Other mythicists also base their arguments on Ryle's work. See particularly T. R. Sarbin, "The Scientific Status of the Mental Illness Metaphor," in S. C. Plog and R. B. Edgerton (eds.), *Changing Perspective in Mental Illness* (New York: Holt, Rinehart and Winston, 1969), pp. 9–31.
32. For an explicit argument that mind words are not referential see D. Dennett, *Content and Consciousness* (London: Routledge & Kegan Paul, 1969), chap. 1.
33. Szasz, *The Manufacture of Madness,* p. 167.
34. See *The Manufacture of Illness.* See also Szasz's *Ideology and Insanity,* p. 19: "The term 'bodily illness' refers to physiological occurrences"; and p. 23: "We call people physically ill when their body functioning violates certain anatomical and physiological norms; similarly we call people mentally ill when their conduct violates certain ethical, political, and social norms." Despite the considerable literature in the philosophy of medicine since these passages were written, Szasz clings to this by now obviously inadequate account of illness as deviation. See his "The Concept of Mental Illness," in Caplan et al. (eds.), p. 471.
35. The ordinary language conceptions of illness and health are explored in G. H. Von Wright, *The Varieties of Goodness* (London: Routledge & Kegan Paul, 1963), pp. 50–61; and in L. S. King, "What is Disease?" pp. 193–203. The relation of illness to incapacitation is also suggested in Joel Feinberg, *Doing and Deserving* (Princeton, N.J.: Princeton University Press, 1970), pp. 253–60.
36. Szasz, *Law, Liberty, and Psychiatry,* p. 25.

37. All quotes are from *Ideology and Insanity,* pp. 191–6.
38. Peters, *The Concept of Motivation* (London: Routledge & Kegan Paul, 1958). See Szasz, *The Myth of Mental Illness,* esp. p. 88, and chap. 10, for his explicit reliance on Peters.
39. One of the reasons for this is the idea Szasz quotes from Peters: Movements "cannot be characterized as intelligent or unintelligent, correct or incorrect, efficient or inefficient." One may only describe *actions* with such adjectives (Peters, *The Concept of Motivation,* p. 15, quoted in *The Myth of Mental Illness,* p. 171). Since one of the principal requirements for using the identity sign is that the expressions referring to the same thing be substitutable for one another without change of truth value, one cannot identify action with movements. But this argument goes only against *identifying* mental entities with physical ones; it says nothing about correlating the two and calling one the cause of the other, for there is no substitutability requirement for the names of effects and their causes.
40. An informative summary of the recent evidence that some forms of schizophrenia may have a genetic etiology is L. L. Heston's "The Genetics of Schizophrenic and Schizoid Disease," *Science,* vol. 167(1970): 249–56.
41. Szasz, *Ideology and Insanity,* p. 15.
42. H. Putnam, "Brains and Behavior," in R. J. Butler (ed.), *Analytical Philosophy,* 2d ser. (Oxford: Blackwell Publisher, 1965), p. 6. Putnam uses the concept of disease as an example of a much more general point, namely, that the meaning of "natural kind" words, such as water, gold, or red (or polio) is not fixed by operational tests based on contemporary knowledge, but presupposes a hidden nature that we know with increasing precision with the advancement of science. See his "The Meaning of 'Meaning,' " in H. Feigl and M. Scriven (eds.), *Language, Mind and Knowledge,* Minnesota Studies in the Philosophy of Science, vol. 7 (Minneapolis: University of Minnesota Press, 1975), pp. 131–93.
43. Quine, "On What There Is," in *Logical Point of View,* p. 19.
44. Manfred Bleuler, "Researches and Changes in Concepts in the Study of Schizophrenia," *Bulletin of the Isaac Ray Medical Library,* vol. 3(1955): 42–5.
45. Levin, "Concept of Mental Illness," p. 363.
46. For further argument and citations, see Moore, "Moral Reality," *Wisconsin Law Review* (1982): 1061–1156.
47. Szasz, *Law, Liberty, and Psychiatry,* p. 18.
48. Szasz, *The Myth of Mental Illness,* p. 131.
49. Szasz, *The Manufacture of Madness,* pp. 122–3. See also *Ideology and Insanity,* p. 204: "Most psychiatric diagnoses may be used, and are used, as invectives: their aim is to degrade – and, hence, socially constrain – the person diagnosed." Laing makes the same objection in numerous places in his work. E.g., *The Politics of Experience,* pp. 121–2.
50. Szasz, *Law, Liberty, and Psychiatry,* p. 205. See also p. 19: "The new label 'mental illness' (and its variants) became only a substitute for the abandoned words of denigration."

51. For a review of the passing of the emotivist and prescriptivist traditions in metaethics, see Moore, "Moral Reality."
52. J. L. Austin, *How To Do Things With Words* (Cambridge, Mass.: Harvard University Press, 1961).
53. M. S. Moore, "Some Myths About 'Mental Illness,'" *Inquiry*, vol. 18(1975): 259.
54. Szasz, "The Concept of Mental Illness," in Caplan et al. (eds.), p. 459.
55. Ibid., p. 473.
56. F. A. Gerbode, Book Review, *Santa Clara Lawyer*, vol. 13(1973): 622. For statements of each of these positions as a result of some version of the myth argument, see T. Szasz, "Psychiatry, Ethics and the Criminal Law," *Columbia Law Review*, vol. 58(1958): 183–98; J. H. Hardisty, "Mental Illness: A Legal Fiction," *Washington Law Review*, vol. 48(1973): 735–62; Szasz, *Psychiatric Justice* (New York: Macmillan, 1965); G. Alexander and T. Szasz, "From Contract to Status via Psychiatry," *Santa Clara Lawyer*, vol. 13(1973): 537–59; R. Roth, M. Dayley, and J. Lerner, "Into the Abyss: Psychiatric Reliability, and Emergency Commitment Statutes," *Santa Clara Lawyer,* vol. 13(1973): 400–66; L. V. Kaplan, "Civil Commitment 'As You Like It,'" *Boston University Law Review*, vol. 49(1969): 14–45; A. T. Elliott, "Procedures of Involuntary Commitment on the Basis of Alleged Mental Illness," *University of Colorado Law Review*, vol. 42(1970): 231–69, esp. p. 231; B. Ennis, *Prisoners of Psychiatry* (New York: Harcourt Brace Jovanovich, 1972). American courts have begun to accept such conclusions of the myth argument. See *Lessard v. Schmidt*, 349 F. Supp. 1078 (E. D. Wis. 1972), vacated, 414 U.S. 473, 94 S.Ct. 713, 38 L.Ed.2nd 661 (1974), and *State ex rel Hawks v. Lazaro*, 202 S.E.2d 109 (W. Va. 1974), holding unconstitutional the Wisconsin and West Virginia civil commitment statutes; *United States v. Brawner*, 471 F.2d 969, 985–6, 995 (D.C. Cir. 1972), where the Court of Appeals for the District of Columbia gave more than sympathetic consideration to eliminating mental illness as an excuse in the criminal law.

5. The Concept of Mental Illness

1. Lexical and stipulative definitions are discussed in Richard Robinson, *Definition* (Oxford: Oxford University Press [Clarendon Press], 1950).
2. Sir James Stephen, *A History of the Criminal Law of England*, vol. 2 (London: Macmillan, 1883), pp. 128–9.
3. One apparent avenue that might seem tempting is to discern that the proper subject of the predicates "is ill" and "is sick" is neither minds nor bodies, but persons and that accordingly, one need not ask what sorts of things minds are to understand the concept of mental illness, because a sick mind is not involved, only a sick person. Although I believe "is ill" to be a predicate whose proper subject is persons, the conclusion allowing one to avoid the sticky question of the ontological status of mental entities does not follow; for unless one abandons entirely the notion of mental illness, and speaks only of illness as such, one will still need to mark off those illnesses that are mental

from those that are not. Presumably this would be done either in terms of mental symptoms or mental causes, or both. In any case, one will inextricably be bound up in saying something about the nature of mental causes, as opposed to physical ones, or symptoms manifested "in the mind" as opposed to physiologically. The "person-is-primitive" strategy of P. F. Strawson (*Individuals* [London: Methuen & Co., 1959]) fails to avoid the mind/body problem, for understanding mental illness as well as more generally.

4. Thus, the repeated use of character words as examples in a behavioral view of mind such as in Gilbert Ryle, *The Concept of Mind* (London: Hutchinson, 1949). Mental illness was also used by Ryle as a seemingly obvious example of the correctness of the behaviorist view. See ibid., p. 21: "For all that we can tell [in a nonbehaviorist account] the inner lives of persons who are classed as idiots or lunatics are as rational as those of anyone else. Perhaps only their overt behavior is disappointing."

5. See the research study conducted by the National Opinion Research Center of the University of Chicago in the mid-1950s, in which a significant percentage of the thirty-five hundred interviewees thought both present and former mental patients to be quite different and unpredictable. S. A. Star, "The Public's Idea About Mental Illness," presented in 1955 to the annual meeting of the National Association of Mental Health, Indianapolis. Reprinted in part in R. C. Donnelly, J. Goldstein, and R. D. Schwartz (eds.), *Criminal Law* (New York: Free Press, 1962), pp. 818–20.

6. See L. S. King, "What Is Disease?" *Philosophy of Science*, vol. 21(1954): 195: "Ordinarily statistics alone cannot label any part of the data as 'diseased.' When we apply statistical methods we already have in mind the idea of health." See also the excellent discussion of this point in Stephen J. Morse, "Crazy Behavior, Morals and Science: An Analysis of Mental Health Law," *Southern California Law Review*, vol. 51(1978): 569.

7. See L. E. Hinsie and R. J. Campbell, *Psychiatric Dictionary*, 3d ed. (New York: Oxford University Press, 1960), defining psychosis as a disorder but not a disease.

8. L. S. King, "What Is Disease?" p. 197.

9. See generally Hilary Putnam, "Dreaming and Depth Grammar," in R. J. Butler (ed.), *Analytical Philosophy*, 1st ser. (Oxford: Blackwell Publisher, 1962), pp. 36–48; and Putnam, "Brains and Behavior," in R. J. Butler (ed.), *Analytical Philosophy*, 2d ser. (Oxford: Blackwell Publisher, 1965), pp. 1–20, wherein Putnam rejects the analysis of the meaning of disease words as being simply a cluster of symptoms, even if the causes are unknown.

10. Again, this does not mean that physical deviation is a sufficient criterion of having a heart disease any more than it is of being ill in general. Abnormal physical structures of a particular organ will constitute a disease of that organ only if those structures impair the functioning of the organ.

11. Other distinctions between illness and disease not here germane would include the fact that "ill" is predicated principally of persons whereas "diseased" will be predicated of any living system. We readily talk of plants being diseased and of there being plant diseases; we do not talk of a plant being ill.

Using ill also seems to involve us more often in acts of evaluation than use of disease, suggested by phrases such as being in "ill health" and the proverbial ill wind that blows no good, when "ill" is used simultaneously with "poor" and "bad." On this last distinction, see Christopher Boorse, "On the Distinction Between Disease and Illness," *Philosophy and Public Affairs,* vol. 5(1975): 49–68. Reprinted in A. L. Caplan, H. T. Engelhardt, and J. J. McCartney (eds.), *Concepts of Health and Disease* (Reading, Mass.: Addison-Wesley, 1981).

12. Psychiatrists have had an unfortunate tendency to regard as mental illness all and only those conditions listed as a mental disorder in DSM-II (*Diagnostic and Statistical Manual of Mental Disorders,* 2d ed. [Washington, D.C.: (American Psychiatric Association 1968]). This would make our concept of illness (here, mental illness) dependent on our empirical success in isolating syndromes and their causes. Our ideas about who is ill or sick do not depend on particular schemes of classification, as many psychiatrists have come to recognize. See E. W. Busse, "The Presidential Address: There Are Decisions to be Made," *American Journal of Psychiatry,* vol. 129(1972): 1–9. See also the good discussion of this point, and of the way in which DSM-III handles it, in Robert L. Spitzer and Jean Endicott, "Medical and Mental Disorder: Proposed Definition and Criteria," in R. L. Spitzer and D. F. Klein (eds.), *Critical Issues in Psychiatric Diagnosis* (New York: Raven Press, 1978), pp. 15–39, esp. pp. 30–1.

13. Louis Swartz, " 'Mental Disease': The Groundwork for Legal Analysis and Legislative Action," *University of Pennsylvania Law Review,* vol. 111(1963): 404. Despite the quoted language, Swartz goes on to develop a redefinition of disease based on the values of avoiding pain and death.

14. Aubrey Lewis ("Health as a Social Concept," *British Journal of Sociology,* vol. 4[1953]: 109–24) early on advanced the view Swartz adopts, distinguishing part dysfunction (as illness) from total malfunctioning (as badness). Lewis's later views are set forth in his *The State of Psychiatry* (New York: Science House, 1967).

15. Boorse, "Disease and Illness," in Caplan et al. (eds.), p. 552 (emphasis in original). Boorse elaborates his views—about the value-free nature of function assignments in biology and the consequently value-free nature of our concepts of health and illness—in "Wright on Functions," *Philosophical Review,* vol. 85 (1976): 70–86, and in "Health as a Theoretical Concept," *Philosophy of Science,* vol. 44(1977): 542–73. Boorse argues (1) that we *can* assign functions relative to end states ("goals" for Boorse) that the organism in fact pursues; (2) that we *do* assign functions in biology in just this value-free way, the organizing end state being survival of the organism and of the species; and (3) that the functional impairment that is the essence of both illness and disease is an impairment of these survival-based functions. It is the third of these premises that I find troubling, for the functional impairment that entitles us to label another as mentally ill seems to have little to do with survival. Rather, the functions we assign to various perceptual states, to pain, to imagination, and so forth are those effects such states usually have that causally contribute to

persons having the wide behavioral repertoire that we think they should have. The behavioral capacities we use as the basis for giving the mind a functional organization do not consist in some monotonous seeking of survival; rather, such behavioral repertoires consist in all the behaviors we can imagine would be intelligible means to intelligible ends. This involves a value judgment of the type I later call the "thin theory of the good." (Boorse himself appears to abandon survival and reproduction as the end state by which we assign *mental* functions, in "What a Theory of Mental Health Should Be," *Journal of Theory of Social Behavior*, vol. 6[1976]: 61–84.)

16. See Donald Klein, "A Proposed Definition of Mental Illness," in Spitzer and Klein (eds.), pp. 41–71, who recognizes the dependence on evolutionary theory of his own value-free definition of mental illness.

17. J. G. Scadding, "Diagnosis: The Clinician and the Computer," *Lancet*, vol. 2(1967): 877–82; R. E. Kendell, "The Concept of Disease and Its Implications for Psychiatry," *British Journal of Psychiatry*, vol. 127(1975): 305–15.

18. Joseph Margolis, "The Concept of Disease," *Journal of Medicine and Philosophy*, vol. 1(1976): 238–55. Reprinted in Caplan et al. (eds.), pp. 561–77, quotation on p. 570 (emphasis in the original).

19. This is a classically Freudian hypothesis. For a comparatively modern statement, see Menninger, Mayer, and Pruyser, *The Vital Balance, The Life Process in Mental Health and Illness* (New York: Viking Press, 1963).

20. *Durham v. United States*, 214 F.2d 862, 875 (D.C. Cir. 1954).

21. Thomas Szasz, *Ideology and Insanity: Essays on the Psychiatric Dehumanization of Man* (Garden City, N.Y.: Doubleday, 1970), pp. 12–24.

22. See Harvey Mullane, "Psychoanalytic Explanation and Rationality," *Journal of Philosophy*, vol. 68(1971): 413–26, who characterizes the neurotic as "irrational because what he does is regularly and systematically self-defeating."

23. This analysis of mental illness as lack of rationality is derived from my article, "Mental Illness and Responsibility," *Bulletin of the Menninger Clinic*, vol. 39(1975): 308–28. Other analyses of mental illness as irrationality are Herbert Fingarette, "Insanity and Responsibility," *Inquiry*, vol. 15(1972): 6–29; Fingarette, *The Meaning of Criminal Insanity* (Berkeley: University of California Press, 1972); Joel Feinberg, "What Is So Special About Mental Illness?" in his *Doing and Deserving* (Princeton, N.J.: Princeton University Press, 1970), pp. 272–92.

24. Star, "The Public's Idea." See also Robert Waelder, "Psychiatry and the Problem of Criminal Responsibility," *University of Pennsylvania Law Review*, vol. 101(1952): 378–90, who on p. 384 notes a "common core" to the concept of mental illness centered on "conditions in which the sense of reality is crudely impaired, and inaccessible to the corrective influence of experience—for example, when people are confused or disoriented or suffer from hallucinations or delusions. That is the case in organic psychoses, in schizophrenia, in manic-depressive psychosis. Their characterization as diseases of the mind is not open to reasonable doubt."

25. The Declaration of Hawaii, a kind of code of ethics for the profession adopted by the World Psychiatric Association, proclaims that psychiatric

treatment is forbidden in the absence of illness (as reported in the *Times*, [London] September 1, 1977). This is to adopt this "trigger for treatment" rationale for redefining the phrase mental illness.
26. E. Jellinek, *The Disease Concept of Alcoholism* (New Brunswick, N.J.: Rutgers Center of Alcohol Studies Publications, 1960), pp. 58–9.
27. F. K. Taylor, "A Logical Analysis of the Medicopsychological Concept of Disease," *Psychological Medicine*, vol. 1(1971): 356–65.
28. E. W. Busse, "The Presidential Address."
29. Talcott Parsons, *The Social System* (New York: Free Press, 1951), pp. 428–79.
30. Robert Veatch, "The Medical Model: Its Nature and Problems," *The Hastings Center Studies*, vol. 1(1973): 59–76. Reprinted in Caplan et al. (eds.), pp. 523–44, quotation on p. 530.
31. See Swartz, "Mental Disease," pp. 400–1: "The nomenclature criterion of disease is a variant of the treatment criterion. Its proponents argue that *mental disease* should be defined as that which comes within the classificatory system of accepted psychiatric nomenclature ... But again the definition is circular. What should be included in psychiatric nomenclature? The only answer is *mental disease.*"
32. See, e.g., the definition by Spitzer and Endicott, in "Medical and Mental Disorder."
33. John Rawls, *A Theory of Justice* (Cambridge, Mass.: Harvard University Press, 1971).
34. Ibid., p. 92.
35. See Spitzer and Endicott, "Medical and Mental Disorder." Spitzer discusses the history of his definition not only in this article, but also in Robert Spitzer and Janet Williams, "The Definition and Diagnosis of Mental Disorder," in W. R. Gove (ed.), *Deviance and Mental Illness* (Beverly Hills, Calif.: Sage, 1982), pp. 15–31. I twice commented on this definition as it progressed, once informally in response to a letter by Spitzer and once more formally at the 1977 annual convention of the American Psychopathological Association.
36. Aristotle, *Topics*, book 6, trans. and ed. E. S. Foster (Cambridge, Mass.: Harvard University Press, 1960).
37. Spitzer and Endicott, "Medical and Mental Disorder," p. 18.
38. Ibid., p. 36.
39. Ibid., p. 23.
40. Ibid., p. 24.
41. See Scadding, "Diagnosis."
42. Spitzer and Endicott, "Medical and Mental Disorder," p. 34.
43. Ibid., p. 26.
44. Max Friedemann, "Cleptomania: The Analytic and Forensic Aspects," *Psychoanalytic Review*, vol. 17(1930): 452–70.
45. Quoted in Spitzer and Williams, "Definition and Diagnosis," p. 19.
46. Even a fully worked out thin theory of the good, with a specific taxonomy of primary goods, would not (yet) yield a crisp definition of mental illness. The reason for this is that giving a functional organization to the mind is not *simply* to specify the end state toward which all functions contribute. One

459

also needs a lot of factual information on how the mind works, information of which we as yet have little. B. A. Farrell nicely puts this last point: "Psychiatrists and others have been liable . . . to take a short cut . . . They go hunting for definitions. This strategy is wrong, principally because psychiatry has not yet reached the stage where it is in a position to offer a suitable definition. . . . Psychiatrists need much more knowledge from the relevant basic sciences—knowledge about human functioning, about the psychological and neurochemical machinery involved in it—before they will be able to formulate with objective precision and with general agreement the standards of functioning and dysfunctioning which they require to demarcate the boundaries of the mentally ill." Farrell, "Mental Illness: A Conceptual Analysis," *Psychological Medicine,* vol. 9(1979): 33–4.

47. Spitzer and Endicott, "Medical and Mental Disorder," p. 29.
48. Ibid., p. 23.

6. The Legal Concept of Sanity

1. *Regina v. M'Naghten,* 10 Clark and F. 200, 8 Eng. Rep. 718 (1843).
2. Abraham Goldstein, *The Insanity Defense* (New Haven, Conn.: Yale University Press, 1967), p. 45.
3. *Parsons v. State,* 81 Ala. 577, 597, 2 So. 854, 866–67 (1887).
4. Goldstein, *The Insanity Defense,* pp. 67–79.
5. American Law Institute, Model Penal Code, sec. 4.01, Proposed Official Draft, 1962.
6. *Durham v. United States,* 214 F.2d 862 (D.C. Cir. 1954).
7. *Carter v. United States,* 252 F. 2d 608, 617 (D.C. Cir. 1957).
8. For a clear separation of these, see Henry Weihofen, "The Definition of Mental Illness," *Ohio State Law Journal,* vol. 21(1960): 1–16.
9. In book 3, chap. 1 of the *Nicomachean Ethics,* Aristotle subdivides actions that may be regarded as involuntary (and thus excused) into two classes, those done in ignorance and those done under compulsion:

"Virtue or excellence is, as we have seen, concerned with emotions and actions. When these are voluntary, we receive praise and blame; when involuntary, we are pardoned and sometimes even pitied. Therefore, it is, I dare say, indispensable for a student of virtue to differentiate between voluntary and involuntary actions . . .

. . . It is of course generally recognized that actions done under constraint or due to ignorance are involuntary. An act is done under constraint when the initiative or source of motion comes from without. It is the kind of act in which the agent or the person acted upon contributes nothing . . .

. . . Ignorance in moral choice does not make an act involuntary — it makes it wicked; nor does ignorance of the universal, for that invites reproach; rather it is ignorance of the particulars which constitute the circumstances and the issues involved in the action . . .

. . . As ignorance is possible with regard to all these factors which constitute an action, a man who acts in ignorance of any one of them is considered as acting involuntarily, especially if he is ignorant of the most important

factors. The most important factors are the thing or person affected by the action and the result." *Nichomachean Ethics,* trans. Martin Ostwald (New York: Bobbs-Merrill, 1962), pp. 52–7.
10. I am indebted to Joel Feinberg ("What Is so Special About Mental Illness?" in his *Doing and Deserving* [Princeton, N.J.: Princeton University Press, 1970], pp. 272–92) for seeing this general point.
11. 3 Add. Eccl. Rep. 79. Lord Erskine in his eloquent defense in *Hadfield's Case,* 27 How. St. Tr. 1281, 1314 (1800) asserted that "delusion . . . where there is no frenzy or raving madness, is the true character of insanity."
12. Mistake of law is only partly available as an excuse in criminal law. "Ignorance of the law is no excuse" is an old maxim sufficiently riddled with exceptions that it is difficult to say what is the general rule and what is the exception.
13. In *Commonwealth v. Rogers,* 7 Metc. 500 (Mass. 1844), Ray's views were presented at the trial by Ray himself; among a number of other tests, Chief Justice Shaw, presiding at the trial, told the jury that they were to find "whether the prisoner in committing the homicide acted from an irresistible and uncontrollable impulse," paraphrasing rather closely Ray's earlier language that some mentally ill persons are "irresistibly impelled to the commission of criminal acts." See Ray, *A Treatise on the Medical Jurisprudence of Insanity* (Boston: Little, Brown, 1838), sec. 187.
14. Joe Goldstein and Jay Katz assume that mental illness negates intention in their well-known and polemical "Abolish the Insanity Defense – Why Not?" *Yale Law Journal,* vol. 72(1963): 853–76. Norval Morris also assumes that "in the broad run of cases" when the defense of insanity is successfully raised the presence or absence of intention should be the real issue, because mental illness excuses only by negating intentionality of action. Morris, *Madness and the Criminal Law* (Chicago: University of Chicago Press, 1982), particularly pp. 54–5, 65–6.
15. Evidence of mental illness is used to negate not only intention, but also premeditation and deliberation in murder trials and (in California until very recently) malice as well. "Diminished capacity" is the general name for this allowance of psychiatric testimony to rebut various *mens rea* elements of the prosecution's case in chief. For a good review of this, see Stephen Morse, "Diminished Capacity: A Moral and Legal Conundrum," *International Journal of Law and Psychiatry,* vol. 2(1979): 271–98.
16. Ray, *Medical Jurisprudence of Insanity.*
17. J. Biggs, *The Guilty Mind* (New York: Harcourt Brace, 1955), pp. 100–2. See also Bernard Diamond, "Isaac Ray and the Trial of Daniel M'Naghten," *American Journal of Psychiatry,* vol. 112(1956): 651–6.
18. See n. 13, this chapter.
19. Ray, *Medical Jurisprudence of Insanity,* sec. 31.
20. Theodore Reik, "The Doe-Ray Correspondence: A Pioneer Collaboration in the Jurisprudence of Mental Disease," *Yale Law Journal,* vol. 63(1953): 187.
21. Ibid.
22. *State v. Pike,* 49 N.H. 399, 442 (1869). This notion of mental disease as

physical cause made the irresponsibility of the mentally ill self-evident to many other nineteenth-century judges as well. See, for example, *Commonwealth v. Mosler*, 4 Pa. St. 264 (1846), in which Chief Justice Gibson spoke of "an unseen ligament pressing on the mind, drawing it to consequences which it sees but cannot avoid."

23. *State v. Pike*, 49 N.H. at 442 (1869).
24. See particularly Daniel Dennett, "Mechanism and Responsibility," in T. Honderich (ed.), *Essays on Freedom of Action* (London: Routledge & Kegan Paul, 1973), pp. 157–85.
25. *Boardman v. Woodman*, 47 N.H. 120, 148 (1865) (Doe in dissent).
26. Reik, "Doe-Ray Correspondence," p. 187.
27. *State v. Pike*, 49 N.H. at 442 (1869).
28. The "verdict" of the state hospital psychiatrists in New Hampshire has in practice been accepted as authoritative regarding the mental illness of any individual accused. See J. P. Reid, "The Working of the New Hampshire Doctrine of Criminal Insanity," *University of Miami Law Review*, vol. 15(1960): 14–58.
29. Ibid., p. 19.
30. *Durham v. United States*, 214 F.2d at 847–75 (D.C. Cir. 1954).
31. Group for the Advancement of Psychiatry, *Criminal Responsibility and Psychiatric Expert Testimony*. G.A.P. Report No. 26, 1954.
32. *Blocker v. United States*, 274 F.2d 572, 573 (D.C. Cir. 1959).
33. *Blocker v. United States*, 288 F.2d 853, 860 (D.C. Cir. 1961).
34. *Carter v. United States*, 252 F.2d 608, 617 (D.C. Cir. 1957).
35. See *McDonald v. United States*, 312 F.2d 847, 851 (D.C. Cir. 1962). In explaining the *McDonald* decision some years afterward, Judge Bazelon noted that "by casting the test wholly in terms of mental illness [in *Durham*] we had unwittingly turned the question of responsibility over to the psychiatric profession . . . [In *McDonald*] we made 'mental illness' a legal term of art for the purposes of the insanity defense and told juries and judges that they could find mental illness when the psychiatrists found none." Bazelon, "New Gods for Old: 'Efficient' Courts in a Democratic Society," *New York University Law Review*, vol. 46(1971): 658–9.
36. *McDonald v. United States*, 312 F.2d at 851 (D.C. Cir. 1962).
37. Judge Bazelon himself came to recognize this. In his opinion in *United States v. Brawner*, 471 F.2d 969, 1011 (D.C. Cir. 1972), he noted: "The definition of mental disease adopted in *McDonald* rendered our test, in almost every significant respect, identical to the ALI test."
38. *United States v. Brawner*.
39. Thomas Szasz, with his usual penchant for hyperbole, attacked the product requirement as "unadulterated nonsense." "Psychiatry, Ethics and the Criminal Law," *Columbia Law Review*, vol. 58(1958): 183–98.
40. In *Carter v. United States*, 252 F.2d 608 (D.C. Cir. 1957), the court analyzed the causal relationship to be that of sine qua non familiar throughout the law: "But for the disease the act would not have been committed."
41. One knows this because in *Stewart v. United States*, 214 F.2d 879 (D.C. Cir.

1954), decided only two weeks after *Durham,* Judge Bazelon reversed a trial court instruction that had equated mental illness with brain disease.
42. *Carter v. United States,* 252 F.2d at 617 (D.C. Cir. 1957).
43. *Washington v. United States,* 370 F.2d 444 (D.C. Cir. 1967).
44. *United States v. Brawner,* 471 F.2d at 1029 (D.C. Cir. 1972). Cf. Alan Stone, *Mental Health and Law: A System in Transition* (Rockville, Md.: Center for Crime and Delinquency, National Institute of Mental Health, 1975), p. 226. "Psychiatry failed Judge Bazelon because like all of the social and behavioral sciences it lacks a concept of an evil-meaning mind as a cause."
45. C. S. Lewis, "The Humanitarian Theory of Punishment," *Res Judicatae,* vol. 6(1953): 224–30.
46. Herbert Morris has thoughtfully defended a more sophisticated version of the rehabilitative ideal that seeks to meet two of these three objections. In "A Paternalistic Theory of Punishment," *American Philosophical Quarterly,* vol. 18(1981): 263, Morris articulates a theory that successfully avoids the third danger (of excessive or cruel "treatments") and partly meets the second, or libertarian, objection. Morris's theory runs into more serious difficulty in accommodating itself to our intuitions about desert, because: (1) unaddressed is the objection that criminals do not deserve paternalistic concern in competition with other groups, and (2) unaccounted for is our practice of punishing offenders who are already repentant ("reformed") or are incapable of being made repentant ("unreformable").
47. "Real moral qualities" are not so strange as the name may seem to some. Desert is no stranger as a property than is merit, injustice, courage, or greediness. Objectivism about all such properties is defended in M. S. Moore, "Moral Reality," *Wisconsin Law Review* (1982): 1061–1156.
48. See Margaret Jane Radin, "Cruel Punishment and Respect for Persons: Super Due Process for Death," *Southern California Law Review,* vol. 53(1981): 1169–73.
49. The main problem with the pure utilitarian theory of punishment is that it potentially sacrifices the innocent in order to achieve a collective good. The main problem with the pure retributivist theory of punishment is that it potentially requires punishment of the guilty even if no further good is achieved by doing so. (Each of these problems is discussed shortly.) The unnamed and unclaimed mixed theory would have both of these problems.
50. For two somewhat different versions of this branch of the mixed theory, see H. L. A. Hart, *Punishment and Responsibility* (Oxford: Oxford University Press, 1968), and Herbert Packer, *The Limits of the Criminal Sanction* (Palo Alto, Calif.: Stanford University Press, 1968).
51. See Andrew Von Hirsch, *Doing Justice: The Choice of Punishments* (New York: Hill and Wang, 1976), who in chap. 6 distinguishes this second form of the mixed theory from the first.
52. For other counterexamples, see Michael Moore, "Mental Illness and Responsibility," *Bulletin of the Menninger Clinic,* vol. 39(1975): 308–28.
53. The Australian philosopher, J. J. C. Smart, is one of the few utilitarians willing to make this move. See J. J. C. Smart and B. Williams, *Utilitarianism:*

For and Against (Cambridge: Cambridge University Press, 1973), pp. 67–73. This has earned Smart the following entry in Dan Dennett's humorous glossary of terms constructed out of philosophers' names: "Outsmart, v. To embrace the conclusion of one's opponent's *reductio ad absurdum* argument. (As in) 'They thought they had me, but I outsmarted them. I agreed that it was sometimes just to hang an innocent man.' " D. Dennett and K. Lambert (eds.), *The Philosophical Lexicon*, 7th ed. (Published privately, 1978), p. 8.

54. The classic defense is John Rawls's "Two Concepts of Rules," *Philosophical Review*, vol. 64(1955): 3–32.
55. The best-known thought experiment of this kind is Kant's: "Even if a civil society were to dissolve itself by common agreement of all its members (for example, if the people inhabiting an island decided to separate and disperse themselves around the world), the last murderer remaining in prison must first be executed, so that everyone will duly receive what his actions are worth and so that the blood-guilt thereof will not be fixed on the people because they failed to insist on carrying out the punishment; for if they fail to do so, they may be regarded as accomplices in this public violation of legal justice." I. Kant, *The Metaphysical Elements of Justice*, trans. J. Ladd (Indianapolis: Bobbs-Merrill, 1965), p. 102.
56. *State v. Chaney*, 477 P.2d 441 (Alaska 1970).
57. Hugo Bedau, "Retribution and the Theory of Punishment," *Journal of Philosophy*, vol. 75(1978): 601–20.
58. This view of justification of any ethical principles is defended in John Rawls's *A Theory of Justice* (Cambridge, Mass.: Harvard University Press, 1971), sec. 4, 9, 87, and is elaborated on at some length in Moore, "Moral Reality."
59. *Durham v. United States*, 214 F.2d, at 876 (D.C. Cir. 1954).
60. *Royal Commission on Capital Punishment 1953 Report*, sec. 322 (London: 1953).
61. See A. Goldstein, *The Insanity Defence*, pp. 59–62, where he reports a "quite widespread feeling among psychiatrists that all psychotics should be regarded as insane." See also J. M. Livermore and P. E. Meehl, "The Virtues of M'Naghten," *Minnesota Law Review*, vol. 51(1967): 789–856, where on p. 804 they conclude that "the criminal law has usually used the term [mental disease] in what one writer [Waelder, quoted in n. 24 of chap. 5] has called its core concept."

7. Does the Unconscious Exist?

1. Ernst Nagel, "Methodological Issues in Psychoanalytic Theory," in S. Hook (ed.), *Psychoanalysis, Scientific Method, and Philosophy* (New York: New York University Press, 1959), p. 47.
2. Fyodor Dostoevsky, *The Eternal Husband* (London: Heinemann, 1950), p. 124.
3. Freud, "The Unconscious," in vol. 4 of *Collected Papers* (New York: Basic Books, 1959), pp. 98–136. See p. 104: "In psycho-analysis there is no choice for us but to declare mental processes to be in themselves unconscious, and to compare the perception of them by consciousness with the perception of the

outside world through the sense-organs; we even hope to extract some fresh knowledge from the comparison. The psycho-analytic assumption of unconscious mental activity seems to be an extension of the corrections begun by Kant in regard to our views of external perception. Just as Kant warned us not to overlook the fact that our perception is subjectively conditioned and must not be regarded as identical with the phenomena perceived but never really discerned, so psycho-analysis bids us not to set conscious perception in the place of the unconscious mental process which is its object. The mental, like the physical, is not necessarily in reality just what it appears to us to be. It is, however, satisfactory to find that the correction of inner perception does not present difficulties so great as that of outer perception—that the inner object is less hard to discern truly than is the outside world."

4. The analogy to Kant is pursued in Ilham Dilman, "The Unconscious," *Mind*, vol. 68(1959): 446–73.
5. B. F. Skinner, "Critique of Psychoanalytic Concepts and Theories," in H. Feigl and M. Scriven (eds.), *The Foundations of Science and the Concepts of Psychology and Psychoanalysis,* Minnesota Studies in the Philosophy of Science, vol. 1 (Minneapolis: University of Minnesota Press, 1956), pp. 85–6.
6. Michael Scriven, "A Study of Radical Behaviorism," in Feigl and Scriven (eds.), pp. 88–130.
7. David Levin, "Picturing the Freudian Unconscious," *The Psychoanalytic Review*, vol. 68(1981): 259.
8. Ibid., p. 258. For some related explication of Merleau-Ponty's notion of body (or "flesh"), see Paul Ricoeur, *Freud and Philosophy* (New Haven, Conn.: Yale University Press, 1970), p. 382.
9. Freud, "The Unconscious," in vol. 4, *Collected Papers*, p. 101.
10. J. Laird, "Is the Conception of the Unconscious of Value in Psychology?" *Mind*, vol. 31(1922): 434–5.
11. G. C. Field, "Is the Conception of the Unconscious of Value in Psychology?" *Mind*, vol. 31(1922): 413–14.
12. Freud, "A Note on the Unconscious in Psycho-Analysis," in vol. 12 of *The Standard Edition of the Complete Psychological Works of Sigmund Freud* (London: Hogarth Press, 1958), p. 263.
13. Freud, "Introductory Lectures on Psycho-analysis," in vol. 15 of *The Standard Edition*, p. 22.
14. Freud, "The Unconscious," in vol. 14 of *The Standard Edition*, p. 167.
15. Freud was not above attacking a logical argument by psychologizing. He believed that the criticism depended "either on convention or on emotional factors" ("The Ego and the Id," in vol 19 of *The Standard Edition*, p. 16). By the latter, he meant our inability to accept the fact that man "is not even master in his own house" ("Introductory Lectures," in vol. 16 of *The Standard Edition*, p. 285), which, when added to the Copernican and Darwinian insights, is just too much for the human ego to stand. Freud thought that it was from this emotional prejudice about our importance in the universe that the "general revolt" against psychoanalysis arose (ibid.).
16. Freud, "Introductory Lectures," in vol. 16 of *The Standard Edition*, p. 277.

17. Freud, "The Unconscious," in vol. 14 of *The Standard Edition*, p. 167.
18. In looking back at his discovery of the unconscious, Freud said, "Everywhere I seemed to discern motives and tendencies analogous to those of everyday life" ("On the History of the Psychoanalytic Movement," in vol. 14 of *The Standard Edition*, p. 11). See also Freud, "The Unconscious," in vol. 14 of *The Standard Edition*, p. 168: "All the categories which we employ to describe conscious mental acts, such as ideas, purposes, resolutions and so on, can be applied to them [unconscious mental acts]. Indeed, we are obliged to say of some of these latent states that the only respect in which they differ from conscious ones is precisely in the absence of consciousness."
19. Gilbert Ryle, *The Concept of Mind* (London: Hutchinson, 1949).
20. For development of the parallel between these ontological divides, see M. Moore, "Moral Reality," *Wisconsin Law Review* (1982): 1061–1156.
21. Frederick Siegler, "Unconscious Intentions," *Inquiry*, vol. 10(1967): p. 257.
22. The claim of privileged access often is taken to be much stronger than that of noninferential and nonobservational knowledge; often the claims I call those of incorrigibility and self-intimation are included as claims of privileged access. See W. Alston, "Varieties of Privileged Access," *American Philosophical Quarterly*, vol. 8(1971): 223–41, for a lucid distinguishing of a wide variety of epistemic claims going under this label.
23. Some, such as Alston, "Varieties of Privileged Access, and R. Audi, "The Limits of Self-Knowledge," *Canadian Journal of Philosophy*, vol. 4(1974): 253–67, would distinguish incorrigibility from infallibility, and both from indubitability. An even weaker sense of incorrigibility is explored by Rorty, "Incorrigibility as the Mark of the Mental," *Journal of Philosophy*, vol. 67(1970): 399–424. The three distinct claims discussed in the text will suffice for my purposes, and I shall ignore these further nuances of this much-explored question.
24. The term "self-intimating" is Gilbert Ryle's, *Concept of Mind*. See, generally, Audi, "The Epistemic Authority of the First Person," *Personalist*, vol. 56(1975): 5–15.
25. Siegler, "Unconscious Intentions," p. 256.
26. Ibid.
27. Quoted in Ilham Dilman, "Is the Unconscious a Theoretical Construct?" *Monist*, vol. 56(1972): 325.
28. See, e.g., Arthur Pap, "On the Empirical Interpretation of Psychoanalytic Concepts," in S. Hook (ed.), pp. 283–97.
29. See the quotations in chap. 3, the subsection entitled "Freud's nontheoretical uses of unconscious."
30. For somewhat similar interpretations of psychoanalysis emphasizing the role of memory, see B. F. McGuiness, "I Know What I Want," *Proceedings of the Aristotelian Society*, vol. 57(1957): 305–20; Alisdair MacIntyre, *The Unconscious* (London: Routledge & Kegan Paul, 1958), chap. 4; L. W. Beck, "Conscious and Unconscious Motives," *Mind*, vol. 75(1966): 155–79; I. Dilman, n. 27, this chapter; and S. Hampshire, "Disposition and Memory," *International Journal of Psycho-Analysis*, vol. 42(1963): 59–68. Reprinted in his

Freedom of Mind (Princeton, N.J.: Princeton University Press, 1971), pp. 160–82. As pointed out by Morris Eagle, "Validation of Motivational Formulations: Acknowledgement as a Criterion," in B. B. Rubinstein (ed.), *Psychoanalysis and Contemporary Science*, vol. 2(1973): 265–75, one would not want to say that actual recapture of memories of certain mental states is a necessary condition for those states' existence, as this would disallow far too many states that we are reasonably certain exist (because of other evidence).

31. Only if one imposed a strong demand that the objects of a person's desires be *consistent* would the incorrigibility thesis be a general argument against there being unconscious mental states. Yet it is just with regard to unconscious mental states that we are most willing to countenance unresolved conflict.
32. Richard Peters, *The Concept of Motivation* (London: Routledge & Kegan Paul, 1958), p. 61.
33. Freud, "Introductory Lectures," in vol. 15 of *The Standard Edition*, pp. 261–3.
34. A point defended in N. S. Sutherland, "Motives as Explanations," *Mind*, vol. 69(1959): 145–59.
35. On the theoretical nature of the concept of desire, see Richard Brandt and Jaegwon Kim, "Wants as Explanations of Actions," *Journal of Philosophy*, vol. 60(1963): 425–35.
36. Nagel, "Methodological Issues," p. 45.
37. Ibid.
38. Ibid.
39. Perhaps what Nagel had in mind here is that the subject *believes* that the object of his wishes is impossible of attainment; that, accordingly, the actor could not have believed that his acts will get him what he wants; and that therefore the wish cannot have been the motive for his adult behavior. This argument, which I make in chap. 8, does not show that "unconscious wish" or "unconscious motive" is nonsense; it shows only that often unconscious wishes are *nonmotivational* causes of behavior in Freud's theory.
40. Adopted here is Quine's notion of ontological commitment whereby a willingness to paraphrase away betrays that there is no commitment to a thing by the speech so eliminated. See W. V. Quine, "On What There Is," in his *From a Logical Point of View* (Cambridge, Mass.: Harvard University Press, 1953).
41. Freud, "The Unconscious," in vol. 4 of *Collected Papers*, p. 102.
42. Freud, "Introductory Lectures," in vol. 16 of *The Standard Edition*, p. 257.
43. Ibid., p. 278.
44. T. R. Miles, *Eliminating the Unconscious* (Oxford: Pergamon Press, 1966), p. 86.
45. Nagel, "Methodological Issues," p. 47.
46. Jean Schimek, "A Critical Re-examination of Freud's Concept of Unconscious Mental Representation," *International Review of Psycho-Analysis*, vol. 2(1975): 184.
47. Ibid., p. 183.
48. Ibid.

49. Ibid.
50. Miles, *Eliminating the Unconscious*.
51. MacIntyre, *The Unconscious*.
52. Dilman, "The Unconscious" and "Is the Unconscious a Theoretical Construct?"
53. See Roy Schafer, *A New Language for Psychoanalysis* (New Haven, Conn.: Yale University Press, 1976); W. W. Meissner, "Metapsychology – Who Needs It?" *Journal of the American Psychoanalytic Association*, vol. 29(1981): 921–38. A representative sampling of antimetapsychological views will be found in the essays in Merton Gill and Philip Holzman (eds.), *Psychology versus Metapsychology* (New York: International Universities Press, 1976). A review of the critical literature is Robert Holt, "The Death and the Transfiguration of the Metapsychology," *International Review of Psychoanalysis*, vol. 8(1981): 129–43.
54. Dilman, "The Unconscious," p. 455.
55. Ibid., p. 454.
56. Dilman, "Is the Unconscious a Theoretical Construct?" p. 339.
57. Dilman, "The Unconscious," p. 454.
58. Freud, *The Ego and the Id*, vol. 19 of *The Standard Edition*, p. 8.
59. Schafer, *New Language for Psychoanalysis*. For an excellent review of Schafer along the lines suggested in the text, see Roderick Anscombe, "Referring to the Unconscious: A Philosophical Critique of Schafer's Action Language," *International Journal of Psycho-Analysis*, vol. 62(1981): 225–41.
60. Daniel Dennett, *Content and Consciousness* (London: Routledge & Kegan Paul, 1969), pp. 90–6.
61. Ibid., p. 93.
62. Ibid.
63. Ibid., pp. 93–4.
64. See the papers cited in n. 53, this chapter. See also H. J. Home, "The Concept of Mind," *International Journal of Psychoanalysis*, vol. 47(1966): 42–9.
65. This separation, characteristic of logical positivist thinking about science, is reviewed and attacked in F. Suppe (ed.), *The Structure of Scientific Theories*, 2d ed. (Urbana: University of Illinois Press, 1977). See particularly Suppe's introduction, pp. 45–9, and 66–86, wherein he concludes that "the observational-theoretical distinction obviously is untenable."
66. I. Matte-Blanco, *The Unconscious as Infinite Sets* (London: Duckworth, 1975).
67. Eric Rayner, "Infinite Experiences, Affects and the Characteristics of the Unconscious," *International Journal of Psycho-Analysis*, vol. 62(1981): 409.
68. Freud, *An Outline of Psychoanalysis* (New York: Norton, 1949), p. 13.
69. Stephen Morse, "Failed Explanations and Criminal Responsibility: Experts and the Unconscious," *Virginia Law Review*, vol. 68(1982): 1014.
70. Ibid., pp. 996–1003.
71. Adolf Grunbaum, "Is Freudian Psychoanalytic Theory Pseudo-Scientific by Karl Popper's Criterion of Demarcation?" *American Philosophical Quarterly*, vol. 16(1979): 131–41; A. Grunbaum, "Can Psychoanalytic Theory Be Co-

gently Tested on 'The Couch'?" In L. Laudan (ed.), *Mind and Medicine: Problems of Explanation and Evaluation in Psychiatry and the Biomedical Sciences* (Berkeley: University of California Press, 1982).
72. For an early beginning, see W. Dement, "Experimental Dream Studies," *Science and Psychoanalysis*, vol. 7(1964): 129–62, 176–77.

8. The Nature of Psychoanalytic Explanation

1. See A. Flew, "Psychoanalytic Explanation," *Analysis*, vol. 10(1949): 8–15; reprinted in M. MacDonald (ed.), *Philosophy and Analysis* (Oxford: Blackwell Publisher, 1954); A. Flew, "Motives and the Unconscious," in *The Foundations of Science and the Concepts of Psychology and Psychoanalysis*, Minnesota Studies in the Philosophy of Science, vol. 1 (Minneapolis: University of Minnesota Press, 1956), pp. 155–73; R. Peters, *The Concept of Motivation* (London: Routledge & Kegan Paul, 1958); A. MacIntyre, *The Unconscious* (London: Routledge & Kegan Paul, 1958); J. Ehrenwald, "Cause, Purpose and Meaning in Psychosomatic Medicine," *Journal of Experimental and Clinical Psychopathology*, vol. 11(1950): 164–73; A. R. Louch, *Explanation and Human Action* (Berkeley: University of California Press, 1969); Roy Schafer, *A New Language for Psychoanalysis* (New Haven, Conn.: Yale University Press, 1976). Others have adopted a modified stance urging the value of the purely causal aspects of the theory. See M. Sherwood, *The Logic of Explanation in Psychoanalysis* (New York: Academic Press, 1969); P. Ricoeur, *Freud and Philosophy* (New Haven, Conn.: Yale University Press, 1970); and M. Eagle, "A Critical Examination of Motivational Explanation in Psychoanalysis," *Psychoanalysis and Contemporary Thought*, vol. 3(1980): 329–80; reprinted in L. Laudan (ed.), *Mind and Medicine: Problems of Explanation in Psychiatry and the Biomedical Sciences* (Berkeley: University of California Press, 1982).
2. Indeed, Freud complained late in life about the lack of any revision of the theory of dreams: "The analysts behave as though they had no more to say about dreams, as though there was nothing more to be added to the theory of dreams." S. Freud, *New Introductory Lectures on Psycho-Analysis*, vol. 22 of *The Standard Edition of the Complete Psychological Works of Sigmund Freud* (London: Hogarth Press, 1968), p. 8. For a contemporary example of the degree to which the psychoanalytic dream theory remains where Freud left it in 1900, see H. Nagera (ed.), *Basic Psychoanalytic Concepts on the Theory of Dreams* (New York: Basic Books, 1969). See also R. Fliess, *The Revival of Interest in the Dream: A Critical Study of Post-Freudian Psychoanalytic Contributions* (New York: International Universities Press, 1953), for a summary of developments in psychoanalytic dream theory between Freud and the 1950s.
3. Michael Scriven, for example, at times a severe critic of the theory, nonetheless considers Freud's dream theory to be a "brilliant conception." See M. Scriven, "The Experimental Investigation of Psychoanalysis," in S. Hook (ed.), *Psychoanalysis, Scientific Method, and Philosophy* (New York: New York University Press, 1959), p. 250.

4. From the preface to the third, revised English edition of *The Interpretation of Dreams*, vols. 4 and 5 of *The Standard Edition*, p. xxxii, written by Freud in 1931: "This book, with the new contribution to psychology which surprised the world when it was published, remains essentially unaltered. It contains, even according to my present-day judgment, the most valuable of all the discoveries it has been my good fortune to make. Insight such as this falls to one's lot but once in a lifetime."
5. See the review by Talcott Parsons in *Daedalus*, vol. 103(1973): 91–6.
6. Freud, *Interpretation of Dreams*, vol. 4 of *The Standard Edition*, p. 96.
7. Freud, *Introductory Lectures on Psycho-Analysis*, vol. 15 of *The Standard Edition*, p. 106.
8. Ibid., p. 94.
9. Freud's "psychic determinism" is a postulate he relies on throughout the whole of psychoanalytic theory, not merely as a justification for trying to find meaning in dreams. A slip of the tongue, for example, could not in principle be explained adequately in terms of fatigue or other physical predispositions, even if those dispositions were sufficient causes: "Even though it may have been given a physiological explanation," the slips would "remain a chance event from the psychological point of view" (*Introductory Lectures*, vol. 15 of *The Standard Edition*, p. 32). Contrary to what Freud sometimes thought, such a postulate of psychic determinism does not follow from a determinist world view and cannot be supported by it alone. Thus, Freud's claim that anyone who believes that parapraxes are simply accidental "has thrown overboard the whole *Weltanschauung* of science" (ibid., p. 28), or the more contemporary claim that the interpretation of dreams as wish fulfillments "is based on a deterministic assumption that everything has a cause and an effect" (B. B. Wolman, *The Unconscious Mind* [Englewood Cliffs, N.J.: Prentice-Hall, 1968], p. 22), is simply wrong. For a more explicit separation of psychic determinism from ordinary scientific determinism, see Wesley Salmon, "Psychoanalytic Theory and Evidence," in S. Hook (ed.), pp. 252–67.
10. Freud, *Introductory Lectures*, vol. 15 of *The Standard Edition*, p. 85.
11. Freud, *Interpretation of Dreams*, vol. 5 of *The Standard Edition*, p. 512.
12. Ibid., p. 506.
13. Freud, *Introductory Lectures*, vol. 15 of *The Standard Edition*, p. 120. Freud's more typical formulation is to treat the latent dream thoughts as "carriers" of the meaning: "It is from these dream thoughts and not from a dream's manifest content that we disentangle its meaning." Freud, *Interpretation of Dreams*, vol. 4 of *The Standard Edition*, p. 277. R. M. Jones comes to a conclusion regarding dream thoughts similar to that discussed in the text in "Dream Interpretation and the Psychology of Dreaming," *Journal of the American Psychoanalytic Association*, vol. 13(1965): 304–19.
14. One may have noticed that there is a fourth motivational explanation in the exposition of Freud's dream theory presented here, namely, that we have motives for selectively reporting our dreams. I have ignored such motives because they are not part of the psychoanalytic explanation of dreams but are given to explain our act of relating a dream in a particular way at a later

time. Furthermore, discussion of such motives would involve an analysis of the important idea of *resistance*, an idea having far-reaching implications throughout psychoanalytic theory, not just for dreams.
15. Freud, *Interpretation of Dreams*, vol. 5 of *The Standard Edition*, p. 630.
16. Freud, *Interpretation of Dreams*, vol. 4 of *The Standard Edition*, p. 268 (emphasis in the original).
17. Ibid., p. 267.
18. Ibid., p. 234 (emphasis in the original).
19. S. Freud, *The Origins of Psychoanalysis; Letters to Wilhelm Fliess, Drafts, and Notes, 1887–1902* (New York: Basic Books, 1954), letter 108.
20. Freud's apparent reason for adopting this postulate of a wish to sleep was to maintain the parallel he thought existed between neurotic symptoms and dreams. Freud thought that "a symptom is not merely the expression of a realized unconscious wish; a wish from the preconscious which is fulfilled by the same symptoms must also be present" (*Interpretation of Dreams*, vol. 5 of *The Standard Edition*, p. 569). Accordingly, if dreams were to be "overdetermined" in this way, Freud needed to postulate some preconscious wish as motivating the dream along with the unconscious wish from childhood. Dreams as well as neurotic symptoms could then be seen as "compromise formations" between opposed wishes belonging to different topographical systems.
21. Ibid., p. 571.
22. Freud uses all such terms in speaking of the desire to sleep. See "The Theory of Dreams," in vol. 4 of *Collected Papers* (New York: Basic Books, 1959), pp. 137, 139 (the intention to sleep); *Interpretation of Dreams*, vol. 4 of *The Standard Edition*, pp. 233–4 (wish, purpose, and motive).
23. Freud, *Interpretation of Dreams*, vol. 4 of *The Standard Edition*, p. 123. See also Freud's *Introductory Lectures*, vol. 15 of *The Standard Edition*, pp. 128–9, and the *New Introductory Lectures*, vol. 22 of *The Standard Edition*, pp. 16, 129–30, for further explicit discussion of the function of dreaming.
24. E. L. Hartmann, *The Functions of Sleep* (New Haven, Conn.: Yale University Press, 1973).
25. Freud, *Interpretation of Dreams*, vol. 5 of *The Standard Edition*, p. 573.
26. M. H. Hollender, "Is the Wish to Sleep a Universal Motive for Dreaming?" *Journal of the American Psychoanalytic Association*, vol. 10(1962): 323–8. Hollender's insightful article is critical of the wish-to-sleep notion because he is unwilling to make the hypothesis stated here.
27. R. M. Jones, "The Psychoanalytic Theory of Dreaming–1968," *Journal of Nervous and Mental Disease*, vol. 147(1968): 587–604.
28. See W. Dement, "Experimental Dream Studies," *Science and Psychoanalysis*, vol. 7(1964): 132. In his attempt to restate the psychoanalytic theory of dreams, Dement mixes the two idioms as thoroughly as did Freud: "If by certain processes the instigated dream can then deal with the stimulus, it forestalls arousal and facilitates a return to deeper sleep, thus promoting the continuation of sleep which, it is assumed, the organism needs and desires. This is what is usually meant by the 'guardian of sleep' function of the dream,

the motivating power of which is the wish to sleep, which in turn is assumed to arise out of a physiological need for sleep as well as perhaps an additional psychological need for sleep in the sense of withdrawing from the daily struggles and frustrations of the waking life."

29. James Strachey, "Introduction to Freud," *Interpretation of Dreams*, vol. 4 of *The Standard Edition*, p. xix.
30. See Dement, "Experimental Dream Studies"; and more recently, S. Fisher and R. Greenberg, *The Scientific Credibility of Freud's Theories and Therapy* (New York: Basic Books, 1977), chap. 2. See also R. M. Jones, *The New Psychology of Dreaming* (New York: Grune & Stratton, 1970), pp. 20–2.
31. Freud, *New Introductory Lectures*, vol. 22 of *The Standard Edition*, p. 29. Freud was dealing here not with counterexamples to the wish to sleep, but with counterexamples to the unconscious wish fantasized as fulfilled in the dream.
32. This functional interpretation applies equally well to the third wish Freud sometimes posited to explain dreams. The unconscious wish from childhood (the first wish), Freud thought, created tension that the dreaming subject, because he wished to sleep (the second wish), wished to discharge (the third wish). This "wished-for instinctual satisfaction" or discharge of psychic tension (*New Introductory Lectures*, vol. 22 of *The Standard Edition*, p. 19) is a third wish Freud sometimes posits. Like the wish to sleep itself, however, Freud needs only to assert that the *function* of dreams is to discharge such tension and, by such discharge, keep the dreamer asleep (which itself promotes health). There is no more evidence of a wish for discharge than there is of a wish to sleep, whereas everything Freud seemingly wanted to assert can in both cases be conveyed in the language of function. Those who test the guardian-of-sleep hypothesis quite rightly construe this part of it as discharge *function* of dreams, not as a wish for discharge. See, e.g., Fisher and Greenberg, *Scientific Credibility*, pp. 46–62; B. Lerner, "Dream Function Reconsidered," *Journal of Abnormal Psychology*, vol. 72(1967): 85–100. See also L. Breger, "Function of Dreams," *Journal of Abnormal Psychology Monographs*, vol. 72(1967): 5, who interprets Freud as holding that "the function of dreams is to provide discharge for unconscious impulses" before rejecting the hypothesis as incompatible with the evidence.
33. Freud, *Interpretation of Dreams*, vol. 4 of *The Standard Edition*, pp. 118–19 (emphasis in the original).
34. Ibid., p. 117.
35. Ibid., p. 120.
36. Jones, "Dream Interpretation," on pp. 314–15, also notes that not a single dream reported in *The Interpretation of Dreams* is explained by reference to such a wish.
37. Roy Schafer, *New Language for Psychoanalysis*.
38. Ibid., p. 139 (citing certain action theorists, such as G. E. M. Anscombe, for whom reasons are crucial in understanding intentional action).
39. Ibid., p. 148. See generally chap. 7, "Claimed and Disclaimed Actions." In addition to his misconception of action, Schafer's position here results to

some extent from the (potential) therapeutic efficacy of getting patients in analysis to view their dreams, slips, etc., as actions they performed. Freud also on occasion adopted such a therapeutic viewpoint. (See "Moral Responsibility for the Content of Dreams," in vol. 5 of *Collected Papers* (New York: Basic Books, 1959), p. 155, where Freud urges that we view dreams as actions for which we are responsible: "Obviously one must hold oneself responsible for the evil impulses of one's dreams. In what other way can one deal with them?" A concept (re)defined because of its therapeutic efficacy is, of course, beside the point if one wants to know whether a dream is an action according to our ordinary conception of an action.

40. See E. D'Arcy, *Human Acts* (Oxford: Oxford University Press [Clarendon Press], 1963). The incorporation of consequences in descriptions of actions has been, for obvious reasons, of much concern to lawyers. See J. Austin, *Lectures on Jurisprudence* (London: J. Murray, 1869), p. 427; J. Salmond, *Jurisprudence*, 11th ed. (London: Sweet and Maxwell, 1957), pp. 400–2.
41. See G. E. M. Anscombe, *Intention*, 2d ed. (Ithaca, N.Y.: Cornell University Press, 1963), pp. 84–9. ("A great many of our descriptions of events effected by human beings are *formally* descriptions of executed intentions.")
42. This feature of conventionally complex action descriptions was taken by many, following the later Wittgenstein, to provide the key to understanding human action as such. See, e.g., A. I. Melden, "Action," *Philosophical Review*, vol. 65(1956): 523–41; Winch, *The Idea of a Social Science* (London: Routledge & Kegan Paul, 1958), particularly pp. 24–33, 45–54; and Peters, *The Concept of Motivation*. Louch forcefully counters this analysis as an adequate analysis of *action* (as opposed to some species of complex action) in chap. 9 of his *Explanation and Human Action*.
43. See A. Danto, "Basic Actions," *American Philosophical Quarterly*, vol. 2(1965): 141–48.
44. One might be tempted to say that one does do an even more basic action here, namely, moving all those muscles necessary to move one's arm. Yet significantly, this is not the way we think of this act. Most of us, without special training, do not know how to move "just those muscles" as a basic act; we can do so only as a complex act, i.e., we do so *by moving our arm*. (On this, see Melden, *Free Action* [London: Routledge & Kegan Paul, 1961].) The notion of a basic act depends importantly on what an agent *knows* how to do directly, i.e., without doing something else first.
45. Notice that it would be awkward to make "dreaming" into a complex action verb to cover such cases.
46. L. Wittgenstein, *Philosophical Investigations*, 2d ed. (Oxford: Blackwell Publisher, 1958), p. 161e.
47. Goldman, *A Theory of Human Action* (Englewood Cliffs, N.J.: Prentice-Hall, 1970), pp. 49–63.
48. The philosophy-of-action literature is rich with attempts to get around this problem. See R. Chisholm, "The Descriptive Element in the Concept of Action," *Journal of Philosophy*, vol. 61(1964): 613–25 (first noticing the problem); Goldman, *Theory of Human Action*, pp. 61–3 (requiring that belief/de-

sire sets cause basic acts "in a certain characteristic way," of which, Goldman claims, we are intuitively aware); D. Davidson, "Freedom to Act," in T. Honderich (ed.), *Essays on Freedom of Action* (London: Routledge & Kegan Paul, 1973), pp. 137–56 (surveying others' attempts before despairing "of spelling out . . . the way in which attitudes must cause actions"); I. Thalberg, *Perception, Emotion and Action* (New Haven, Conn.: Yale University Press, 1977), pp. 56–62; D. F. Pears, "The Appropriate Causation of Intentional Basic Actions," *Critica*, vol. 7(1975): 39–69; C. Peacocke, "Deviant Causal Chains," *Midwest Studies in Philosophy*, vol. 4(1979): 123–55.

49. See, e.g., Pears, "Appropriate Causation."
50. S. Freud, "Moral Responsibility for the Content of Dreams," in vol. 5 of *Collected Papers*, pp. 154–7.
51. See Irving Thalberg, "Freud's Anatomies of the Self," in R. Wollheim (ed.), *Freud: A Collection of Critical Essays* (Garden City, N.Y.: Doubleday [Anchor Books], 1974); Ronald de Sousa, "Rational Homunculi," in A. Rorty (ed.), *The Identities of Persons* (Berkeley: University of California Press, 1976), pp. 217–38.
52. I shall later argue against the fragmentation-of-self notion in Freudian metapsychology. See chap. 11.
53. To show this conclusively, one would have to work out a full-fledged theory of action and show that dreaming does not fit within it. If one gives up on refining a causal theory of action, one might revert to the epistemic criterion suggested in chap. 2. Dreaming might then be defined as an unconscious action, if one's memory allowed one to know noninferentially that one tried to produce a dream. Rarely, however, does Freud even attempt to have his patients recapture in their memory that they *tried* to produce a dream. I pursue this in chap. 9, concluding that for almost all dreams the requisite memories are not present. (Robert Shope comes to a similar conclusion in "Freud's Concepts of Meaning," *Psychoanalysis and Contemporary Science*, vol. 2[1973]: 276–303.) Rather, Freud and more contemporary analysts simply assume that if they have discovered unconscious wishes explaining an event, then that event can be viewed as an action.
54. Freud, *Interpretation of Dreams*, vol. 4 of *The Standard Edition*, p. 151.
55. One thing that is clear is that we cannot always ascribe a belief-that-q to some subject just because he believes both p and $p \supset q$. If we were justified in doing this, then we would always know all the logical implications of our beliefs. Yet we plainly do not know all such implications, as our difficulties in finding the solutions to logical proofs and mathematical puzzles illustrate.
56. The "Metapsychological Supplement" is in vol. 14 of *The Standard Edition*, pp. 222–35.
57. Ibid., p. 229.
58. Ibid., pp. 226–31.
59. Flew, "Motives and the Unconscious," p. 164. For a contrary view, urging that dreams, parapraxes, and symptoms are not actions, see F. Cioffi, "Wollheim on Freud," *Inquiry*, vol. 15(1972): 171–230, esp. pp. 178–81.
60. As noted earlier (n. 39, this chapter), the therapeutic efficacy of getting pa-

tients to view their dreams as actions for which they are responsible is no justification for saying that dreams are (really) actions. Peter Alexander has concluded that "the typical Freudian mode of explanation of neurotic symptoms is in terms of reasons." Alexander, "Wishes, Symptoms and Actions," *Aristotelian Society Supplementary Volume,* vol. 48(1974): 126. Alexander appears to believe that we should so classify Freudian explanations because "we may, by coming to think of a piece of our behavior as not, after all, just caused but done for a reason, be enabled to control it" (ibid., p. 126). Such enlarging of our control is a desirable consequence one may achieve in successful therapy by convincing a patient he dreams for reasons; that does not mean, however, that in the past, before he got such control, he dreamed for reasons.

61. Theodore Mischel, "Concerning Rational Behaviour and Psychoanalytic Explanation," *Mind,* vol. 74(1965): 75. Richard Wollheim is another philosopher who is quite willing to attribute wildly irrational beliefs to neurotics in order to "discover" a complete practical syllogism for such persons. Wollheim, *Sigmund Freud* (New York: Viking Press, 1971), pp. 91–4.
62. Mischel, "Rational Behaviour," p. 75.
63. See particularly, Arthur Collins, "Unconscious Belief," *Journal of Philosophy,* vol. 66(1969): 667–80. See also D. C. Dennett, *Brainstorms* (Montgomery, Vt.: Bradford Books, 1978), p. 285, where Dennett concludes that "there is no objectively satisfiable sufficient condition for an entity's *really* having beliefs."
64. J. Balmuth, "Psychoanalytic Explanation," *Mind,* vol. 74(1965): 229–35. (Balmuth is discussing symptoms and not dreams, but presumably his point would be the same.)
65. Various senses in which a dream or symptom could express a wish (and still not be motivated by it) are explored in Robert Shope, "The Psychoanalytic Theories of Wish-Fulfillment and Meaning," *Inquiry,* vol. 10(1967): 427–38. On the same point, see also Peter Alexander, "Psychoanalysis and the Explanation of Behaviour," *Mind,* vol. 80(1971): 391–402, esp. 399–400.
66. See n. 32, this chapter.
67. Gary Fuller considers and rejects a number of such substituted practical syllogisms for neurotic symptoms in "Freudian Explanations, Rational Explanation, and Meaning," *Philosophy Research Archives,* vol. 3(1977): 813–31.
68. Wittgenstein, for one, so interpreted what Freud had done: "If I take any one of the dream reports . . . which Freud gives, I can by the use of free association arrive at the same results as those he reaches in his analysis – although it was not my dream. And the association will proceed through my own experiences and so on. The fact is that whenever you are preoccupied with something, with some trouble or with some problem which is a big thing in your life – as sex is, for instance – then no matter what you start from the association will lead finally and inevitably back to that same theme. Freud remarks on how, after the analysis of it, the dream appears so very logical. And of course it does. You could start with any of the objects on this table – which certainly are not put there through your dream activity – and you could find

that they all could be connected in a pattern like that; and the pattern would be logical in the same way. One may be able to discover certain things about oneself by this sort of free association, but it does not explain why the dream occurred." L. Wittgenstein, *Lectures and Conversations* (Berkeley: University of California Press, 1970), pp. 50–1. See generally Robert Steele, "Psychoanalysis and Hermeneutics," *International Review of Psycho-Analysis,* vol. 6(1979): 389–411, for a systematic development of this view of Freud's theory.

69. "Suppose I have a picture-puzzle, a rebus, in front of me. It depicts a house with a boat on its roof, a single letter of the alphabet, the figure of a running man whose head has been conjured away, and so on. Now I might be misled into raising objections and declaring that the picture as a whole and its component parts are nonsensical. A boat has no business to be on the roof of a house, and a headless man cannot run. Moreover, the man is bigger than the house, and if the whole picture is intended to represent a landscape, letters of the alphabet are out of place because such objects do not occur in nature. But obviously we can only form a proper judgment of the rebus if we put aside criticisms such as these of the whole composition and its parts and if, instead, we try to replace each separate element by a syllable or word that can be represented by that element in some way or other. The words which are put together in this way are no longer nonsensical but form a poetical phrase of the greatest beauty and significance. A dream is a picture-puzzle of this sort." Freud, *Interpretation of Dreams,* vol. 4 of *The Standard Edition,* pp. 277–8.
70. Ibid., p. 41. Jones, "Dream Intrepretation," documents Freud's explanatory (as well as his interpretive) intent in dream theory.
71. Freud, *Interpretation of Dreams,* vol. 4 of *The Standard Edition,* p. 136.
72. Ibid., vol. 4, p. 308.
73. Ibid., vol. 5, p. 339.
74. Ibid., vol. 5, p. 490.
75. Ibid., vol. 5, pp. 470–1.
76. Ibid., vol. 4, p. 141.
77. Ibid., vol. 5, p. 339.
78. Ibid., vol. 4, p. 267 (emphasis in the original).
79. The reasons given here for reconstruing the motives of distortion as functions do *not* include the lack of intelligibility of distortion as a motive; the phenomena of resistance and self-deception show us that often in waking life we do perform actions with distortion as our (unconscious) motive. In such cases the avoidance of pain is both the function served by our behavior and the motive that causes it.
80. There has been a burgeoning literature on whether the unconscious wishes with which Freudians explain parapraxes and neurotic symptoms operate as reasons or only as mental causes. For a defense of the view that Freud's explanations of symptoms and parapraxes are not in terms of reasons, see Robert Shope, "Theories of Wish-Fulfillment and Meaning," pp. 421–38; Shope, "The Significance of Freud for Modern Philosophy of Mind," in

Philosophy of Mind, vol. 4 (Dordrecht: Reidel, 1982); Gary Fuller, "Freudian Explanations," pp. 813–31; Peter Alexander, "Rational Behavior and Psychoanalytic Explanation," *Mind,* vol. 71(1962): 328–41; P. Alexander, "Psychoanalysis and the Explanation of Behaviour," pp. 391–402; and for an early version, Richard Peters, *The Concept of Motivation.*

81. Freud, *New Introductory Lectures,* vol. 22 of *The Standard Edition,* p. 81.
82. See P. Alexander, "Cause and Cure in Psychotherapy," *Aristotelian Society Supplementary Volume,* vol. 29(1955): 25–42, who interprets the theory causally and thus construes the therapy as indoctrination.

9. Increased Responsibility

1. As noted in chap. 2, this implication amounts to the trivial truth that acting (for a reason) is acting. As was also noted in chap. 2, this implication from acting for reasons to acting cannot be made into some criterion of when one performs an action.
2. Anscombe would say an action is necessarily intentional under that description of it for which there is a reason-giving explanation. G. E. M. Anscombe, *Intention,* 2d ed. (Ithaca, N.Y.: Cornell University Press, 1963). This implication holds true in the knowledge theory of intention as well: If a person acts for a reason in doing action *A,* that means that he believes that *A* will get him the object of his desires; he has such a belief only if he knows that he is doing *A* to begin with, and such knowledge is the criterion of intentional in the knowledge theory of intention I adopted in chap. 2.
3. S. Freud, *The Psychopathology of Everyday Life,* vol. 6 of *The Standard Edition of the Complete Psychological Works of Sigmund Freud* (London: Hogarth Press, 1960).
4. Ibid., p. 167.
5. Ibid., p. 183.
6. Ibid., p. 185.
7. Ibid., p. 201.
8. Ibid., p. 174.
9. Ibid., p. 168.
10. S. Freud, "Fragment of an Analysis of a Case of Hysteria," in vol. 7 of *The Standard Edition,* pp. 3–122.
11. Ibid., p. 42.
12. Ibid., p. 43, n. 1.
13. See T. Szasz, *Law, Liberty, and Psychiatry* (New York: Macmillan, 1968), pp. 123–37.
14. Ibid., p. 135.
15. Ibid., p. 137 (emphasis in original).
16. Ibid., p. 135.
17. R. Schafer, *A New Language for Psychoanalysis* (New Haven, Conn.: Yale University Press, 1976).
18. Representative of this tradition are: A. Flew, "Psychoanalytic Explanation," *Analysis,* vol. 10(1949): pp. 8–15; Flew, "Motives and the Unconscious," in Feigl and Scriven (eds.), *The Foundations of Science and the Concepts of*

Psychology and Psychoanalysis, Minnesota Studies in the Philosophy of Science, vol. 1 (Minneapolis: University of Minnesota Press, 1956), pp. 155–73; A. MacIntyre, *The Unconscious* (London: Routledge & Kegan Paul, 1958); Richard Wollheim, *Sigmund Freud* (New York: Viking Press, 1971); Theodore Mischel, "Concerning Rational Behaviour and Psychoanalytic Explanation," *Mind,* vol. 74(1965): 71–8; Mischel, "Understanding Neurotic Behavior: From 'Mechanism' to 'Intentionality,'" in T. Mischel (ed.), *Understanding Other Persons* (Oxford: Blackwell Publisher, 1974), pp. 216–59; Peter Alexander, "Wishes, Symptoms and Actions," *Aristotelian Society Supplementary Volume,* vol. 48(1974): 119–34; J. Balmuth, "Psychoanalytic Explanation," *Mind,* vol. 74(1965): 229–35.

19. Although Freud's theory of dreams attempts both to interpret dreams and to explain them, it is necessary to separate these two tasks in order to understand the implications that Freud's theory could have for reconceptualizing dreams as actions. For the separation of these two tasks, see Jones, "Dream Interpretation and the Psychology of Dreaming," *Journal of the American Psychoanalytic Association,* vol. 13(1965): 304–19.
20. For an explication of the notion of an intention *in* a statute, painting, or dream, see M. S. Moore, "The Semantics of Judging," *Southern California Law Review,* vol. 54(1981): 151–294, esp. pp. 258–62. See also Donald Gustafson, "On Unconscious Intentions," *Philosophy,* vol. 48(1973): 178–82.
21. For a historical analysis of repression in Freud's thought, see Theodore Mischel, "Understanding Neurotic Behavior." Mischel urges that Freud began with an Intentional account of repression as an act a person performs for reasons, shifted midcareer into a mechanistic account, and returned in the 1920s to the Intentional account. Mischel himself believes, contrary to the text, that repression is an act for reasons.
22. 298 F. 145 (S.D. N.Y. 1924).
23. Only if "copying" were thought to be an intentionally complex act description (so that a copier must intentionally copy to copy) would one need to speak of unconscious knowledge here. In such a case, *two* knowledge questions would be pertinent to the issue of whether the defendant copied: (1) Did the defendant know he was performing the basic acts in question; and (2) did the defendant know that he was copying by doing the basic acts he was doing. Copy as used in the Copyright Act (17 U.S.C. Sec. 106 [Supp. III 1979]) is not used as an intentionally complex action verb. Hence, one only need ask the first knowledge question in order to decide whether the defendant copied. And as to that question, on the facts of *Dillingham* the defendant unquestionably copied because he consciously knew he was performing those basic acts that constituted copying.
24. Conscious knowledge, as used here and in chap. 3, involves either conscious experience or the disposition to have such experience if one's mind is directed to the question of whether one was acting. In Freudian terms, both conscious and preconscious knowledge are included here.
25. This is what I call the pretheoretical unconscious in chap. 3, which consists of material that is hard to recapture but potentially recapturable by memory.

26. Memory is particularly crucial here for the reason set forth in the text: Personal identity is tied up with memory, and so, therefore, is personal agency, the concept that lies at the heart of human action. Although one might well develop a theory about unconscious actions that would not itself be in terms of a person's first-person awareness (see chap. 7), what the theory would be about would remain the unconscious actions we can potentially remember.

   Although Freud hoped that his concepts such as that of an unconscious action would eventually be explained by some all-encompassing physical theory of the mind, his insights, he thought, could and should be judged independently of any such integration. His essential insight about the unconscious was the claim of extended memory: that one can remember far more than one would have thought prior to psychoanalysis. As Freud rather dramatically noted, "The property of being conscious or not is in the last resort our one beacon-light in the darkness of depth-psychology." S. Freud, *The Ego and the Id*, in vol. 19 of *The Standard Edition*, p. 18.
27. "What, then, must we do in order to replace what is unconscious in our patients by what is conscious? There was a time when we thought this was a very simple matter: all that was necessary was for us to discover this unconscious material and communicate it to the patient. But we know already that this was a short-sighted error. *Our* knowledge about the unconscious material is not equivalent to *his* knowledge . . . [w]e must look for it in his memory." S. Freud, *Introductory Lectures on Psycho-Analysis*, vol. 16 of *The Standard Edition*, p. 436 (emphasis in original).
28. Ibid., p. 102.
29. Ibid., p. 103.
30. John Locke made the most famous argument for the connection between memory and personhood. For an excellent discussion of Locke's views in this regard, and a modern, more limited restatement of them, see D. Wiggins, "Locke, Butler and the Stream of Consciousness: And Men as Natural Kind," in A. Rorty (ed.), *The Identities of Persons* (Berkeley: University of California Press, 1976).
31. On the idea of memory extending well beyond remembrances of what was consciously known but then forgotten, see M. Williams, *Groundless Belief* (Princeton, N.J.: Princeton University Press, 1977), pp. 90–1.
32. Frank Cioffi, "Wollheim on Freud," *Inquiry*, vol. 15(1972): 181. Cioffi later elaborated on his objections to an actor's belated recognition of his agency. Conceding that such belated recapture is possible about unconscious emotions, Cioffi asks: "But what of the hidden *actions* to which Freud is so often committed? Would we allow that a claim about what an hysteric was unconsciously doing at a certain time, e.g. inducing headaches or nausea, could be settled by what she 'would feel if this or that were to happen?' . . . A patient might ultimately come to realize that she *harboured* a particular unconscious impulse, for example, a defloration or pregnancy fantasy . . . but what of the relation between the impulse and its supposed manifestations, e.g. migraine, vomiting, i.e. its efficacy in producing symptoms, dreams, errors? Could she

'realize' this, too, in the same way? What we need in the case of claims that phenomena like these are to be ascribed to an unconscious motive is not mere evidence of possession but evidence of implementation. And this the patient's subsequent introspection is in no position to give us." Cioffi, "Wishes, Symptoms and Actions," *Aristotelian Society Supplementary Volume,* vol. 48(1974): 113.

Cioffi seems to think that we cannot recapture an experience of agency in the same way we can recapture an experience of an emotion. Yet why not? Why is it not at least possible that a person can come to see that he was acting in the same way that he can come to see that he was angry? For conscious actions and conscious emotions one has noninductive awareness that one is acting or that one is, e.g., angry. The concept of an unconscious action only requires that such privileged access is deferred until a later time.

It will *not* do, as Peter Alexander does (in "Wishes, Symptoms, and Actions," pp. 131–2), to argue that we do not possess noninductive knowledge even of our normal, conscious actions. Alexander confuses our knowing the reason for which we act with knowing that we act. The reason for which we act is a causal question on which we have no privileged access; whether we act, the only issue here relevant, is a question on which we do have such privileged access.

33. A broader concept of the person, and thus a broader notion of personal agency and of action, is discussed in the last section of this chapter.
34. This illegitimate inference seems to be the basis for Schafer's conclusion, similar to Freud's, that "thinking is a kind of action engaged in by persons. We are responsible for all our thoughts, including as Freud pointed out, our dreams." R. Schafer, *New Language for Psychoanalysis,* p. 148.
35. Robert Shope also applies this account of action to Freudian examples. He concludes that because the actors lack knowledge (or even potential recall) that they have done something, what they have done is not to be considered an action. Shope, "Freud's Concepts of Meaning," *Psychoanalysis and Contemporary Science,* vol. 2(1973): 276–303.
36. Wollheim, *Sigmund Freud,* p. 78.
37. Ibid., pp. 82–3.
38. "Knowledge is not always the same as knowledge: there are different sorts of knowledge, which are far from equivalent psychologically... If the doctor transfers his knowledge to the patient as a piece of information, it... does not have the result of removing the symptoms.... The patient knows after this what he did not know before – the sense of his symptom; yet he knows it just as little as he did. Thus we learn that there is more than one kind of ignorance. We shall need to have a somewhat deeper understanding of psychology to show us in what these differences consist. But our thesis that the symptoms vanish when their sense is known remains true in spite of this. All we have to add is that the knowledge must rest on an internal change in the patient such as can only be brought about by a piece of psychical work with a particular aim. We are faced here by problems which will presently be

brought together into the *dynamics* of the construction of the symptoms." Freud, *Introductory Lectures*, vol. 16 of *The Standard Edition*, p. 281 (emphasis in original) (footnote omitted).
39. Cioffi, "Wishes, Symptoms and Actions," p. 114.
40. In his informative paper on what one can do in the way of basic actions, Arthur Danto appears to merge these two questions. Danto, "What We Can Do," *Journal of Philosophy*, vol. 60(1963): 435–45. He argues that one can do some basic act, for example, wiggling one's ears, only if one knows one can do it. His essential point is that the power and the knowledge of that power to do some basic act cannot be separated. This is true and forms the basis for one of the arguments in the text; yet it is also important to see that there are many things no amount of training can ever give one the power to do because they are beyond human capacity. As a basic action, one cannot make a tree fall over although as a complex action one can, of course, "fell a tree." Contrary to Freud's suggestions, many of the symptoms Freud examines cannot be basic actions on this fundamental ground that *no one* could perform them as basic actions.
41. This is from the case study of Elizabeth Von R., from *Studies on Hysteria, The Standard Edition*, vol. 2 at p. 166.
42. S. Freud, *New Introductory Lectures on Psychoanalysis*, vol. 22 of *The Standard Edition*, p. 19.
43. Freud, *Introductory Lectures*, vol. 16 of *The Standard Edition*, p. 261.
44. Ibid., pp. 261–2.
45. Freud, *Psychopathology of Everyday Life*, vol. 6 of *The Standard Edition*, pp. 175–6.
46. Freud, *Introductory Lectures*, vol. 16 of *The Standard Edition*, pp. 262–3.
47. See, e.g., Antony Flew, "Motives and the Unconscious"; Stuart Hampshire, "Disposition and Memory," *International Journal of Psycho-Analysis*, vol. 42(1963): 59–68.
48. F. Siegler, "Unconscious Intentions," *Inquiry*, vol. 10(1967): 251–67.
49. This is one of the main points developed in chap. 8 as to why psychoanalytic explanations are not reason giving in form.
50. Theodore Mischel, "Concerning Rational Behavior," appears to believe one should attribute such irrational beliefs to the woman in this example.
51. Theodore Dreiser, *An American Tragedy* (New York: Boni and Liveright, 1925).
52. Ibid., vol. 2, pp. 77–8.
53. Ibid., vol. 2, p. 388.
54. Ibid.
55. D. Dennett, *Content and Consciousness* (London: Routledge & Kegan Paul, 1969), pp. 114–31. (Dennett is talking about awareness, but similar remarks would apply to belief.)
56. See, e.g., R. Gregory, *Eye and Brain* (New York: McGraw-Hill, 1966).
57. This is the artificial intelligence approach to mental states. One suspends the question of whether the system really has such input subsystems and postulates them wherever it is predictively useful. See M. Arbib, *The Metaphorical*

Brain (New York: Wiley, 1972). See generally D. Dennett, "Intentional Systems," in *Brainstorms* (Montgomery, Vt.: Bradford Books, 1978).
58. See A. Goldstein, *The Insanity Defense* (New Haven, Conn.: Yale University Press, 1967), pp. 49–50, 56–7. The American Law Institute explicitly adopted this rejection of propositional knowledge as sufficient for sanity with its language of "appreciate." Model Penal Code sec. 4.01 (Proposed Official Draft, 1962).
59. See n. 38, this chapter.
60. S. Freud, "Notes upon a Case of Obsessional Neurosis," in vol. 10 of *The Standard Edition,* p. 196, n. 1 (emphasis in original) (hereafter cited as Freud, "The Rat-Man").
61. Ibid., pp. 195–6.
62. As Bentham recognized, one may be quite repelled by a particular action, yet nonetheless adopt that action as one's chosen means to some end one wants more. Such an intention is not even an oblique intention, but a direct (if mediate) intention. J. Bentham, *An Introduction to the Principles of Morals and Legislation* (New York: Hafner Press, 1948), p. 84. (First published Oxford: Clarendon Press, 1876.)
63. See Harvey Mullane, "Unconscious Emotion," *Theoria,* vol. 31(1965): 181–90; M. Fox, "On Unconscious Emotions," *Philosophy and Phenomenological Research,* vol. 34(1973): 151–70.
64. See the discussion of this point in chap. 8, n. 55.
65. See, e.g., W. F. LaFave and A. W. Scott, *Criminal Law* (St. Paul: West, 1972), sec. 59.
66. See H. Morris, "Punishment for Thoughts," in his *Guilt and Innocence* (Los Angeles: University of California Press, 1976).
67. If a person thinks this not to be true, it may be due to his *anger* at being hurt – an anger considerably diminished if someone only *tried* to hurt him. Such anger, however, is not to be confused with moral insight. For a contrary view of this much-discussed ethical issue, see T. Nagel, "Moral Luck," in his *Mortal Questions* (Princeton, N.J.: Princeton University Press, 1979).
68. C. Brenner, *An Elementary Textbook of Psychoanalysis,* rev. ed. (New York: International Universities Press, 1973), p. 135.
69. Freud, *New Introductory Lectures,* vol. 22 of *The Standard Edition,* p. 29.
70. The point so relied on by Ernst Nagel in his general attack on Freud's unconscious mental states. See chap. 7.
71. Freud, *Introductory Lectures,* vol. 16 of *The Standard Edition,* pp. 264–9.
72. Ibid., pp. 267–8.
73. Anscombe, *Intention.*
74. See, e.g., Model Penal Code, sec. 5.01(1) (Proposed Official Draft, 1962). The Model Penal Code provision is a proposal rather than a restatement of existing criminal law doctrine. The impossibility doctrines of the decided cases are a jumble of inconsistent results.
75. Freud, *Introductory Lectures,* vol. 16 of *The Standard Edition,* p. 267.
76. Often when Freud is unable to produce such beliefs from the extended memory of his patients, he posits an unconscious knowledge of symbolism that

one uses when one dreams as well as in the formation of symptoms. "The dreamer has a symbolic mode of expression at his disposal which he does not know in waking life and does not recognize." Freud, *Introductory Lectures,* vol. 15 of *The Standard Edition,* p. 165. These symbolic transformations "are not freshly made on each occasion; they lie ready to hand and are complete, once and for all." Ibid.

Such beliefs in a "universal" symbolism are not mental states of the person, even if such states exist; for as Freud admits, they are even outside the domain of extended memory.

77. Gary Fuller, "Freudian Explanations, Rational Explanation, and Meaning," *Philosophy Research Archives,* vol. 3(1977): 827.
78. J. Balmuth, "Psychoanalytic Explanation," p. 233 (emphasis added).
79. Richard Wollheim makes a beginning in this direction in his account of fantasy as it developed in Freud's thinking. According to Wollheim, fantasy became for Freud "the portrayal or representations of a desire come true, that is, of a desire realized . . . against the background of certain beliefs. Accordingly, it marked an increasing recognition on Freud's part of the importance of belief alongside desire when he came to connect symptoms with phantasies." *Sigmund Freud,* pp. 93–4.

What Wollheim seems to have in mind here is that Freud's developed view was that the repressed desire caused the neurotic to have those beliefs necessary to make his symptoms into an action for reasons. In Dora's case, for example, her sexual love for Herr K. causes her to believe that she had been deflowered by him; this belief (fantasy) then allows her to express her love for Herr K. as a pregnancy, which in turn gets expressed as a hysterical attack of appendicitis because of Dora's further "association" (believed identification?) of appendicitis with pregnancy.

These beliefs, like so many in Freud, cry out for some substantiating evidence. Without such evidence, Wollheim's theoretical adjustments are as suspect as Freud's.

80. Freud, *Interpretation of Dreams,* vol. 4 of *The Standard Edition,* p. 67.
81. Freud, *Psychopathology of Everyday Life,* vol. 6 of *The Standard Edition,* p. 153.
82. This would remain true even if one subscribed to Freud's view that "the unconscious is the true psychical reality." Freud, *The Interpretation of Dreams,* vol. 5 of *The Standard Edition,* p. 613. Even if all conscious mental states are caused by unconscious ones, as Freud thought, this would not mean that people do not have either conscious knowledge or ignorance, as the case may be. To explain a phenomenon is not to explain it away.
83. See J. Rawls, *A Theory of Justice* (Cambridge, Mass.: Harvard University Press, 1971), sec. 4, 7, and 9 for a defense of this view of justification. One need not be apologetic about the seeming circularity of such a coherence view of justification of moral principles, for it is no worse than in the coherence view of justification of factual judgments. For the parallel, see M. S. Moore, "Moral Reality," *Wisconsin Law Review* (1982): 1061–1156.
84. "I think . . . that the Roman emperor was in the wrong, when he had one of

his subjects executed because he had dreamt of murdering the emperor... Would it not be right to bear in mind Plato's dictum that the virtuous man is content to *dream* what a wicked man really *does?*" Freud, *The Interpretation of Dreams,* vol. 5 of *The Standard Edition,* p. 620 (emphasis in original).
85. See Model Penal Code, sec. 2.01 (Proposed Official Draft, 1962); *Fain v. Commonwealth,* 78 Ky. 183 (1879); *People v. Newton,* 8 Cal. App. 3d 359, 87 Cal. Rptr. 394 (1970).
86. Model Penal Code, sec 2.01(2)(c) (Proposed Official Draft, 1962).
87. See *Fisher v. Dillingham,* 298 F. 145, 148 (S.D. N.Y. 1924) (dictum, the issue of willfulness was not before the court).
88. H. L. A. Hart, *Punishment and Responsibility* (Oxford: Oxford University Press, 1968), p. 177.
89. J. Rawls, *Theory of Justice,* sec. 38.
90. For arguments connecting the principle of responsibility to a more basic principle of liberty, see Hart, *Punishment and Responsibility,* p. 181; Rawls, *Theory of Justice,* p. 241.
91. In the discussion of the practical syllogism in chap. 1 it was assumed that the major premise was the content of a desire. It is more in accordance with Aristotle's own examples to use a moral norm as the major premise, so that one might reason: (1) One ought not to kill; (2) this proposed action is a killing; (3) therefore, this ought not to be done. In such cases one reaches a conclusion about the moral worth of a particular action by showing that the moral norm is applicable to the proposed action. The effect of the unconscious here can be to blind the actor to the moral quality of action.
92. The law has long reflected this moral requirement in those early versions of its tests for the responsibility of children and the insane that required knowledge of right and wrong. See chap. 6. For utilitarian reasons the law has not been so kind to sane adults of different cultures, it being expedient to adopt the maxim that "ignorance of the law is no excuse."
93. Dennett reaches this conclusion by somewhat similar reasoning. D. Dennett, *Brainstorms* (Montgomery, Vt.: Bradford Books, 1978). Dennett argues, first, that "if one is incapable of 'listening to reason' in some matter, one cannot be held responsible for it"; second, that only those capable of giving reasons for their actions can be reasoned with beforehand about them; and third, that only those conscious of what they are doing can give reasons for doing it. Ibid., pp. 282–3. Dennett's moral dialogue as the prerequisite of responsibility bears some similarity to the moral inference drawing of the text.
94. Stuart Hampshire argues persuasively that we all have this task responsibility to know ourselves and to do better. *Thought and Action* (New York: Viking Press, 1960).
95. See R. Schafer, *New Language for Psychoanalysis,* pp. 152–4; T. Szasz, *Law, Liberty, and Psychiatry,* pp. 135–7.
96. S. Freud, "Moral Responsibility for the Content of Dreams," in vol. 19 of *The Standard Edition,* p. 131.
97. Ibid., p. 133.
98. Ibid., pp. 133–4 (emphasis added).

99. Freud, *Interpretation of Dreams*, vol. 5 of *The Standard Edition*, p. 621.
100. Ibid., p. 620.
101. Freud, *Psychopathology of Everyday Life*, vol. 6 of *The Standard Edition*, pp. 152–3.
102. Freud, "Case of Hysteria," in vol. 7 of *The Standard Edition*, p. 42.
103. For a contrary view, see Herbert Fingarette, "Psychoanalytic Perspectives on Moral Guilt and Responsibility: A Re-evaluation," *Philosophy and Phenomenological Research*, vol. 16(1955): 18–36. Fingarette's conclusion is that "the wish is, in a sense, *morally* the act." Ibid., p. 24 (emphasis in original). He arrives at this conclusion by noting, correctly, that one may feel as guilty about a wish as about an act and, incorrectly, by urging that one is responsible morally if one *accepts* responsibility, which one does when one feels guilt.

   There is simply no reason to follow Fingarette and to confuse the conditions under which one may fairly be blamed or punished (*being* responsible) with the conditions under which one feels guilty (*feeling* responsible). One may feel guilty for surviving harms suffered by others, but one is not therefore responsible for those harms.
104. Freud, "The Rat-Man," note 60, this chapter, p. 185.
105. Even Freud recognized that this responsibility for being the sort of person who has such wishes may be slight, because one may also have countervailing wishes to be moral that are even stronger: "Actions and consciously expressed opinions are as a rule enough for practical purposes in judging men's characters. Actions deserve to be considered first and foremost; for many impulses which force their way through to consciousness are even then brought to nothing by the real forces of mental life before they can mature into deeds." Freud, *Interpretation of Dreams*, vol. 5 of *The Standard Edition*, p. 621.
106. I am indebted to Alan Garfinkel for clarifying this example with me.
107. E.g., *People v. Decina*, 2 N.Y. 2d 133, 138 N.E. 2d 799, 157 N.Y. S. 2d 558 (1956).
108. See R. Schafer, *New Language for Psychoanalysis*, p. 54.
109. P. F. Strawson once urged that a person is an individual of whom one predicates both physical and mental properties. *Individuals* (London: Methuen & Co., 1959).
110. It is doubtful whether even this is possible. If a transcendental argument will ever work, it should work for the concept of a person. How, indeed, would we do without the concept of our selves?

10. Decreased Responsibility

1. 171 F. Supp. 474 (E.D. Mich. 1959), *rev'd*, 282 F. 2d 450 (6th Cir. 1960).
2. 282 F. 2d at 463.
3. Ibid.
4. Each of these factors has at one time or another been presented as the key to understanding why the mentally ill are excused for their wrongful acts. For a discussion of these factors in that context, see M. S. Moore, "Mental Illness and Responsibility," *Bulletin of the Menninger Clinic*, vol. 39(1975): 308–28.
5. 282 F. 2d at 454–5, n. 2.

6. Hospers, "Meaning and Free Will," *Philosophy and Phenomenological Research,* vol. 10(1950): p. 318. Hospers later seems to have modified this position. See Hospers, "What Means This Freedom?" in R. Abelson (ed.), *Ethics and MetaEthics* (New York: St. Martin's Press, 1963), pp. 507–23.
7. Hospers, "Meaning and Free Will," p. 321.
8. Ibid., p. 325.
9. For some suggestions in this regard that do not lead one to hard determinism, see M. Brand (ed.), *The Nature of Human Action* (Glenview, Ill.: Scott, Foresman, 1970), pp. 123–216.
10. Karl Menninger, *The Crime of Punishment* (New York: Viking Press, 1968), p. 118. As Alan Stone has recently reminded us, it is not only Freudian psychiatrists who are hard determinists: "Generations of American psychiatrists have tried to find ways around what more and more of them came to recognize as problematic and embarrassing. The most well-known and beloved American popularizer of Freud's ideas, Karl Menninger, was moved to wonder, *Whatever became of sin?* But it is not just psychoanalysis in modern psychiatry that called into question the ideal of a free moral agent. All of the dominant conceptual paradigms of modern psychiatry, biological, behavioral, psychodynamic, and social, conflict with traditional ideas about free moral agents . . . At least for psychiatrists who explain behavior in terms of biological transmethylation, reinforcement schedules, defective superegos, and demographic trends, there is still no convincing resolution of this problem." Stone, "Psychiatry and Morality." Delivered as the Tanner Lectures, Department of Philosophy, Stanford University, spring 1982, pp. 9–10.
11. Bernard Diamond, "With Malice Aforethought," *Archives of Criminal Psychodynamics,* vol. 2(1957): 27.
12. David Louisell and Bernard Diamond, "Law and Psychiatry: Detente, Entente, or Concomitance?" *Cornell Law Quarterly,* vol. 50(1965): 219. Others have also noted the seeming presupposition of freedom involved in psychotherapy. Thus Wilber Katz, for example, found this to be a "paradox between psychological determination and the notion of 'effort' which patients (and everyone else) must make in order to grow in responsibility." Katz, "Law, Psychiatry and Free Will," *University of Chicago Law Review,* vol. 22(1955): 401. See also Michael Basch, "Psychic Determinism and Freedom of the Will," *International Review of Psycho-Analysis,* vol. 5(1978): 257–64, wherein Basch attempts to explain away such freedom as an illusion that may make people feel better.
13. Franz Alexander and Hugo Staub, *The Criminal, the Judge, and the Public: A Psychological Analysis* (New York: Macmillan, 1931), pp. 72–3.
14. 171 F. Supp. 474, 479–80 (partially quoting Jerome Hall, "Psychiatry and Criminal Responsibility," *Yale Law Journal,* vol. 65[1956]: 761–5).
15. Katz, "Law, Psychiatry and Free Will," p. 400. Katz goes on to assert that "the area of free choice is far more limited than the area assumed by common sense notions of moral responsibility." Ibid., p. 401.
16. Glueck, *Law and Psychiatry: Cold War or Entente Cordiale?* (Baltimore: Johns Hopkins University Press, 1962), p. 12.

17. Ibid.
18. Ibid., p. 13.
19. Stephen Morse, "Failed Explanations and Criminal Responsibility: Experts and the Unconscious," *Virginia Law Review*, vol. 68(1982): 971–1084. See particularly pp. 1030–9. The phrase "selective determinism" comes from P. Hollander, "Sociology, Selective Determinism, and the Rise of Expectations," *American Sociologist*, vol. 8(1973): 147–53.
20. Morse, "Failed Explanations" p. 1030. For an example of a selective determinist in law, see Norval Morris, *Madness and the Criminal Law* (Chicago: University of Chicago Press, 1982), especially pp. 61–4. Morris assumes that it makes sense to speak of factors (such as social adversity or psychosis) as having varying degrees of "potency" or "pressure" toward criminality, and thus that there are corresponding degrees of free choice.
21. E.g., David Bazelon, "The Morality of the Criminal Law," *Southern California Law Review*, vol. 49(1976): 385–405.
22. See, e.g., Morton White, *Foundations of Historical Knowledge* (New York: Harper & Row, 1965), chap. 4.
23. Morse, "Failed Explanations," p. 1031. See also Stephen Morse, "Crazy Behavior, Morals and Science: An Analysis of Mental Health Law," *Southern California Law Review*, vol. 51(1978): 564–6 for further elucidation of the idea of a predisposing cause.
24. Morse, "Failed Explanations," pp. 1031–3.
25. Carl Hempel, *Aspects of Scientific Explanation* (New York: Free Press, 1965), pp. 381–412.
26. Sheldon Glueck appears to take this position, for he buttresses his "more-or-less" causation with the findings of recent physics: "In recent years even physical science has rejected a rigid and inflexible cause-and-effect determinism for a theory of 'indeterminacy' or probability." Glueck, *Law and Psychiatry*, pp. 15–16.
27. Richard Bonnie and Christopher Slobogin, "The Role of Mental Health Professionals in the Criminal Process: The Case for Informed Speculation," *Virginia Law Review*, vol. 66(1980): 427–522.
28. Morse, "Failed Explanations," p. 1027.
29. Bonnie and Slobogin, "Mental Health Professionals," pp. 488–92 (see particularly p. 492, n. 198).
30. Freud, "Some Additional Notes on Dream-Interpretation as a Whole," in vol. 19 of *The Standard Edition of the Complete Psychological Works of Sigmund Freud* (London: Hogarth Press, 1961), p. 133.
31. The example is from Joel Feinberg, "Causing Voluntary Actions," in his *Doing and Deserving* (Princeton, N.J.: Princeton University Press, 1970), pp. 152–86.
32. Bernard Diamond is a self-confessed manipulator of legal standards of the type mentioned in the text. See Diamond, "Criminal Responsibility of the Mentally Ill," *Stanford Law Review*, vol. 14(1961): 59–86.
33. James's forthright repudiation of determinism on moral grounds should give anyone pause who has some allegiance to the idea of objective truth in

science: "If a certain formula for expressing the nature of the world violates my moral demand, I shall feel as free to throw it overboard, or at least to doubt it, as if it disappointed my demand for uniformity of sequence, for example: the one demand being, so far as I can see, quite as subjective and emotional as the other is." *The Will to Believe* (New York: Longman, 1898), p. 147.

34. The "by-and-large" qualification of the text is made because another thing a compatibilist must do is to show that determinism is compatible with the principle that punishment is unjust unless the actor "could have done other than he did." See the articles collected in Brand (ed.), *Nature of Human Action,* for this kind of reconciliation.

35. Hospers, "Meaning and Free Will," p. 325.

36. E.g., Norman Malcolm, "The Conceivability of Mechanism," *The Philosophical Review,* vol. 77(1968): 45–72; Richard Taylor, *Action and Purpose* (Englewood Cliffs, N.J.: Prentice-Hall, 1966); A. I. Melden, *Free Action* (London: Routledge & Kegan Paul, 1961). For a criticism of this point of view, see D. W. Hamlyn, "Causality and Human Behaviour," in N. Care and C. Landesman (eds.), *Readings in the Theory of Action* (Bloomington: Indiana University Press, 1968), pp. 48–67.

37. Moritz Schlick, "Causality in Everyday Life and in Recent Science," *University of California Publications in Philosophy,* vol. 15(1932): 99–125. Reprinted in H. Morris (ed.), *Freedom and Responsibility* (Stanford, Calif.: Stanford University Press, 1961), pp. 292–303.

38. A. J. Ayer, "Freedom and Necessity," *Polemic,* vol. 5(1946): 36–44.

39. M. Schlick, "Causality," in Morris (ed.), pp. 298–9.

40. M. Schlick, *Problems of Ethics* (New York: Dover, 1961), p. 147.

41. With the caveat expressed in chap. 2, that if one distinguishes appetitive character from evaluational character, the former may act as a compulsion. The distinction is from Gary Watson, "Free Agency," *Journal of Philosophy,* vol. 72(1975): 205–20.

42. For an attempt to revive the long-criticized concept of a volition, see Lawrence Davis, *Theory of Action* (Englewood Cliffs, N.J.: Prentice-Hall, 1979).

43. Hospers, "Meaning and Free Will," reprinted in H. Morris (ed.), *Freedom and Responsibility* (Stanford, Calif.: Stanford University Press, 1961), p. 465.

44. David Rapaport, "On the Psychoanalytic Theory of Motivation," in 1960 *Nebraska Symposium on Motivation* (Lincoln: University of Nebraska Press, 1960), p. 187.

45. In 1945, an American Bar Association Committee warned that the spread of psychoanalytic doctrines "calls for careful consideration" because such doctrines "tend toward determinism." 70 A.B.A. Rep. 338, 339 (1945). See generally Morse, "Failed Explanations." Even the American Psychiatric Association has recently recognized that the deterministic assumptions of many psychiatrists may prevent them from giving helpful testimony on the volitional impairment of the mentally ill: "The line between an irresistible impulse and an impulse not resisted is probably no sharper than that between twilight and dusk. Psychiatry is a deterministic discipline that views all hu-

man behavior as, to a good extent, 'caused.' The concept of volition is the subject of some disagreement among psychiatrists. Many psychiatrists therefore believe that psychiatric testimony (particularly that of a conclusory nature) about volition is more likely to produce confusion for jurors than is psychiatric testimony relevant to a defendant's appreciation or understanding." American Psychiatric Association, *Statement on the Insanity Defense* (Washington, D.C.: 1983), p. 10.
46. 282 F.2d at 454–5; see n. 2, this chapter.
47. Lawyers and psychiatrists have often assumed that mental illness is an excuse because it shows an action not to have been intentional. See, e.g., Goldstein and Katz, "Abolish the Insanity Defense–Why Not?" *Yale Law Journal*, vol. 72(1963): 853–76. This, however, is false, as we have seen in chap. 6. It is also false that mental illness negates specific intent, as traditional versions of the diminished capacity defense assume. See P. Arenella, "The Diminished Capacity and Diminished Responsibility Defense: Two Children of a Doomed Marriage," *Columbia Law Review*, vol. 77(1977): 827–65; Morse, "Diminished Capacity: A Moral and Legal Conundrum," *International Journal of Law and Psychiatry*, vol. 2(1979): 271–98.
48. American Law Institute, Model Penal Code, sec. 2.02(7) (Proposed Official Draft, 1962), defines willful blindness as having awareness of a "high probability" of a fact's existence unless the actor "actually believes that it does not exist."
49. One has two choices if one is certain the actor believed not-*p*: either give up the idea that his beliefs are consistent or say that he does not believe that *p*. It is contradictory to assert:

   1. $\sim[B(p) \cdot B(\sim p)]$ and
   2. $B(p)$ and
   3. $B(\sim p)$

   If one is sure 3 is true, and is unwilling to give up 1, then 2 must yield.
50. Now one can give up the first premise in n. 49, this chapter, in order to remain free of contradiction. We are plainly more willing to ascribe contradictory beliefs to another if one of those beliefs is unconscious.
51. This problem was addressed earlier in chap. 9. Then, however, the fact verified by common sense was that the actor was ignorant. Here, the commonsense position is that the actor knows the fact. In each case, the problem is reconciling the supposed psychoanalytic insight with the commonsense position.

    One contradicts the other unless different meanings of believe or know are being used. Without a different sense of B, $B(p)$ is the contradictory of $\sim B(p)$.
52. Richard Peters, *The Concept of Motivation* (London: Routledge & Kegan Paul, 1958), p. 58.
53. Ibid, p. 60.
54. 282 F. 2d at 463.
55. I explore the reasons for this in "Individuating Intentions in the Criminal Law," currently unpublished. Given the fine-grained modes of individuating intentions yielded by *de dicto* interpretations of the objects of intentions,

judges must have the freedom to include many intentions not literally covered by a statute. Unless they do this, many quite culpable criminals would not be covered by criminal statutes prohibiting certain intentions.
56. Note, "Why Do Criminal Attempts Fail? A New Defense." *Yale Law Journal*, vol. 70(1960): 160–9.
57. See Harvey Mullane, "Psychoanalytic Explanation and Rationality," *Journal of Philosophy*, vol. 68(1971): 413–26; see more generally Moore, "Mental Illness and Responsibility."
58. Freud, "Notes upon a Case of Obessional Neurosis," in *Three Case Histories* (New York: Macmillan, 1963).
59. Ibid., p. 27.
60. Ibid., p. 28.
61. Ibid., p. 34.
62. This problem pervades David Blumenfeld's attempt to liken unconscious mental states to coercion ("Free Action and Unconscious Motivation," *Monist*, vol. 56[1972]: 426–43). Blumenfeld imagines a neurotic who forms an impulse to kill dogs as a defense against anxiety. In such a case, Blumenfeld tells us: "The neurotic finds himself in a state of literal panic. He can avoid intense anxiety only by killing dogs. Like the man who is coerced, he experiences great danger unless he does this. Further, like the man who is coerced, the neurotic does not choose the fact that it is just this (symptomatic) action which will relieve him. Both find themselves facing a painful alternative, if they do not follow a certain course of action and both have the elimination of danger as their sole aim." Ibid., p. 441. The problem here is that the neurotic does not have the elimination of anxiety or danger as his sole aim, in the sense that he is not reasoning practically with this as his major premise. He may be caused to act by his anxiety, but he is not acting with the elimination of that anxiety as his reason. He is thus not *coerced* by the unconscious desires that stand behind his impulse to kill, even if (by hypothesis) he is *caused* to act by them.
63. Freud, "Case of Obsessional Neurosis," in *Three Case Histories*, p. 26.
64. This latter interpretation was suggested to me by Howard Shevrin, then on the Menninger Foundation staff, with whom I once jointly taught this case. This interpretation, unlike that of the Menninger Foundation psychiatrists whose reports were introduced into evidence in the case, maintains the proportionality between the level of guilt and the badness of the wish, a proportion some claim to be a hidden feature of Freud's treatment of unconscious emotions. See Sachs, "On Freud's Doctrine of the Emotions," in R. Wollheim (ed.), *Freud, A Collection of Critical Essays* (Garden City, N.Y.: Doubleday [Anchor Press], 1974), pp. 132–46.
65. See, e.g., Field, "Is the Conception of the Unconscious of Value in Psychology?" *Mind*, vol. 31(1922): 413–14: "When I reflect on what I mean by a wish or an emotion or feeling, I can only find that I know and think of them simply as different forms of consciousness."
66. S. Freud, "The Unconscious," in vol. 14 of *The Standard Edition*, p. 177.
67. Ibid.

68. "Strictly speaking, then, and although no fault can be found with the linguistic usage, there are no unconscious affects as there are unconscious ideas. But there may very well be in the system Ucs. affect structures which, like others, become conscious. The whole difference arises from the fact that ideas are cathexes—basically of memory-traces—whilst affects and emotions correspond to processes of discharge, the final manifestations of which are perceived as feelings." Ibid., p. 178.
69. See Harvey Mullane, "Unconscious Emotion," *Theoria*, vol. 31(1965): 181–90; Michael Fox, "On Unconscious Emotions," *Philosophy and Phenomenological Research*, vol. 34(1973): 151–70.
70. See Max Friedemann, "Cleptomania: The Analytic and Forensic Aspects," *Psychoanalytic Review*, vol. 17(1930): 452: "The cleptomaniac act in its purest form is an impulsive act . . . the chief goal being not the acquisition of a stolen object but the satisfaction of a repressed urge . . . it is symbolic in character; i.e., the apparent rational act signifies quite another element than that objective expressed by the act. It is just this symbolic character and its derivation from the unconscious which constitutes its essential nature."
71. Blumenfeld, "Free Action," p. 435.
72. Ibid., p. 436.
73. A split that is increasingly emphasized within the theory's practitioners themselves. See the collection of essays in M. Gill and P. Holzman (eds.), *Psychology versus Metapsychology* (New York: International Universities Press, 1976).
74. Ricoeur, *Freud and Philosophy* (New Haven, Conn.: Yale University Press, 1970).
75. Flew, "Motives and the Unconscious," in H. Feigl and M. Scriven (eds.), *The Foundations of Science and the Concepts of Psychology and Psychoanalysis*, Minnesota Studies in the Philosophy of Science, vol. 1 (Minneapolis: University of Minnesota Press, 1956), pp. 155–73.
76. Fingarette, *The Self in Transformation* (New York: Harper & Row, 1963), chap. 1.
77. Freud, "The Unconscious," in vol. 14 of *The Standard Edition*, p. 168.
78. Freud, "On the History of the Psychoanalytic Movement," in vol. 14 of *The Standard Edition*, p. 11.

11. The Unity of the Self

1. Thomas Schelling, "The Intimate Contest for Self-Command," *The Public Interest*, vol. 60(1980): 95–6.
2. For an analysis of conflicting emotions beginning with the idea of ambivalence, see Patricia Greenspan, "A Case of Mixed Feelings: Ambivalence and the Logic of Emotion," in A. Rorty (ed.), *Explaining Emotions* (Berkeley: University of California Press, 1980), pp. 233–50.
3. See generally Jacob Arlow and Charles Brenner, *Psychoanalytic Concepts and the Structural Theory* (New York: International Universities Press, 1964).
4. On the intelligibility of desire, see A. J. Watt, "The Intelligibility of Wants," *Mind*, vol. 81(1972): 553–61. On the rationality of belief, see R. J. Acker-

mann, *Belief and Knowledge* (Garden City, N.Y.: Doubleday [Anchor Books], 1972). On the proportionality of emotions, see David Sachs, "On Freud's Doctrine of Emotions," in R. Wollheim (ed.), *Freud: A Collection of Critical Essays* (Garden City, N.Y.: Doubleday [Anchor Books], 1974), pp. 132–46.

5. D. Bannister, "Psychology as an Exercise in Paradox." *Bulletin of the British Psychological Society,* vol. 19(1966): 21–6. Reprinted in Brian Foss (ed.), *New Horizons in Psychology* (Baltimore: Penguin Books, 1966), p. 363.

6. Morris Eagle, "Anatomy of the Self in Psychoanalytic Theory," in M. Ruse (ed.), *Nature Animated,* vol. 2 (Dordrecht: Reidel, 1982).

7. Daniel Dennett, *Content and Consciousness* (New York: Humanities Press, 1969), pp. 90–6.

8. Eagle, "Anatomy of the Self," in Ruse (ed.). Donald Davidson urges that discovery of simple causal efficacy of an unconscious, conflicting desire is enough to require a psychological theorist to posit substructures of the mind. Without causal agency and practical reason, however, Davidson is clear that these substructures are not to be thought of as personlike agencies. Davidson, "Paradoxes of Irrationality," in R. Wollheim and J. Hopkins (eds.), *Philosophical Essays on Freud* (Cambridge: Cambridge University Press, 1982), pp. 289–305.

9. Eagle, "Anatomy of the Self," in Ruse (ed.). Compare David Pears, "Motivated Irrationality, Freudian Theory and Cognitive Dissonance," in R. Wollheim and J. Hopkins (eds.), pp. 264–88. Pears views self-deception as but part of a larger group of phenomena, all of which (for Pears) suggest some hypothesis of a divided mind.

10. Freud, *Dora: An Analysis of a Case of Hysteria* (New York: Collier Books, 1963), p. 96.

11. On multiple personalities generally, see Morton Prince, *Dissociation of a Personality* (London: Longmans Green, 1930); and A. M. Ludwig, M. M. Brandsma, C. B. Wilbur, F. Bendfeldt, and D. H. Jameson, "The Objective Study of a Multiple Personality," *Archives of General Psychiatry,* vol. 26(1972): 298–310.

12. Freud, *Introductory Lectures on Psycho-Analysis,* vol. 16 of *The Standard Edition of the Complete Psychological Works of Sigmund Freud,* p. 285.

13. See Baruch Brody, *Identity and Essence* (Princeton, N.J.: Princeton University Press, 1980), for a summary of the now voluminous literature on personal identity.

14. See Freud, "A Note on the Unconscious in Psycho-Analysis," in vol. 4 of *Collected Papers* (New York: Basic Books, 1959), where on p. 29 he notes that "the index-value of the unconscious has far outgrown its importance as a property."

15. Freud, *The Ego and the Id,* in vol. 19 of the *Standard Edition.*

16. Irving Thalberg, "Freud's Anatomies of the Self," in R. Wollheim (ed.), *Freud: A Collection of Critical Essays* (Garden City, N.Y.: Doubleday [Anchor Books], 1974), p. 161.

17. Roy Schafer, *A New Language for Psychoanalysis* (New Haven, Conn.: Yale University Press, 1976).

18. Bernard Williams, *Problems of the Self* (Cambridge: Cambridge University Press, 1973), pp. 15–18.
19. Morris Eagle, "Anatomy of the Self," in Ruse (ed.), takes up this suggestion.
20. See A. M. Ludwig et al., "Study of a Multiple Personality."
21. W. S. Taylor and M. F. Martin, "Multiple Personality," *Journal of Abnormal Social Psychology,* vol. 39(1944): 281–300, distinguish coconscious personalities existing simultaneously from alternating personalities, which appear only in sequence over time.
22. Therapy for such persons is usually thought to involve a "merging" or a "fusion" of the separate personalities into one. Such fusion involves the disappearance of the memory blockage and the character discontinuities. See Ludwig et al., "Study of a Multiple Personality." Insofar as such fusion involves recapture of the memories of what one felt and did while in different personalities, as Morton Prince claimed in his classic study, *Dissociation of a Personality,* one could even urge that one and the same person was there all of the time. For then there would be not only spatiotemporal continuity, but also a restoration of the experience of unity, another of the three major criteria for personal identity. As Prince described one of his successfully cured patient's remembrances: "These different states seem to her to be very largely difference of moods. She regrets them, but does not attempt to excuse them, because, as she says, 'After all, it is always myself.' " Ibid., p. 525.
23. Eagle ends his paper urging that his "main position . . . is that while most of us may be assured of numerical unity (that is, one self per body), as far as the issue of integration is concerned, unity of self and of personality is a developmental integrative achievement in which we are not all equally successful." Morris Eagle, "Anatomy of the Self," in Ruse (ed.).
24. These two senses of the unity of the self correspond, respectively, to Morris Eagle's "unity of the self" and "unity of personality." Ibid.
25. R. D. Laing, *The Divided Self* (London: Tavistock, 1960).
26. Heinz Kohut, *The Analysis of Self* (New York: International Universities Press, 1971); Kohut, *The Restoration of the Self* (New York: International Universities Press, 1977).
27. Eventually published as "A Project for a Scientific Psychology," in vol. 1 of *The Standard Edition,* pp. 283–397.
28. Freud, *An Outline of Psychoanalysis* (New York: Norton, 1949), p. 13.
29. W. Ronald D. Fairbairn, *An Object-Relations Theory of the Personality* (New York: Basic Books, 1954). Because "from a practical psychotherapeutic standpoint the analysis of 'impulses' considered apart from structures proves itself a singularly sterile procedure" (p. 85), Fairbairn sought to replace Freud's "psychology of impulses" with his own object-relations theory. Fairbairn subdivided the psyche into "three separate egos–(1) a central ego (the 'I'), (2) a libidinal ego, and (3) an aggressive, persecutory ego," which Fairbairn called "the internal saboteur" (p. 101). What Fairbairn hoped to gain from this reconceptualization of psychic structure was a better description of the conflicts experienced by his patients. What he perceived was that such a description could be better only if one gave up Freud's concept of the id, the

highly energized but objectless motivator of all behavior. One gets a better description of conflict, in other words, if one gives up the simultaneous demand that the substructures in conflict also represent the connection of body to mind.
30. Daniel Dennett, *Brainstorms* (Montgomery, Vt.: Bradford Books, 1978), pp. 80–1.

Conclusion

1. "Audience Commentary," in R. L. Spitzer and D. F. Klein, *Critical Issues in Psychiatric Diagnosis* (New York: Raven Press, 1978), p. 105.
2. I have in mind both Ronald Dworkin's arguments about the place of moral principles in any adequate theory of law (*Taking Rights Seriously* [Cambridge, Mass.: Harvard University Press, 1978]) and my own beginnings in working out the role of values in a theory of adjudication. Moore, "The Semantics of Judging," *Southern California Law Review*, vol. 54(1981): 151–294; Moore, "Moral Reality," *Wisconsin Law Review* (1982): 1061–1156.
3. On the inseparability of philosophical and psychological theories of perception, see George Pitcher, *A Theory of Perception* (Princeton, N.J.: Princeton University Press, 1971).
4. "Regimented" is a term I have borrowed from Willard Quine (*Word and Object* [Cambridge, Mass.: MIT Press, 1960]), who speaks of *regimenting* natural languages so as to give systematic exposition of them.
5. B. F. Skinner, *Beyond Freedom and Dignity* (New York: Knopf, 1971), p. 200.

References

Abelson, R. (ed.). *Ethics and MetaEthics.* New York: St. Martin's Press, 1963.
Abrams, Samuel. The Psychoanalytic Unconscious. In M. Kanzel (ed.), *The Unconscious Today.* New York: International Universities Press, 1971.
Ackerman, Bruce. Law and the Modern Mind. *Daedalus,* vol. 103(1974): 119–30.
Ackermann, R. J. *Belief and Knowledge.* Garden City, N. Y.: Doubleday (Anchor Books), 1972.
Alexander, Franz, and Hugo Staub. *The Criminal, the Judge, and the Public: A Psychological Analysis.* New York: Macmillan, 1931.
Alexander, G., and T. Szasz. From Contract to Status via Psychiatry. *Santa Clara Lawyer,* vol. 13(1973): 537–59.
Alexander, Peter. Wishes, Symptoms and Actions. *Aristotelian Society Supplementary Volume,* vol. 48(1974): 119–134.
Alexander, Peter. Psychoanalysis and the Explanation of Behaviour. *Mind,* vol. 80(1971): 391–402.
Alexander, Peter. Rational Behaviour and Psychoanalytic Explanation. *Mind,* vol. 71(1962): 326–41.
Alexander, Peter. Cause and Cure in Psychotherapy. *Aristotelian Society Supplementary Volume,* vol. 29(1955): 25–42.
Alston, W. Varieties of Privileged Access. *American Philosophical Quarterly,* vol. 8(1971): 223–41.
American Bar Association, 70 A.B.A. Rep. 338, 339 (1945).
American Law Institute. Model Penal Code, Proposed Official Draft. Philadelphia: 1962.
American Psychiatric Association. *Statement on the Insanity Defense.* Washington, D.C., 1983.
American Psychiatric Association. *Diagnostic and Statistical Manual of Mental Disorders,* 2d ed. Washington, D.C.: 1968; 3d ed.: 1980.
Anscombe, G. E. M. *Intention,* 2d ed. Ithaca, N.Y.: Cornell University Press, 1963.
Anscombe, Roderick. Referring to the Unconscious: A Philosophical Critique of Schafer's Action Language. *International Journal of Psycho-Analysis,* vol. 62(1981): 225–41.
Apel, K. O. The Erklären-Verstehen Controversy in the Philosophy of the Natural

References

and Human Sciences. In G. Fløistad (ed.), *Contemporary Philosophy.* The Hague: Martinus Nijhoff, 1982.

Arbib, M. *The Metaphorical Brain.* New York: Wiley, 1972.

Arenella, Peter. The Diminished Capacity and Diminished Responsibility Defense: Two Children of a Doomed Marriage. *Columbia Law Review,* vol. 77(1977): 827–865.

Aristotle. *Nicomachean Ethics,* book 3, chap. 1. In R. McKeon (ed.), *Introduction to Aristotle.* Chicago: University of Chicago Press, 1973.

Aristotle. *Nichomachean Ethics.* Translated by Martin Ostwald. New York: Bobbs-Merrill, 1962.

Aristotle. *Topics,* book 6. Translated and edited by E. S. Forster. Cambridge, Mass.: Harvard University Press, 1960.

Arlow, Jacob, and Charles Brenner. *Psychoanalytic Concepts and the Structural Theory.* New York: International Universities Press, 1964.

Audi, Robert. The Epistemic Authority of the First Person. *Personalist,* vol. 56(1975): 5–15.

Audi, Robert. The Limits of Self-Knowledge. *Canadian Journal of Philosophy,* vol. 4(1974): 253–67.

Audi, Robert. Moral Responsibility, Freedom and Compulsion. *American Philosophical Quarterly,* vol. 11(1974): 1–14.

Austin, John. *Lectures on Jurisprudence.* London: J. Murray, 1869.

Austin, J. L. *How to Do Things With Words.* Cambridge, Mass.: Harvard University Press, 1961.

Austin, J. L. A Plea for Excuses. *Proceedings of the Aristotelian Society,* vol. 57(1956): 1–30.

Ayer, A. J. *Language, Truth and Logic,* 2d ed. New York: Dover, 1952.

Ayer, A. J. Freedom and Necessity. *Polemic,* vol. 5(1946): 36–44.

Baier, Kurt. Action and Responsibility. In M. Brand (ed.), *The Nature of Human Action.* Glenview, Ill.: Scott, Foresman, 1970.

Balmuth, J. Psychoanalytic Explanation. *Mind,* vol. 74(1965): 229–35.

Bannister, D. Psychology as an Exercise in Paradox. *Bulletin of the British Psychological Society,* vol. 19(1966): 21–6. Reprinted in Brian Foss (ed.), *New Horizons in Psychology.* Baltimore: Penguin Books, 1966.

Basch, Michael. Psychic Determinism and Freedom of the Will. *International Review of Psycho-Analysis,* vol. 5(1978): 257–64.

Bazelon, David. The Morality of the Criminal Law. *Southern California Law Review,* vol. 49(1976): 385–405.

Bazelon, David. New Gods for Old: "Efficient" Courts in a Democratic Society. *New York University Law Review,* vol. 46(1971): 658–59.

Beck, L. W. Conscious and Unconscious Motives. *Mind,* vol. 75(1966): 155–79.

Becker, L. E. Durham Revisited. *Psychiatric Annals,* vol. 3(1973): 16–49.

Bedau, Hugo. Retribution and the Theory of Punishment. *Journal of Philosophy,* vol. 75(1978): 601–20.

Benditt, Theodore. *Law as Rule and Principle.* Stanford, Calif: Stanford University Press, 1978.

Benedict, Ruth. *Patterns of Culture.* 2d ed. Boston: Houghton Mifflin, 1959.

References

Benn, Stanley. Rights. In P. Edwards (ed.), *The Encyclopedia of Philosophy*, vol. 7. New York: Macmillan, 1957.
Benn, Stanley, and Richard Peters. *Social Principles and the Democratic State*. London: Allen & Unwin, 1959.
Bentham, Jeremy. *An Introduction to the Principles of Morals and Legislation*. New York: Hafner Press, 1948. First published Oxford: Clarendon Press, 1876.
Biggs, J. *The Guilty Mind*. New York: Harcourt Brace, 1955.
Bishin, W., and C. Stone. *Law, Language and Ethics*. Mineola, N.Y.: Foundation Press, 1972.
Bleicher, Josef. *Contemporary Hermeneutics*. London: Routledge & Kegan Paul, 1980.
Bleuler, Manfred. Researches and Changes in Concepts in the Study of Schizophrenia. *Bulletin of the Isaac Ray Medical Library*, vol. 3(1955): 42–5.
Blumenfeld, David. Free Action and Unconscious Motivation. *Monist*, vol. 56(1972): 426–43.
Bonnie, Richard, and Christopher Slobogin. The Role of Mental Health Professionals in the Criminal Process: The Case for Informed Speculation. *Virginia Law Review*, vol. 66(1980): 427–522.
Boorse, Christopher. On the Distinction Between Disease and Illness. *Philosophy and Public Affairs*, vol. 5(1975): 49–68. Reprinted in A. L. Caplan, H. T. Engelhardt, and J. J. McCartney (eds.), *Concepts of Health and Disease*. Reading, Mass.: Addison-Wesley, 1981.
Boorse, Christopher. Health as a Theoretical Concept. *Philosophy of Science*, vol. 44(1977): 542–73.
Boorse, Christopher. Wright on Functions. *Philosophical Review*, vol. 85(1976): 70–86.
Boorse, Christopher. What a Theory of Mental Health Should Be. *Journal of Theory of Social Behaviour*, vol. 6(1976): 61–84.
Braginsky, B. M., O. D. Braginsky, and K. Ring. *Methods of Madness: The Mental Hospital as Last Resort*. New York: Holt, Rinehart and Winston, 1969.
Brand, M. (ed.). *The Nature of Human Action*. Glenview, Ill.: Scott, Foresman, 1970.
Brandt, Richard. *A Theory of the Good and the Right*. Oxford: Oxford University Press (Clarendon Press), 1979.
Brandt, Richard, and Jaegwon Kim. Wants as Explanations of Actions. *Journal of Philosophy*, vol. 60(1963): 425–35.
Breger, L. Function of Dreams. *Journal of Abnormal Psychology Monographs*, vol. 72(1967): 1–28.
Brenner, C. *An Elementary Textbook of Psychoanalysis*, rev. ed. New York: International Universities Press, 1973.
Brentano, Franz. *Psychologie vom Empirischen Standpunkt*. Leipzig: 1874. Selection translated in R. Chisholm (ed.), *Realism and the Background of Phenomenology*. Glencoe, Ill.: Free Press, 1960.
Brody, Baruch. *Identity and Essence*. Princeton, N.J.: Princeton University Press, 1980.

References

Brown, Norman. *Love's Body*. New York: Random House (Vintage Books), 1968.
Brown, Norman. *Life Against Death*. Middletown, Conn.: Wesleyan University Press, 1959.
Buhler, C. *Values in Psychotherapy*. New York: Free Press, 1962.
Busse, E. W. The Presidential Address: There Are Decisions to be Made. *American Journal of Psychiatry*, vol. 129(1972): 1–9.
Butler, Samuel. *Erewhon*. London: Trübner, 1872.
Calabresi, G., and A. D. Melamed. Property Rules, Liability Rules, and Inalienability: One View of the Cathedral. *Harvard Law Review*, vol. 85(1972): 1089–1128.
Canfield, John. Teleological Explanations in Biology. *British Journal for the Philosophy of Science*, vol. 13(1963): 285–95.
Caplan, A. L., H. T. Englehardt, and J. J. McCartney (eds.). *Concepts of Health and Disease*. Reading, Mass.: Addison-Wesley, 1981.
Carnap, Rudolph. Psychology in Physical Language. In A. J. Ayer (ed.), *Logical Positivism*. New York: Free Press, 1959.
Chisholm, Roderick. The Descriptive Element in the Concept of Action. *Journal of Philosophy*, vol. 61(1964): 613–25.
Chisholm, Roderick. *Perceiving: A Philosophical Study*. Ithaca, N.Y.: Cornell University Press, 1957.
Chomsky, Noam. *Rules and Representations*. New York: Columbia University Press, 1980.
Cioffi, F. Wishes, Symptoms and Actions. *Aristotelian Society Supplementary Volume*, vol. 48(1974): 97–118.
Cioffi, F. Wollheim on Freud. *Inquiry*, vol. 15(1972): 171–230.
Cohen, Felix. Transcendental Nonsense and the Functional Approach. *Columbia Law Review*, vol. 35(1935): 809–49.
Cohen, Jonathan. Teleological Explanation. *Proceedings of the Aristotelian Society*, vol. 51(1955): 255–92.
Collingwood, R. G. *The Idea of History*. Oxford: Oxford University Press, 1946.
Collins, Arthur. Unconscious Belief. *Journal of Philosophy*, vol. 66(1969): 667–80.
Cooter, Robert. Justice and Mathematics: Two Simple Ideas. In Roger Skurski (ed.), *New Directions in Economic Justice*. South Bend, Ind.: University of Notre Dame Press, 1983.
Cornman, James. Intentionality and Intensionality. *Philosophical Quarterly*, vol. 12(1962): 44–52.
Danto, Arthur. Basic Actions. *American Philosophical Quarterly*, vol. 2(1965): 141–8.
Danto, Arthur. What We Can Do. *Journal of Philosophy*, vol. 60(1963): 435–45.
D'Arcy, E. *Human Acts*. Oxford: Oxford University Press (Clarendon Press), 1963.
Davidson, Donald. Paradoxes of Irrationality. In R. Wollheim and J. Hopkins (eds.), *Philosophical Essays on Freud*. Cambridge: Cambridge University Press, 1982.
Davidson, Donald. *Actions and Events*. Oxford: Oxford University Press, 1980.
Davidson, Donald. Freedom to Act. In T. Honderich (ed.), *Essays on Freedom of Action*. London: Routledge & Kegan Paul, 1973.
Davidson, Henry A. The Psychiatrist's Role in the Administration of Criminal

References

Justice. In R. W. Nice (ed.), *Criminal Psychology.* New York: Philosophical Library, 1962.
Davis, Lawrence. *Theory of Action.* Englewood Cliffs, N.J.: Prentice-Hall, 1979.
Dement, W. Experimental Dream Studies. *Science and Psychoanalysis,* vol. 7(1964): 129–77.
Dennett, Daniel C. *Brainstorms.* Montgomery, Vt.: Bradford Books, 1978.
Dennett, D. The Conditions of Personhood. In A. O. Rorty (ed.), *The Identities of Persons.* Berkeley: University of California Press, 1976. Reprinted in D. C. Dennett, *Brainstorms.* Montgomery, Vt.: Bradford Books, 1978.
Dennett, D. Intentional Systems. *Journal of Philosophy,* vol. 68(1971): 87–106. Reprinted in D. C. Dennett, *Brainstorms.* Montgomery, Vt.: Bradford Books, 1978.
Dennett, Daniel. Mechanism and Responsibility. In T. Honderich (ed.), *Essays on Freedom of Action.* London: Routledge & Kegan Paul, 1973.
Dennett, Daniel. *Content and Consciousness.* London: Routledge & Kegan Paul, 1969.
Dennett, Daniel, and K. Lambert (eds.). *The Philosophical Lexicon,* 7th ed. Published privately, 1978.
de Sousa, Ronald. The Rationality of Emotions. In A. Rorty (ed.), *Explaining Emotions.* Berkeley: University of California Press, 1980.
de Sousa, Ronald. Rational Homunculi. In A. Rorty (ed.), *The Identities of Persons.* Berkeley: University of California Press, 1976.
de Sousa, Ronald. The Politics of Mental Illness. *Inquiry,* vol. 15(1972): 187–201.
Dewey, John. *Human Nature and Conduct.* New York: Holt, Rinehart and Winston, 1922.
Diamond, Bernard. Criminal Responsibility of the Mentally Ill. *Stanford Law Review,* vol. 14(1961): 59–86.
Diamond, Bernard. With Malice Aforethought. *Archives of Criminal Psychodynamics,* vol. 2(1957): 1–45.
Diamond, Bernard. Isaac Ray and the Trial of Daniel M'Naghten. *American Journal of Psychiatry,* vol. 112(1956): 651–6.
Dilman, Ilham. Is the Unconscious a Theoretical Construct? *Monist,* vol. 56(1972): 313–42.
Dilman, Ilham. The Unconscious. *Mind,* vol. 68(1959): 446–73.
Dostoevsky, Fyodor. *The Eternal Husband.* London: Heinemann, 1950.
Dray, William. *Laws and Explanation in History.* Oxford: Oxford University Press, 1957.
Dreiser, Theodore. *An American Tragedy.* New York: Boni and Liveright, 1925.
Dworkin, Ronald. *Taking Rights Seriously.* Cambridge, Mass.: Harvard University Press, 1978.
Dworkin, Ronald. Lord Devlin and the Enforcement of Morals. *Yale Law Journal,* vol. 75(1966): 986–1005.
Eagle, Morris. Anatomy of the Self in Psychoanalytic Theory. In M. Ruse (ed.), *Nature Animated,* vol. 2. Dordrecht: Reidel, 1982.
Eagle, Morris. A Critical Examination of Motivational Explanation in Psychoanalysis. *Psychoanalysis and Contemporary Thought,* vol. 3(1980): 329–80.

References

Reprinted in L. Laudan (ed.), *Mind and Medicine: Problems of Explanation and Evaluation in Psychiatry and the Biomedical Sciences*. Berkeley: University of California Press, 1982.

Eagle, Morris. Validation of Motivational Formulations: Acknowledgment as a Criterion. In B. B. Rubinstein (ed.), *Psychoanalysis and Contemporary Science*, vol. 2(1973): 265–75.

Ehrenwald, J. Cause, Purpose and Meaning in Psychosomatic Medicine. *Journal of Experimental and Clinical Psychopathology*, vol. 11(1950): 164–73.

Elliott, A. T. Procedures of Involuntary Commitment on the Basis of Alleged Mental Illness. *University of Colorado Law Review*, vol. 42(1970): 231–69.

Ellis, Albert. An Operational Reformulation of Some of the Basic Principles of Psychoanalysis. In H. Feigl and M. Scriven (eds.), *The Foundations of Science and the Concepts of Psychology and Psychoanalysis*. Minnesota Studies in the Philosophy of Science, vol. 1. Minneapolis: University of Minnesota Press, 1956.

Ennis, B. *Prisoners of Psychiatry*. New York: Harcourt Brace Jovanovich, 1972.

Epstein, I. (ed.). *Babylonian Talmud, Baba Kamma*. London: Soncino Press, 1935.

Epstein, Richard. Possession as the Root of all Title. *Georgia Law Review*, vol. 13(1979): 1221–43.

Erskine, Lord. *Hadfield's Case*. 27 How. St. Tr. 1281, 1314 (1800).

Esterson, A., and R. D. Laing. *Sanity, Madness and the Family*, 2d ed. Harmondsworth: Penguin Books, 1970.

Fairbairn, W. Ronald D. *An Object-Relations Theory of the Personality*. New York: Basic Books, 1954.

Farrell, B. A. Mental Illness: A Conceptual Analysis. *Psychological Medicine*, vol. 9(1979): 21–35.

Fay, Brian. Practical Reasoning, Rationality, and the Explanation of Intentional Action. *Journal of the Theory of Social Behavior*, vol. 8(1977): 77–101.

Feinberg, Joel. *Doing and Deserving*. Princeton, N.J.: Princeton University Press, 1970.

Fenichel, Otto. *The Psychoanalytic Theory of Neurosis*. New York: Norton, 1945.

Field, G. C. Is the Conception of the Unconscious of Value in Psychology? *Mind*, vol. 31(1922): 413–23.

Fingarette, Herbert. Insanity and Responsibility. *Inquiry*, vol. 15(1972): 6–29.

Fingarette, Herbert. *The Meaning of Criminal Insanity*. Berkeley: University of California Press, 1972.

Fingarette, Herbert. *The Self in Transformation*. New York: Harper & Row, 1963.

Fingarette, Herbert. Psychoanalytic Perspectives on Moral Guilt and Responsibility: A Re-evaluation. *Philosophy and Phenomenological Research*, vol. 16(1955): 18–36.

Fisher, Seymour, and Roger Greenberg. *The Scientific Credibility of Freud's Theories and Therapy*. New York: Basic Books, 1977.

Fleming, B. On Intention. *Philosophical Review*, vol. 73(1964): 301–20.

Fletcher, George. *Rethinking Criminal Law*. Boston: Little, Brown, 1978.

Flew, Antony. *Crime or Disease?* London: Macmillan Press, 1973.

References

Flew, Antony. Motives and the Unconscious. In H. Feigl and M. Scriven (eds.), *The Foundations of Science and the Concepts of Psychology and Psychoanalysis.* Minnesota Studies in the Philosophy of Science, vol. 1. Minneapolis: University of Minnesota Press, 1956.

Flew, Antony. Psychoanalytic Explanation. *Analysis,* vol. 10(1949): 8–15. Reprinted in M. MacDonald (ed.), *Philosophy and Analysis.* Oxford: Blackwell Publisher, 1954.

Fliess, R. *The Revival of Interest in the Dream: A Critical Study of Post-Freudian Psychoanalytic Contributions.* New York: International Universities Press, 1953.

Fodor, Jerry. *The Language of Thought.* New York: Crowell, 1975.

Fox, Michael. On Unconscious Emotions. *Philosophy and Phenomenological Research,* vol. 34(1973): 151–70.

Frankfurt, Harry. Coercion and Moral Responsibility. In T. Honderich (ed.), *Essays in Freedom of Action.* London: Routledge & Kegan Paul, 1973.

Frankfurt, Harry. Freedom of the Will and the Concept of a Person. *Journal of Philosophy,* vol. 68(1971): 5–20.

Frege, G. Uber Sinn und Bedeutung. *Zeitschrift für Philosophie und Philosophische Kritik,* vol. 100(1892): 25–50. Translated and reprinted in H. Feigl and W. Sellars (eds.), *Readings in Philosophical Analysis.* New York: Appleton-Century-Crofts, 1949, and in P. T. Geach and M. Black (eds.), *The Philosophical Writings of Gottlob Frege.* Oxford: Blackwell Publisher, 1960.

French, Peter. The Corporation as a Moral Person. *American Philosophical Quarterly,* vol. 16(1979): 207–15.

Freud, Sigmund. *New Introductory Lectures on Psychoanalysis.* Translated and edited by James Strachey. New York: Norton, 1965. First published New York: Norton, 1933. Translated by W. J. H. Sprout.

Freud, Sigmund. *Dora: An Analysis of a Case of Hysteria.* New York: Collier Books, 1963.

Freud, Sigmund. *The Problem of Anxiety.* New York: Norton, 1963.

Freud, Sigmund. *Three Case Histories.* New York: Macmillan, 1963.

Freud, Sigmund. *The Ego and the Id.* New York: Norton, 1960. (First published in 1923.)

Freud, Sigmund. *Collected Papers,* vols. 4 and 5. Vol. 5 edited by James Strachey. New York: Basic Books, 1959.

Freud, Sigmund. *The Origins of Psychoanalysis; Letters to Wilhelm Fliess, Drafts and Notes, 1887–1902.* New York: Basic Books, 1954.

Freud, Sigmund. *Introductory Lectures on Psychoanalysis.* Written and delivered in 1915 and 1917, first translated and published in America as *A General Introduction to Psychoanalysis* (New York: Washington Square Press, 1952).

Freud, Sigmund. *An Outline of Psychoanalysis.* New York: Norton, 1949.

Freud, Sigmund. *The Standard Edition of the Complete Psychological Works of Sigmund Freud.* 24 vols. Edited by James Strachey, in collaboration with Anna Freud, assisted by Alix Strachey and Alan Tyson. London: Hogarth Press, 1953–1975.

Fried, Charles. *Contract as Promise.* Cambridge, Mass.: Harvard University Press, 1981.

References

Fried, Charles. Right and Wrong: Preliminary Considerations. *Journal of Legal Studies,* vol. 5(1976): 165–200.
Friedemann, Max. Cleptomania: The Analytic and Forensic Aspects. *Psychoanalytic Review,* vol. 17(1930): 452–70.
Fromm, Erich. *The Sane Society.* New York: Fawcett, 1951.
Fromm, Erich. *Man for Himself: An Enquiry Into the Psychology of Ethics.* New York: Fawcett, 1947.
Fuller, Gary. Freudian Explanations, Rational Explanation, and Meaning. *Philosophy Research Archives,* vol. 3(1977): 813–31.
Fuller, Lon. *The Morality of Law,* 2d ed. New Haven, Conn.: Yale University Press, 1969.
Garfinkel, Alan. *Forms of Explanation.* New Haven, Conn.: Yale University Press, 1980.
Gerbode, F. A. Book Review. *Santa Clara Lawyer,* vol. 13(1973): 616–22.
Gewirth, Alan. The Basis and Content of Human Rights. In J. R. Pennock and J. W. Chapman (eds.), *Human Rights. Nomos,* vol. 23(1981): 119–47.
Gill, Merton, and Philip Holzman (eds.). *Psychology versus Meta-psychology.* New York: International Universities Press, 1976.
Glueck, Sheldon. *Law and Psychiatry: Cold War or Entente Cordiale?* Baltimore: Johns Hopkins University Press, 1962.
Goble, Frank. *The Third Force.* New York: Grossman, 1970.
Goldman, Alvin. *A Theory of Human Action.* Englewood Cliffs, N.J.: Prentice-Hall, 1970.
Goldstein, Abraham. *The Insanity Defense.* New Haven, Conn.: Yale University Press, 1967.
Goldstein, Joe, and Jay Katz. Abolish the Insanity Defense—Why Not? *Yale Law Journal,* vol. 72(1963): 853–76.
Goslin, J. Mental Causes and Fear. *Mind,* vol. 71(1962): 289–306.
Gove, W. R. (ed.). *Deviance and Mental Illness.* Beverly Hills, Calif.: Sage, 1982.
Greenspan, Patricia. A Case of Mixed Feelings: Ambivalence and the Logic of Emotion. In A. Rorty (ed.), *Explaining Emotions.* Berkeley: University of California Press, 1980.
Gregory, R. L. *Eye and Brain.* New York: McGraw-Hill, 1966.
Grice, G. R. Motive and Reason. In J. Raz (ed.), *Practical Reasoning.* Oxford: Oxford University Press, 1978.
Grice, H. P. Meaning. *Philosophical Review,* vol. 66(1957): 377–88.
Group for the Advancement of Psychiatry. *Criminal Responsibility and Psychiatric Expert Testimony.* G.A.P. Report No. 26, 1954.
Grunbaum, Adolf. Can Psychoanalytic Theory Be Cogently Tested on "The Couch"? In L. Laudan (ed.), *Mind and Medicine: Problems of Explanation and Evaluation in Psychiatry and the Biomedical Sciences.* Berkeley: University of California Press, 1982.
Grunbaum, Adolf. Is Freudian Psychoanalytic Theory Pseudo-Scientific by Karl Popper's Criterion of Demarcation? *American Philosophical Quarterly,* vol. 16(1979): 131–41.

References

Gustafson, Donald. On Unconscious Intentions. *Philosophy,* vol. 48(1973): 178–82.
Hailsham, Lord. *Hyam v. Director of Public Prosecutions.* [1975] A. C. 55 (1974).
Hale, M. *Select Pleas of the Crown,* vol. 1. London: Selden Society, 1887.
Hall, Jerome. *General Principles of Criminal Law,* 2d. ed. New York: Bobbs-Merrill, 1960.
Hall, Jerome. Psychiatry and Criminal Responsibility. *Yale Law Journal,* vol. 65(1956): 761–85.
Halleck, Seymour. *Psychiatry and the Dilemmas of Crime.* Berkeley: University of California Press, 1971.
Hamlyn, D. W. Causality and Human Behavior. In N. Care and C. Landesman (eds.), *Readings in the Theory of Action.* Bloomington: Indiana University Press, 1968.
Hampshire, Stuart. Disposition and Memory. *International Journal of Psycho-Analysis,* vol. 42(1963): 59–68. Reprinted in Hampshire, *Freedom of Mind.* Princeton: Princeton University Press, 1971.
Hampshire, Stuart. *Thought and Action.* New York: Viking Press, 1960.
Hardisty, J. H. Mental Illness: A Legal Fiction. *Washington Law Review,* vol. 48(1973): 735–62.
Hare, R. M. *Freedom and Reason.* Oxford: Oxford University Press, 1963.
Hare, R. M. *The Language of Morals.* Oxford: Oxford University Press (Clarendon Press), 1952.
Hart, H. L. A. *Punishment and Responsibility.* Oxford: Oxford University Press, 1968.
Hart, H. L. A. Definition and Theory in Jurisprudence. *Law Quarterly Review,* vol. 70(1954): 37–60.
Hart, H. L. A. The Ascription of Responsibility and Rights. *Proceedings of the Aristotelian Society,* vol. 49(1949): 171–94.
Hart, H. L. A., and A. M. Honore. *Causation in the Law.* Oxford: Oxford University Press, 1959.
Hartmann, E. L. *The Functions of Sleep.* New Haven, Conn.: Yale University Press, 1973.
Hartmann, Heinz. Psychoanalysis as a Scientific Theory. In S. Hook (ed.), *Psychoanalysis, Scientific Method, and Philosophy.* New York: New York University Press, 1959.
Hartmann, Heinz. Psychoanalysis and the Concept of Health. *International Journal of Psychoanalysis,* vol. 20(1939): 308–21.
Hayward, M., and J. E. Taylor. A Schizophrenic Patient Describes the Action of Intensive Psychotherapy. *Psychiatric Quarterly,* vol. 30(1956): 211–48.
Heidegger, Martin. *Being and Time.* Translated by John Macquarrie and Edward Robinson. New York: Harper & Row, 1962.
Hempel, Carl. Rational Action. *Proceedings and Addresses of the American Philosophical Association,* vol. 35(1962): 5–23. Reprinted in N. S. Care and C. Landesman (eds.), *Readings in the Theory of Action.* Bloomington: Indiana University Press, 1968.
Hempel, Carl. *Aspects of Scientific Explanation.* New York: Free Press, 1965.

References

Herbert, A. P. *Uncommon Law,* 7th ed. London: Methuen & Co., 1952.
Heston, L. L. The Genetics of Schizophrenic and Schizoid Disease. *Science,* vol. 167(1970): 249–56.
Hinsie, L. E., and R. J. Campbell. *Psychiatric Dictionary,* 3rd ed. New York: Oxford University Press, 1960.
Hohfeld, W. *Fundamental Legal Conceptions.* New Haven, Conn.: Yale University Press, 1923.
Hollander, P. Sociology, Selective Determinism, and the Rise of Expectations. *American Sociologist,* vol. 8(1973): 147–53.
Hollender, M. H. Is the Wish to Sleep a Universal Motive for Dreaming? *Journal of the American Psychoanalytic Association,* vol. 10(1962): 323–8.
Holmes, Oliver Wendell, Jr. *The Common Law.* Edited by Mark deWolfe Howe. Boston: Little, Brown, 1963.
Holt, Robert. The Death and the Transfiguration of the Metapsychology. *International Review of Psychoanalysis,* vol. 8(1981): 129–43.
Home, H. J. The Concept of Mind. *International Journal of Psychoanalysis,* vol. 47(1966): 42–9.
Hospers, John. What Means This Freedom? In R. Abelson (ed.), *Ethics and Meta-Ethics.* New York: St. Martin's Press, 1963.
Hospers, John. Meaning and Free Will. *Philosophy and Phenomenological Research,* vol. 10(1950): 307–30. Reprinted in H. Morris (ed.), *Freedom and Responsibility.* Stanford, Calif.: Stanford University Press, 1961.
Hull, Clark. *Principles of Behavior.* New York: Appleton-Century-Crofts, 1966.
Ingber, Stanley. Book Review. *UCLA Law Review,* vol. 27(1980): 816–48.
Jahoda, Marie. *Current Concepts of Positive Mental Health.* New York: Basic Books, 1958.
James, William. *The Will to Believe.* New York: Longman, 1898.
Jellinek, E. *The Disease Concept of Alcoholism.* New Brunswick, N.J.: Rutgers Center of Alcohol Studies Publications, 1960.
Jones, Ernest. Rationalization in Everyday Life. *Journal of Abnormal Psychology,* vol. 3(1908): 161–9.
Jones, R. M. *The New Psychology of Dreaming.* New York: Grune & Stratton, 1970.
Jones, R. M. The Psychoanalytic Theory of Dreaming–1968. *Journal of Nervous and Mental Disease,* vol. 147(1968): 587–604.
Jones, R. M. Dream Interpretation and the Psychology of Dreaming. *Journal of the American Psychoanalytic Association,* vol. 13(1965): 304–19.
Kant, I. *The Metaphysical Elements of Justice.* Translated by J. Ladd. Indianapolis: Bobbs-Merrill, 1965.
Kaplan, L. V. Civil Commitment "As You Like It." *Boston University Law Review,* vol. 49(1969): 14–45.
Katz, Wilber. Law, Psychiatry and Free Will. *University of Chicago Law Review,* vol. 22(1955): 397–404.
Kendell, R. E. The Concept of Disease and Its Implications for Psychiatry. *British Journal of Psychiatry,* vol. 127(1975): 305–15.

References

Kenny, Anthony. Mental Health in Plato's *Republic*. *Proceedings of the British Academy*, vol. 55(1969): 229–53.
Kenny, Anthony. Intention and Purpose. *Journal of Philosophy*, vol. 63(1966): 642–51.
Kenny, Anthony. *Action, Emotion, and Will*. London: Routledge & Kegan Paul, 1963.
Kerner, George. Passions and the Cognitive Foundations of Ethics. *Philosophy and Phenomenological Research*, vol. 31(1970): 177–92.
King, L. S. What Is Disease? *Philosophy of Science*, vol. 21(1954): 193–203.
Klein, Donald. A Proposed Definition of Mental Illness. In R. L. Spitzer and D. F. Klein (eds.), *Critical Issues in Psychiatric Diagnosis*. New York: Raven Press, 1978.
Kohut, Heinz. *The Restoration of the Self*. New York: International Universities Press, 1977.
Kohut, Heinz. *The Analysis of Self*. New York: International Universities Press, 1971.
Kubie, Lawrence. *Practical and Theoretical Aspects of Psychoanalysis*. New York: International Universities Press, 1950.
Ladd, John. Morality and the Ideal of Rationality in Formal Organizations. *Monist*, vol. 54(1970): 488–516.
LaFave, W. F., and A. W. Scott. *Criminal Law*. St. Paul: West, 1972.
Laing, R. D. *The Politics of Experience*. New York: Ballantine Books, 1967.
Laing, R. D. *The Divided Self*. London: Tavistock, 1960.
Laird, J. Is the Conception of the Unconscious of Value in Psychology? *Mind*, vol. 31(1922): 433–42.
Lerner, B. Dream Function Reconsidered. *Journal of Abnormal Psychology*, vol. 72(1967): 85–100.
Levin, David. Picturing the Freudian Unconscious. *The Psychoanalytic Review*, vol. 68(1981): 255–63.
Levin, David Michael. The Concept of Mental Illness: Working Through the Myths. *Inquiry*, vol. 19(1976): 360–5.
Lewis, Aubrey. *The State of Psychiatry*. New York: Science House, 1967.
Lewis, Aubrey. Health as a Social Concept. *British Journal of Sociology*, vol. 4(1953): 109–24.
Lewis, C. S. The Humanitarian Theory of Punishment. *Res Judicatae*, vol. 6(1953): 224–30.
Livermore, J. M., and P. E. Meehl. The Virtues of M'Naghten. *Minnesota Law Review*, vol. 51(1967): 789–856.
Locke, D. Intention and Intentional Action. In J. J. MacIntosh and S. Coval (eds.), *The Business of Reason*. New York: Humanities Press, 1969.
Locke, John. *An Essay Concerning Human Understanding*, book 2, chap. 27. New York: Dover, 1959.
Locke, John. *Two Treatises of Government*. New York: Hafner Press, 1956.
Louch, A. R. *Explanation and Human Action*. Berkeley: University of California Press, 1966.

References

Louisell, David, and Bernard Diamond. Law and Psychiatry: Detente, Entente, or Concomitance? *Cornell Law Quarterly*, vol. 50(1965): 217–34.
Ludwig, A. M., M. M. Brandsma, C. B. Wilbur, F. Bendfeldt, and D. H. Jameson. The Objective Study of a Multiple Personality. *Archives of General Psychiatry*, vol. 26(1972): 298–310.
MacIntyre, Alisdair. *The Unconscious*. London: Routledge & Kegan Paul, 1958.
Mackie, J. L. The Grounds of Responsibility. In P. M. S. Hacker and J. Raz (eds.), *Law, Morality and Society*. Oxford: Oxford University Press, 1977.
Malcolm, Norman. *Problems of Mind*. New York: Harper & Row, 1971.
Malcolm, Norman. The Conceivability of Mechanism. *The Philosophical Review*, vol. 77(1968): 45–72
Malcolm, Norman. Behaviorism as a Philosophy of Psychology. In T. W. Wann (ed.), *Behaviorism and Phenomenology*. Chicago: University of Chicago Press, 1964.
Mapel, Brenda M. Philosophical Criticism of Behaviorism: An Analysis. *Behaviorism*, vol. 5(1977): 17–32.
Marcuse, Herbert. *Eros and Civilization*. Boston: Beacon Press, 1955.
Margolis, Joseph. The Concept of Disease. *Journal of Medicine and Philosophy*, vol. 1(1976): 238–55. Reprinted in A. L. Caplan, H. T. Engelhardt, and J. J. McCartney (eds.), *Concepts of Health and Disease*. Reading, Mass.: Addison-Wesley, 1981.
Martin, Michael. Interpreting Skinner. *Behaviorism*, vol. 6(1978): 129–38.
Martin, Rex. *Historical Explanation: Re-enactment and Practical Inference*. Ithaca, N.Y.: Cornell University Press, 1977.
Maslow, Abraham, and Bela Mittelmann. *Principles of Abnormal Psychiatry: The Dynamics of Psychic Illness*, rev. ed. New York: Harper & Row, 1951.
Matte-Blanco, I. *The Unconscious as Infinite Sets*. London: Duckworth, 1975.
May, Rollo. The Work and Training of the Psychological Therapist. In M. H. Krout (ed.), *Psychology, Psychiatry and the Public Interest*. Minneapolis: University of Minnesota Press, 1956.
McGuiness, B. F. I Know What I Want. *Proceedings of the Aristotelian Society*, vol. 57(1957): 305–20.
Meiland, J. W. *The Nature of Intention*. London: Methuen & Co., 1970.
Meissner, W. W. Metapsychology – Who Needs It? *Journal of the American Psychoanalytic Association*, vol. 29(1981): 921–38.
Melden, A. I. *Rights and Persons*. Berkeley: University of California Press, 1977.
Melden, A. I. Action. *Philosophical Review*, vol. 65(1956): 523–41. Reprinted in M. Brand (ed.), *The Nature of Human Action*. Glenview, Ill.: Scott, Foresman, 1970.
Melden, A. I. *Free Action*. London: Routledge & Kegan Paul, 1961.
Menninger, Karl. *The Crime of Punishment*. New York: Viking Press, 1968.
Menninger, Karl. *The Human Mind*. New York: Knopf, 1961.
Menninger, Karl, Martin Mayer, and Paul Pruyser. *The Vital Balance: The Life Process in Mental Health and Illness*. New York: Viking Press, 1963.
Michaelman, Frank. Property, Utility and Fairness; Comments on the Ethical

References

Foundations of "Just Compensation" Law. *Harvard Law Review*, vol. 80(1967): 1165–1258.
Miles, T. R. *Eliminating the Unconscious*. Oxford: Pergamon Press, 1966.
Mill, John Stuart. *A System of Logic*. London: Longman Group, 1965. First published London: J. W. Parker & Son, 1843.
Mill, John Stuart. *On Liberty*. Arlington Heights, Ill.: AHM Publishing, 1947. First published London: J. W. Parker & Son, 1859.
Mischel, T. Understanding Neurotic Behaviour: From 'Mechanism' to 'Intentionality.' In T. Mischel (ed.), *Understanding Other Persons*. Oxford: Blackwell Publisher, 1974.
Mischel, T. Concerning Rational Behaviour and Psychoanalytic Explanation. *Mind*, vol. 74(1965): 71–8.
Moore, G. E. *Principia Ethica*. Cambridge: Cambridge University Press, 1903.
Moore, Michael S. Moral Reality. *Wisconsin Law Review* (1982): 1061–1156.
Moore, Michael S. Closet Retributivism. *Cites* (spring-summer, 1982): 5–15.
Moore, Michael S. The Semantics of Judging. *Southern California Law Review*, vol. 54(1981): 151–294.
Moore, Michael S. Mental Illness and Responsibility. *Bulletin of the Menninger Clinic*, vol. 39(1975): 308–28.
Moore, Michael S. Some Myths About "Mental Illness." *Inquiry*, vol. 18(1975): 233–65.
Moore, Michael S. Individuating Intentions in the Criminal Law. Unpublished paper.
Morris, Herbert. A Paternalistic Theory of Punishment. *American Philosophical Quarterly*, vol. 18(1981): 263–71.
Morris, Herbert. *Guilt and Innocence*. Los Angeles: University of California Press, 1976.
Morris, Herbert. Moral and Non-Moral Guilt. Unpublished manuscript, 1980.
Morris, Norval. *Madness and the Criminal Law*. Chicago: University of Chicago Press, 1982.
Morse, Stephen. Failed Explanations and Criminal Responsibility: Experts and the Unconscious. *Virginia Law Review*, vol. 68(1982): 971–1084.
Morse, Stephen. Diminished Capacity: A Moral and Legal Conundrum. *International Journal of Law and Psychiatry*, vol. 2(1979): 271–98.
Morse, Stephen J. Crazy Behavior, Morals and Science: An Analysis of Mental Health Law. *Southern California Law Review*, vol. 51(1978): 527–654.
Mullane, Harvey. Psychoanalytic Explanation and Rationality. *Journal of Philosophy*, vol. 68(1971): 413–26.
Mullane, Harvey. Unconscious Emotion. *Theoria*, vol. 31(1965): 181–90.
Nagel, Ernst. *The Structure of Science*. New York: Harcourt Brace & World, 1961.
Nagel, Ernst. Methodological Issues in Psychoanalytic Theory. In S. Hook (ed.), *Psychoanalysis, Scientific Method, and Philosophy*. New York: New York University Press, 1959.
Nagel, Thomas. *Mortal Questions*. Princeton, N.J.: Princeton University Press, 1979.

References

Nagera, H. (ed.). *Basic Psychoanalytic Concepts of the Theory of Dreams.* New York: Basic Books, 1969.
Nietzsche, Friedrich. *On the Genealogy of Morals.* Translated by W. Kaufmann. New York: Random House, 1967.
Notes and Comments, Why Do Criminal Attempts Fail? A New Defense. *Yale Law Journal,* vol. 70(1960): 160–69.
Nozick, Robert. *Anarchy, State and Utopia.* New York: Basic Books, 1974.
Nozick, Robert. Coercion. In S. Morgenbesser, P. Suppes, and M. White (eds.), *Philosophy, Science and Method.* New York: St. Martin's Press, 1969.
Nussbaum, Martha. *Aristotle's De Moto Animalum.* Princeton, N.J.: Princeton University Press, 1977.
Oakeshott, Michael. *Experience and its Modes.* Cambridge: Cambridge University Press, 1933.
Packer, Herbert. *The Limits of the Criminal Sanction.* Palo Alto, Calif.: Stanford University Press, 1968.
Pap, Arthur. On the Empirical Interpretation of Psychoanalytic Concepts. In S. Hook (ed.), *Psychoanalysis, Scientific Method, and Philosophy.* New York: New York University Press, 1959.
Parsons, Talcott. Review. *Daedalus,* vol. 103(1973): 91–6.
Parsons, Talcott. *The Social System.* New York: Free Press, 1951.
Peacocke, C. Deviant Causal Chains. *Midwest Studies in Philosophy,* vol. 4(1979): 123–55.
Pears, David. Motivated Irrationality, Freudian Theory and Cognitive Dissonance. In R. Wollheim and J. Hopkins (eds.), *Philosophical Essays on Freud.* Cambridge: Cambridge University Press, 1982.
Pears, D. F. The Appropriate Causation of Intentional Basic Actions. *Critica,* vol. 7(1975): 39–69.
Peters, Richard. Motivation, Emotion, and Schemes of Common Sense. In T. Mischel (ed.), *Human Action.* New York: Academic Press, 1969.
Peters, Richard. More About Motives. *Mind,* vol. 76(1967): 92–97.
Peters, Richard. *The Concept of Motivation.* London: Routledge & Kegan Paul, 1958.
Pitcher, George. *A Theory of Perception.* Princeton, N.J.: Princeton University Press, 1971.
Plato, *Republic.* In E. Hamilton and H. Cairns (eds.), *The Collected Dialogues of Plato.* Princeton, N.J.: Princeton University Press, 1961.
Platt, A., and B. Diamond. The Origins of the "Right and Wrong" Test of Criminal Responsibility and Its Subsequent Development in the United States: An Historical View. *California Law Review,* vol. 54(1966): 1227–60.
Prince, Morton. *Dissociation of a Personality.* London: Longmans Green, 1930.
Prosser, William. *Handbook of the Law of Torts,* 4th ed. St. Paul: West, 1971.
Putnam, Hilary. *Mind, Language and Reality.* Cambridge: Cambridge University Press, 1975.
Putnam, Hilary. The Meaning of "Meaning." In H. Feigl and M. Scriven (eds.), *Language, Mind and Knowledge.* Minnesota Studies in the Philosophy of Science, vol. 7. Minneapolis: University of Minnesota Press, 1975.

References

Putnam, Hilary. Brains and Behavior. In R. J. Butler (ed.), *Analytical Philosophy,* 2d ser. Oxford: Blackwell Publisher, 1965.
Putnam, Hilary. Dreaming and Depth Grammar. In R. J. Butler (ed.), *Analytical Philosophy,* 1st ser. Oxford: Blackwell Publisher, 1962.
Quine, W. V. *Philosophy of Logic.* Englewood Cliffs, N.J.: Prentice-Hall, 1970.
Quine, W. V. *Ontological Relativity and Other Essays.* New York: Columbia University Press, 1969.
Quine, W. V. *Word and Object.* Cambridge, Mass.: MIT Press, 1960.
Quine, W. V. *From A Logical Point of View.* Cambridge, Mass.: Harvard University Press, 1953.
Rabin, Robert (ed.). *Perspectives on Tort Law.* Boston: Little, Brown, 1976.
Radin, Margaret Jane. Property and Personhood. *Stanford Law Review,* vol. 34(1982): 957–1015.
Radin, Margaret Jane. Cruel Punishment and Respect for Persons: Super Due Process for Death. *Southern California Law Review,* vol. 53(1981): 1143–85.
Rapaport, David. On the Psychoanalytic Theory of Motivation. In 1960 *Nebraska Symposium on Motivation.* Lincoln: University of Nebraska Press, 1960.
Rawls, John. *A Theory of Justice.* Cambridge, Mass.: Harvard University Press, 1971.
Rawls, John. Two Concepts of Rules. *Philosophical Review,* vol. 64(1955): 3–32.
Ray, Isaac. *A Treatise on the Medical Jurisprudence of Insanity.* Boston: Little, Brown, 1838.
Rayner, Eric. Infinite Experiences, Affects and the Characteristics of the Unconscious. *International Journal of Psycho-Analysis,* vol. 62(1981): 403–12.
Raz, Joseph (ed.). *Practical Reasoning.* Oxford: Oxford University Press, 1978.
Redlich, F. C. The Concept of Health in Psychiatry. In A. H. Leighton, J. A. Clausen, and R. N. Wilson (eds.), *Explorations in Social Psychiatry.* New York: Basic Books, 1957.
Reid, J. P. The Working of the New Hampshire Doctrine of Criminal Insanity. *University of Miami Law Review,* vol. 15(1960): 14–58.
Reik, Theodore. The Doe-Ray Correspondence: A Pioneer Collaboration in the Jurisprudence of Mental Disease. *Yale Law Journal,* vol. 63(1953): 183–96.
Ricoeur, P. *Freud and Philosophy.* New Haven, Conn.: Yale University Press, 1970.
Riviere, Joan. The Unconscious Phantasy of an Inner World. In M. Klein, P. Heimann, and R. E. Money-Kyrle (eds.), *New Directions in Psychoanalysis.* New York: Basic Books, 1955.
Robinson, Richard. *Definition.* Oxford: Oxford University Press (Clarendon Press), 1950.
Roche, Philip. *The Criminal Mind.* New York: Wiley, 1958.
Rorty, Richard. *Philosophy as the Mirror of Nature.* Princeton, N.J.: Princeton University Press, 1979.
Rorty, Richard. Incorrigibility as the Mark of the Mental. *Journal of Philosophy,* vol. 67(1970): 399–424.
Rosenberg, A. Causation and Teleology in Contemporary Philosophy of Science. In

References

G. Fløistad (ed.), *Contemporary Philosophy: A New Science*. The Hague: Martinus Nijhoff, 1982.

Ross, Alf. Tu-Tu. *Harvard Law Review*, vol. 70(1957): 812–25.

Roth, R., M. Dayley, and J. Lerner. Into the Abyss: Psychiatric Reliability, and Emergency Commitment Statutes. *Santa Clara Lawyer*, vol. 13(1973): 400–66.

Royal Commission on Capital Punishment 1953 Report, sec. 322. London: 1953.

Royko, Mike. As reported in *Kansas City Star*, June 22, 1975.

Ryle, Gilbert. *The Concept of Mind*. London: Hutchinson, 1949.

Sachs, David. On Freud's Doctrine of the Emotions. In R. Wollheim (ed.), *Freud, A Collection of Critical Essays*. Garden City, N.Y.: Doubleday (Anchor Press), 1974.

Salmon, Wesley. Psychoanalytic Theory and Evidence. In S. Hook (ed.), *Psychoanalysis, Scientific Method, and Philosophy*. New York: New York University Press, 1959.

Salmond, J. *Jurisprudence*, 11th ed. London: Sweet and Maxwell, 1957.

Sarbin, T. R. The Scientific Status of the Mental Illness Metaphor. In S. C. Plog and R. B. Edgerton (eds.), *Changing Perspectives in Mental Illness*. New York: Holt, Rinehart and Winston, 1969.

Scadding, J. G. Diagnosis: The Clinician and the Computer. *Lancet*, vol. 2(1967): 877–82.

Schafer, Roy. *A New Language for Psychoanalysis*. New Haven, Conn.: Yale University Press, 1976.

Scheff, Thomas. *Being Mentally Ill: A Sociological Theory*. Chicago: Aldine, 1966.

Schelling, Thomas. The Intimate Contest for Self-Command. *The Public Interest*, vol. 60(1980): 94–118.

Schimek, Jean. A Critical Re-examination of Freud's Concept of Unconscious Mental Representation. *International Review of Psycho-Analysis*, vol. 2(1975): 171–87.

Schlick, Moritz. *Problems of Ethics*. New York: Dover, 1961.

Schlick, Moritz. Causality in Everyday Life and in Recent Science. *University of California Publications in Philosophy*, vol. 15(1932): 99–125. Reprinted in H. Morris (ed.), *Freedom and Responsibility*. Stanford, Calif.: Stanford University Press, 1961.

Scriven, M. The Experimental Investigation of Psychoanalysis. In S. Hook (ed.), *Psychoanalysis, Scientific Method, and Philosophy*. New York: New York University Press, 1959.

Scriven, M. A Study of Radical Behaviorism. In H. Feigl and M. Scriven (eds.), *The Foundations of Science and the Concepts of Psychology and Psychoanalysis*. Minnesota Studies in the Philosophy of Science, vol. 1. Minneapolis: University of Minnesota Press, 1956.

Scruton, Roger. Emotion, Practical Knowledge and Common Culture. In A. Rorty (ed.), *Explaining Emotions*. Berkeley: University of California Press, 1980.

Sherwood, Michael. *The Logic of Explanation in Psychoanalysis*. New York: Academic Press, 1969.

References

Shope, Robert. The Significance of Freud for Modern Philosophy of Mind. In *Philosophy of Mind*, vol. 4. Dordrecht: Reidel, 1982.
Shope, Robert. Freud's Concepts of Meaning. *Psychoanalysis and Contemporary Science*, vol. 2(1973): 276–303.
Shope, Robert. The Psychoanalytic Theories of Wish-Fulfillment and Meaning. *Inquiry*, vol. 10(1967): 276–303.
Siegler, Frederick. Unconscious Intentions. *Inquiry*, vol. 10(1967): 51–67.
Skinner, B. F. *About Behaviorism*. New York: Knopf, 1974.
Skinner, B. F. *Beyond Freedom and Dignity*. New York: Knopf, 1971.
Skinner, B. F. Critique of Psychoanalytic Concepts and Theories. In H. Feigl and M. Scriven (eds.), *The Foundations of Science and the Concepts of Psychology and Psychoanalysis*. Minnesota Studies in the Philosophy of Science, vol. 1. Minneapolis: University of Minnesota Press, 1956.
Smart, J. J. C., and B. Williams. *Utilitarianism: For and Against*. Cambridge: Cambridge University Press, 1973.
Smyth, T. W. Unconscious Desires and the Meaning of "Desire." *Monist*, vol. 56(1972): 413–26.
Spitzer, Robert, and Janet Williams. The Definition and Diagnosis of Mental Disorder. In W. R. Gove (ed.), *Deviance and Mental Illness*. Beverly Hills, Calif.: Sage, 1982.
Spitzer, Robert L., and Jean Endicott. Medical and Mental Disorder: Proposed Definition and Criteria. In R. L. Spitzer and D. F. Klein (eds.), *Critical Issues in Psychiatric Diagnosis*. New York: Raven Press, 1978.
Spitzer, R. L., and D. F. Klein (eds.), *Critical Issues in Psychiatric Diagnosis*. New York: Raven Press, 1978.
Star, S. A. The Public's Idea About Mental Illness. Presented in 1955 to the annual meeting of the National Association of Mental Health, Indianapolis. Reprinted in part in R. C. Donnelly, J. Goldstein, and R. D. Schwartz (eds.), *Criminal Law*. New York: Free Press, 1962.
Steele, Robert. Psychoanalysis and Hermeneutics. *International Review of Psycho-Analysis*, vol. 6(1979): 389–411.
Stephen, Sir James. *A History of the Criminal Law of England*, vol. 2. London: Macmillan, 1883.
Stevenson, C. L. *Ethics and Language*. New Haven, Conn.: Yale University Press, 1944.
Stone, Alan. Psychiatry and Morality. Delivered as the Tanner Lectures, Department of Philosophy, Stanford University, spring, 1982.
Stone, Alan. *Mental Health and Law: A System in Transition*. Rockville, Md.: Center for Crime and Delinquency, National Institute of Mental Health, 1975.
Stone, Alan. Psychiatry Kills: A Critical Evaluation of Dr. Thomas Szasz. *Journal of Psychiatry and Law*, vol. 1(1973): 23–37.
Stone, Christopher D. Corporate Accountability in Law and Morals. In J. Houck and O. Williams (eds.), *The Judaeo-Christian Vision and the Modern Business Corporation*. Notre Dame, Ind.: University of Notre Dame Press, 1982.

References

Strawson, P. F. *Individuals.* London: Methuen & Co., 1959.

Suppe, F. (ed.), *The Structure of Scientific Theories,* 2d ed. Urbana: University of Illinois Press, 1977.

Sutherland, N. S. Motives as Explanations. *Mind,* vol. 68(1959): 145–59.

Swartz, Louis. "Mental Disease": The Groundwork for Legal Analysis and Legislative Action. *University of Pennsylvania Law Review,* vol. 111(1963): 389–420.

Szasz, Thomas. The Concept of Mental Illness: Explanation or Justification? In H. T. Engelhardt and S. F. Spicker (eds.), *Mental Health: Philosophical Perspectives.* Dordrecht: Reidel, 1978. Reprinted in A. L. Caplan, H. T. Engelhardt, and J. J. McCartney (eds.), *Concepts of Health and Disease.* Reading, Mass.: Addison-Wesley, 1981.

Szasz, Thomas. *Ideology and Insanity: Essays on the Psychiatric Dehumanization of Man.* Garden City, N.Y.: Doubleday, 1970.

Szasz, Thomas. *The Manufacture of Madness.* New York: Harper & Row, 1970.

Szasz, Thomas. *Law, Liberty, and Psychiatry.* New York: Macmillan, 1968.

Szasz, Thomas. *Psychiatric Justice.* New York: Macmillan, 1965.

Szasz, Thomas. *The Myth of Mental Illness.* New York: Harper & Row, 1961.

Szasz, Thomas. Psychiatry, Ethics and the Criminal Law. *Columbia Law Review,* vol. 58(1958): 183–98.

Taylor, Charles. Responsibility for Self. In A. Rorty (ed.), *The Identities of Persons.* Berkeley: University of California Press, 1976.

Taylor, Charles. *The Explanation of Behavior.* New York: Humanities Press, 1964.

Taylor, F. K. A Logical Analysis of the Medicopsychological Concept of Disease. *Psychological Medicine,* vol. 1(1971): 356–65.

Taylor, Richard. *Action and Purpose.* Englewood Cliffs, N.J.: Prentice-Hall, 1966.

Taylor, W. S., and M. F. Martin. Multiple Personality. *Journal of Abnormal Social Psychology,* vol. 39(1944): 281–300.

Thalberg, Irving. *Perception, Emotion and Action.* New Haven, Conn.: Yale University Press, 1977.

Thalberg, Irving. Freud's Anatomies of the Self. In R. Wollheim (ed.), *Freud: A Collection of Critical Essays.* Garden City, N.Y.: Doubleday (Anchor Books), 1974.

Twining, William. *Karl Llewellyn and The Realist Movement.* London: Weidenfeld and Nicolson, 1973.

Urmson, J. O. *The Emotive Theory of Ethics.* Oxford: Oxford University Press, 1968.

Veatch, Robert. The Medical Model: Its Nature and Problems. *The Hastings Center Studies,* vol. 1(1973): 59–76. Reprinted in A. L. Caplan, H. T. Engelhardt, and J. J. McCartney (eds.), *Concepts of Health and Disease.* Reading, Mass.: Addison-Wesley, 1981.

Von Hirsch, Andrew. *Doing Justice: The Choice of Punishments.* New York: Hill and Wang, 1976.

Von Wright, George Hendrik. *Explanation and Understanding.* Ithaca, N.Y.: Cornell University Press, 1973.

References

Von Wright, George Hendrik. *The Varieties of Goodness.* London: Routledge & Kegan Paul, 1963.
Waelder, Robert. Psychiatry and the Problem of Criminal Responsibility. *University of Pennsylvania Law Review,* vol. 101(1952): 378–90.
Watson, Gary. Free Agency. *Journal of Philosophy,* vol. 72(1975): 205–20.
Watt, A. J. The Intelligibility of Wants. *Mind,* vol. 81(1972): 553–61.
Weihofen, Henry. The Definition of Mental Illness. *Ohio State Law Journal,* vol. 21(1960): 1–16.
White, G. *Patterns of American Legal Thought.* Indianapolis: Bobbs-Merrill, 1978.
White, Morton. *Foundations of Historical Knowledge.* New York: Harper & Row, 1965.
Whiteback, Caroline. A Theory of Health. In A. L. Caplan, H. T. Engelhardt, and J. J. McCartney (eds.), *Concepts of Health and Disease.* Reading, Mass.: Addison-Wesley, 1981.
Wiggins, David. *Sameness and Substance.* Cambridge, Mass.: Harvard University Press, 1980.
Wiggins, David. Locke, Butler and the Stream of Consciousness: And Men as Natural Kind. In A. Rorty (ed.), *The Identities of Persons.* Berkeley: University of California Press, 1976.
Wigmore, H. *Evidence,* vol. 1, 3d ed. Boston: Little Brown, 1940.
Williams, Bernard. *Problems of the Self.* Cambridge: Cambridge University Press, 1973.
Williams, Glanville. *Criminal Law: The General Part,* 2d ed. London: Stevens and Sons, 1961.
Williams, Michael. *Groundless Belief.* Princeton, N.J.: Princeton University Press, 1977.
Winch, Peter. *The Idea of a Social Science.* London: Routledge & Kegan Paul, 1958.
Wittgenstein, L. *Lectures and Conversations.* Berkeley: University of California Press, 1970.
Wittgenstein, Ludwig. *Philosophical Investigations,* 2d ed. Oxford: Blackwell Publisher, 1958.
Wollheim, Richard. *Sigmund Freud.* New York: Viking Press, 1971.
Wolman, B. B. *The Unconscious Mind.* Englewood Cliffs, N.J.: Prentice-Hall, 1968.
Wootton, Barbara. *Social Science and Social Pathology.* New York: Macmillan, 1959.
Wright, L. Functions. *Philosophical Review,* vol. 82(1973): 139–68.
Year Books of Edward II. *Year Book Series,* vol. 5. Edited by W. C. Ballard, F. W. Maitland, and L. W. V. Harcourt. London: Selden Society, 1909.

Index

accident, 4, 45, 67, 70, 110, 140, 311–14, 318, 321, 324, 346, 383, 438–9n103
accountability, 50, 51, 100, 140
action, 3, 4, 5, 9–16, 18–23, 26, 30–4, 42, 45, 47, 48, 50, 52–5, 57–9, 61, 63–85, 89, 96, 100–2, 105, 108, 109, 111, 117, 140–2, 145, 148, 161, 168, 173, 178, 180, 185, 194, 195, 225, 244, 253, 254, 262–4, 274–7, 279, 281, 288, 289, 291–6, 298, 300–1, 307, 308, 309, 311–14, 316, 318–27, 332–5, 339, 341, 345, 348, 349, 351–5, 359–63, 370, 371, 374, 378, 379, 382, 383, 392, 394, 395, 399, 402, 403, 424, 425, 454n39; basic, 68, 69, 72–7, 79, 80, 99, 108, 111, 148, 149, 151, 292, 293, 314–21, 332, 344, 361–3, 451n134, 473n44, 481n40; causal theory of, 71, 72, 74, 78; causes of, 11, 15, 20, 23, 31, 33, 36–7, 188, 232, 251; complex, 76, 77, 109, 111, 148, 173, 292, 293, 314, 319, 320, 322, 327, 344, 362; conscious, 315, 319, 326, 338, 339, 364, 382, 402; consciously executed, 31, 316, 319; consciously intentional, 4, 339, 383; consciously unintentional, 142, 339; free, 363; intelligible, 30, 196; intentional, 13, 47, 51, 52, 54, 59, 72, 76, 77, 79, 80, 87, 90, 108, 111, 124, 140, 142, 151, 262, 307, 310, 311, 321–33, 338, 339, 342, 345, 347, 350, 351, 365, 368, 369, 370, 372, 374, 377, 382, 383, 404; intentionally complex, 79–80, 109; involuntary, 58, 87, 225; irrational, 17, 162, 197; mental, 74, 340, 382, 413; minimally rational, 19; from motives, 47, 309; physical, 340; purposive, 37; rational, 15, 30, 170, 179, 197, 232, 299, 301, 365, 393; for reasons, 16, 22, 34, 75, 88, 92, 95, 96, 100, 101, 160, 163, 172, 226, 265, 295, 298, 299, 301, 319, 325, 335, 341, 342, 402, 404, 424; simple (*see also* basic), 56, 57, 68, 75; theory of, 16, 45, 77, 292, 293, 294; uncaused, 33, 352–4; unconscious, 315–17, 321, 325, 338–41, 382, 383, 394, 403, 479n26, 479–80n32; from unconscious motives, 265; unconsciously intentional, 323, 325, 326, 331, 338, 341; unintentional, 79, 83, 151, 262, 311, 312, 322, 323, 325, 338, 366, 383; voluntary, 53, 58, 59, 70, 194, 298, 321
action description, 68, 75, 76, 292, 310, 366, 369, 370, 478n23
action/intention predicates, 168, 366
actor, *see* agents
addiction, 108, 125, 202, 205, 364
Aeschylus, 381
affect, 277, 305, 307, 377, 378
agents (*see also* persons, as rational, autonomous agents), 2, 9, 10, 13, 14, 19–22, 24–6, 30–2, 50, 55, 58, 70–2, 74, 75, 96, 101, 102, 109, 161, 162, 197, 225, 262, 264, 402; accountable, 51, 52, 93, 99, 113, 140, 221, 222; autonomous, 2, 97, 100, 109, 111, 362, 423, 424, 425; free, 219; intelligent, 42, 301; irrational, 162, 366, 374, 383; moral, 2–3, 50, 61–6, 217, 244, 245; minimally rational, 160; nonaccountable, 113; nonmoral, 342; rational, 2, 10, 13, 19, 66, 83, 97, 100, 101, 106, 111, 114, 160, 244, 298, 373, 383, 394, 423, 424, 425; uncaused, 109; unified, 295, 387
aim *see* end; object, of instincts
akrasia, *see* will, weakness of
Alexander, Franz, 353
amentia, 297
American Law Institute, 219
American legal realism (*see also* functionalism, in law), 46, 47

514

Index

American Psychiatric Association, 200, 211, 215, 418
American Psychopathological Association, 416
Andrews, Judge, 46
animal, 22, 37, 51, 62, 63, 65, 66, 91, 93, 178, 218, 223, 245, 335, 373
animism, 26, 63, 245, 295, 359
Anscombe, G.E.M., 76, 77, 80, 334
anxiety, 302, 307, 330, 378
appetitive part of mind, 117, 144, 195
Aristotle, 13, 14, 27, 72, 85, 87, 95, 110, 117, 118, 119, 206, 208, 221, 391
Arlow, Jacob, 144
artificial intelligence, 21, 35, 145, 277, 278, 392, 413, 414, 425
ascriptivism, 45, 47
attempt, 331–4, 335, 336, 337, 339, 341, 347, 350, 369, 371, 372, 373, 383; conscious, 338; unconscious, 334, 335, 337, 338, 340, 383
Austin, J.L., 116, 179
Austin, John, 71, 72
autonomy, 5, 62, 95, 100, 108–12, 126, 145, 196, 353, 361, 362, 383, 403, 416, 423, 425
average reasonable person, 57, 58, 83, 84, 111–12.
Ayer, A.J., 362

Balmuth, J., 300, 337
basic actions, *see* action, basic
Bazelon, David, 224, 231, 244
Bedau, Hugo, 242
behavior (*see also* action), 9, 14, 18, 19, 22, 25, 32, 33, 35–9, 41, 43, 61, 119, 147, 158, 160, 161, 164, 167, 168, 171, 172, 174, 183, 184, 196, 213, 219, 251, 254, 255, 257–9, 263, 265, 266, 268, 270, 271, 283, 285, 299, 300, 311, 313, 316, 317, 319, 322, 324, 336, 337, 341, 343, 347, 349, 353, 355, 363, 364, 366, 373, 378, 383, 396, 397, 402, 403, 404, 405, 406, 407, 420, 424, 425; accidental, 313; causation of, 1, 16, 35, 39, 171, 225, 231, 352, 356–60, 364, 379, 380, 382, 393, 394, 403, 425; goal directed, 28, 40, 159, 161, 162; human, theory of, 21, 232, 271; intentional, 22; involuntary, 46, 298, 300, 307; irrational, 115, 205, 207; meaningful, 173, 292; minimally rational, 160; motivated, 40, 159, 313, 364; neurotic, 299, 337; nonconsciously directed, 73, 74; purposive, 39, 160; rational, 160, 206, 208, 245; rule following, 20, 43, 161, 162; theory of, 201, 250, 272, 352, 381, 417; unintelligible, 196; violent, 123; voluntary, 40, 42, 307
behavioral construct, *see* entities
behaviorism, 2, 23, 33, 36–8, 70, 146, 148, 162, 184, 257, 261, 268–70, 359, 363, 364, 381, 382, 414; logical, 36, 138, 167, 183; methodological, 36; philosophical, 36–9; radical, 249, 251, 425
belief, 9, 12, 13, 15, 16, 19, 20, 22, 24, 30, 31, 34–9, 41, 42, 55, 58, 64, 71, 72, 85, 86, 88, 93, 100, 104–6, 107, 165, 168, 174, 176, 183, 215, 223, 245, 256–62, 264, 265, 288, 293–5, 297–301, 307, 308, 311, 314, 325, 326, 328, 330, 334–8, 362, 363, 364, 367, 378, 383, 389, 403, 408, 418, 419; behavioral sense of, 329, conscious, 135, 161, 258, 265, 337, 367, 375, 376, 401; delusional, 418, 419; factual, 105, 106, 207, 209; inconsistent, 105, 389; intelligible, 105, 390; irrational, 10, 19, 162, 163, 164, 207, 208, 299, 300, 302, 326, 328, 373, 419; means/ends, 105, 313, 324; mistaken, 367, 368; moral, 13, 101–4, 106, 207, 208, 372; obsessive, 377; ontological status of, 23–5; paranoid, 419; rational, 19, 20, 66, 95, 101, 102, 104–6, 160, 163, 178, 197, 245, 325; repressed, 134, 337; unconscious, 161, 162, 164, 257, 258, 264, 301, 317, 335–7, 339, 341, 367, 368, 375, 376, 383, 452n22; unintelligible, 168
belief/desire set, 10–12, 14–19, 22, 23, 32, 61, 63, 71, 72, 74, 75, 77, 78, 81, 101, 110, 145, 160, 162, 197, 293, 294, 300–2, 314, 354, 362, 370
Benedict, Ruth, 121
Benn, Stanley, 92, 95
Bentham, Jeremy, 77–9, 92, 222
Bernheim, 316
Beverly's case, 66
Blackstone, 63
blame, 5, 45, 46, 50–2, 58, 63, 110, 142, 202, 223, 234, 244, 342, 352, 361, 373
Bleuler, Manfred, 175, 178
Blumenfeld, David, 379, 380
body, 135, 165, 170, 173, 184, 187–93, 206, 208, 209, 252, 277, 279, 316, 348, 352; number of persons per, 387, 392, 396, 398, 399, 403, 405, 410; structure, 186
Bonnie, Richard, 359
Boorse, Christopher, 115, 192, 431–2n54
Bracton, 66
Braginsky, B.M., 159, 160, 161, 162
Braginsky, O.D., 159
brain, 34, 36, 139, 174, 225, 226, 231,

515

Index

brain (cont.)
254, 277–9, 328, 393, 397, 403, 413, 415, 425; disease, 188, 195, 224, 226; events, 25, 166, 172, 174; physiology, 261, 278, 280, 284, 413, 425; processes, 271; states, 34, 35, 38, 136, 138, 349, 361, 418

Brenner, Charles, 144
Brentano, Franz, 23, 135
Brown, Norman, 142
Burger, Warren, 229

Camus, Albert, 74
capacity to reason, *see* reasoning faculty
Cardozo, Benjamin, 60
Carnap, Rudolph, 37
categorical imperative, 62
category difference, 37, 120, 166, 171–3, 275, 276, 354, 355, 432n62
category mistake, 35, 64, 164, 165, 166, 169, 171, 172, 180, 272, 354
causal agency, 70, 73, 95, 100, 108, 109, 114, 138, 145, 146, 196, 250, 394, 397; personal, 55, 56, 70, 72, 75, 225, 292, 314, 316, 317, 362
causal connection, 30, 31, 50, 55, 232, 271, 290; between dreaming and sleeping, 287, 288, 289; between functional processes and end states, 27, 288, 308, 392; between mental states and behavior, 258, 265, 321, 324, 394; between physiological states and actions, 354
causal laws, 27, 352, 353, 354, 362, 423
causal order, 362
causal powers, 72, 99, 108, 109, 114, 146, 147, 249, 361, 362, 394, 395, 423, 424
causal relations, 32, 57, 72, 358
causation, 50, 51–9, 71–2, 80, 81, 109, 111, 189, 192, 214, 230, 231, 264, 290, 303, 331, 334, 335, 355, 356, 359, 360, 361, 364, 365, 373, 374; degrees of, 356, 357, 358, 360; event or state, 55, 72, 362; mental state, 75, 77, 293, 294, 314, 325, 347, 351, 359, 370, 393; physical theory of, 231; predisposing, 356, 357, 358; psychological theory of, 231
cause, 4, 12, 32, 309, 382; of action, 11, 15, 18, 23, 31, 36, 147, 173, 188, 263, 316, 325, 335, 355, 361, 376, 395, 399; of behavior, 16, 35, 39, 43, 140, 147, 172, 174, 178, 225, 226, 230, 251, 270, 290, 353, 363, 364, 365, 379, 382, 403, 425; behavioristic, 360; direct, 57, 59; of dream content, 284, 290, 302–5, 307, 308, 318; of dreaming, 309, 313, 314; of events, 15, 292, 294, 309; external, 272, 361; environmental, 36, 363, 364, 425; factual, 54–8; final, 27; of harm, 331, 332, 339, 343, 346; internal, 361; intervening, 58, 59; mechanical, 32, 33, 37, 165, 166, 171, 173, 226, 231, 232, 281, 354, 383; mental, 16, 165, 195, 211, 219, 282, 354, 382, 428n13; of mental illness, 195; motivational, 291; paramechanical, 166, 171, 232, physical, 40, 170, 186, 187–8, 195, 211, 225, 226, 349, 418; physiological, 272, 360; proximate, 46, 54, 57–9; psychoanalytic, 360; superseding, 58

censor, 114, 267, 307, 395, 401, 404
character, 52, 83, 88, 89, 103, 106, 107, 109–11, 309, 345, 347, 361, 363, 364, 380, 397, 399, 401, 405, 406, 407, 424; acting in, 397, 405; acting out of, 111, 405; intelligible, 390, 391, 397, 401, 404, 405, 407; radically disunified, 406, 411; structure, 103, 146, 390, 400, 404, 407; traits, 171, 172, 185, 196, 363, 409, 410
children, 51, 62, 64–6, 84, 93, 96, 99, 178, 218, 221, 223, 235, 245, 342, 345, 373, 406
choice (*see also* action; determinism; volition), 84, 87, 89, 91–3, 107, 178, 349, 352, 354, 361–3, 365, 375, 378, 379, 383, 440n122; capacity for, 225, 355; free, 352–4; purposive, 355; rational, 93, 160
Chomsky, Noam, 139
Cioffi, Frank, 317, 320
civil commitment, 155, 217
Coke, Lord, 64, 66
Collingwood, R.G., 21
community of subagents, *see* person, as community of selves
compatibilism, *see* determinism, soft
complex action, *see* action, complex; action, intentionally complex
compulsion, 361, 363–5, 373, 375, 380, 381, 383; inner psychological, 110, 214, 330, 333, 351, 376–9, 422; as legal or moral excuse, 65, 86, 88, 89, 108, 111, 221–3, 230, 330, 362, 374; unconscious, 272
computer, 21, 22, 414
concepts, 2, 5, 9, 36, 41, 349; biological, 269; legal, 3, 44, 45, 47, 60; medical, 115; mental, 2, 26, 254; moral, 3, 47, 60, 115, 120, 124, 349; observational, 272; personal, 2; physical, 277; physiological, 36; psychological, 35–6, 211, 269; theoretical, 272

516

Index

conflict, intrapersonal, 136, 137, 143, 387–91, 393, 394, 401, 413, 415, 417, 422; irrational, 102; phenomenology of, 414, 415; principles for subdividing the mind, 390, 393, 397, 399, 400, 401, 411, 413

consciousness, 126, 136, 143, 144, 149, 161–3, 252–4, 267, 273, 274, 278, 279, 298, 339, 341, 372, 382, 399, 400; as awareness, 317, 413; of matters of fact, 128, 340; of one's behavior, 251, 341; of one's mental states, 127, 128, 129, 131–3, 252, 254, 260, 263, 265, 272, 283, 299, 316, 403; part of mind, 399, 411; as process, 253; as state of an individual (stream of consciousness), 126, 127, 130, 135, 141, 145, 152, 256, 339, 396, 399

contents, 37; of beliefs and desires, 10–11, 13, 14, 16, 24, 160, 261, 297; of brain states, 35; of dreams (see also dreams), 282, 285, 286, 290, 291, 296, 302, 303, 308, 343; of mental states, 148, 261, 269, 289, 389; of mind, 128, 137, 185

contract law, 57, 60, 99, 103, 108, 110

corporate self, see self, as a corporation of subpersonal agents

corporation, 46, 47, 62–5.

crazy, see insanity, as madness or craziness, the common view

criminal conduct, see behavior, criminal

criminal law, 3, 52–4, 57, 60, 61, 68, 73, 77, 79–83, 86, 87, 103, 104, 106, 108, 126, 151, 194, 217, 218, 220, 221, 223, 233, 243, 245, 329, 331, 332, 334, 353, 364, 420

culpability, 51, 53, 54, 62, 64, 79, 83, 84, 86, 90, 151, 221, 245, 329, 331, 332, 342, 366, 369, 370, 372; legal, 64, 80, 81, 104, 125; moral, 52, 64, 77, 244

Danto, Arthur, 68
Davidson, Donald, 12, 56–7
defense mechanism, 402, 409, 413
definition, 200, 201, 202, 204; descriptive, 200; lexical, 182, 198, 203; normative, 200; ostensive, 157; stipulative, 182, 198, 199, 203, 205
Dennett, Daniel, 21, 22, 274, 275, 328, 392, 414
Dershowitz, Alan, 372
Descartes, 164, 183, 254
desert, 142, 235, 236, 237, 240, 243–5, 340
desire (see also wish), 9, 12, 13, 15, 16, 20, 22, 26, 30, 31, 34, 35, 37–9, 41, 42, 55, 64, 71, 72, 74, 89, 106, 107, 109, 111, 143, 147, 168, 174, 195, 215, 254–62, 264, 265, 290, 293, 296, 299, 301, 307, 311, 314, 318, 322, 324–6, 328, 335, 337, 347, 362, 363, 364, 366, 371, 372, 376, 377, 380, 390, 391, 403; compulsive, 378; conflicting, 389; conscious, 133, 258, 381, 401; intelligible, 10, 19, 20, 95, 102, 160, 197, 206, 207, 216; irrational, 373; ontological status of, 23–5; rational, 101–4, 197; repressed, 306, 337, 379; second-order, 109–10, 152, 300; transitive ordering of, 103, 105, 160, 206, 207, 408; unconscious, 140, 161, 162, 164, 197, 250, 258, 264, 273, 311, 312, 333, 350, 351, 368, 370, 373, 379, 380, 381, 393–6, 402, 452n22; unintelligible, 19, 168, 207

determinism, 1, 33, 35, 36, 114, 115, 174, 231, 282, 342, 352–5, 357, 358, 360, 362, 373, 421, 442n3, 488–9n45; hard, 349, 352, 355, 357, 360, 380; psychiatric, 1, 115; psychic, 232; selective, 355; soft, 361

deterrence (see also punishment), 233, 236, 241, 242

deviant causal chain, 72, 294

Dew v. Clark, 221

Dewey, John, 45

diagnostic categories, 417

Diamond, Bernard, 352

Dilman, Ilham, 272–5

Dilthey, Wilhelm, 21

diminished capacity defense, 222, 365, 416n15

disease, 116, 119, 125, 157, 174, 187, 188, 189, 191, 192, 193, 194, 200, 213, 218, 225, 226, 227, 230, 231, 418, 419, 456–7n11; disability as a criterion of, 194, 211, 214–16; disadvantage as a criterion of, 211, 213–15; distress as a criterion of, 211, 214–16

displacement, see dream work

disposition, 36–8, 128, 148, 165, 171, 183, 214, 232, 249, 254, 261, 326, 353

dissociation, 364, 368, 410

distortion, see dream work

disunity of self, see self, disunity of

Doe, Justice, 223–8

Dostoevsky, Fyodor, 250, 252, 254

Dray, William, 21

dream memories, 283, 305

dream work, 285, 297, 302–4, 320, 402, 410, 476n79; as a process, 285, 303–6, 308

dreams, 20, 138, 140, 141, 143, 282–309, 311–15, 317, 318, 322, 333, 336, 338, 340, 343–5, 347, 348, 382, 394, 396,

517

Index

dreams (cont.)
401–3, 471n20, 474n53; anxiety, 303, 318, 336; causal theory of, 306; of convenience, 293; counterwish, 295, 296, 303; etiology of, 382; as expressions of wishes, 301–3, 402, 403; Freud's theory of, 280, 282–7, 298, 301–3, 311, 314, 402; function of, 288, 289, 309, 324; latent thoughts, 283–5, 290, 291, 304, 306, 307; manifest content of, 283–5, 290, 291, 303–6, 401, 403; meaning of, 290, 302, 335; physiology of, 280, 305; psychoanalytic theory of, 4, 281, 282, 288, 303; punishment, 303

Dreiser, Theodore, 89, 294, 327
drives, 39, 274, 353, 364, 377, 383, 412; instinctual, 40–3, 123, 231, 364, 365, 422; primitive, 33; unconscious, 141, 351, 365

Droysen, 21
dualism, 148, 165, 254; Cartesian, 164, 167, 183; Kantian, 354; linguistic, 354; metaphysical, 254
duress, 108, 151, 219, 221, 223, 379
Durham experiment, *see* insanity tests
Durham v. United States, 223, 224, 228, 230, 231, 244
duty, 59–60, 91–3, 342; legal, 51, 92; moral, 51
dysfunction, *see* functional impairment
dyscontrol, 123

Eagle, Morris, 391, 394, 395
egalitarianism, 94, 96
ego, 114, 119, 123, 143–7, 149, 151, 267, 294, 295, 343, 353, 359, 390–3, 400, 401, 404, 406, 407, 410–15
egoism, 151, 152
emotion, 89, 112, 184, 252, 257, 259, 314, 346, 354, 363, 377–9, 381, 389, 390, 418; conflicting, 389, 400; rationality of, 107; unconscious, 330, 377, 378
emotional appreciation, 329, 330, 368
emotional states, 110, 208, 298, 347
emotivism, 46, 47, 179
empiricism, 416
end, 12, 13, 20, 27, 74, 75, 104, 117, 178, 198, 209, 260, 328, 331, 333, 334, 374, 394; intelligible, 13, 19, 66, 101, 102, 105; irrational, 197
end state, 26–32, 190, 192, 193, 208, 210, 213, 215, 287, 288, 392
energy, 42, 43, 123, 274; drive, 40; Freud's theory, 135; instinctual, 144; psychic, 39, 40, 41, 42, 231, 300, 301; psychological, 122
entities, abstract, 157, 158; behavioral constructs, 250, 270; concrete, 157; differences in ontological status of, 165, 250; fictional, 270; mental, 174; ontological status of mental, 164, 165, 167, 455–6n3; theoretical, 183, 250, 271–3, 276, 298

epistemic claims, 185, 255–6, 266
epistemic features, 254, 291, 325
epistemological relativity, 176
epistemology, 106, 175, 177, 180
Epstein, Richard, 98
equality, *see* rights, to equality
ethical relativism, 120
ethics, 181, 191, 192, 210, 243; naturalist, 117–19, 191; objectivist, 116, 117, 120, 207, 208, 235
excuse, 3, 51, 52, 79, 84–90; legal, 1, 65, 84–90, 100, 105, 108, 110, 141, 151, 218, 219, 223, 224, 226–31, 233, 243, 244, 245, 341, 351, 356, 358–60, 362, 364, 366, 367, 373, 374, 378–80, 383; moral, 1, 85, 141, 145, 177, 220–4, 226, 230, 231, 243–5, 341, 351, 356, 358, 359, 362, 364, 366, 373–5, 379, 380, 383
existential psychiatry, 175
experience, 258, 259; childhood, 354, conscious, 253, 254, 318, 348, 378; mental, 168, 185, 186, 254; of inner phenomenology, 127, 129
explanation, 2, 4, 17, 18, 20, 22, 26–9, 32, 33, 270, 298, 309; action/intention mode of, 168; behaviorist, 36; causal, 15, 21, 39–40, 89, 198, 303, 305, 309, 314; Freudian, 298, 299, 300, 313, 335, 376; functional, 2, 26, 27, 29, 32, 282, 285, 287, 288, 314; hermeneutic interpretation as, 2, 15, 22; historical, 21; in terms of the unconscious, 161; mechanistic, 32–3, 36, 39, 43; mental cause, 2, 15, 16, 18, 89, 285, 347; mental state, 311, 314, 324; mentalistic, 35, 36; motivational, 10, 15–16, 30, 266, 281, 282, 285–8, 291, 294, 298, 303, 308, 309; neurophysiological, 34–5, 36; nonmechanistic, 171; nonmotivational, causal, 291; physiological, 174; probabilistic, 356, 357; psychoanalytic, 4, 5, 281, 298, 299, 309, 313, 314, 335, 337, 356, 370; reason-giving, 2, 9–15, 16–23, 25–6, 30–7, 39, 43, 71, 74, 75, 79, 80, 81, 100, 101, 105, 173, 174, 196, 298, 301, 313, 324, 376, 425; teleological, 23, 26, 39; unconscious mental state, 313, 314, 332, 335, 351, 356, 365, 366, 368, 382, 383, 424
extended memory, *see* memory, extended
extensional language, 173, 275, 430n48

518

Index

Fairbairn, W. Ronald D., 414
fantasy, 285, 286, 295–7, 299, 301–3, 308, 336, 344, 483n79
feeling, 252, 273
Field, G.C., 254
Fingarette, Herbert, 382
Fisher v. Dillingham, 315
Fletcher, George, 45, 84, 87
Flew, Antony, 298, 300, 382
forces, 274, 336, 352
forensic psychiatry, 224, 422
Frankfurt, Harry, 110
free association, 257, 283, 290, 291, 295, 302, 303
freedom, 354, 356, 365, 379, 425; degrees of, 357, 373; as uncaused agency, 361, 362, 373
Frege, Gottlob, 158, 278
French, Peter, 64, 90
Freud, Sigmund, 4, 12, 20, 35, 39, 40, 41, 43, 113, 115, 118, 119, 122, 126, 127, 129–40, 142–7, 201, 250, 252–5, 257, 262, 263, 265–72, 276–80, 282–5, 287–92, 294–8, 300–8, 310–14, 316, 318–26, 328, 329, 332, 333, 335, 338, 340, 341, 343, 344, 346, 347, 359, 364, 370, 372, 374–8, 382, 383, 387, 388, 390–7, 399–404, 407, 409, 411–16, 419, 425
Freudian psychoanalytic theory, 126, 266, 267
Freudians, 35, 41, 119, 122, 139, 146, 149, 292, 294, 332, 343, 352, 376, 402
Friedemann, Max, 214
Fromm, Erich, 117–20, 123, 179, 201, 204, 205, 206, 209
Fuller, Gary, 336
Fuller, Lon, 60–2, 92–3
function, 4, 27, 28, 30, 31; aggregation of, 147; assignments, 193, 208, 412, 413, 457–8n15; as effect (contrast end), 96, 190; natural, 193; statements, 28, 30, 431–2n54
function/structure correlation (*see also* mind/brain correlations), 393, 403
functional attributions, 26, 28, 30, 31, 285, 287, 288
functional explanations, *see* explanation, functional
functional impairment, 189, 192, 193, 195, 206, 207, 209, 210, 215, 457–8n15; behavioral, 215; mental, 208; of the organism, 211, 213, 216; psychological, 215
functional organization, 28, 29, 146, 147, 206, 209, 215, 278, 392, 393, 412, 413, 414, 415, 417

functionalism, as a theory of mind, 35, 136, 145, 148, 167, 183, 258, 392; in law, 46, 47

Garfinkel, Alan, 33, 35
gatekeepers, 267, 395
Genesis, 64
Gide, André, 74
Glueck, Sheldon, 355, 373
Goldman, Alvin, 71, 72, 293, 294
Goldstein, Abraham, 219
Goldstein, Kurt, 118
good, collective or social, 236; full theory of, 209, 210, 216; for humans, 117, 118, 191, 422; life, 208, 210; thin theory of, 191, 208, 209, 210, 215, 216, 459–60n46.
Group for the Advancement of Psychiatry, 228
Grunbaum, Adolf, 280
guardians, 404

Hale, Sir Matthew, 66
Hand, Learned, 82, 83, 315
happiness, 117, 119, 120, 190, 201, 206
Hare, R.M., 119
harm, 45, 47, 50–8, 62, 65, 80, 81, 82, 104, 105, 151, 236, 240, 310, 311, 331, 339, 341, 343, 346, 373
Hart, H.L.A., 45, 49–51, 58–9, 71, 79, 83, 92, 341, 342, 352
Hartmann, Heinz, 119, 146
health, 29, 115, 116, 119, 120, 122, 155, 167, 186, 190, 194, 443n7; expansive view of, 118, 210, 267; as goodness, 113, 116, 118, 124, 191, 210; as human flourishing, 116, 118, 190; as not being ill, 190, 191; physical, 209, 392; psychological, 118; as proper functioning, 190, 191, 209, 210; as a system's end state, 28, 208, 287, 288, 308, 392;
Hebraic Law, 66
Heidegger, Martin, 110
Hempel, Carl, 21, 27, 356
Herbert, A.P. 111
hermeneutic interpretation (*see also* explanation, hermeneutic interpretation as), 22, 203
Hohfeld, W., 44, 60
Holmes, O.W., 62–3, 70
homeostatic balance (*see also* end state), 29, 193, 392
homuncili, *see* subpersonal agents
Honore, A.M., 58–9
Horney, Karen, 118
Hospers, John, 351, 352, 361, 363, 364
Hull, Clark, 37

519

Index

Hume, David, 54, 57, 72, 74, 144, 290
hysteria, 161, 166, 170, 171, 172, 321, 322, 332

id, 114, 119, 143–7, 149, 151, 267, 294, 295, 337, 343, 359, 390, 391, 399, 401, 404, 406, 407, 410, 411, 412, 414, 415
idealism, 165
identity, numerical, 398, 404; of personalities, 404; qualitative, 398, 399, 404, 405; personal, 399, 400, 407, 408
identity of indiscernibles principle, 404
ignorance, 65, 85, 86, 222, 223, 230, 341, 366, 367, 368, 380, 395; emotional, 368; of fact, 221; of law, 221; veil of, 209
illness (*see also* mental illness), 116, 119, 121–5, 155, 161, 167, 168, 170, 174, 182, 191, 201–4, 207, 208, 211, 216, 217, 229, 232, 422, 443n7, 456–7n11, 457–8n15; as badness, 113, 120, 121, 191; expansive view of, 115, 210, 267; functional, 188; ordinary concept of, 186–95, 205, 213; physical, 157, 169, 173, 188, 229; physically caused, 166; unhappiness as, 118
incompetency, 155, 181
incorrigibility, 185, 225, 256, 261–5, 317
indeterminism, 109, 110
infallibility, *see* incorrigibility
inference (*see also* practical reasoning, practical syllogism), 13, 14, 17, 21, 22, 62, 64, 65, 106, 278, 325, 328, 330, 342, 348, 367, 381
information processing, 328, 348, 403
Ingber, Stanley, 46
insane human beings, 51, 64, 65, 66, 93, 96, 99, 101, 177, 178, 223, 233, 235, 243, 244, 245, 342, 359, 373, 374
insanity (*see also* mental illness; madness), 49, 121, 175, 176–8, 183, 218, 225, 227, 421; definition of legal, 220, 222, 223, 225, 226, 227, 229, 230, 243, 245, 422; legal, 65, 66, 219, 220, 221, 222, 224, 228, 229, 230; legal concept of, 3, 217–246; legal definition of, 422; as madness or craziness, the common view, 3, 176, 198, 245; psychiatric definition of, 232, 233
insanity defense, 66, 156, 181, 218, 225, 228, 244, 329, 365, 377, 421
insanity tests, 155, 218–20, 245; American Law Institute test, 219–20, 222, 230; *Durham* test (District of Columbia), 220, 223, 224, 228, 229, 230, 232; good and evil test, 64, 66; irresistible impulse test, 119, 220, 221, 222, 224, 230, 377, 422; M'Naghten test (rules), 66, 218–24, 226, 230, 245, 329; New Hampshire test, 220, 223, 224, 232
instinct, 43, 122, 123, 134–6, 138, 139, 143, 377, 382, 391, 401; Freud's theory of, 39–41, 135, 136, 400, 413; repressed, 142, 280
instinctual drives, *see* drives, instinctual
intelligent functioning, 138, 139, 144, 168, 169, 250, 277, 397, 403.
intention, 3, 34, 44, 47, 48, 52, 53, 59, 71, 75–7, 81, 100, 102, 103, 105, 140, 143, 145, 148, 168, 183, 209, 223, 255, 256, 264, 282, 287, 291, 292, 294, 311, 313, 341, 343, 400, 489–90n55; causal theory of, 78; conscious, 141, 142, 254, 338, 339; purposive theory of, 78; reflexive, 99, theory of, 77, 78; unconscious, 141, 325, 339, 340, 383
Intentional discourse, 38, 173, 261, 381, 382, 425
intentionality, 21, 79, 222, 226, 324, 365
Intentionality, 274, 275, 277, 354, 430n.46,47
interests, 93, 96, 152
interpretation (*see also* explanation, hermeneutic interpretation as), 4, 18, 19, 20, 22; of action, 335; of behavior, 314; of beliefs and desires, 25, 26, of dreams, 291, 313, 318; meaning, 20, 21; non-causal, 21; of utterances, 25, 26
irrationality (*see also* appetitive part of mind), 115, 159, 160, 178, 179, 206, 207, 214, 215, 244, 245, 278, 299, 326, 365, 373, 389
irresistible impulse test, *see* insanity tests

James, William, 360
Jellinek, E., 200
Jones, Ernest, 12
just deserts, 3, 237, 238, 240, 241, 394
justice, 46, 240; corrective, 48; distributive, 149, 152, 235; social, 155; theory of, 208
justification, 2, 12, 51, 52, 84, 91, 94, 95, 107, 151, 221

Kant, Immanuel, 62, 95
Katz, Wilbur, 355
Kepler, 363
Klein, Donald, 124
kleptomaniac, 174, 213, 214, 378, 379
knowledge (*see also* privileged access; emotional appreciation; self-intimation), 73–4, 85, 86, 105, 106, 259, 326, 329, 338, 339, 365, 395, 403; behavioral sense of, 328; of causal connections, 258, 264,

Index

357; conscious, 315, 321, 322, 325, 342, 361, 366, 383; factual, 342; first-person, of mental states, 37, 162, 184, 255, 263, 264, 307; of good and evil, 64; of mental states, 34, 255, 256, 262, 402; moral, 219, 221, 222, 223, 342; noninferential, 128, 256, 274; nonobservational, 128, 129, 257, 361; objective, 176, 331; propositional, 329, 330, 368; third-person, of mental states, 255; unconscious, 315, 321, 325, 326, 338, 341, 361
Kohut, Heinz, 408, 415
Korsakoff's syndrome, 170

labeling theory, 120, 121
Ladd, John, 64
LaFave, W.F., 81
Laing, R.D. 162, 163, 175, 177, 408
Laird, J., 254
language of thought, 25
latent dream thoughts, *see* dreams, latent thoughts
law of torts, 52–4, 57, 59, 60, 73, 79, 81–3, 188, 217
legal persons, *see* persons, legal
legal realism, *see* American legal realism
legal responsibiity, *see* responsibility, legal
Leibniz, Gottfried, 404
Leibniz's Law, 399
Levin, David, 157, 175, 251, 252
Levin, Judge, 353
Lewis, C.S., 235
liability, 2, 50, 51, 53, 63, 80, 84, 110, 111; legal, 2, 44, 48, 49, 51–4, 57, 61, 62, 70, 77, 83, 124, 141, 151, 222, 229, 341, 371
libertarianism, 94
liberty, *see* rights, to liberty
linguistic turn, 254, 354
linguistics, 139, 278
"little agents," *see* subpersonal agents
"little people," *see* subpersonal agents
Locke, John, 44, 56, 72, 98, 99, 108, 149, 316, 348, 405, 408
logic, 10, 13, 14, 85, 278
logical positivism, *see* positivism
Louch, A.R., 12
Louisell, David, 352

McDonald v. United States, 230, 462n35
MacIntyre, Alisdair, 270
Mackie, J.L., 71, 72
madness (*see also* insanity; mental illness), 198, 207, 215, 313; the extended view, 3, 124, 126, 155, 204
Malcolm, Norman, 37

mandatory commitment statutes, 244
Margolis, Joseph, 193
Maslow, Abraham, 118
materialism, 148, 167
Matte-Blanco, I., 278
May, Rollo, 118
meaning, 19, 116, 121, 179, 194, 203, 204, 230, 275, 276, 281, 282, 283; of an action, 20; of behavior, 18, 313, 314; of concepts, 44, 46; of dreams, 284, 290, 291, 302, 304, 305, 335; of illness, disease or disorder, 212, 213; of mental terms, 256, 257, 259, 266; theory of, 38, 257, 258
means/end calculation, *see* practical reasoning
mechanism, 33, 35, 37
mechanistic explanation, *see* explanation, mechanistic
medicine, 115, 126, 191, 192, 210
Melden, A.I., 20, 76, 97
memory, 66, 133, 134, 138, 170, 257, 283, 290, 295, 304, 305, 307, 315–18, 320, 324, 335, 338, 348, 361, 400, 408, 478n26; extended, 134, 137, 139, 141, 162, 250, 257, 260, 273, 317, 325, 326, 329, 338, 339, 341, 342, 348, 359, 402, 403, 413, 442n2, 482–3n76
Menninger, Karl, 119, 122, 123, 204, 205, 352
mental cause explanation, *see* explanation, mental cause
mental defect, 220, 225, 228, 229, 230
mental disease (*see also* mental illness), 119, 156, 172, 193, 198, 200, 211, 215, 219, 220, 224, 225, 227–30, 417, 418; deviance as, 120–4
mental entities, *see* entities, mental
mental health, 115, 122, 159, 177, 179, 201, 208, 210, 392, 444n18; as human flourishing, 113, 116, 117, 201; moral goodness as, 116–20, 179
mental illness (*see also* mental disease), 46, 47, 65, 66, 121, 122, 124, 155–60, 162, 164, 166–71, 173–5, 177–82, 184–6, 188, 206, 207, 208, 211, 215, 216, 218–32, 243, 245, 275, 417, 419, 457n12, 459–60n46; extended psychiatric view of, 249; legal definition of, 217, 224, 228, 232, 233, 244, 424; moral badness as, 114, 116, 120, 122, 123; ontological status of, 156–9; ordinary concept of, 184, 186, ;195–8, 209, 210, 232; psychiatric definition of, 3, 198–204, 205, 224, 233, 424; as social deviance, 113, 121;
mental life, 267, 279, 351, 388, 402

Index

mental processes, 266, 271, 275, 417
mental representation (*see also* object), 135, 269, 270
mental states (*see also* knowledge, of mental states), 2, 12, 15, 21, 23, 32, 35–8, 43, 50, 52–4, 67, 71, 77–84, 115, 126, 129, 131, 137, 138, 139, 141, 148, 152, 183–5, 208, 253, 256, 258, 260–2, 266, 269, 273, 274, 277–9, 293, 294, 301, 302, 311, 314, 324, 326, 327, 329, 332, 334, 348, 349, 371, 372, 388, 389, 404, 408, 409, 415; aggregation of, 136, 390–3, 397, 399, 400, 402, 405, 411, 412; conflicting, 136, 140, 143, 144, 336, 372, 388, 389, 390, 391, 393, 394, 397, 400, 409; conscious, 129, 139, 251, 255, 260, 272, 278, 317, 349, 393, 411; ego-alien, 143, 391, 393, 401, 408, 410; function of, 391, 392, 398, 400, 411, 412; as functional states, 254, 258; ontological status of, 254; as physical states, 254; unconscious, 67, 129, 131–6, 138–40, 142, 250–8, 260, 261, 265, 266, 267, 269, 272, 276, 280, 310, 312, 322, 324, 325, 331, 332, 334, 335, 336, 344, 345, 349, 351, 359, 365, 366, 368, 370–4, 377, 379, 381–3, 388, 393–6, 400, 401, 402, 409, 410, 490n62
mental terms, 38, 165, 173, 183, 184, 253, 254, 255, 257, 260, 291, 330, 337
mentalistic language, 146, 184, 195, 260, 274, 275, 276, 281, 382
Merleau-Ponty, Maurice, 251
metaphysics, 147, 152, 254, 277, 349, 398, 399, 405, 420, 421
metapsychology, 271, 272, 273, 275, 373, 419, 425 developmental (*see also* metapsychology, genetic), 138, 266–71; dynamic, 41, 43, 134, 136, 137, 139, 140, 271, 272, 382, 402; economic, 41, 43, 139, 271, 272, 274, 377, 382, 383, 402, 413; Freud's, 122, 130, 201, 250, 267, 268, 274, 276, 277, 278, 279, 280, 295, 364; genetic (*see also* metapsychology, developmental), 138, 268, 270, 279; Intentionalistic, 274; structural, 143, 146, 147, 271, 372, 387, 391, 393, 397, 400, 410–13; topographical, 134, 136, 137, 139, 143, 271, 272, 297, 372, 387, 393, 397, 400, 410–13
methodological behaviorism, *see* behaviorism, methodological
Miles, T.R., 270
Mill, John Stuart, 31, 71, 72, 96
mind (*see also* dualism), 1, 2, 25, 31, 112, 116, 117, 119, 128, 135, 137, 143, 144, 166–9, 174, 183, 185, 203, 208, 219, 225, 229, 252, 255, 256, 272, 277, 278, 317, 392, 415; artificial intelligence view of, 414–15; functional organization of, 5, 136, 146, 206, 208, 209, 215, 337, 387, 393, 413; as functional states of a physical system, 167, 183; functional subdivision of, 145, 146, 404; legal view of, 2, 4, 112, 126, 137, 139, 140, 249, 267; ontological status of, 165, 166, 183; ordinary meaning of, 182–6, 261; psychiatric theory of, 2; sick, 166, 167, 184; state of, 30, 50, 81–4, 255, 324, 332, 367; theory of, 1, 2, 35, 254, 258, 271, 273, 274, 275, 279, 422
mind/body problem, 148, 413, 418
mind/body relationship, 184, 254, 278, 279, 398, 406, 413, 415
mind/brain correlations (*see also* function/structure correlations), 139
mind/brain identity, 139, 183
Mischel, Theodore, 299, 313
mistake, 341, 366, 367, 368
Mittelmann, Bela, 118
M'Naghten case, *see Regina v. M'Naghten*
M'Naghten test, *see* insanity tests
Model Penal Code, 70, 86, 219, 367
Molière, 284
Moore, G.E., 47, 119, 120
moral agent, *see* agent, moral
moral judgments, 46, 62, 120, 124, 126, 177, 180, 191, 193, 214, 216, 343
moral knowledge, *see* knowledge, moral
moral paradigm, 220, 221, 245
moral philosophy, 5, 45, 46, 214, 216
moral principles, 52, 60, 64, 243, 244, 340, 341, 349
moral theories, 48, 49, 60, 80, 149, 150, 151, 209, 423, 425
moral utterances, 45, 46, 120
morals, 1, 48, 52, 57, 67, 70, 77, 81, 99, 109, 115, 137, 150, 152, 205, 221, 225, 309, 341, 347, 353, 354, 360, 399, 405, 406, 420, 421, 422; medicalization of (*see also* psychiatric turn), 116, 119, 124, 126, 210
Morse, Stephen, 279, 335, 358, 359
Moslem law, 65
motivation, 2, 39, 140, 159, 294, 366, 371; conscious, 231; theory of, 39, 41, 42, 104; ultimate, 135; unconscious, 231, 365
motives (*see also* reasons, for action), 10–11, 12, 18, 23, 26, 31, 35, 39–43, 45, 47, 88, 101, 102, 144, 146, 168, 184, 185, 249, 253, 262, 265, 269, 281, 282, 285–90, 292, 295, 296, 300, 302, 307, 309, 313, 343, 346, 382, 401; con-

Index

scious, 262, 263, 264, 266, 370; intelligible, 262; mixed, 11, 26, 263; possible, 19, 30, 428–9n22; rational, 214; unconscious, 140, 253, 257, 262–6, 269–70, 282, 304, 309, 313, 370
movement, 254; accidental, 322, bodily, 34, 37, 67, 69, 70–4, 77, 80, 173, 225, 226, 293, 294, 312, 321, 339, 341, 346, 349, 454n39; involuntary, 142; mechanical, 275, 281; voluntary, 56
multiple personalities, 149, 150, 397, 399, 401, 403–8, 411, 422, 493n22
multiple selves, 148, 149, 151, 388, 389, 390, 393, 395, 397, 407, 408
multiple-selves thesis, 387, 392, 450n129

Nagel, Ernst, 32, 147, 249, 252, 266, 269, 271
natural law, 49, 60, 227
natural rights theory, 98
naturalistic ethics, *see* ethics, naturalist
naturalistic fallacy, 119
negligence, 49, 77, 81–3, 106, 331, 342, 343
neurophysiology, 82, 250, 271; as a discipline, 35
neurosis (*see also* symptoms, neurotic), 123, 143, 323, 324, 336, 374, 376, 378, 413, 444n20
New Hampshire experiment, *see* insanity tests, New Hampshire test
New Hampshire test, *see* insanity tests, New Hampshire test
Nicholl, Sir John, 221
Nietzsche, Friedrich, 52, 143
nominalism, 157
norm, 120, 121; legal, 62, 65, 85, 90, 92, 93; moral, 60, 62, 64, 65, 85, 90, 92, 93, 120; physiological, 169, 186
Nozick, Robert, 98

Oakeshott, Michael, 21
object (*see also* contents), 43; of belief, 24–6, 102, 105, 300, 330, of desire, 15, 24–6, 102, 260, 333, 391, 394; *ding-an-sich*, 251; of instincts, 40, 41, 43, 135; intensional, 260, 330, 378; Intentional, 23, 260; linguistic, 23–5; of mental states, 24, 25, 37, 260; propositional, 102, 103, 105, 107, 260; of utterance, 26; of wishes, 266, 270, 289, 297, 300
objectivist ethics, *see* ethics, objectivist
obligation, 50, 52, 91–3;; contractual, 60, 181; legal, 51, 60–2, 65; moral, 51, 60, 62, 65
obsessional neurosis, *see* neurosis

ontological commitment, 137, 157, 158, 267, 408, 411
ontology, 156–8, 258, 276
Orestes, 381
original position, 209
orthodox psychiatry, 158, 160, 171, 172, 178, 179
ostensive definition, *see* definition, ostensive
ostensive reference, *see* reference
overdetermination, 11, 56, 306

pain, 129, 259, 260, 274–6
pain avoidance, 37, 306, 308, 314
Palsgraf v. Long Island R.R., 46, 60
parapraxes, 140, 141, 143, 308, 309, 311, 313–15, 317–20, 322, 323, 336, 338, 340, 343, 347, 348, 382, 394, 402
Parsons, Talcott, 124, 202
passions, *see* appetitive part of mind
perceptions, 183, 328, 341, 348
person (*see also* identity, personal), 1, 2, 32, 35, 119, 133, 138, 142, 145–50, 165, 168–70, 173, 178, 181, 183, 188–90, 192, 193, 206, 208, 212, 215, 219, 226, 235, 245, 274, 276, 277, 278, 298, 348, 396–9, 404–7, 409–11, 415, 421; as community of selves, 3, 4, 142, 397; fragmented, 307; functional organization of, 392; legal, 2, 46–50, 90, 91, 217; legal view of, 2, 3, 5, 44–112, 113–14, 126, 137, 139, 140, 267, 268, 383, 387, 422, 423, 424; Lockean conception of, 348, 349; as mind and body, 349; moral, 46, 48, 49, 64, 311; as practical reasoner, 3, 14, 49, 53, 54, 57, 61, 82, 84, 91, 93–7, 99, 100, 108, 364; psychiatric view of, 2, 113–152, 419, 422–4; as rational, autonomous agent, 2, 3, 5, 49, 62, 86, 96–9, 106, 108–12, 354, 361, 362, 383, 389, 416, 418, 423, 425; theory of, 1, 2, 382, 417, 419, 423; the unconscious and subpersonal agents as, 250, 267, 387, 391, 395, 398, 410; as unified agent, 3, 4, 387, 406, 415
personality (*see also* multiple personality), 122, 123, 352, 395, 404, 405, 407–12
personality dysfunction, 123
personhood, 9, 14, 62–4, 66, 94, 178, 373, 406
Peters, Richard S., 20, 30, 37, 42, 43, 74, 76, 173, 174, 262, 370
phenomenology, 22, 249, 251
philosophy of action, 5, 34, 68, 148, 292
philosophy of law, 5, 423
philosophy of mind, 5, 34, 148, 184, 254, 392, 423
philosophy of science, 5, 54, 423

523

Index

physical states and processes, 32, 34, 139, 148, 254, 275, 277, 279, 281, 352
physical systems, 167, 183
physicalism, 33, 165, 183, 359
physiological psychology, 2, 364
physiology, 34, 139, 259, 269, 276, 278, 354, 359, 414
pictoral representation, *see* mental representation
Plato, 116, 117, 144, 145, 414
Pollard v. United States, 350, 351, 353, 364, 366, 368, 370, 371
positivism, 37, 38, 60, 259, 420
Powell v. Texas, 125
practical inference, *see* practical reasoning; inference.
practical reason, 2, 9 13, 14, 33, 54–7, 59, 62, 64, 67, 77, 78, 90, 95, 99, 100, 138, 145–7, 250, 394
practical reasoner (*see also* person, as practical reasoner), 2, 13, 14, 49, 52–4, 58, 61, 62, 65, 83, 90, 92, 93, 95–7, 100
practical reasoning, 14, 16, 17, 21, 25, 55, 59, 61, 63, 64, 66, 74–9, 81, 85–7, 93, 95, 101, 104, 105, 108, 114, 207, 208, 245, 295, 301, 307, 308, 326, 363, 364, 376, 380, 381, 428n17, 492n8
practical syllogism, 10, 13, 14, 16–19, 61, 63, 71, 76, 77, 81, 83, 90, 101, 102, 108, 160, 244, 287, 293, 295–300, 302, 303, 324, 326, 332, 338, 380, 399
praise, 5, 45, 142, 373
preconscious, 130, 132, 135, 137, 288, 297, 411
prescriptivism, 46, 47
primary goods, 209
primary process, 115, 141, 277, 326
privileged access, 128, 129, 133, 137, 184, 185, 256, 258, 272, 274–277, 316, 317, 348, 377; deferred, 257, 291, 317, 348
property law, 48, 98, 99
Prosser, William, 188
psyche, 117, 144, 279, 414
psychiatric turn, 115, 210
psychic determinism, *see* determinism, psychic
psychoanalysis, 282, 283, 292, 298, 313, 335, 339, 369, 404, 406, 407, 409, 410, 419; clinical, 119, 145, 272, 273, 281, 284, 285, 305, 309, 316, 318, 322, 325, 360, 396; theoretical, 280, 281, 309
psychoanalytic explanations, *see* explanation, psychoanalytic
psychoanalytic theory, 20, 43, 152, 295, 309, 312, 317, 326, 365, 381, 387, 388, 391, 396, 398, 399, 401, 402, 406, 408, 409, 411, 414, 415

psychopathology, 228–9, 355
psychosis, 119, 123, 177, 198, 203, 245, 364
punishment, 48, 51, 53, 62, 63, 65, 81, 92, 103, 111, 124, 125, 126, 141, 142, 151, 156, 181, 195, 221, 223, 227, 233–43, 313, 332, 338, 341, 353, 371, 372; mixed theory, 237, 238, 240–4; retributive theory, 235–7, 240, 242–4; utilitarian theory, 236–40, 242–4
purpose (*see also* end), 37; as end, 26, 63, 81, 96, 334, 382; as function or effect, 26, 28

Quine, W.V., 37, 156, 158, 175, 278

radical psychiatry, 155–60, 164, 167, 170, 177–80, 249
Rapaport, David, 35, 39–43, 271, 279, 364
Rat-Man, 345, 374–7
rational agent, *see* agent, rational
rational consumer, 388, 390, 395, 397, 399
rational part of mind, *see* reasoning faculty
rationality, 3, 5, 11, 62, 64–6, 86, 95, 100, 102–5, 107, 108, 112–15, 117, 126, 141, 145, 159, 161, 162, 164, 168, 171, 178, 180, 196, 206, 207, 209, 223, 365, 393, 394, 406, 419, 424, 425
rationalization, 10–13, 15–20, 23, 75, 101, 102, 105, 294, 296, 303, 352
Rawls, John, 95, 208–9, 341
Ray, Isaac, 221, 224–6
Rayner, Eric, 278
realism, 176
reason-giving explanation; *see* explanation, reason-giving
reasoning faculty, 117, 144, 170, 195, 379; defect of, 196, 218, 219, 222, 232
reasons, 12, 15, 16, 19, 20, 26, 30, 31, 33, 37, 43, 74, 75, 100, 226, 274, 318, 338, 349, 376; for action, 2–3, 9–15, 17, 20, 21, 32, 40–2, 64, 81, 88–90, 140, 160, 173, 196, 258, 259, 262, 264, 265, 281, 298, 299, 314, 324, 326, 332, 335, 347, 371, 380, 390; conscious, 339, 369, 370; causally operative, 21; for action, unconscious, 4, 140, 300, 313, 314, 337, 340, 369, 370, 376; intelligible, 101, 373, 390, 395; moral, 92; rational, 141, 373
Redlich, F.C., 118, 119
reductionism, *see* physicalism; behavioralism; mechanism
reduction, definitional, 279; of explanations, 33, 39; of mental states, 35, 37, 39, 400; of moral concepts to medical

524

Index

concepts, 124; of personal agency to event causation, 362; of psychological concepts, 36, 37, 39–43, 433n67
reference, 24, 156, 158, 159, 165, 166, 167, 183
Regina v. M'Naghten, 221, 224
rehabilitation, 233, 234, 236, 241, 244
relativism, *see* ethical relativism; epistemological relativism
repression, 25, 129, 131, 134–6, 138–40, 143–6, 276, 306, 308, 314, 335, 337, 395, 400, 402, 409
resistance, 143, 145, 403
responsibility, 1, 2, 3, 5, 43, 45, 47–53, 62–68, 91, 99, 115, 126, 145, 178, 181, 202, 205, 212, 231, 250, 309, 317, 322, 343, 347–50, 352, 360, 363, 382, 404–6, 485n104, n105; causal, 50, 51, 59, 73, 75, 225–6, 292, 345; decreased, 271, 350, 352, 355, 365, 371, 372, 374, 381, 383; extended, 381, 383; for one's character, 253, 309, 345, 347; legal, 2, 4, 47, 61, 65, 77, 90, 100, 102, 104–7, 110, 111, 113, 140–2, 150–2, 217–22, 224–30, 232, 244, 245, 346, 353, 423, 424; moral, 2, 4, 48, 50, 52, 53, 58, 59, 65, 69, 77, 110, 111, 113, 124, 125, 140–2, 150–2, 177, 221–6, 232, 244, 245, 294, 309, 310, 311, 313, 327, 329–32, 338–42, 344, 345, 349, 351–61, 364, 369, 373, 375, 379, 380, 424; prospective, 50–2, 344, 346, 347; retrospective, 50–4, 344, 345, 346
retributivism, *see* punishment
reward, 110, 142
Ricoeur, Paul, 382
rights, 3, 5, 48, 51, 126, 142, 145, 146, 152, 181, 209, 250, 406; animal, 91; basic, 94; civil, 181; contract, 94, 97–100, 141; correlative, 91; desert, 94, 102, 110, 141; to equality, 47, 48, 91, 94–7; human, 94; legal, 2, 44, 47, 48, 49, 90–100, 104, 107, 111, 113, 149, 156, 178, 217, 423; to liberty, 47, 48, 91, 94–97, 99, 126, 209; moral, 2, 47, 90–100, 111, 113, 149, 178, 349; natural, 48, 94; personal, 94, 97; prima facie, 95, 100; property, 47, 48, 91, 94, 97–100, 103, 141, 150
Ring, K., 159
Riviere, Joan, 142
Robinson v. California, 125
Roche, Philip, 121
Rogers, Carl, 118
Roman law, 66, 90
Rorty, Richard, 22
Russell, Bertrand, 278

Ryle, Gilbert, 37, 38, 148, 164–5, 167, 168, 171–3, 254, 259, 284

sane human beings, 221, 223, 406
sanity, 114, 141, 183
Sartre, J.P., 109, 110, 381
Schafer, Roy, 274, 275, 292, 294, 298, 300, 313, 348, 402
Scheff, Tom, 121
Schelling, Thomas, 388–91, 393–6, 399, 407
Schimek, Jean, 269, 270
schizophrenia, 159, 161–3, 166, 171–5, 177, 178, 197, 198
Schlick, Moritz, 362, 363
Scott, A.W., 81
Scriven, Michael, 251
secondary process, 115
self, 110, 142, 143, 150, 151, 225, 292; anthropomorphic subdivisions of, 267; continuity of, 103; as a corporation of subpersonal agents, 287; disunity of, 5, 138, 147, 148, 387, 398, 399, 400, 401, 403, 405–7, 409–13, 424; extended, physical, 349; fragmentation of, 4, 295; personal, 295, 316, 329, 359, 405, 425; structural subdivisions of, 410; topographical subdivisions of, 410; as unitary agent, 295; unity of, 5, 142, 148–52, 295, 394, 398, 404–6, 408, 413
self-control, 219, 417; impairment of, 222, 229, 230
self-deception, 150, 295, 331, 368, 395, 403
self-defense, 221, 223
self-determination, 111
self-identity, 133, 408
self-interest, 115, 151, 152
self-intimation, 185, 186, 255, 256, 258, 260, 261, 265, 317, 320
sensations, 183, 259
sense of a word, 158, 254, 259
sickness, 115, 116, 119, 122, 124, 187, 188, 189
sick people, 113, 155, 181, 205, 215, 245
sick role, 124, 125, 199, 202, 212
Siegler, F.A., 254–6, 258
Skinner, B.F., 36, 38, 82, 146, 251, 425, 433n67
sleep, 284, 286–8, 295
Slobogin, Christopher, 359
social contract, 234
social deviance, 115, 121, 122
social gain (from punishment), 236–42
sociobiology, 425
sociopath, 228, 229, 355
Socrates, 144

Index

Spitzer, Robert, 210–16
split brain, 397, 399, 403
State v. Chaney, 241
State v. Pike, 227
State v. Sikora, 141
Staub, Hugo, 353
Stephen, Sir James, 182
stimuli, 36, 37, 39, 135, 138, 270, 284, 287, 328
Stone, Christopher, 46, 47
structuralism, 295, 307, 359
subagency, *see* subpersonal agency
subagent, *see* subpersonal agents
subpersonal agency, 145, 146, 307, 308, 359, 394, 410
subpersonal agents (*see also* person), 145, 151, 295, 401, 402, 414, 424; as persons or other selves, 295, 359, 372, 392, 395, 396
substance, 167, 168
substitutivity of identicals principle, 260
superego, 143–7, 267, 295, 359, 404, 406, 407, 410, 411, 414, 415
supervenient attitude (toward dreams), 318, 338, 401
Swartz, Louis, 191, 192
Sydenham, 417
symbolic representation, *see* mental representation
symptoms, 157, 163, 164, 166, 171, 174, 175, 187, 188, 194, 195, 198, 215, 221, 222, 227, 309, 314, 329, 333, 336, 340, 348, 374, 382, 417, 418; neurotic, 143, 274, 282, 307, 308, 311–13, 315, 317, 319, 320–3, 336, 338, 345, 347, 394, 395, 401, 402, 471n20; physical, 186, 321; psychological, 211, 418
System Csc, 143, 372
System Pcs, 143
System Ucs, 114, 134, 136, 140, 143, 250, 267, 273, 372, 400, 406
Szasz, Thomas, 3, 46, 155–62, 165–7, 169, 171–4, 177–81, 186, 195, 249, 312, 313, 354

Taylor, F. Kaupl, 200
Taylor, Richard, 56–7
Thalberg, Irving, 146, 401
thinking, 14, 277, 278, 280, 292, 353, 359, 402
Tracy, Justice, 66
transference, 257
Trieb, see instinct
Tyler, Dr., 225

unconscious, 3, 4, 43, 74, 113, 115, 119, 126, 133, 134, 140, 141, 142, 424, 477n65, 464–5n3; as an aggregation of mental states or functions, 136, 137, 250; animistic, 114, 138, 250, 267; behaviorist, 138, 250, 268, 269; descriptive sense (Freud's), 129, 130, 131; dynamic sense, 129–32, 134, 135, 137–9, 142, 143; economic sense, 138; as entity, 249, 267–8, 272–3, 275, 280; Freudian, 250, 271, 272, 275–7, 311, 348, 359, 360, 363, 364, 382, 393, 395, 399, 411; Freud's nontheoretical concept, 129–34; Freud's theory of, 250, 251; functional definition of, 137; ontological status of, 267–80; part of mind, 266, 270, 274, 278, 310, 315, 316, 319, 329, 331, 332, 337, 342, 352, 353, 356, 361, 366, 368, 373, 379, 383, 387, 394, 402, 417, 422; physiological, 138, 139, 250, 271; psychological theory of, 139; pretheoretical (ordinary discourse sense), 126–9, 137–9, 250, 251, 273, 276, 402; as property, 250, 251, 267, 273, 280, 400; topographical sense, 129, 134–9
unconscious process, 249, 253, 265
unconsciousness, 341, 377, 393, 396
unified agent, *see* self, unity of
United States vs. Carroll Towing Co., 82
universal symbolism, 335
utilitarianism (*see also* punishment), 48, 82, 98, 235, 239, 372
utility, 240, 242

value, 104, 191–4, 206–10, 216, 236, 254
Veatch, Robert, 202
verification, 255, 257
verificationism, 37, 256
verstehen, 21
virtue, 116–18, 119, 120, 209, 343, 345
volition (*see also* will), 68, 70–1, 363
volitional incapacity (*see also* functional impairment), 219, 222, 232, 235
Von Wright, G.H., 22, 23

watchman (Freud's), 401
Weber, Max, 21
Weintraub, Chief Justice, 141
will (*see also* volition), 1, 70–1, 74, 99, 107, 108, 141, 145, 195, 225; acts of, 352, 363; conscious, 4, 351; free, 1, 65, 109, 231, 232, 352, 360, 373, 421, 423; weakness of, 16, 391, 428n17
willful blindness, 86, 331, 367, 489n48
Williams, Bernard, 404
Winch, Peter, 20
Wisdom, John, 256
wishes (*see also* desire), 252, 253, 269, 282,

526

Index

287, 290, 294–6, 298, 299, 301, 305, 313, 320, 344, 485n105; causally operative, 309, 318, 321–2, 403; conscious, 266, 290, 300; expressed by behavior, 300, 337; expressed by dreams, 285, 301, 303, 309, 336; motivational, 270; preconscious, 285–6, 287, 323; repressed, 266, 284, 285, 290, 291, 307; second-order, 300; to sleep, 285–8, 291, 323, 324, 402, 471n20; unconscious, 253, 257, 262, 266, 267, 270, 274, 284–6, 290–3, 297, 300, 301, 303, 304, 313, 314, 318, 321–2, 337, 345, 370, 375, 377, 394, 402, 403

wish fulfillment in dreams, 266, 284, 285, 290, 291–301, 302, 303, 304, 306, 307, 318, 322, 332–3, 402

Wittgenstein, Ludwig, 20, 69, 70, 74, 97, 149, 254, 293

Wollheim, Richard, 318, 319